Understanding Pharmacology in Nursing Practice

Ehsan Khan • Pauline Hood

Editors

Understanding Pharmacology in Nursing Practice

Second Edition

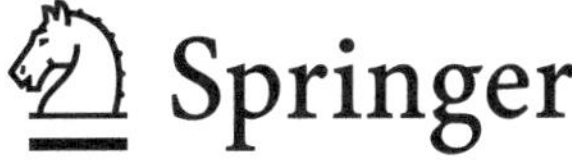 Springer

Editors
Ehsan Khan
Faculty of Nursing Midwifery
and Palliative Care
King's College London
London, UK

Pauline Hood (Retired)
Faculty of Nursing Midwifery
and Palliative Care
King's College London
London, UK

ISBN 978-3-032-03963-7   ISBN 978-3-032-03964-4   (eBook)
https://doi.org/10.1007/978-3-032-03964-4

This Springer imprint is published by the registered company Springer Nature Switzerland AG
The registered company address is: Gewerbestrasse 11, 6330 Cham, Switzerland

If disposing of this product, please recycle the paper.

Preface

Pharmacology is a vital biomedical science that has made, and continues to make, a profound contribution to health care. Indeed, it is no exaggeration to state that juxtaposed with advances in medical care, the evolution of pharmacology has transformed patient care and outcome. Equally, as biomedical science progresses, this compels healthcare professionals to be knowledgeable, informed, and aware of the significance of pharmacology in practice, be it hospital or community centred.

The nurse's role with medication management is prominent. Nurses must, therefore, have a robust comprehension of pharmacology. Consequently, providing pharmacology education for both pre- and post-qualification nurses is essential.

There are numerous elements that influence a patient's or service user's medication management. The practitioners involved in the process of prescribing, administering, monitoring, and assessing outcome are obliged not just to have an understanding and allegiance to medication policies and procedures but also to be person-centred and sensitive to an individual's personal circumstances. This includes; addressing the patient's personal expectations of the medication, explaining the practical aspects of the medication regimen, elucidating the need to monitor the medications impact, and explaining the need for follow-up care. Appreciating and responding to a person's views and concerns may also facilitate concordance with a medication regimen and is, therefore, an important activity.

Fundamentally, whether prescribing, administering, or monitoring medication, a nurse's contribution is pivotal. Therefore, while identifying and exploring the principles of pharmacology alongside a comprehensive explanation of systemic pharmacology applied to clinical practice, this second edition of the book additionally acknowledges and discusses the challenges and the role of the nurse and pharmacology.

While recognising the increasing complexity of therapeutic pharmacology, it is envisaged that this book provides a strong knowledge platform that empowers the nurse to confidently deliver safe, effective pharmaceutical care in practice.

London, UK Ehsan Khan
London, UK Pauline Hood

Contents

Challenges in Nursing Pharmacology

1

Marlon Bernardo

Learning Outcomes

After reading this chapter, you will be able to:

- Appreciate the challenges that exist in teaching pharmacology to nursing students.
- Have an understanding of strategies improve pharmacology education in nursing curricula.

Pharmacology is a cornerstone of nursing education, where nurses play a critical role in patient care and medication administration. The Nursing and Midwifery Council (2023) emphasises the necessity of nursing curricula to provide learning opportunities that align with the required proficiencies and programme outcomes, including safe and effective administration of medications. The significance of pharmacology in nursing education is underscored by several key factors such as patient safety, clinical decision-making, interdisciplinary collaboration, and professional competence. Nevertheless, teaching and learning pharmacology within nursing education presents several challenges. This chapter delves into four key challenges that nursing students encounter during their pharmacology studies, including the inherent fear of nursing students towards biosciences, poor spiralling of biosciences in nursing curricula, getting the language and detail right, and teaching pharmacology and medication management.

M. Bernardo (✉)
King's College London, London, UK
e-mail: marlon.bernardo@kcl.ac.uk

E. Khan, P. Hood (eds.), *Understanding Pharmacology in Nursing Practice*,
https://doi.org/10.1007/978-3-032-03964-4_1

1.1 Inherent Fear of Nursing Students Towards Biosciences

In nursing, bioscience encompasses foundational biological knowledge, including anatomy, physiology, pathophysiology, and pharmacology. This knowledge is essential for understanding the human body and its functions, and for providing effective and safe patient care. While nursing students recognise the importance of bioscience within the nursing programme, studies consistently reveal that many students perceive bioscience education as anxiety-provoking. This anxiety is often attributed to the difficulty and complexity of the subject matter, and it even exists before students begin formal university studies (Craft et al. 2013; Malik et al. 2018; McVicar et al. 2015). The inherent fear of nursing students towards biosciences is a multifaceted issue stemming from various psychological and educational factors.

Nursing students often fear biosciences due to the perceived complexity of the subject, previous negative experiences, inadequate preparation, and anxiety. For example, a student who struggled with secondary school biology might enter the nursing programme with a mindset that they are not 'science-minded', creating a mental block, making it difficult for them to engage with bioscience subjects. They may carry this belief into their nursing studies, believing they are not capable of understanding complex scientific concepts. Another student might have had a negative experience with a previous science teacher who made the subject seem overly complicated and unapproachable. This experience can lead to a persistent fear of bioscience courses.

Students who feel inadequately prepared often experience heightened levels of anxiety. For instance, a student who did not take advanced science courses in school might feel unprepared for the rigorous bioscience curriculum within the nursing programme. This lack of preparation can cause significant anxiety, leading them to avoid studying or participating in class. Additionally, a student who feels overwhelmed by the volume of information in a pharmacology course might experience anxiety that prevents them from asking questions or seeking help, resulting in poor performance with exams and assignments.

In terms of educational factors, the learning environment and assessment methods may contribute to this inherent fear towards biosciences. The shift towards blended learning environments has introduced additional challenges. Blended learning employs a combination of face-to-face learning experiences and online activities to deliver learning (Advance HE n.d.), and this approach has gained popularity especially during and after the COVID-19 pandemic. Many students struggle with the transition from traditional methods to more contemporary blended models, leaving them feeling unsupported in their learning and contributing to their anxiety. Students have expressed a need for more interactive and supportive teaching approaches in bioscience courses, such as what Koch et al. (2020) highlighted in their study that blended learning could potentially disadvantage nursing students. A student who is not familiar with online learning platforms might struggle with the transition to a blended learning environment. They might find it difficult to navigate the technology, access resources, or participate in online discussions, leading to feelings of isolation and anxiety. Students from under represented groups might face additional challenges in blended learning environments due to a lack of access to reliable internet or technology. This can create a significant barrier to their learning and contribute to their anxiety about bioscience courses.

High-stakes exams can contribute to fear and anxiety among nursing students. For example, a final exam in a pathophysiology course that determines a large portion of the student's grade can create significant pressure. Students may fear that one poor performance could jeopardise their academic progress, leading to increased stress and anxiety. The lack of formative assessments, such as quizzes and practice tests, may also result in uncertainty about their knowledge and increased fear of failing. Students may feel they have not had enough opportunities to practice and receive feedback prior to taking their summative assessments.

1.2 Poor Spiralling of Biosciences in Nursing Curricula

Spiralling refers to the pedagogical approach that sequentially revisits key concepts over time with increasing levels of complexity throughout the curriculum. This approach emphasises building upon previous learning, allowing nursing students to deepen their understanding of essential topics as they progress through their education. By integrating a spiralling curriculum, educators aim to foster a comprehensive mastery of both foundational and advanced concepts necessary for effective nursing practice. A central component of this approach is the recognition that nursing education encompasses various competencies, including clinical skills, theoretical knowledge, and critical thinking. Each of these elements can be revisited in a structured manner to reinforce learning. For instance, a nursing student might begin with basic anatomy and physiology in their first academic year, and as they advance, they revisit these topics alongside related subjects, such as pharmacology or pathophysiology.

The spiralling of biosciences in nursing curricula has been a topic of concern for many educators and students. Poor spiralling can lead to significant challenges that impact student learning, retention, and overall performance in these critical courses. Key challenges associated with the ineffective integration of biosciences into nursing curricula include insufficient curriculum time, ineffective teaching methods, and theory-practice misalignment.

Biosciences often receive limited time within nursing programmes, which is insufficient for students to grasp complex concepts. The reduction in the biosciences taught in nursing programmes can be traced back to the 1980s when the psychosocial aspects of patient care were given much greater attention in an effort to define the distinctive role of nursing within the healthcare system. In the UK, a survey conducted by Taylor et al. (2015) confirms a wide variation in the teaching hours of biosciences across higher education institutions, representing only 0.4 to 2.4% of the total time in a pre-registration nursing programme. Previous studies have also shown that the number of biosciences taught is insufficient (Davis 2010; McVicar et al. 2010), posing significant challenges for nursing students to understand and apply bioscientific concepts in clinical practice.

Teaching biosciences encompasses a range of challenges related to teaching methods that can significantly impact student learning outcomes. Large group lectures are common practice in teaching biosciences (Taylor et al. 2015), but may not be the most effective way to teach challenging bioscience concepts. Such large class sizes may lead to a reliance on traditional lecturing methods rather than active engagement. In some countries, there are classroom sessions and laboratory components in teaching biosciences such as in anatomy and physiology. Nursing students are given opportunities to study the human body and bodily functions with the use of cadavers in a laboratory setting. However, this may not be practical in some institutions due to financial and resource constraints. These systemic challenges can make it difficult for educators to deliver high-quality bioscience education that meets the needs of nursing students.

The theory-practice misalignment is one of the most persistent challenges in teaching biosciences. Nursing students often struggle to connect theoretical bioscience knowledge with clinical practice, which can undermine their confidence and application in real-world scenarios. Craft et al. (2017) discovered that nursing students believe that pharmacology should relate to bioscience, and bioscience should relate to nursing. This suggests that students continue to encounter challenges in translating bioscience knowledge into the clinical environment. For example, students might learn about pharmacokinetics in isolation without seeing its application in patient care. Additionally, a course on anatomy might focus heavily on memorising parts of the body without connecting this knowledge to real-life nursing scenarios. There is a lack of contextualised theoretical integration resulting to students feeling inadequate and ill-prepared for their clinical practice.

1.3 Getting the Language and Detail Right

Another significant challenge among nursing students is the complex language and comprehensive detail. Pharmacology involves a vast array of complex terms and nomenclature that can be daunting for nursing students. The names of drugs, their classifications, mechanisms of action, and adverse effects are often derived from Latin or Greek roots, making them difficult to understand and remember. Many drugs have lengthy and intricate names that are challenging to pronounce and remember, and their names can vary across regions, further overwhelming students (Moloney et al. 2020). For instance, a commonly used analgesic is referred in the UK as 'paracetamol', while in the USA, it is known as 'acetaminophen'. Despite these variations, both names refer to the same chemical compound: N-(4-Hydroxyphenyl)-acetamide. Drugs are categorised into various classes based on their therapeutic effects, mechanisms of action, or chemical structure. Beta-blockers, for example, are used to manage hypertension and heart conditions, but understanding the nuances between different beta-blockers can be challenging. Learning how drugs interact with the body at a molecular level requires understanding complex biological processes, which can be learnt from other biosciences such as microbiology and biochemistry.

Aside from the complex language, nursing students often face information overload due to the sheer volume of material they need to learn in pharmacology. Students often encounter excessive information regarding pharmacodynamics, pharmacokinetics, drug interactions, and nursing considerations, all compressed into a limited timeframe and leading to cognitive overload. Finding the right level of detail is crucial as too much detail can overwhelm students, while too little can leave them unprepared for clinical practice. A typical pharmacology course covers numerous drugs, each with unique properties and uses, which can be overwhelming. In an effort to enhance the course, Phillips and Ford (2021) initiated a quality improvement project. They streamlined pharmacology with physiology and pathophysiology content and concentrated on commonly prescribed medications. Consequently, the authors noticed an increase in student engagement and a reduction in study time.

Lecturers may also have limited time to present vast amounts of information, leading to dense and fast-paced lectures. In a typical pharmacology lecture, a lecturer may cover several drug classes, their mechanism of action, adverse effects, and interactions within a short period. For instance, a lecture on cardiovascular drugs might include beta-blockers, ACE inhibitors, diuretics, and calcium channel blockers, each with detailed pharmacokinetics and pharmacodynamics. Students might struggle to keep up with the pace and retain the information presented. Another contributory factor for information overload is that pharmacology is often taught alongside other demanding bioscience courses or nursing-specific modules. Balancing the workload from multiple courses is undeniably a challenge among students.

1.4   Teaching Pharmacology and Medication Management

It is crucial to distinguish between pharmacology and medication management, as nursing students frequently confuse these two terms. Pharmacology is the science that studies how drugs interact with living organisms, encompassing the understanding of drug properties, mechanisms of action, therapeutic effects, adverse effects, and potential risks. Medication management involves the practical aspects of administering medications to patients, ensuring the correct dosage, timing, route of administration, monitoring for adverse effects, and educating patients about their medications. Pharmacology and medication management are closely related fields, but they have distinct areas of focus. Pharmacology delves into the biological and chemical aspects of drugs, while medication management focuses on ensuring the safe and effective use of medications in clinical settings.

One common misunderstanding among students, on one hand, is about the scope of pharmacology. Some students might think pharmacology is only about memorising drug names and dosages, rather than understanding the underlying principles of drug action. For example, they might focus on rote memorisation of 'ibuprofen', but without understanding why this nonsteroidal anti-inflammatory drug for reducing inflammation and pain is effective for certain conditions and not to others. The understanding of medication management, on the other hand, is often limited and focused on oral medications only, as noted in the study by Moloney et al. (2020) of final year nursing students. They might be well-versed in administering oral medications like tablets and capsules but lack knowledge and experience about other routes of administration. For instance, they might know how to give a patient oral antibiotics but struggle with intravenous (IV) administration, which requires understanding of IV compatibility, infusion rates, and monitoring for adverse reactions.

Nursing students often face the challenge of integrating pharmacological knowledge and applying it to clinical settings. It is crucial that they must combine their understanding of pharmacology with practical medication management skills for effective patient care. However, evidence suggests that nursing students struggle to apply theoretical knowledge gained in classroom settings to real-world clinical scenarios (Phillips and Ford 2021; Preston et al. 2019). For example, a student might understand the pharmacological action of anticoagulants like warfarin but struggle with the practical aspects of monitoring a patient's International Normalised Ratio (INR) levels and reporting it to the prescriber for possible dose adjustments. Applying pharmacological knowledge to clinical practice involves considering patient-specific factors such as age, weight, comorbidities, and other medications. This requires critical thinking and clinical decision-making abilities. Nursing students must be able to assess patient conditions, interpret clinical data, and make informed decisions about medication management. For instance, when administering antibiotics to a patient with renal impairment, a nursing student must consider how the patient's condition influences drug metabolism and excretion, which may necessitate a different administration method or a lower dosage. These are few examples, underscoring the importance of integrating and applying pharmacology knowledge and medication management skills.

1.5 Meeting the Challenges in Nursing Pharmacology

To effectively address the challenges nursing students face in pharmacology, a student-centred approach is essential. This approach focuses on the needs, experiences, and active participation of students in their learning process. The student-centred approach includes creating supportive learning environments, engaging with opportunities for practical applications, and ensuring active participation and reflection.

Creating supportive learning environments, such as study groups and mentorship opportunities with other students, encourages them to collaborate, share knowledge, and support one another. Peer support, along with assistance from family and faculty, can help alleviate anxiety and build confidence (Al-Najdi et al. 2025; Frangieh et al. 2024). Students should consider utilising the diverse support services offered by universities, including tutoring, online and in-person forums with fellow students and academic staff, and counselling and mental health services. To address the challenges posed by the shift towards blended learning environments, universities provide short courses and support from relevant professional services and library staff to help students develop and enhance their computer literacy. These resources can help students manage stress and overcome challenges related to pharmacology and other academic demands of the nursing programme. Practical applications of the knowledge gained in nursing pharmacology are paramount, particularly since medication management is a key competency for nurses (NMC 2018). Students are given the opportunities to apply their pharmacological knowledge both in a simulated clinical environment and real-world settings. In these opportunities, students can practice administering medications, monitoring patients, educating them about their treatments, and collaborating with other members of the healthcare team. It is essential for students to be proactive learners during clinical placements where they interact with trained staff, who play a vital role in helping students navigate complex clinical situations and develop critical thinking skills. Additionally, students are encouraged to collaborate with other members of the multidisciplinary team, such as the pharmacist and doctors, to gain a comprehensive understanding of pharmacology and medication management in clinical practice.

This student-centred approach to meeting the challenges in nursing pharmacology would be incomplete without emphasising the importance of students' active participation and reflection. Active involvement in the learning process goes beyond passive information absorption; it involves engaging with it through various activities. Students should actively participate in learning through discussions, group projects, or activities during seminar sessions, as well as interactive lectures that promote teamwork and collaboration and deepen their understanding of pharmacological concepts. Students must also regularly assess their comprehension and identify areas for improvement. Self-assessment tools like reflective journals can aid students in tracking their progress and setting achievable goals. As highlighted by the NMC (2023), students must be empowered and supported to become reflective and lifelong learners. This approach would enable them to take charge of their learning even after completing their university education.

1.6 Conclusion

This chapter introduces four key challenges that nursing students encounter while studying pharmacology. These challenges encompass the inherent fear of nursing students towards biosciences, the poor integration of biosciences into nursing curricula, the difficulty in grasping the language and intricate details, and the challenges of teaching pharmacology and medication management. Nursing students often harbour a fear of biosciences due to its perceived complexity, past negative experiences, inadequate preparation, and anxiety. Additionally, the blended learning environment and high-stake assessment methods contribute to this apprehension. The poor integration of biosciences into nursing curricula presents significant challenges, including insufficient curriculum time, ineffective teaching methods, and a misalignment between theory and practice. Another crucial challenge for nursing students is the overwhelming language and comprehensive details associated with pharmacology. Lastly, students struggle to integrate and apply pharmacological knowledge and medication management skills into real-world clinical scenarios.

To address these challenges effectively, a multifaceted approach is necessary. This approach should encompass supportive learning environments, well-designed teaching strategies, and opportunities for practical application. By comprehending and overcoming these obstacles, educators can empower nursing students to succeed in their pharmacology courses and develop the necessary competencies to become proficient healthcare professionals.

Multiple Choice Questions

1. Many students perceive bioscience education as anxiety-provoking. The following scenarios can help students alleviate this anxiety, except for which one?
   (a) Engaging in peer mentoring programmes where more experienced students can help new students.
   (b) Acknowledging that this is a valid feeling and that there are available supports to help cope with the academic demands.
   (c) Reading the recommended textbooks and materials before attending a lecture.
   (d) None of the above
2. Spiralling of biosciences in nursing curricula is an important pedagogical approach in nursing education. The following statements is correct, except for which one? Spiralling…
   (a) Fosters limited mastery of foundational concepts for effective nursing practice.
   (b) Emphasises on building what has been previously learnt.
   (c) Revisits key nursing concepts over time throughout the curriculum.
   (d) Enables nursing students to deepen their understanding of fundamental topics.
3. Pharmacology and medication management are closely related fields, but with different areas of focus. Which of the following statements is correct?
   (a) Pharmacology involves administering the correct medication and monitoring for adverse reactions.
   (b) Medication management aims to ensure the safe and effective use of medications.
   (c) Medication management deals with the studies of how medications are absorbed in the body.
   (d) Pharmacology focuses on ensuring the correct dosage, timing, and route of administration.
4. Which of the following scenarios best describes medication management?
   (a) Measuring a patient's blood pressure before administering anti-hypertensive medication.
   (b) Providing health education to a patient who is being discharged with multiple medications.
   (c) Ensuring the correct needle size is used in administering a subcutaneous injection.
   (d) All of the above

5. A student-centred approach is essential to meeting the challenges in nursing pharmacology. The following scenarios exemplify this approach, except for which one?
   (a) A student seeks guidance from the practice supervisor regarding the proper technique for administering intramuscular injections.
   (b) A student shares their lecture notes with a classmate who missed the session.
   (c) A student studies independently without seeking any assistance from anyone at all.
   (d) A student reflects on the feedback given by their practice assessor during clinical placements.

Answers

1. (d)
2. (a)
3. (b)
4. (d)
5. (c)

References

Advance HE (n.d.) Blended Learning. Retrieved March 22, 2025, from https://www.advance-he.ac.uk/knowledge-hub/blended-learning-0

Al-Najdi S, Mansoor A, Al Hayk O, Al-Hashimi N, Ali K, Daud A (2025) Silent struggles: a qualitative study exploring mental health challenges of undergraduate healthcare students. BMC Med Edu 25(1):157. https://doi.org/10.1186/S12909-025-06740-8

Craft J, Hudson P, Plenderleith M, Wirihana L, Gordon C (2013) Commencing nursing students' perceptions and anxiety of bioscience [article]. Nurse Educ Today 33(11):1399–1405. https://doi.org/10.1016/j.nedt.2012.10.020

Craft J, Christensen M, Bakon S, Wirihana L (2017) Advancing student nurse knowledge of the biomedical sciences: a mixed methods study. Nurse Educ Today 48:114–119. https://doi.org/10.1016/j.nedt.2016.10.003

Davis GM (2010) What is provided and what the registered nurse needs — bioscience learning through the pre-registration curriculum. Nurse Educ Today 30(8):707–712. https://doi.org/10.1016/j.nedt.2010.01.008

Frangieh J, Hughes V, Edwards-Capello A, Humphrey KG, Lammey C, Lucas L (2024) Fostering belonging and social connectedness in nursing: Evidence-based strategies: A discussion paper for nurse students, faculty, leaders, and clinical nurses. Nurs Outlook 72(4):102174. https://doi.org/10.1016/j.outlook.2024.102174

Koch J, Ramjan LM, Everett B, Maceri A, Bell K, Salamonson Y (2020) "Sage on the stage or guide on the side"—undergraduate nursing students' experiences and expectations of bioscience tutors in a blended learning curriculum: a qualitative study [article]. J Clin Nurs 29(5–6):863–871. https://doi.org/10.1111/jocn.15140

Malik R, Hussain M, Sarwer H, Afzal M, Gilani SA (2018) Bioscience subjects background and nursing education. Int J Soc Sci Manag 5(3):163–169. https://doi.org/10.3126/IJSSM.V5I3.20605

McVicar A, Clancy J, Mayes N (2010) An exploratory study of the application of biosciences in practice, and implications for pre-qualifying education. Nurse Educ Today 30(7):615–622. https://doi.org/10.1016/j.nedt.2009.12.010

McVicar A, Andrew S, Kemble R (2015) The 'bioscience problem' for nursing students: an integrative review of published evaluations of year 1 bioscience, and proposed directions for curriculum development. Nurse Educ Today 35(3):500–509. https://doi.org/10.1016/j.nedt.2014.11.003

Moloney M, Kingston L, Doody O (2020) Fourth year nursing students' perceptions of their educational preparation in medication management: an interpretative phenomenological study [article]. Nurse Educ Today 92:104512. https://doi.org/10.1016/j.nedt.2020.104512

Nursing & Midwifery Council (2018) Standards of proficiency for registered nurses. https://www.nmc.org.uk/globalassets/sitedocuments/standards/2024/standards-ofproficiency-for-nurses.pdf

Nursing & Midwifery Council (2023) Standards framework for nursing and midwifery education. https://www.nmc.org.uk/globalassets/sitedocuments/standards/2024/standards-framework-for-nursing-and-midwifery-education.pdf

Phillips CJ, Ford K (2021) The next gen pharmacology classroom: a quality improvement approach to transformation [article]. Teach Learn Nurs 16(4):379–383. https://doi.org/10.1016/j.teln.2021.05.009

Preston P, Leone-Sheehan D, Keys B (2019) Nursing student perceptions of pharmacology education and safe medication administration: a qualitative research study [article]. Nurse Educ Today 74:76–81. https://doi.org/10.1016/j.nedt.2018.12.006

Taylor V, Ashelford S, Fell P, Goacher PJ (2015) Biosciences in nurse education: is the curriculum fit for practice? Lecturers' views and recommendations from across the UK [article]. J Clin Nurs 24(19–20):2797–2806. https://doi.org/10.1111/jocn.12880

Pharmacokinetics and Pharmacodynamics

2

Ehsan Khan

Learning Outcomes
At the end of this chapter, you will be able to:

- Describe the processes of pharmacokinetics.
- Identify the pharmacokinetic mechanisms of commonly used medications.
- Appreciate the significance of the physiological status of a patient when administering medication.
- Understand how some drug combinations may be harmful due to possible drug–drug interactions.
- Describe the processes of pharmacodynamics.
- Identify agonistic and antagonistic receptor interactions.

2.1 Introduction

A medication is not just one active chemical, the drug, as medications contain a number of substances that aid both administration and delivery of the chemicals concerned. The quantity of active ingredient (drug) of a medication weight for weight may be relatively low, as the majority of a single medicine consists of numerous materials that include disintegrating agents that assist drug absorption and distribution together with stabilising elements which establish a medication's expiry date. Formulation of a medicine is an important aspect of pharmacology as it has a direct relevance to pharmacokinetics. It is important that the practitioner's involved in prescribing and administering medications have a clear understanding of these concepts, as attempts to adjust the structure of any medication, for example,

E. Khan (✉)
Faculty of Nursing Midwifery and Palliative Care, King's College London, London, UK
e-mail: eu.khan@kcl.ac.uk

E. Khan, P. Hood (eds.), *Understanding Pharmacology in Nursing Practice*,
https://doi.org/10.1007/978-3-032-03964-4_2

crushing tablets or opening capsules, may result in destroying the drug or lead to a suboptimal drug level entering the bloodstream. Therefore, informed administration technique should be employed to ensure the patient receives the correct dosage of a prescribed drug. Details regarding formulation may be found in Chap. 3, which focuses on this salient aspect of pharmaceutical practice.

2.2 Pharmacokinetics

Pharmacokinetics is the study of the effect of the body on the drug; this includes a number of processes that modulate and, in principle, limit access of the drug to its site of action. Most pharmacokinetic processes exist to reduce entry of toxins into the body. Pharmacokinetic processes do not differentiate between toxins and therapeutic substances (drugs). As toxins and drugs are structurally diverse, rather than identifying specific structures as toxins, pharmacokinetic processes protect the body by 'recognising' basic chemical characteristics, of which fat solubility is paramount.

Pharmacokinetics is associated with four main processes:

- *Absorption*
- *Distribution*
- *Metabolism*
- *Elimination/excretion*

2.2.1 Absorption

Drug absorption examines a medication's entry into the bloodstream. Drugs that enter the circulation directly via the intravenous route have a bioavailability of 100%. Bioavailability is the amount of drug that remains available to exert an effect following absorption. For all other routes of administration, a quantity of drug does not enter the bloodstream, resulting in the drug's bioavailability being less than 100%.

The process of absorption starts from swallowing an orally prescribed medication and finishes with absorption of the drug, frequently in the small intestine (Fig. 2.1). Many processes influence the absorption of the drug from the small intestine; the principal features of this process are (Fig. 2.1).

2.2.1.1 Oesophageal Transit

Oesophageal transit is initiated and assisted by swallowing. When taking solid forms of orally prescribed medication, that is, tablets or capsules, taking the medication with water is important. There is no clear consensus or evidence base regarding the optimal volume of liquid to be used when taking tablets; however, it is generally accepted that a volume between 60 mL (minimal) and 150 mL is sufficient. If taking less than this, there is potential for the medicine to get no further than the oesophagus and cause irritation, oesophagitis or in some cases mucosal erosion

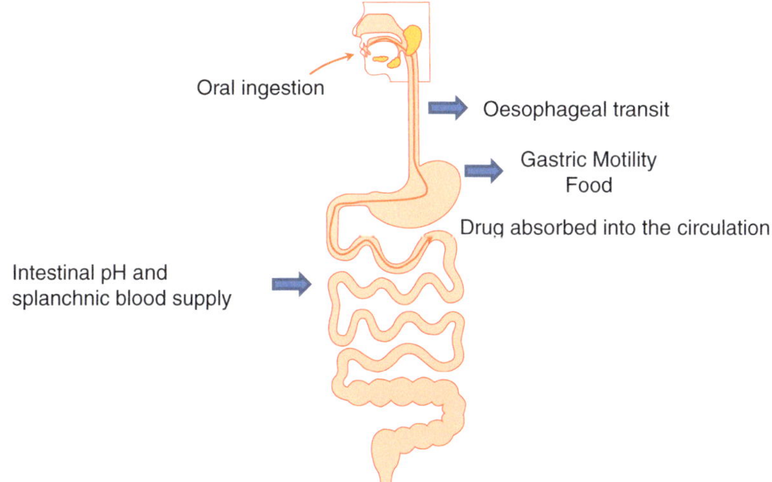

Fig. 2.1 Absorption of oral drugs and influences that modulate this absorption

and strictures (narrowing) of the oesophagus. Medications known to do this include some antimicrobial tablets and capsules, potassium chloride, vitamin C and iron tablets. It is therefore good practice to ensure oral tablets and capsules are taken with adequate amounts of water to ensure that the tablet transits the oesophagus and arrives at the site of absorption. If taking adequate volumes of fluid with oral medication is not feasible, for example, when someone is fluid restricted, then alternative routes of administration should be considered.

2.2.1.2 Food

Movement of substances through the gastrointestinal (GI) tract is dependent upon peristalsis and the fluidity of stomach content. Motility of the stomach and small intestine differ. The more frequently the stomach empties, the faster the medicine can get to the small intestine from where it will be absorbed. Movement of substances from the stomach into the intestine is governed by the pyloric sphincter. When the stomach is empty (starved state), cycles of contractions known as the 'migrating motility complex (MMC)' (Mudie et al. 2010), empty the stomach on average every 1.25–1.5 hours (Janssen et al. 2011). Gastric emptying therefore takes an average of 25 min in the starved state allowing drugs if present to enter the small intestine and be absorbed. In the presence of food, the MMC contractions are inhibited to allow time for food to be digested. In the presence of food, gastric opening time varies greatly from 40 to as long as 200 min (Mudie et al. 2010). In general, fatty meals reduce the frequency of gastric emptying the most. Therefore, food delays absorption of drug in the intestine and consequently delays the onset of a drug's effect. It is, however, important to remember that many drugs need to be taken with food owing to their effects in the stomach, for example, non-steroidal anti-inflammatory drugs.

2.2.1.3 Gastrointestinal Motility

Age and lack of mobility reduce peristalsis and gastric emptying. Peristalsis may also be inhibited by medication; such effects are seen with opioids and anticholinergic drugs. The occurrence of nausea and vomiting also reduces and delays the effects of medication. In such situations, for example, migraine, addition of an anti-emetic with oral pain relief tends to improve the analgesic effect. This is because anti-emetics improve peristalsis and promote the arrival of pain relief at its site of absorption.

If persistent nausea and vomiting occurs when taking oral medication, it may be advisable to utilise a different administration approach such as the intravenous (IV) or intramuscular (IM) route to ensure drug absorption is optimised.

There is a near 100-fold difference between the surface area of the stomach and the small intestine. The structure of the small intestine provides an optimal area for oral drugs to be absorbed, and many oral drugs are specifically designed to be absorbed in this area.

To facilitate absorption, a drug needs to be in a dissolved state when it arrives in the small intestine, and to diffuse across the membrane, the drug must be fat-soluble (Fig. 2.2).

The solubility state of a substance is not constant; it changes according to the pH of its environment. This is because medications are either acidic or basic in nature (Table 2.1). When a basic drug is in a 'basic' or alkaline environment, it becomes lipidic or fat-soluble; similarly, when an acidic drug is in an acidic environment, it becomes lipidic or fat-soluble. To render a drug fat-soluble in the intestine, it would therefore be desirable that the drug is 'basic' in nature, so that it is fat-soluble in the alkaline environment of the intestine; this will aid its absorption through the intestinal wall into the bloodstream. Table 2.1 depicts the acid or base characteristics of some medications. In practice, relatively acidic drugs may also absorb significantly in the alkaline environment of the small intestine. This is because of the large surface area the small intestine presents to the drug, compared to other structures such as the stomach, allowing more drug to be absorbed despite its poor fat solubility.

In addition to the pH effect on lipid solubility, the size of the drug molecule is important in terms of membrane diffusion. The size of a molecule is commonly

Fig. 2.2 Substance movement across a cell wall

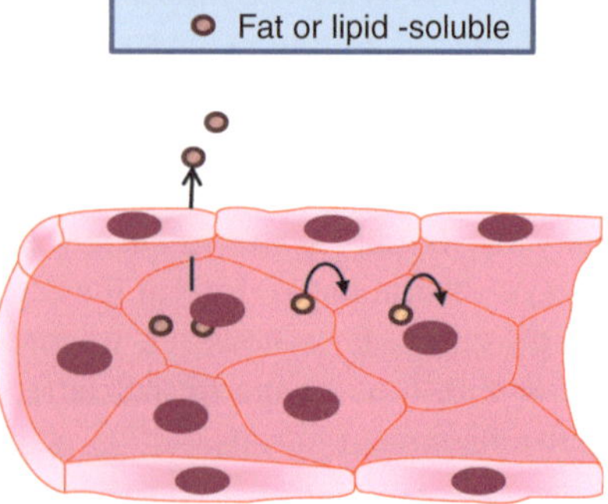

Table 2.1 pH characteristics of some commonly used medications

Drug	Weak base or acid	Source
Amiodarone	Base	Latini et al. (1984)
Lorazepam	Base	Abernethy et al. (1984)
Metoprolol	Base	Cerqueira et al. (1999)
Morphine	Base	Stanski et al. (1978)
Furosemide	Acid	Andreasen et al. (1983)
Phenytoin	Acid	Allen et al. (1979)

measured as its molecular weight which is measured in units of Daltons (Da). A molecular weight below 600 Da is an optimal size for enabling diffusion through a membrane. So, for a drug to diffuse rapidly through a membrane, it should be relatively small in size and be fat-soluble at the site of absorption.

2.2.1.4 Drug Efflux Proteins

Given that fat-soluble substances can gain easy access to the bloodstream by diffusing through cell membranes, the body requires protection from these substances. This is achieved by proteins that are present in barrier membranes such as the gut, lung and nephron epithelia. These proteins remove (efflux) medications from the membrane as they diffuse through it. The epithelial membranes of the intestine possess numerous drug efflux proteins that are found on the surface that faces the intestinal lumen. The function of these proteins is to recognise fat-soluble substances, be they drug or toxin, and repel the substances from the intestinal epithelial membrane or cell back into the intestinal lumen (Fig. 2.3).

There are different types of drug efflux proteins; however, two main types are of clinical importance are P-glycoprotein (Pgp) multidrug resistance-associated protein (MRP) (Khan 2010). Together these drug efflux proteins recognise and remove a large number of drugs (Khan 2002). These proteins are therefore responsible for limiting drug entry into the bloodstream from the intestine, together with limiting drug entry in other organs such as the liver, kidney, lung and brain. The number of these proteins may change with increased drug dosage, thus rendering an initially effective drug regimen eventually ineffective. Consequently, many therapeutic treatments have limited or unsustainable effect owing to the presence and in some cases drug-induced up-regulation (increase) of these proteins (Khan 2006).

Once the drug enters the intestinal epithelium, it gains access to the capillary network inside the small intestine villi, from here it travels to the liver via the portal vein.

The final factor to consider in relation to drug absorption is that of perfusion or blood supply of the absorbing surface. Although this process is really the domain of the next process to be examined, that is, distribution, there is some merit in interlinking the two processes together at this juncture. Intestinal blood supply is derived from the superior mesenteric artery, but the blood flow to this area is not consistent. It increases after meals and significantly reduces during exercise. In addition, when blood pressure is low, blood is shunted away from the mesenteric vasculature

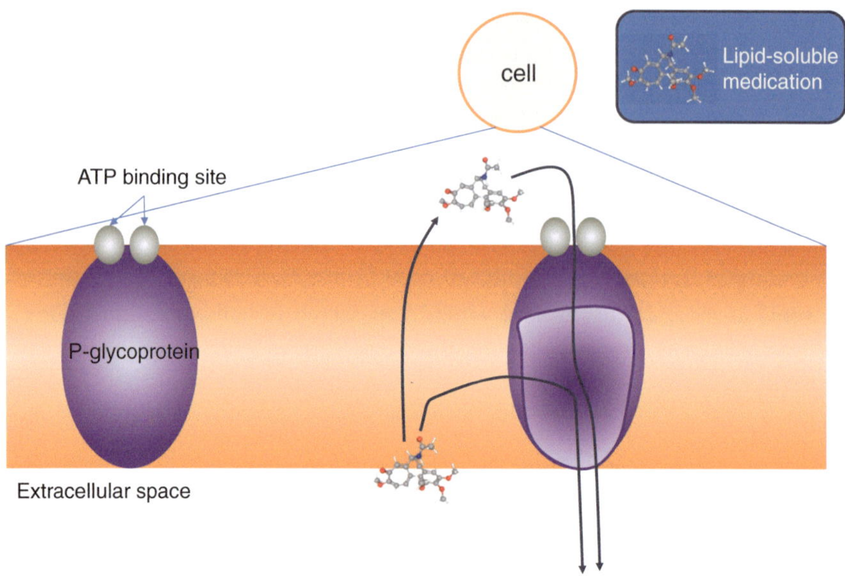

Fig. 2.3 Drug efflux from a membrane

(Steiner et al. 2007) to the core circulation, which mainly consists of the kidneys and brain. This may result in individuals with persistently low blood pressure experiencing impaired drug absorption with oral medication.

2.2.1.5 First-Pass Effect

Blood from the intestine goes straight to the liver via the hepatic portal system; here, absorbed substances are stored and metabolised. Medications also undergo different levels of destruction and activation, a process known as metabolism. The first pass of an absorbed drug from the intestine to the liver is called first-pass effect or hepatic metabolism. First-pass effect is a measure of how much liver enzymes change the drug molecule. First-pass effect has a strong influence on bioavailability of a drug. Drugs that undergo significant first-pass metabolism have low bioavailability. The intravenous route bypasses first-pass effect, as do the highly vascularised buccal and sublingual routes. The benefit of using these routes is their rapid onset of effect, as the drug is not metabolised by the liver. A good example of this process in clinical practice is glyceryl trinitrate (GTN). This anti-angina medication undergoes significant first-pass metabolism in the liver resulting in a bioavailability that is clinically ineffective. However, when GTN is administered by the intravenous or sublingual routes, its bioavailability increases to clinically useful levels.

2.2.1.6 Absorption via Other Routes

Absorption of a drug via other routes depends upon the ease with which the drug separates from its initial formulation. For drugs that are absorbed directly into the bloodstream, for example, IV, the medicine contains little more than a solution of fluid within which the drug is dissolved or suspended. For other routes of administration such as intramuscular (IM) and subcutaneous (SC), the dissolving solution characteristics may govern how fast the drug leaches from the solution into the surrounding circulation and eventually to the central circulation.

2.2.2 Distribution

Distribution of the drug is linked directly to blood flow: the better the blood flow from where the drug is absorbed, the faster the drug enters the circulation and is distributed around the body.

Distribution is an important factor that helps determine the onset of effect of a drug, as most drugs interact with their target inadvertently. Except for antibody-drug conjugate medications so called magic bullet treatments, most medications are administered at a high enough concentration to increase the probability of a drug reaching and binding to its desired target. Drugs that bind specifically to a single or limited number of targets therefore have limited additional effects, and drugs that do not have a specific target have considerably more additional effects.

Drug distribution from the intestine is normally adequate owing to well-perfused mesenteric vasculature. In comparison, other areas such as the skin that has comparatively poor perfusion demonstrates slower absorption and distribution, allowing the drug to have a more prolonged duration of effect. Administration sites used for this approach include transdermal patches and subcutaneous injections.

To help understand drug distribution in some detail, three concepts require defining: plasma protein binding, body compartments and the volume of distribution.

Drugs may circulate bound and unbound to plasma proteins in the bloodstream. Importantly unbound drug, but not bound drug, has a pharmacological effect. As a general rule, drugs that are very hydrophobic or fat-soluble readily bind to plasma proteins. Plasma protein binding affects the drug effect together with the volume of drug within the body. The two proteins of particular importance to plasma protein binding are albumin, the most abundant plasma protein (Day and Myszka 2003), and alpha-1 acid glycoprotein (Fournier et al. 2000). These proteins bind different drugs at the same time. The extent to which a drug is plasma protein bound is an important pharmaceutical assessment during drug development; however, clinically it is normally of little consequence as albumin concentration in the bloodstream is usually 100-fold higher than that of the drug (Day and Myszka 2003). For this reason, even when a person is administered a number of medications that are highly plasma protein bound, there is normally sufficient albumin to bind the drug. Nevertheless, with polypharmacy, poor renal function and reduced albumin levels, the resultant elevated drug concentration in the bloodstream may lead to drug molecules competing for available plasma protein binding sites, which in turn may lead to one drug displacing another from the albumin molecule, resulting in an abnormally elevated level of that drug circulating unbound (pharmacologically active) in the body (Fig. 2.4).

Fig. 2.4 Drugs binding to an albumin molecule in the bloodstream

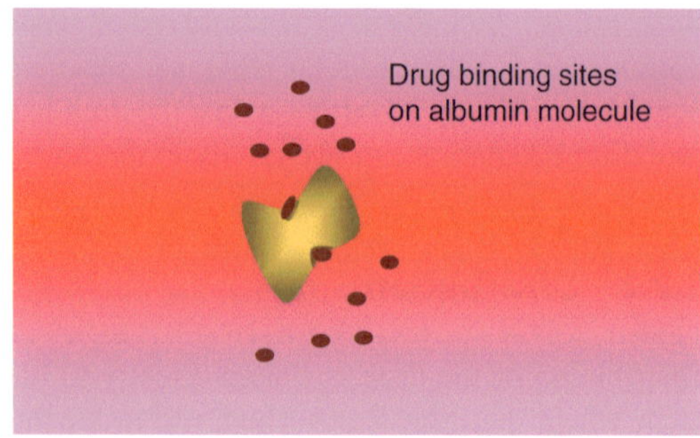

2.2.2.1 Fluid Compartments

Fluid in the body is separated into three areas or compartments.

Fluid is compartmentalised into fluid found in cells (intracellular compartment) and in extracellular compartments. The extracellular compartment includes fluid bathing the cells, the interstitial fluid and the fluid found within the blood vessels, the intravascular compartment.

The intracellular compartment, which is the largest, equals 0.4 × body weight and equates to approximately 28 L.

Extracellular fluid is approximately 0.2 × body weight and accounts for approximately 14 L. Approximately three-fourths of this extracellular fluid is interstitial, approximately 10 L, and the remaining is blood plasma which is about 3.0 L.

Drugs partition into these different compartments depending on concentration and ability to penetrate the membranes of each compartment. Apart from these three fluid compartments, drugs may possess a fourth compartment which is accessible to those drugs that are fat-soluble. This compartment consists of body fat. The extent of absorption and distribution of a drug into the four compartments gives rise to the concept of volume of distribution.

2.2.2.2 Volume of Distribution

Volume of distribution (Vd) is a measure of drug distribution in the body. It is not an actual measure but a virtual or proportionate one. Volume of distribution may be defined as the volume of fluid required (hypothetically) in the body to contain the drug at the same concentration as it is found in the plasma. If the drug remains confined within the blood vessel, then for a 70 kg person with 3.0 L of plasma, the distribution volume of the drug becomes 3.0/70 = 0.042 L/kg or simply put 3 L. As most drugs are not confined to the bloodstream, the extent to which they can distribute into other compartments of the body governs their volume of distribution. Some medications may have a volume of distribution of thousands of litres, which demonstrates that the drug is distributed within most tissues of the body. The Vd of some commonly used medications is given in Table 2.2.

Volume of distribution is linked to fat solubility of a medication. Fat-soluble medications can diffuse through lipid membranes with relative ease. Drugs that are very fat-soluble access most parts of the body, resulting in a large volume of

Table 2.2 Volume of distribution for some common medications

Drug	Vd (L/kg)	References	Fat solubility (Log P)
Simvastatin	124.49 ± 39.76 (with food)	Alakhali et al. (2018)	4.5
Levothyroxine	11–15	Colucci et al. (2013)	1.15
Paracetamol	0.9	Forrest et al. (1982)	0.51
Omeprazole	0.4	Clissold and Campoli-Richards (1986)	1.6

Vd is volume of distribution, Log P is a measure of fat solubility The higher the number, the more fat-soluble the drug

distribution (Table 2.2). Although the drug may potentially access any tissue in the body, fat-soluble drugs tend to accumulate in fat stores, typically in subcutaneous fat. This means that fat-soluble drugs that have a narrow therapeutic margin require a body weight-related adjustment to drug dosage. As a rule, drugs with a large volume of distribution require significant loading before they can have a therapeutic effect. By quickly saturating the fat stores in the body loading a drug helps attain the desired concentration in the blood stream.

The clinical consequence of this is that many fat-soluble drugs take time to achieve a steady-state concentration in the bloodstream resulting in a therapeutic effect, but also once the drug is stopped, it takes time for the drug effect to stop as the drug moves out of the extravascular (fat) stores back into the bloodstream, continuing the drug effect.

2.3 Drug Metabolism

2.3.1 Enzymatic Defence

The concept of enzymatic defence facilitates understanding of how and why the body metabolises medications. To keep the body protected, metabolic enzymes in the liver have to detoxify a large number of different molecules. Given the plethora of chemical structures that can interact with the body, this is a complicated task. The body, however, has an elegant solution to this problem. To be toxic, the substance has to first enter the body. The main factor governing access to the body is fat solubility of the medication. Therefore, for a medication to gain access to the body and exert an effect, it must possess a degree of fat solubility. Most, if not all, drug-detoxifying processes aim to render fat-soluble substances harmless by converting them to more water-soluble structures. Once the substance is rendered water- soluble, the substance cannot exit the bloodstream as it cannot diffuse through cellular membranes. Nearly 75% of medications are rendered ineffective in this manner (Williams et al. 2004). Following metabolism, the drug is said to be eliminated from the system, as it is not available for action, even though it is still physically in the body.

2.3.2 Forms of Drug Metabolism

The conversion of a fat-soluble drug structure to a more water-soluble structure is an example of biotransformation. Biotransformation uses enzymes to transform drugs into products known as metabolites. Drug biotransformation is achieved by two processes: Phase I metabolism that transforms the drug by modifying its structure. Enzymes may catalyse the removal of functional groups that make the drug fat-soluble such as methane (CH3) and add functional groups that make the drug structure more water-soluble such as a hydroxyl ion (OH−). These transformations render the metabolite more water-soluble. Phase II metabolism converts the drug into a more water-soluble form by binding the drug with another water-soluble or polar substance to form a water-soluble complex. This process is known as conjugation.

2.3.3 Phase I Metabolism

Phase 1 metabolism is carried out by a large group of enzymes known as cytochrome P450 (CYP) (Table 2.3). Reactions catalysed by these enzymes result in cleaving of the drug molecule, making the resultant molecule, the metabolite more polar (Guengerich 2008) subsequently rendering the drug more water-soluble (Fig. 2.5a).

Approximately 75% of frequently prescribed drugs are metabolised by the CYP enzyme system (Williams et al. 2004; Guengerich 2008). Of these, CYP3A4 is the most important as it is involved in metabolising approximately 50–65% of all medications prescribed (Anzenbacher and Anzenbacherova 2001; Zhou 2009). In relation to drug metabolism, the other important CYP is CYP 2D6 that is involved in metabolising medications related to mental health treatment (Johnson et al. 2006; Zhou 2009). Usefully CYP3A4 is the most abundant liver enzyme accounting for approximately 30% of all CYPS expressed in the liver (Shimada et al. 1994). In contrast 2D6 only accounts for 2% of the average CYP content of the liver (Shimada et al. 1994).

2.3.4 Phase II Metabolism

Phase II metabolism results in the addition of water-soluble (charged/polar) molecules to the drug molecule by enzymes known as transferases. These additions are known as conjugations and molecules that are added are known as conjugates.

Table 2.3 Nomenclature of CYP enzymes

Enzyme name	Family	Subtype	Gene
CYP1A1	1	A	1
CYP3A4	3	A	4

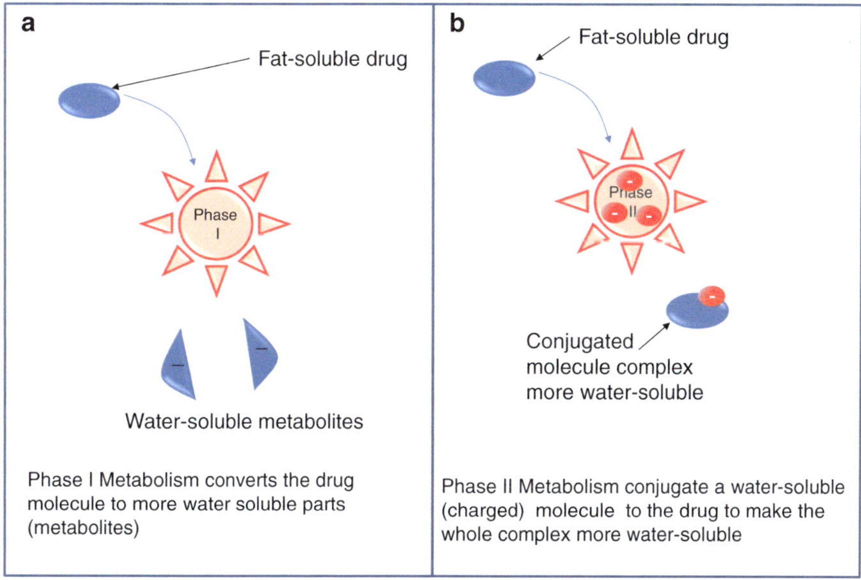

Fig. 2.5 (**a**) Phase 1 metabolism converts the drug molecule to more water soluble parts (metabolites). (**b**) Phase 2 Metabolism conjugate a water-soluble (charged) molecule to the drug to make the whole complex more water-soluble

Conjugates include substances such as glucuronic acid, sulphate or glycine. Conjugation may occur with the unchanged drug or a Phase I metabolite. The charge of the conjugate renders the drug-conjugate complex more water-soluble, assisting in its clearance from the body (Fig. 2.5b).

Medications may undergo Phase I or Phase II or both forms of metabolism.

2.3.5 Phase III Metabolism

Phase III metabolism refers to drug efflux proteins.

Co-localisation of biotransformation Phase I and II enzymes and drug efflux proteins greatly enhances drug metabolism and protection of the body. This is particularly true for co-localisation of the drug efflux protein P-glycoprotein and CYP3A4. P-glycoprotein stops drugs diffusing through barrier membranes, such as is found in the small intestine membrane increasing the exposure of the drug to CYP3A4 giving it repeated opportunities to metabolise the drug. This effect is aided by the fact that P-glycoprotein and CYP3A4 possess similar substrate (substance that interacts with a protein/enzyme) specificities (drug binding profiles).

The presence of both Phase I and Phase II enzymes is not restricted to the liver, as they are found in other locations, for example, the intestine, capillary endothelium, kidney and spleen.

Drug-enzyme interactions may be of three different forms:

- Substrates, drug is metabolised and converted by enzyme.
- Inhibitors, drug inhibits the function of the enzyme but is not converted.
- Inducers, the presence of drug increases the expression of the enzyme.

2.3.6 Enzyme Substrates

Substrate interactions are common and aim to biotransform the drug to a more water-soluble substance rendering the drug harmless. Although this may be the aim of biotransformation, many substrates are converted to an active metabolite by Phase I metabolism. Therefore, in many cases, the drug entering the body may have limited therapeutic effect until it has been converted by metabolic enzymes. Drugs that utilise endogenous (substances produced by the body) enzymes to transform them from relatively inert to more active forms are known as pro-drugs. Common examples of such prodrugs are angiotensin-converting enzyme inhibitors such as enalapril and the vasodilator glyceryl trinitrate (GTN).

Other substrates may be active in their own right, but the activity of their metabolite is clinically more significant than the parent drug. This is true for morphine, in that the morphine-6-glucoronide metabolite (Phase II metabolite) is more active than morphine and is responsible for the full effect of the opioid; likewise, codeine owes much of its analgesic activity to CYP2D6-mediated conversion to morphine (Lötsch 2005). Similarly, the metabolite of spironolactone, canrenone, is responsible for much of spironolactone's therapeutic effect (Li et al. 2016).

2.3.6.1 Clinical Importance of Substrate Interactions

Competition of drugs for the same enzyme may lead to impaired substrate metabolism, leading to an elevated unchanged drug concentration that has the potential to harm the patient. Conversely potent metabolites produced by biotransformation may lose their therapeutic effect following liver dysfunction, owing to a lack of conversion of the drug to the more effective metabolite.

2.3.7 Enzyme Inhibitors

Some medications interact with metabolic enzymes and inhibit their function. These medications are known as inhibitors as they are not converted by the enzyme. This inhibition may be a result of direct enzyme inhibition or by the reduction of the expression (downregulation) of the enzyme (Lown et al. 1997).

The large number of enzyme inhibitors identified (Khan 2002) has clinical significance. If a drug in a multidrug regimen is an enzyme inhibitor and another drug in the regimen is biotransformed by the same enzyme, this may lead to an elevation of co-administered drug.

Such clinically important interactions include systemic azole antifungals such as fluconazole, the macrolide antibiotic erythromycin, a number of protease inhibitors such as ritonavir and calcium channels blockers including the dihydropyridine L-type calcium ion channel blockers (felodipine) and other L-type calcium ion channel blockers such as verapamil. Other naturally occurring inhibitors include chemical components of grapefruit juice such as flavanone that inhibit CYP3A4 (Guengerich 2008).

2.3.8   Enzyme Inducers

Some drugs trigger the production of enzymes; these medications are known as *inducers*. Strong inducers for CYP3A enzymes include the endothelin inhibitor, bosentan as well as other medications such as carbamazepine, phenytoin, rifampicin and the herbal therapy St John's Wort and some weak inducers including dexamethasone, quinine and terbinafine (Polasek et al. 2011). Administration of these drugs within a polypharmacy regimen may lead to loss of effect of some drugs as the increased level of CYP3A4 may increase the metabolism of co-administered drug rendering it ineffective.

In summary, Phase I and II a drug metabolism aims to transforms drugs into more water-soluble substances or metabolites. Owing to their water solubility, these metabolites cannot leave the bloodstream which results in eliminating their therapeutic effect. Eventually these metabolites are removed or excreted from the body typically by the kidney. As there is a finite amount of Phase I and II enzymes in the body, there is a risk that a person prescribed polypharmacy may saturate these enzymes resulting in an increase in unchanged drug in the bloodstream. This may be further complicated by inclusion of a known enzyme inhibiting drug.

2.4   Clearance

Drug clearance is the process by which drugs, or their metabolites, are removed from the body. Although there are many organs that contribute to this process, the route of clearance is primarily determined by drug molecule size. The kidney eliminates drugs which have a molecular weight below 300, and the liver via the bile (biliary) typically removes drugs above this molecular weight (Table 2.4). The lung is the main route of excretion for volatile gases such as inhalation anaesthetics and alcohol.

Table 2.4 An example of how drug clearance relates to molecular weight

Drug	Molecular weight (MWt)	Excretion
Erythromycin	733.29	Biliary
Paracetamol	151.163	Renal
Bisoprolol	325.443	Renal
Metronidazole	171.15	Renal ~70%
Cyclosporine	1202	Biliary

2.4.1 Renal Clearance

The kidney provides the main excretory pathway for medication. This is because biotransformation renders drugs water-soluble, consequently keeping the drug (metabolite) in the bloodstream. Eventually, the metabolites pass via the glomerulus into the renal ultrafiltrate, where again due to water solubility, they are not reabsorbed by nephron reabsorption, ultimately leading to the biotransformed drug/metabolite being voided in the urine.

Another reason renal clearance is common is because of drug size (Table 2.4). Membrane permeability is enhanced by small molecular size; therefore, to enhance absorption, most orally administered drugs have a molecular weight <300 resulting in them being cleared by the kidney.

Kidney excretion of drugs depends upon four processes: filtration, formation of a concentration gradient, tubular reabsorption and active tubular secretion.

Renal filtration is dependent on blood pressure which determines the glomerular filtration rate (GFR). Generally plasma protein bound drugs are not filtered by the glomerulus. Only unbound drugs, changed or unchanged, enter the ultrafiltrate via the glomerulus. Deteriorating renal function with concomitant reduction in GFR may therefore diminish drug clearance. Importantly, it is known that age is associated with a reduction in GFR. Approximately from the age of 70, the GFR may fall to below the recognised threshold for chronic kidney disease of 60 mL/min/1.73 m^2 (Delanaye et al. 2012). It is important, therefore, that caution is employed when treating an older person taking a number of medicines, as their renal function may compromise therapeutic safety.

2.4.1.1 Formation of the Concentration Gradient

The proximal convoluted tubule reabsorbs about two-thirds of water from the ultrafiltrate. This increases the concentration of the drug in the ultrafiltrate generating a concentration gradient that favours unchanged (fat-soluble) drug movement out of the lumen of the proximal tubule (Fig. 2.6). Conversely, when more water is passed in the urine such as with diuretic use, the lower concentration gradient results in more drug being excreted by the kidney. The percentage of unchanged drug present in the ultrafiltrate is an important clinical value, as it determines the potential for drug interactions in the presence of renal dysfunction.

A second site of reabsorption in the nephron is the collecting duct (Fig. 2.6). Unlike the proximal convoluted tubule that has an increased surface area, reabsorption in the collecting duct is dependent on antiduiretic hormone (ADH) that regulates the collecting duct's ability to concentrate the ultrafiltrate to form urine. Increased water absorption in the collecting duct concentrates the ultrafiltrate and increases drug diffusion from nephron to bloodstream.

Active Tubular Secretion: To guard against the reabsorption of drugs, a process known as active tubular secretion exists in the nephron. Active tubular secretion results from the nephron epithelium expressing a large number of different drug efflux transporter proteins such as P-glycoprotein and multidrug resistance-related

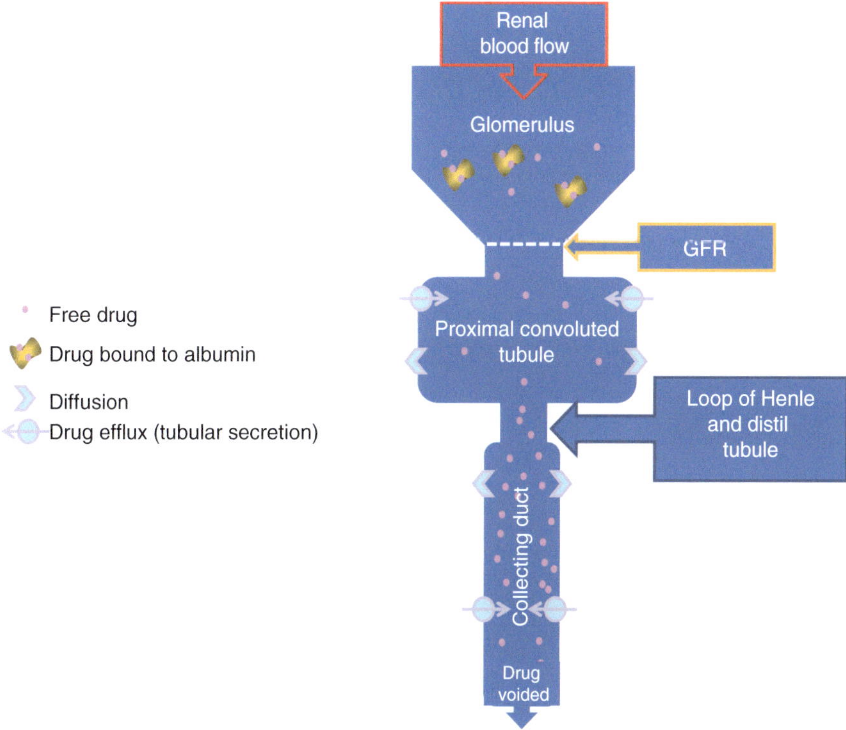

Fig. 2.6 Main factors influencing renal drug clearance

protein in the luminal membranes of the proximal tubule and collecting duct (Fig. 2.6). These efflux pumps actively transporting the drug back into the ultrafiltrate as it diffuses into the epithelial cells of the nephronal tubule wall. In these locations, drug efflux transporters are an important site of drug-drug interaction in the kidney. For example, the use of non-warfarin oral anticoagulant dabigatran is contraindicated when patients have poor a GFR and are also taking a medication that may inhibit Pgp such as ketoconazole and omeprazole. This balance of drug clearance can also be affected by a variation in filtrate pH that will affect fat solubility of some drugs. Fat solubility is modulated by the ionisation (charged) state of the drug (Fig. 2.7a, b), which in turn may be altered by changes in pH. Drugs that change renal pH may change drug reabsorption in the collecting duct and convoluted tubules. Diet may also change pH in the urine; for example, meat renders urine acidic, whereas vegetables render urine alkaline.

Blood pressure is possibly the most important factor that governs renal filtration and therefore drug clearance. It is pharmacologically important to monitor renal function; this is of particular importance when individuals are prescribed polypharmacy as reduction in the GFR may significantly alter drug clearance.

a   Ionization.

Elements have different numbers of electrons that rotate around the nucleus in different energy layers or shells. Apart from the first energy layer or shell, all other shells can take a maximum of 8 electrons. A number of elements have only one electron in their outer most shell such as in the case of sodium and potassium. These elements can easily lose their outermost electron to other elements that only need one electron to complete the 8 electrons in their outermost shell, such as chlorine

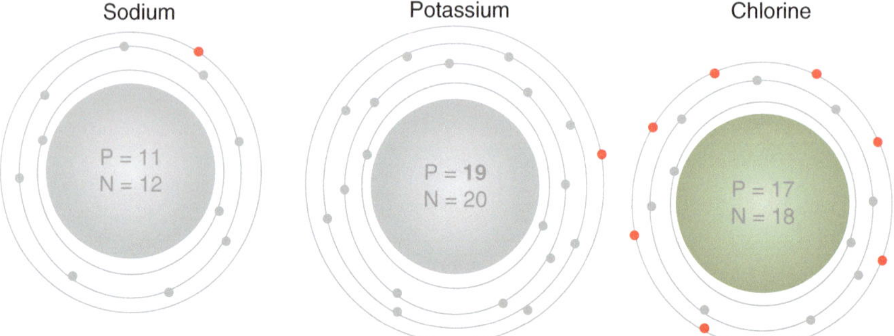

When sodium or potassium lose an electron in such a manner they have one more proton in the nucleus than negatively charged electrons surrounding it. This results in the atom having a net positive charge which is denoted as a superscripted + sign above the element's name (Na^+ or K^+). Similarly Chlorine that has gained an electron to complete its outermost electron shell has one more electron than number of protons in its nucleus. Therefore it has a net negative charge on the atom denoted by a negative sign superscripted next to the atom name (Cl^-). These charged or ionised forms of atoms are called ions.

b   pH, ionisation and fat solubility

Drugs may be weak acids or weak bases.
An acid is a molecule that can donate a positive charge in water rendering it an anion, (ionised with a negative charge).
Weak basic drugs can gain a hydrogen ion (proton) in water rendering them a cation.

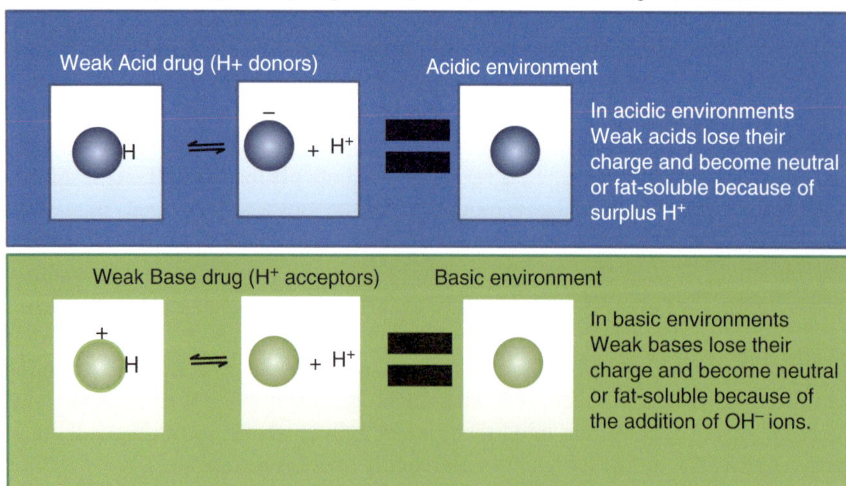

Fig. 2.7 (**a** and **b**) Ionisation panel

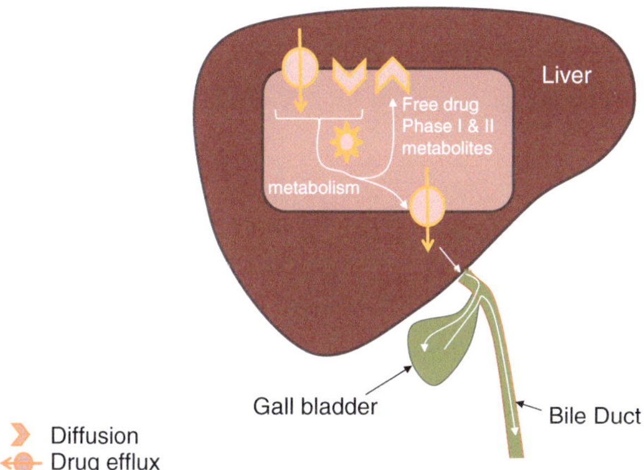

Fig. 2.8 Drug clearance in the liver

2.4.2   Liver Clearance

Drugs may enter the hepatocyte (liver cell) by passive diffusion and as these cells also possess drug efflux proteins, by active transport (secretion) (Shitara et al. 2005; Klaassen and Aleksunes 2010) (Fig. 2.8). In the liver, the drug may be metabolised or pass unchanged through the cell wall. Drug or metabolite may then be secreted in the bile, for excretion via faeces. However, changed and unchanged drug may also re-enter the circulation by passive diffusion (Fig. 2.8).

Bile-secreted conjugated drugs may have their conjugate molecule removed (deconjugation) by intestinal bacteria or flora, releasing the original compound. This medication may be reabsorbed into the bloodstream via the intestine. The possibility of this occurring is determined and quantified during drug development and does not normally pose a problem; however, administration of broad-spectrum antibiotics may reduce gut flora, which in turn may increase drug removal from the body, potentially reducing drug effect.

2.5   Drug Half-Life

The duration of drug effect is dependent upon volume of distribution and drug clearance. Using these two parameters, a measure known as half-life can be calculated. Drug half-life written as $t_{1/2}$ is defined as the time it takes the concentration of drug in the plasma or body to be reduced by half (Fig. 2.9). This is a useful measure as it provides an estimate of how long a drug effect may last.

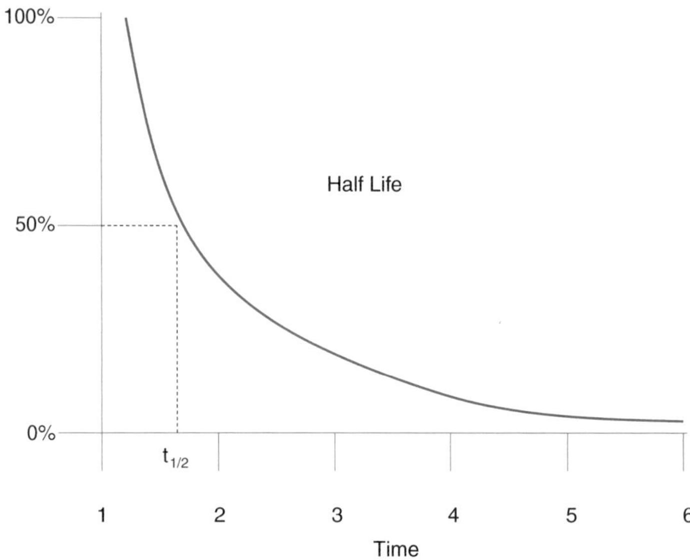

Fig. 2.9 Drug Half life

2.6   Therapeutic Index

This is a measure of the safety margin of a drug. In essence it is a comparison of the quantity of a therapeutic dose of a drug compared to the quantity of drug that would be toxic.

2.7   Pharmacokinetics: Summary

Pharmacokinetic processes influence the impact of a drug in the body. Variations in physicochemical characteristics of the drug or the internal environment of the body may change how a drug interacts passively with the body, as seen with changes in pH altering drug-membrane permeability. Active transport (drug efflux) and enzymatic processes, although many, are potentially saturable, that is, mechanisms that may get overwhelmed with increased drug burden. The liver and renal system are primarily involved in pharmacokinetic processes and certainly, they influence a drug's ultimate efficacy; dysfunction of these organs may influence therapeutic outcome.

Older people are more likely to be receiving polypharmacy and have liver or kidney dysfunction owing to the possible presence of disease- and age-related organ deterioration. Therefore, the older person's medication regimen must to be managed with precise care.

2.8 Pharmacodynamics

Pharmacodynamics is the measure of the drug effect on the body, as such pharmacodynamics relates to the mechanism of action of a medication and the extent of its effect include adverse reactions. Homeostatic processes are modulated by medication to achieve action and effect. To understand how medication achieves this, homeostatic communication in the body is reviewed (Fig. 2.10).

This process will be elaborated with reference to Fig. 2.10, using blood pressure regulation as an example.

Following a reduction in blood pressure (stimulus), the brain initiates the release of a number of substances including hormones as well as chemicals from nerve endings (neurotransmitters). These substances act as the first link in the chain of communication and are known as first messengers (Fig. 2.10). These messengers travel to their site of action, and in this example, these may be the heart, kidney or blood vessel. On arrival, they interact with the organ at a cellular level by interacting or binding with proteins called receptors (Fig. 2.10). The nature of interaction between the first messenger and its receptor depends upon the type of first messenger and the type of receptor that is bound. This is because these interactions determine secondary communications that occur within the cell. These secondary interactions are in turn mediated by receptors and enzymes that modulate chemical reactions within the cell. As these interactions occur following first messenger interaction, these subsequent chemical interactions are known as secondary messenger interactions.

There are a several permutations possible within any system, leading to different effects in different organs. An example of this is adrenaline binding to its receptors

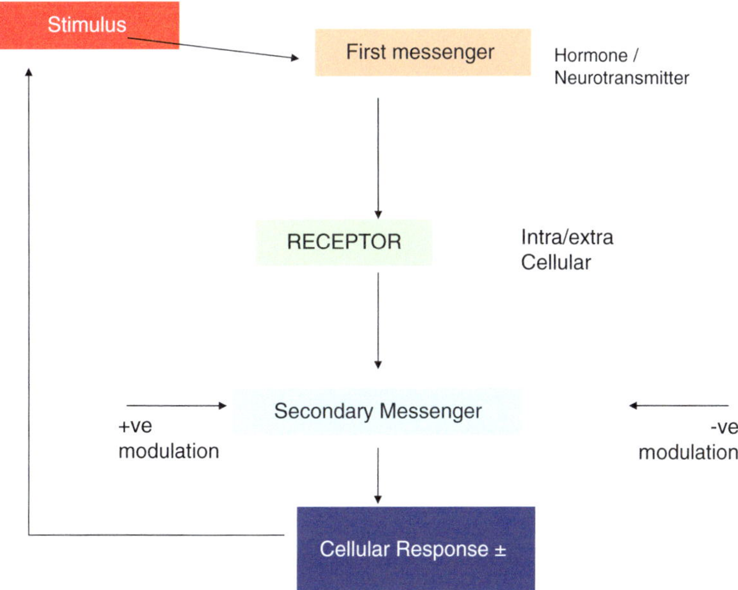

Fig. 2.10 Physiological communication in the body

in the heart, which primarily leads to an increase in function of the heart by excitatory or positive modulation of secondary messenger mechanisms. The response to this is that the heart pumps faster and harder, the effect of which is to increase blood pressure, consequently removing the initial stimulus that initiated the release of the first messenger (Fig. 2.10).

Pharmacologically, medications are designed to modulate first and second messenger interactions, as well as modulate monitoring systems in the body. The target of a medication varies; it may be either an:

- Ion channel
- Transport proteins
- Receptor
- Enzyme
- Cell membrane

2.9 Ion Channels

Ion channels are protein structures that span the membrane (Fig. 2.11). As ions themselves do not penetrate cell membranes, ion channels are needed to enable ion movement across the membrane. Stimuli that open or close ion channels include

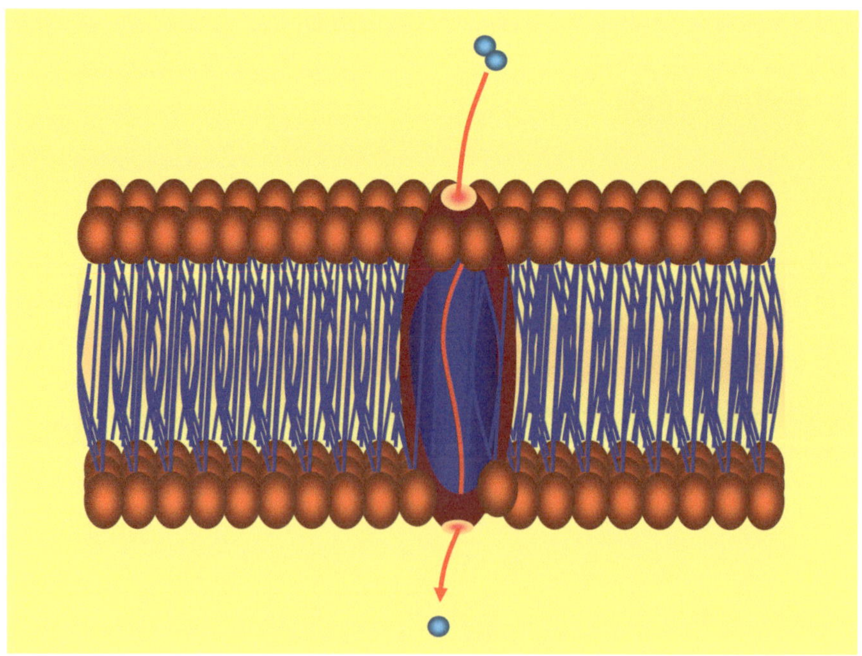

Fig. 2.11 Ion channel (transverse section) of the transmembranous passage affording ions

ligands and voltage. Ion movement through an ion channel is determined by the ion concentration gradient. Ion channels are such that as long as the ion channel is open, ions can flow through them; therefore, ion entry is only limited by the duration of ion channel opening.

Ion channel closing or opening helps control cell function. For example, sodium entry into the cell excites it, leading to contraction in muscles and electrical impulse conduction in a nerve. An example of a drug that impacts on ion channel function in these tissues is lignocaine, which blocks the sodium ion channel, stopping sodium from entering into the cell, and as a consequence reduces muscle excitability and prevents nerve conduction.

2.10 Ligands

A ligand is a drug or endogenous substance which binds to a receptor or other biological molecule and elicits a response (e.g. histamine is a ligand at histamine receptors).

2.11 Transport Proteins

Transport proteins are like ion channels in function in that they enable ion movement across a membrane. However, in addition to ions, transport proteins may also transport other substances such as sugars, amino acids and peptides amongst others. Together these substances are referred to as substrates. When the substrate movement is in accordance with the concentration gradient, the transport is passive (Fig. 2.12). However, if the transport protein moves its substrate against the concentration gradient, then this process is termed active transport. Unlike ion channels, transport proteins are limited by the rate at which they can shuttle their substrates back and forth across the membrane. An example of a medication that inhibits transport proteins is furosemide, which inhibits sodium (and potassium) reabsorption from the nephronal filtrate.

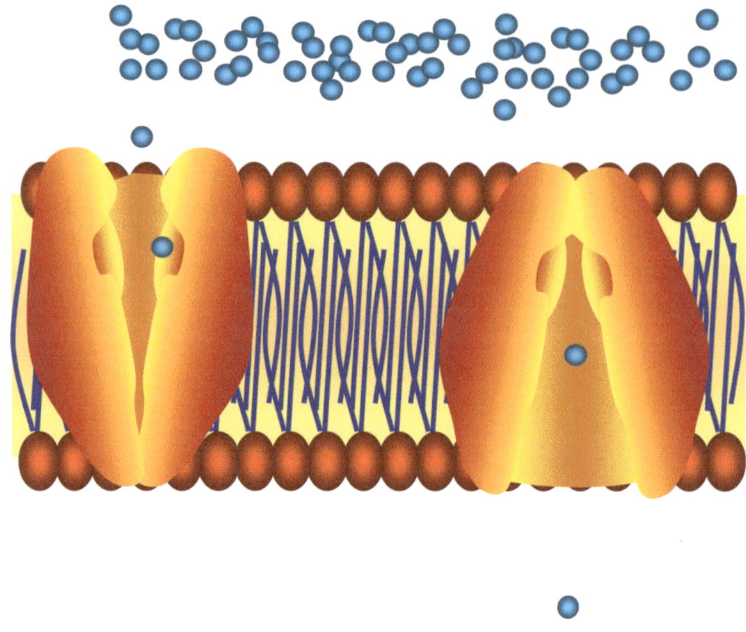

Fig. 2.12 A transport protein transporting ions across the membrane

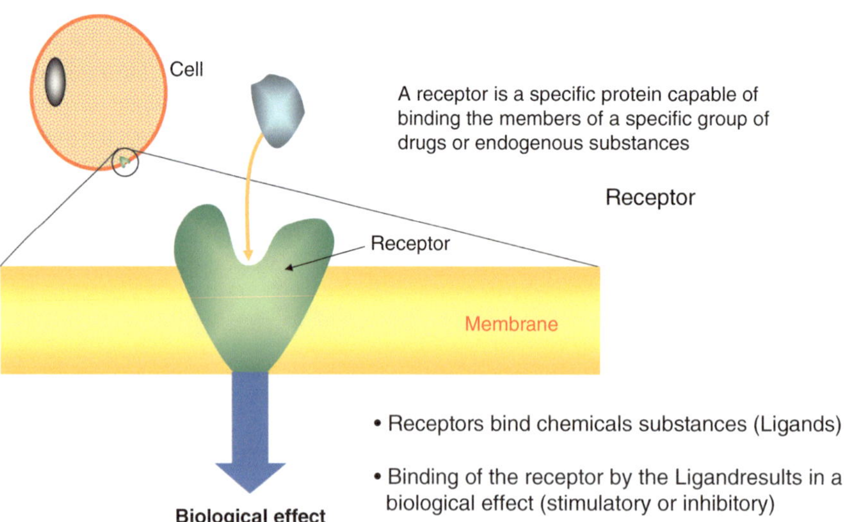

Fig. 2.13 A substance (ligand) binding to its receptor

2.12 Receptor

A receptor is a protein capable of binding the members of a specific group of drugs or endogenous substances (ligands) (Fig. 2.13).

The interaction of a drug with its receptor leads to the pharmacological effect.

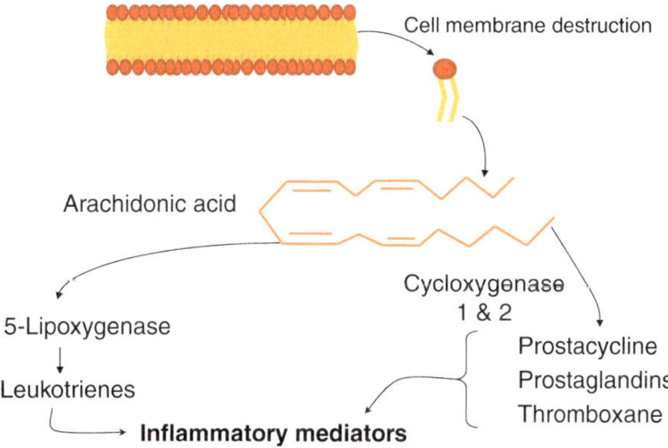

Fig. 2.14 Cyclooxygenase converts arachidonic acid to inflammatory mediators

2.13 Enzymes

Enzymes are chemical catalysts that accelerate biochemical reactions in the body.

There is a diverse array of enzymes in the body and many are probably still unknown. Common examples of enzymes that are pharmacological drug targets include angiotensin-converting enzyme that converts angiotensin I into angiotensin II and the cyclooxygenase enzyme (COX) that converts arachidonic acid into steroidal inflammatory mediators (Fig. 2.14).

2.14 Cell Membranes

Cell membranes may be drug targets involved in the pharmacological effect of some anaesthetics and antibiotics.

2.15 Receptor Theory

Receptors bind substances by weak chemical bonds that are derived from miniscule charges on the ligands and receptor surface. In addition, the ligand must have the right shape to bind to a specific receptor (Fig. 2.15).

2.15.1 Affinity

The characteristics of shape and charge of a ligand give rise to the concept of affinity. The more a ligand's shape fits the binding site of a receptor and the more the charges on the ligand complement those of a receptor binding site, the higher the affinity between the ligand and the receptor. In the example (Fig. 2.16a), the ligand (blue) binds well with the receptor binding site, suggesting the ligand has a high

Fig. 2.15 Ligand shape
and receptor binding

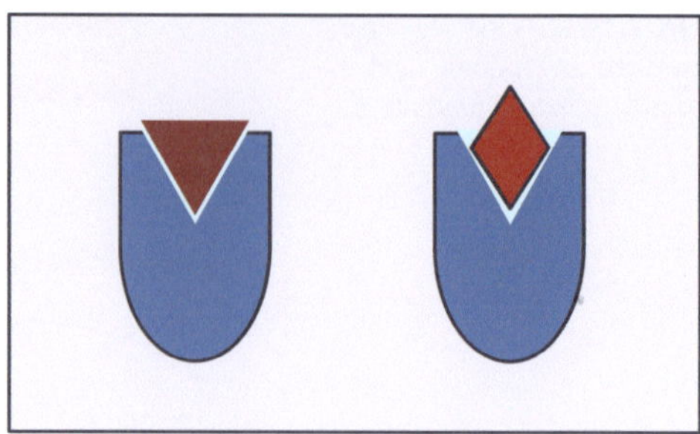

Fig. 2.16 Ligand charge
and morphology determine
receptor affinity

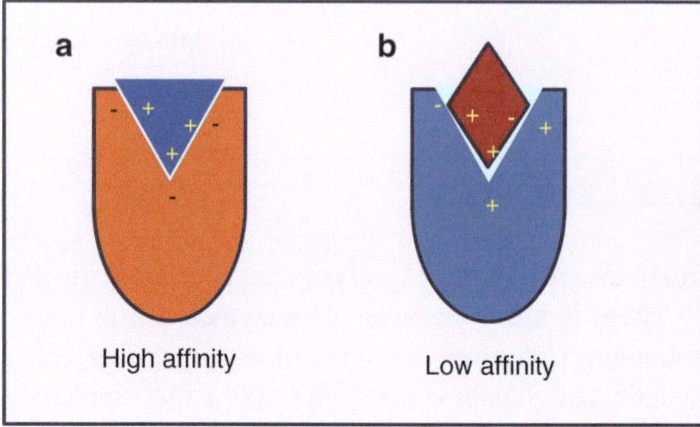

affinity for the receptor. In comparison, if the ligand's shape and charge do not
complement that of the receptor, the ligand will have a low affinity for the receptor
(Fig. 2.16b).

2.16   Drug Interactions with Their Target

There are numerous ways drugs interact with their targets. Using receptors as an
example, for a drug to influence a receptor it has to be able to bind to the receptor
with some affinity.

2.16.1 Agonist

These are drugs that bind with their receptor with high affinity and resulting in high
intrinsic activity, that is, activating the receptor in the manner it would normally be
activated by its normal endogenous ligand.

Therefore agonistic drug interactions mimics the effect of the normal endogenous ligand. When using agonists the number of receptors may reduce over time,
this is known as receptor down regulation.

2.16.2 Antagonists

In these interactions, the drug has a high affinity to allow it to bind to the receptor but binding of the drug to the receptor results in no intrinsic activity.

Binding of the drug to the target therefore results in no effect (the receptor is inhibited).

When using antagonists the number of receptors may increase over time, this is known as receptor up regulation. Antagonism may commonly take on different forms.

2.17   Categories

- A: Competitive antagonists: these compete for the same location on the receptor as its endogenous ligand.
- B: Non-competitive antagonist: these drugs bind to a place other than the endogenous ligand binding site and incapacitate the receptor.
- C: Partial agonists: these act on a receptor but without having maximum effect. Thus reducing the overall effect of the receptor.

2.18   Competitive Antagonism

As the drug and natural ligand compete for the same binding sites, the comparative binding of one compared to the other is determined by the relative affinity of the ligand and drug for the receptor and the concentration of these substances at the receptor (Fig. 2.17).

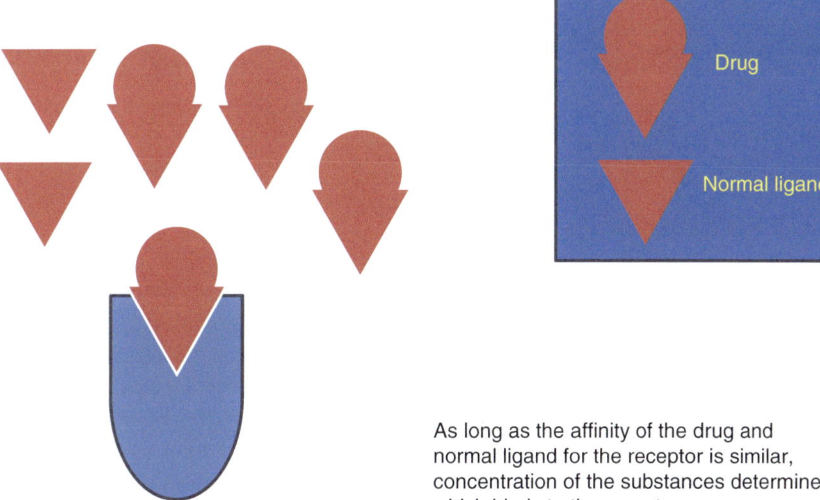

Fig. 2.17 Competitive antagonism, ligand (L) and drug (D) compete for the same receptor site

If the drug and ligand have equal affinities for the receptor, then the binding of the substance is determined by the concentration of the substance at the receptor. The effect of competitive antagonist drugs can be stopped by flooding the system with an agonist targeting the receptor.

2.18.1 Non-competitive Antagonist

In non-competitive antagonism, normal ligand binding to the receptor is not affected (Fig. 2.18). The binding of the drug to the receptor causes a change in the receptor's shape (conformational change), and this influences the chemical effect of the ligand binding to the receptor, resulting in a lack of receptor effect.

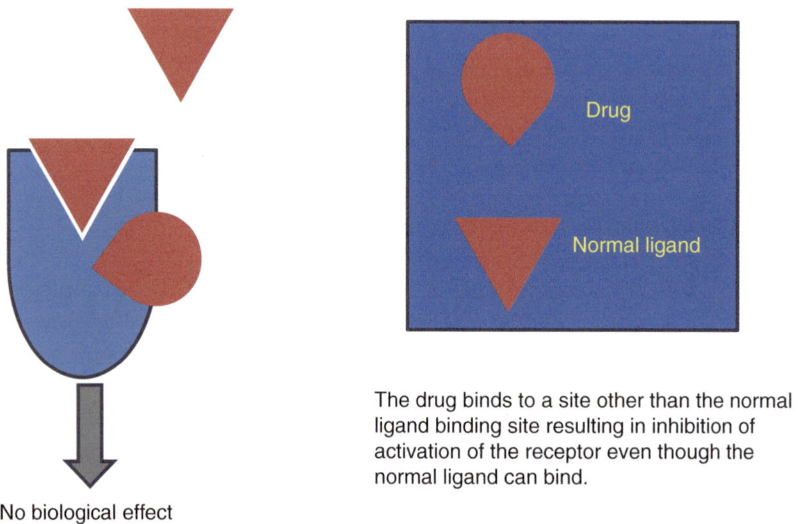

Fig. 2.18 Non-competitive antagonism, with the drug binding to a site other than the normal ligand binding site

2.18.2 Partial Agonists

The term partial agonists may appear as being contrary to antagonism. Partial agonists derive their antagonistic effect from the fact that they partially activate the receptor (agonistic behaviour). This can be explained in terms of intrinsic activity. A drug that has 100% intrinsic activity is a full agonist, whereas a medication that has less than 100% intrinsic activity is a partial agonist. A partial agonist reduces the activity of the receptor, because when a partial agonist is bound to the receptor stimulating it suboptimally, the normal ligand (full agonist) cannot bind and can cause an optimal effect on the receptor. An example of some partial agonists includes the antipsychotic aripiprazole, the opioid buprenorphine and the muscle relaxant suxamethonium.

2.19 Receptor Classification

Receptors are classified in accordance with the natural ligand they bind, e.g. adreno-receptors bind adrenaline, cholinergic receptors bind acetylcholine and dopamine receptors bind dopamine. Given that each receptor type may be associated with different biological effects, receptors have many subtypes. Receptor subtypes help identify the effect a particular receptor may have on the body and conversely describe how a drug would affect the body. Receptor subtypes have a similar general structure with subtle variations, and this allows the body to respond in different ways with the release of a single ligand. An example of this concept is the adrenergic receptor. There are two main subtypes of adrenergic receptors (alpha-and beta-receptors), and in turn these receptors have subtypes, for example, beta-receptors are subdivided into beta-1, beta-2 and beta-3 receptors.

All beta-receptors bind adrenaline (and noradrenaline), but the effect of the receptor subtype differs, with beta-1 receptors having largely stimulatory effects when they bind adrenaline (increased cardiac and brain function), whereas binding of adrenaline to the beta-2 receptor is normally associated with a reduction in stimulation (smooth muscle relaxation in the bronchi, blood vessel and bladder).

2.20 Potency and Efficacy of a Drug

The pharmacodynamics of a drug are assessed in several ways. Two commonly used measures that help assess drug effect are potency and efficacy.

Potency relates to strength of the drug's effect, drugs that a more potent provide a maximal effect (for that drug) at smaller does compared to a drug that is not that potent but the full effect of the drug (its potency) may vary from drug to drug.

Efficacy, which is the more clinically relevant concept, relates to the maximum effect of the drug achievable in the body.

When comparing two drugs the one that demonstrates an effect at a lower dose will typically be more potent, but the drug that provides a greater effect regardless of the drug dose typically has a greater efficacy.

2.21 Summary

Pharmacodynamics is the examination of how a drug interacts with the body. Drugs interfere with homeostatic communication by which they modulate cellular responses and alter organ and/or system function. Drugs interact with the body via drug targets, many of which tend to be proteins that activate or modulate cell function. These proteins include ion channels, membrane transport proteins, receptors and enzymes. Interactions with these proteins may result in inhibition (antagonism) of their function or may enhance or mimic the effect of the protein (agonism). Modulation of these proteins may lead to a retaliatory reaction from the body leading to an increased expression of a drug target (upregulation) when using an antagonist or a downregulation or loss of function of drug target if the drug is an agonist. These effects as well as poor specificity of drugs for their targets, particularly within a similar group of targets, lead to a possibility of side effects occurring while a person is taking the drug and on occasion following cessation of the drug regimen.

Multiple Choice Questions

1. A risk associated with polypharmacy is:
   (a) Obesity
   (b) Drug–drug interaction
   (c) Anorexia
   (d) Urinary retention
2. A non-competitive antagonist:
   (a) Acts on a receptor but without the maximum effect.
   (b) Binds to a site other than the ligand binding site on a target receptor.
   (c) Does not cause any effect on a target receptor.
   (d) Action depends on the time of day the drug is administered.
3. The therapeutic index is:
   (a) The ratio between the lethal dose of a drug and the minimum effective dose of a drug
   (b) The ratio between a drug's efficacy and its bioavailability
   (c) The ratio between the average minimum effective dose of a drug and the average maximum non-toxic dose of a drug
   (d) The ratio between a drug's half-life and the maximum non-toxic dose
4. Pharmacokinetic processes include:
   (a) Inactivation of the drug
   (b) The action and effect of a drug
   (c) The sites and mechanisms of drug action
   (d) Drug potency
5. An agonist is a ligand that has:
   (a) An inhibitory effect on a target receptor
   (b) No effect on a target receptor
   (c) A high affinity for a target receptor with high intrinsic activity
   (d) A high affinity for a target receptor with no intrinsic activity
6. Common drug cytochrome P450 inhibitors include:
   (a) Verapamil
   (b) Dexamethasone
   (c) Tramadol
   (d) Methadone

7. The half-life of a drug can be defined as:
    (a) The time taken for the plasma concentration to increase by half
    (b) Time taken for the plasma concentration of a drug to decrease by half
    (c) The time taken for the drug to be absorbed
    (d) Time taken for the drug to be metabolised
8. A lipid-soluble drug is:
    (a) Water-soluble
    (b) Carries a negative charge
    (c) Carriers a positive charge
    (d) Unionised
9. Which factors affect oral drug absorption:
    (a) Body temperature
    (b) Tachycardia
    (c) Drug solubility
    (d) History of diabetes
10. An antagonist drug:
    (a) Binds to the receptor and mimics the receptor's normal response
    (b) Has no affinity for the binding site
    (c) Binds to the receptor and blocks access by an agonist
    (d) Has no affect

Answers

1. (b)
2. (b)
3. (c)
4. (a)
5. (c)
6. (a)
7. (b)
8. (d)
9. (c)
10. (c)

References

Abernethy DR, Greenblatt DJ, Eshelman FN, Shader RI (1984) Ranitidine does not impair oxidative or conjugative metabolism: noninteraction with antipyrine, diazepam, and lorazepam. Clin Pharmacol Ther 35(2):188–192
Alakhali KM, Vigneshwaran E, Shaik MAA (2018) Effect of food and antacid on simvastatin bioavailability on healthy adult volunteers. J Health Res Rev Dev Ctries 5(1):26–32
Allen JP, Ludden TM, Burrow SR, Clementi WA, Stavchansky SA (1979) Phenytoin cumulation kinetics. Clin Pharmacol Ther 26(4):445–448

Andreasen F, Hansen U, Husted SE, Jansen JA (1983) The pharmacokinetics of frusemide are influenced by age. Br J Clin Pharmacol 16(4):391–397

Anzenbacher P, Anzenbacherova E (2001) Cytochromes P450 and metabolism of xenobiotics. Cell Mol Life Sci 58(5–6):737–747

Cerqueira PM, Cesarino EJ, Mateus FH, Mere Y Jr, Santos SR, Lanchote VL (1999) Enantioselectivity in the steady-state pharmacokinetics of metoprolol in hypertensive patients. Chirality 11(7):591–597

Clissold SP, Campoli-Richards DM (1986) Omeprazole. Drugs 32(1):15–47

Colucci P, Seng Yue C, Ducharme M, Benvenga S (2013) A review of the pharmacokinetics of levothyroxine for the treatment of hypothyroidism. Eur J Endocrinol 9(1):40–47

Day YS, Myszka DG (2003) Characterizing a drug's primary binding site on albumin. J Pharm Sci 92(2):333–343

Delanaye P, Schaeffner E, Ebert N, Cavalier E, Mariat C, Krzesinski JM, Moranne O (2012) Normal reference values for glomerular filtration rate: what do we really know? Nephrol Dial Transplant 27(7):2664–2672

Forrest JA, Clements JA, Prescott LF (1982) Clinical pharmacokinetics of paracetamol. Clin Pharmacokinet 7(2):93–107

Fournier T, Medjoubi-N N, Porquet D (2000) Alpha-1-acid glycoprotein. Biochimica Biophys Acta 1482(1–2):157–171

Guengerich FP (2008) Cytochrome P450 and chemical toxicology. Chem Res Toxicol 21(1):70–83

Janssen P, Vanden Berghe P, Verschueren S, Lehmann A, Depoortere I, Tack J (2011) The role of gastric motility in the control of food intake. Aliment Pharmacol Ther 33(8):880–894

Johnson M, Markham-Abedi C, Susce MT, Murray-Carmichael E, McCollum S, de Leon J (2006) A poor metabolizer for cytochromes P450 2D6 and 2C19: a case report on antidepressant treatment. CNS Spectr 11(10):757–760

Khan EU (2002) The role of P-glycoprotein at the blood-brain barrier. PhD thesis, King's College London (unpublished)

Khan EU (2006) The blood brain barrier: its implications in neurological disease and treatment. Br J Neurosci Nurs 2(1):18–25

Khan EU (2010) Medicine management: pharmacokinetic update for community nurses. Br J Commun Nurs 15(9):436–444

Klaassen CD, Aleksunes LM (2010) Xenobiotic, bile acid, and cholesterol transporters: function and regulation. Pharmacol Rev 62(1):1–96

Latini R, Tognoni G, Kates RE (1984) Clinical pharmacokinetics of amiodarone (weak base). Clin Pharmacokinet 9(2):136–156

Li ZH, Deng Y, Cai HL, Guo ZH, Hou ZY, Wu G, Yan M, Zhang BK (2016) Pharmacokinetic properties and bioequivalence of spironolactone tablets in fasting and fed healthy Chinese male subjects. Int J Clin Pharmacol Ther 54(6):455–461

Lötsch J (2005) Opioid metabolites. J Pain Symptom Manage 29(5 Suppl):S10–S24

Lown KS, Bailey DG, Fontana RJ, Janardan SK, Adair CH, Fortlage LA, Brown MB, Guo W, Watkins PB (1997) Grapefruit juice increases felodipine oral availability in humans by decreasing intestinal CYP3A protein expression. J Clin Investig 99(10):2545–2553

Mudie DM, Amidon GL, Amidon GE (2010) Physiological parameters for oral delivery and in vitro testing. Mol Pharmacol 7(5):1388–1405

Polasek TM, Lin FP, Miners JO, Doogue MP (2011) Perpetrators of pharmacokinetic drug-drug interactions arising from altered cytochrome P450 activity: a criteria-based assessment. Br J Clin Pharmacol 71(5):727–736

Shimada T, Mimura H, Inui Y, Guengerich FP (1994) Interindividual variations in human liver cytochrome P-450 enzymes involved in the oxidation of drugs, carcinogens and toxic chemicals: studies with liver microsomes of 30 Japanese and 30 Caucasians. J Pharmacol Exp Ther 270(1):414–423

Shitara Y, Sato H, Sugiyama Y (2005) Evaluation of drug-drug interaction in the hepatobiliary and renal transport of drugs. Annu Rev Pharmacol Toxicol 45:689–723

Stanski DR, Greenblatt DJ, Lowenstein E (1978) Kinetics of intravenous and intramuscular morphine. Clin Pharmacol Ther 24(1):52–59

Steiner LA, Staender S, Sieber CC, Skarvan K (2007) Effects of simulated hypovolaemia on haemodynamics, left ventricular function, mesenteric blood flow and gastric Pco2. Acta Anaesthesiol Scand 51(2):143–150

Williams JA, Hyland R, Jones BC, Smith DA, Hurst S, Goosen TC, Peterkin V, Koup JR, Ball SE (2004) Drug-drug interactions for UDP-glucuronosyltransferase substrates: a pharmacokinetic explanation for typically observed low exposure (AUCi/AUC) ratios. Drug Metab Dispos 32(11):1201–1208

Zhou S-F (2009) Polymorphism of human cytochrome P450 2D6 and its clinical significance: Part I. Clin Pharmacokinet 48(11):689–723

Drug Formulations

3

Ali A. Dahab

Learning Outcomes
At the end of this chapter, you will be able to:

- Differentiate between active and inactive ingredients in a medication.
- Specify the importance of excipients in medication administration and management.
- Describe the difference between forms of preparation.
- Understand the basic principles of conventional and targeted drug delivery systems.

3.1 Introduction

The goal of drug formulation research and development is to fully utilise all positive properties of existing active drugs as well as developed drug molecules and avoid as many undesired or nonoptimal properties as possible.

In addition to adjusting its activities against patent expirations and the risks of evolving development (Paul et al. 2010; Pammolli et al. 2011), the pharmaceutical industry has chosen formulation research and development as one of its main strategies to enable successful use of drug molecules as widely as possible (Gudiksen et al. 2008; Cavalla 2009). Formulation is an integral part of activities in the phases of drug discovery, development and manufacturing (Fig. 3.1).

A. A. Dahab (✉)
Faculty of Life Science and Medicine, King's College London, London, UK
e-mail: aliadahab@yahoo.co.uk; ali.aboel_dahab@kcl.ac.uk

E. Khan, P. Hood (eds.), *Understanding Pharmacology in Nursing Practice*,
https://doi.org/10.1007/978-3-032-03964-4_3

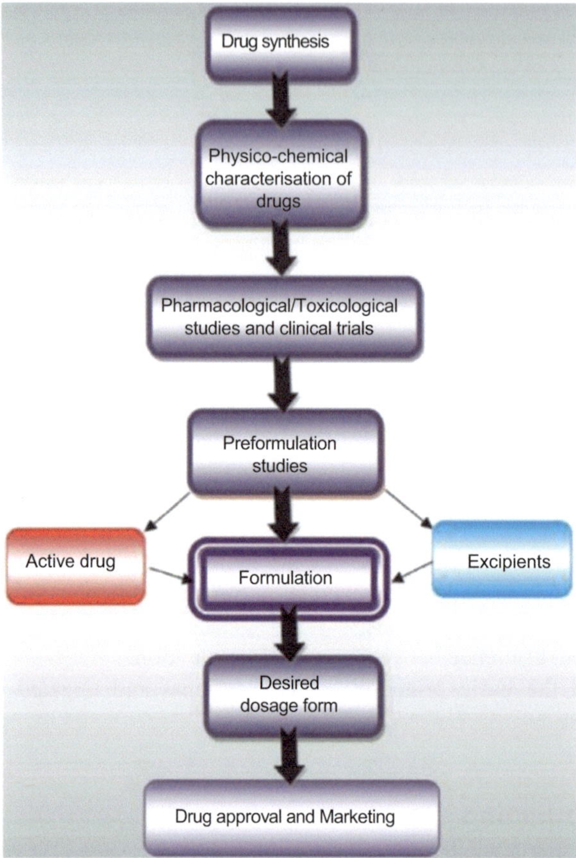

Fig. 3.1 Summary of different phases of new drug development

Therefore, formulation should ensure that a pharmacologically active drug can be synthesised and a medication can be produced, administered and delivered in a desired amount via the route from where it reaches its physiological and pharmacological site of action within the optimal time with the desired therapeutic effect while minimising undesired adverse effects.

The finished dosage form (Fig. 3.2) may be, for example, a modified-release capsule, a standard (conventional) tablet, an orally disintegrating tablet (ODT), gels, or various liquid forms and should be manufactured with appropriate measures of

Fig. 3.2 Various commonly used dosage forms

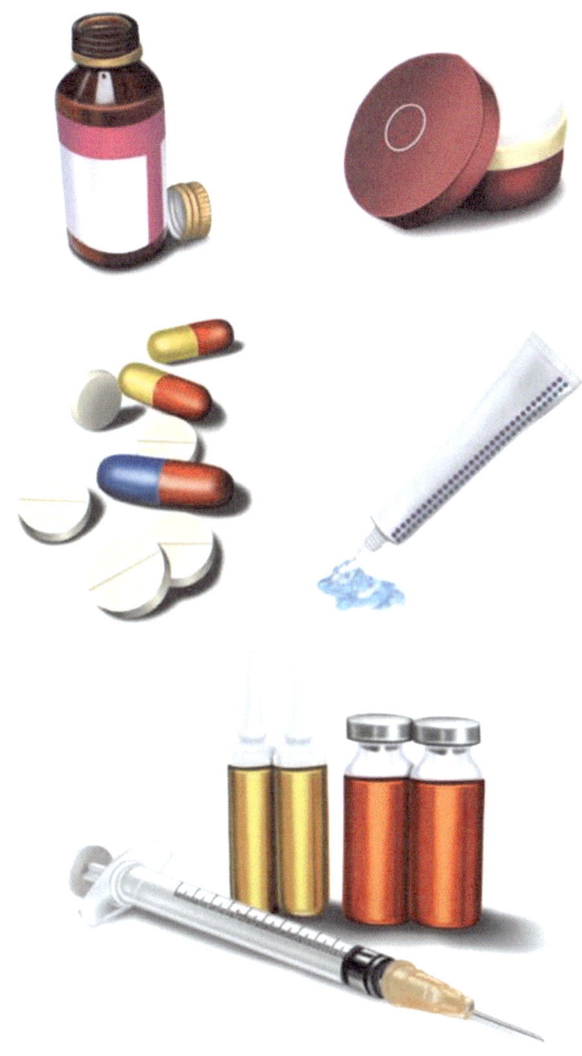

quality control and packaged in containers that maintain product stability. The final product should be labelled to promote correct use and be stored under conditions that contribute to maximum shelf life.

3.2   Necessity for Different Dosage Forms

Owing to the potent nature of most pharmaceutically active agents (drugs), therapeutic doses are present in a medication in the micro and milligram range. It is not possible to safely extract such a small amount of drug from a pure drug stock. This necessitates packaging the drug into a bulkier form known as 'the medicine'. For example, it would not be possible for an untrained person to accurately measure out the required 250 mg of paracetamol and/or 55 mg of caffeine from the bulk material.

Therefore, to make up the dosage unit large enough for ease of handling, solid dosage forms such as tablets and capsules must be prepared with fillers or diluents. In addition to the convenient and safe delivery of small dosage of drugs, dosage forms are needed for other reasons, such as concealing an offensive taste or odour and the protection of drug substances from the destructive influence of the environment, for example, atmospheric oxygen, humidity or gastric acid.

In general, dosage forms are necessary for the safe and efficacious use of drug doses at the various administration sites. Table 3.1 displays a range of drugs with variable doses and dosage forms.

Table 3.1 Dose and dosage forms of some commonly used drugs

Drug	Usual dose (mg)	Common dosage form	Category
Acetaminophen (paracetamol)	250, 1000	Tablets, suspension	Analgesic
Ampicillin	250, 500, 2000	Capsules, IV or IM injections	Antibiotic
Aspirin	75, 300	Tablets	Analgesic
Betaxolol HCl	5–20	Solution and tablets	Antianginal
Clotrimazole	1% w/w	Cream, pessary, solution, lozenge or tablets	Antifungal
Medroxyprogesterone acetate	5, 10/160 mg/mL	Tablets/injectable suspension	Progestin
Methylphenidate HCl	5–20	Solution or tablets	CNS stimulant
Mesoridazine besylate	10, 25, 50	Tablets or IM injection (ampoules)	Antipsychotic
Morphine sulphate	5–30	Oral solutions or tablets	Narcotic analgesic
Nifedipine	10, 30–60	Capsules	Coronary vasodilator
Omeprazole	10, 20, 40	Enteric-coated tablets, capsules, powder for IV injection	Antiulcerative
Quinapril HCl	5,10,20 or 40	Film-coated tablets	Antihypertensive
Chlorazepate dipotassium	5, 10, 20 or 50	Capsules or tablets	Tranquilizer
Buspirone HCl	5, 10, 15, 30	Tablets	Anti-anxiety

(continued)

Table 3.1 (continued)

Drug	Usual dose (mg)	Common dosage form	Category
Enalapril maleate	2.5, 5, 10, 20/1.25 mg/mL	Tablets/IV injection	Antihypertensive
Hydrocodone	5, 10	Tablets, solution	Narcotic analgesic
Prednisolone	1–50/5 mg/mL	Tablets/solution	Adrenocortical steroid
Albuterol sulphate	2–4	Tablets, syrup, inhalants, inhalation capsules	Bronchodilator
Chlorpheniramine maleate	4	Tablets, syrup, injectable solution (IV, IM or SC)	Antihistaminic
Felodipine	2.5	Tablets	Vasodilator
Glyburide	2.5	Tablets	Anti-diabetic
Doxazosin mesylate	1, 2	Tablets	Antihypertensive
Levorphanol tartrate	2	Ampoules	Narcotic analgesic
Prazosin HCl	1, 2	Capsules	Antihypertensive
Risperidone	0.5–2	Orally disintegrating tablets	Antipsychotic
Estropipate	0.625, 1.25, 2.5	Tablets	Oestrogen
Bumetanide	0.5, 1, 2	Tablets	Diuretic
Clonazepam	1	Tablets, orally disintegrating tablets, solution, injectable solution	Anticonvulsant
Ergoloid mesylates	1	Tablet, solution	Cognitive adjuvant
Alprazolam	0.5	Tablets, orally disintegrating tablets	Anti-anxiety
Colchicine	0.6	Tablets	Gout suppressant
Nitroglycerin	0.4	Lingual spray, sublingual tablet, topical ointment, transdermal patch, transmucosal (buccal) tablet	Antianginal
Digoxin	0.25	Tablets, capsules, IV injection	Cardiotonic (maintenance)
Levothyroxine	0.1	Tablets, capsules, suspension	Thyroid
Misoprostol	0.1	Tablets	Antiulcerative, abortifacient
Ethinyl estradiol	0.01, 0.05	Uncoated tablets	Oestrogen

3.3   General Considerations in the Design of Dosage Forms

All aspects of the pharmaceutical design of a medicinal product should be justified scientifically, clinically and ethically. However, in all preformulation studies, after having established that key features, such as bioavailability and clinical efficacy are present, a master formula, which best meets the goals of the product, is selected from various initial formulations of the product. In addition to therapeutic issues, there are other factors that should be considered before formulating the medicinal agent into various dosage forms. Among these factors are the nature of an illness and / or disease and modes of treatment. These factors and the intended target site dictate formulations of certain dosage forms. For example, controlled-release dosage forms that reduce the frequency of administration without sacrificing efficiency are particularly advantageous. In general, all of these factors and routes of administration are taken into consideration when manufacturing a drug into one or more dosage forms. Another element, bioavailability, is influenced by a variety of factors, for example, the method of manufacture or compounding the particle size and crystal form or polymorph of the drug substance and excipients used in formulating the dosage form.

3.4   Drug Stability

Drug stability is the ability of the various pharmaceutical dosage forms to maintain the desirable physical, chemical, therapeutic and microbial properties during the time of storage and usage by the patient. The aim of drug stability studies (Fig. 3.3) is to examine various ways in which drugs (liquids, solids and semi-solid formulations) can lose their activity. In doing so, chemical groups that cause stability problems when present in drug molecules can be identified. Chemically, the structure of a drug may include acids, alcohols, aldehydes, alkaloids, amides, esters, ethers, glycosides, ketones, phenols or salts. Each of these molecules is defined by particular functional groups that have different susceptibilities to chemical degradation. Such degradation can cause lowering or loss of potency, change in physical appearance (e.g. discolouration) and toxicity.

Some degradation products are significantly more toxic than the original therapeutic agent, for example, the antimalarial chloroquine can produce toxic reactions that are attributable to photochemical degradation (Selvaag 1998). Furthermore, physicochemical stability represents a crucial issue with regard to dose and patient care, for example, 5-fluorouracil, carbamazepine, digoxin and theophylline have narrow therapeutic indices, and they need to be carefully titrated for individual patients so that serum levels are neither too high as to be potentially toxic nor too low as to be ineffective.

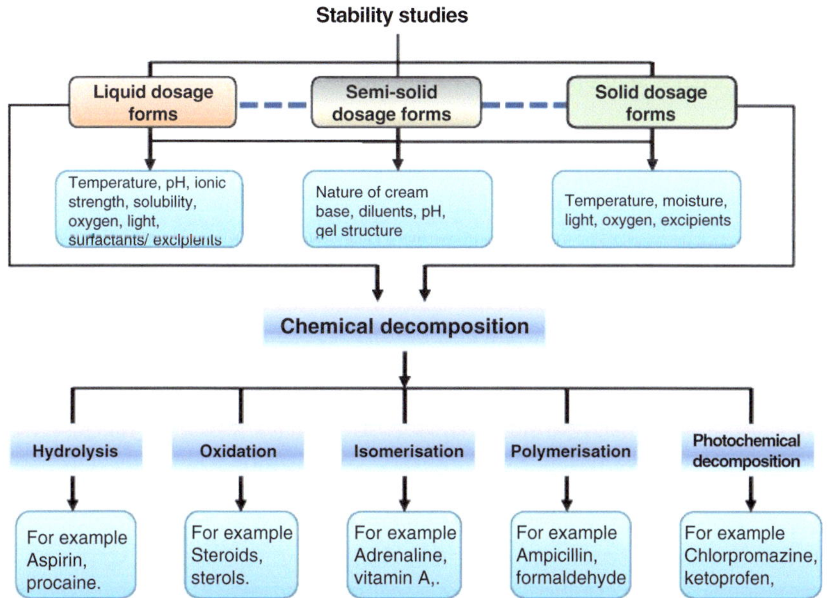

Fig. 3.3 Drug stability studies for various dosage forms

3.5   Product Shelf Life

The stability of a medicinal product is expressed as the manufacturer's shelf life, in which the product is predicted to remain fit for its intended purpose if stored correctly in its closed container. Commonly, this shelf life is defined as the time for the original potency of the active drug to be reduced to 90%. However, time limits may apply especially if the degradation products of a drug are toxic (e.g. tetracycline). Normally, the in-use shelf life may be substantially shorter than the expiry of the unopened product (e.g. morphine sulphate oral solutions have a 90-day shelf life on opening). One of the purposes of primary packaging is to help protect the product and prevent or reduce its degradation or contamination. Therefore, repeated opening for use of pharmaceutical products leads to the exposure of drugs to decomposition factors as mentioned earlier such as moisture, oxygen, light, a rise in temperature and volatilisation (vapourising a dissolved drug), which will affect drug stability and shelf life (Lund 1994).

In general, good practice requires that the storage areas for medicinal products are maintained within acceptable temperature limits for the medicines concerned and that temperatures are monitored regularly to demonstrate that these conditions continue to be met. For temperature-sensitive medicines, it is important that they can be delivered under controlled conditions. Also, temperature monitoring devices used for this purpose should be calibrated regularly, and the temperature in small refrigerators should be checked at least daily. Practically, there should be written procedures in place describing the action to be taken in the event of a loss of control over the storage conditions of temperature-sensitive products, for example, the accidental disconnection or breakdown of a refrigerator.

3.6 Pharmaceutical Excipients

In general, excipients may be defined as the constituents of the pharmaceutical form that is taken by or administered to the patient, other than the active substance. According to the Annex of Directive 2001/83/EC, such constituents may include colourants, preservatives, adjuvants, stabilisers, thickeners, emulsifiers, flavouring and aromatic substances (Brayfield 2017). Table 3.2 presents some of the common excipients used in tablet forms.

In addition to British Pharmacopoeia (2019) and the US Pharmacopoeia (2019), the Handbook of Pharmaceutical Excipients contains monographs for 340 excipients, with each monograph including a 'Safety' section that displays reported adverse reactions. Brayfield (2017) provides safety information about excipients which is a required text for hospital and community pharmacists. Moreover, the monographs for each excipient contain a section on adverse effects reviewed from the literature (Rowe et al. 2009).

Table 3.3 displays some of the common adverse effects of certain excipients. However, not all available data about excipients is published by drug companies.

Table 3.2 Examples of some common excipients used in tablets

Excipient	Use	Examples
Binders, compression aids, granulating agents	Bind the tablet ingredients together giving form and mechanical strength	Gelatin, starches, sugars, sugar alcohols and cellulose derivatives
Colouring agents	Improve acceptability to patients, aid identification and prevent counterfeiting. Increase stability of light-sensitive drugs	Mainly synthetic dyes and natural colours. Compounds that are themselves natural pigments of food may also be used
Diluents	Provide bulk and enable accurate dosing of potent ingredients	Sugar compounds, for example, lactose, dextrin, glucose. Inorganic compounds, for example, silicates, calcium and magnesium salts, etc.
Disintegrants	Aid dispersion of the tablet in the GI tract, releasing the active ingredient and increasing the surface area for dissolution	Compounds which swell or dissolve in water, for example, starch, cellulose derivatives and alginates, crospovidone
Glidants	Improve the flow of powders during tablet manufacturing by reducing friction and adhesion between particles. Also used as anticaking agents	Colloidal anhydrous silicon and other silica compounds

(continued)

Table 3.2 (continued)

Excipient	Use	Examples
Lubricants	Similar action to glidants; however, they may slow disintegration and dissolution. The properties of glidants and lubricants differ, although some compounds, such as starch and talc, have both actions	Stearic acid and its salts (e.g. magnesium stearate)
Preservatives	Antimicrobial preservative, disinfectant, skin penetrant, solvent	Alcohol, benzalkonium chloride, benzoic acid, benzylalcohol
Tablet coatings and films	Protect tablet from the environment (air, light, moisture, stomach), increase the mechanical strength, mask taste and smell, aid swallowing, assist in product identification. Can be used to modify release of the active ingredient. May contain flavours and colourings	Sugar (sucrose) has now been replaced by film coating using natural or synthetic polymers that are insoluble in acid, for example, cellulose acetate phthalate (used for enteric coatings to delay release of the active ingredient)

Table 3.3 Common adverse effects of some commonly used excipients

Excipient	Function	Common adverse effects
Aspartame	Sweetener	Caution in patients with phenylketonuria
Benzalkonium chloride	Preservative	Bronchoconstriction (nebuliser solutions) and ocular toxicity (soft contact lens solutions)
Lactose	Tablet filler	Caution in patients with galactosaemia, glucose-galactose malabsorption syndrome or lactase deficiency
Lanolin (wool fat)	Emulsifier (topical products)	Skin hypersensitivity reactions, caution in patients with known sensitivity
Propyl gallate	Antioxidant	Contact sensitivity and skin reactions
Sesame oil	Oil (injections)	Hypersensitivity reactions reported
Sodium metabisulphite	Antioxidant	Hypersensitivity, including bronchospasm and anaphylaxis, is reported for all sulphites
Tartrazine	Colouring agent	Hypersensitivity and hyperkinetic activity in children

3.7   Identifying Patient Reactions to Excipients in Practice

Drug excipients should be inert; however, they do have the potential to cause adverse effects in sensitive individuals. Identifying such reactions and finding the appropriate safety information will help to ensure a safe outcome for the patient. In many cases when patients experience an adverse reaction to particular drug products, it is important to be aware that adverse reactions are not always due to the active ingredient (Fig. 3.4). They are more likely to occur if the patient has an existing sensitivity to similar ingredients, or is prescribed multiple medications, or when the quantity of

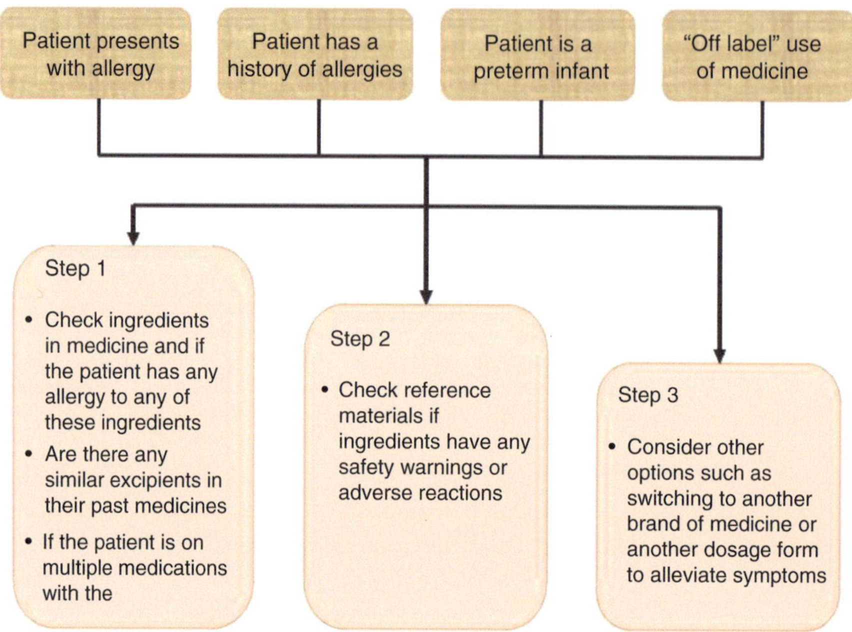

Fig. 3.4 Managing the risk of pharmaceutical excipients in practice

excipients may be high relative to body weight, for example, preterm babies (Valeur et al. 2018). Also, excipients present in a patient's current and past medication history should be considered. This should help to identify which ingredients may be causing the adverse effects.

3.8 Summary

In this chapter, the various aspects of drug formulation and dosage forms can be summarised as:

- The different phases involved in drug development and the reasons that dictate the need for dosage forms, in addition to examples of doses and dosage forms of some commonly used drugs.
- Preformulation is an essential phase in pharmaceutical development; it involves materials research which explores the physicochemical characterisation of the Active Pharmaceutical Ingredients (API) and its compatibility with potential excipient materials in light of the intended route of administration and dosage form.
- There are several considerations that should be taken into account in the design of medicinal products. These include the intended patient, age group, bioavailability aspects and diseases.

- Preformulation studies provide the essential information required for the drug's combination with pharmaceutical ingredients and the preformulation work needed before actual product formulation begins. The effect of physical and chemical properties of the solid state seen in crystals, powders or other forms of both drugs and pharmaceutical excipients on the final product especially dissolution and bioavailability is investigated. These investigations encompass the study of properties such as heat of vaporisation, melting point, dissociation constant and physicochemical stability in general and shelf life.
- Pharmaceutical excipients are essential constituents in medicinal products. They include colouring matters, preservatives, adjuvants, stabilisers, thickeners, emulsifiers, flavouring and aromatic substances. Some excipients cause adverse effects in patients; therefore, managing the risk of pharmaceutical excipients in practice is an important part in patient care. It is important to be aware of these adverse reactions and to follow the correct procedures for their assessment.

3.9   Pharmaceutical Dosage Forms

3.9.1   Introduction

Dosage forms are the means by which drug molecules are delivered to sites of action within the body. They are classified according to their physical state and chemical composition. Dosage forms consist of the active drug and other nontherapeutic substances called the *vehicle* which gives the drugs suitable consistency and may be a solid, semi-solid, liquid or gas. All components in the formulation including the active therapeutic agents, the pharmaceutical ingredients and the packaging materials must be physically and chemically compatible. Also, the product must be effectively packaged and clearly and completely labelled according to legal regulations.

3.9.2   Solid Dosage Forms

The most important pharmaceutical dosage forms are tablets, capsules, granules, powder, dry powder inhalers and chewables. Solid medications may be administered by different routes of administration, such as orally, nasally, rectally, vaginally or topically. However, there are different factors that should be considered when deciding if a solid dosage form is an appropriate choice for a patient. The advantages of solid dosage forms are that they can be self-administered by the patient, are accurate, have longer shelf life and are easier to package, distribute and store. Their disadvantages are that they are not appropriate for unconscious patients or those patients who cannot take the medications orally or nasally. Some solids cause irritation to the GI mucosa (e.g. NSAIDs); moreover, they take longer time to be absorbed by the body, so for immediate action treatments, liquid or injectable medications are the dosage forms of choice.

3.9.3 Capsules

Dosage formulations can be enclosed in various-sized capsules made of hard or soft gelatin shell and be presented as a solid dosage form. Capsules are swallowed whole by the patient with sufficient water. Dosage forms must be left intact, and specific policy and guidelines must be followed if dismantling appears necessary (further detail to follow). Other dosage forms, for example, liquid or suppositories, may be used. The most commonly used capsules are the hard gelatin capsules which are designed to dissolve in the stomach. They contain colourants, for example, dyes and opaquants, for example, titanium dioxide, to make them distinctive, for example, caps and bodies of different colours. Gelatin is subject to microbial decomposition when exposed to moisture, which can affect the rigid shape of the capsules and its content, hence its bioavailability. Also, extreme dryness causes the capsules to become brittle by losing some of its moisture content and crumble when handled. Therefore, it is desirable to store hard gelatin capsules in an environment free from excess humidity or dryness. To avoid the effect of excess moisture especially with hygroscopic drugs, many capsules are packaged along with a small packet of desiccant material such as silica gel, clay or activated carbon.

3.9.4 Tablets

Tablets are solid medications that are compacted into small, formed shapes. The tablet form accounts for approximately 50% of all dosage forms. Tablets are classified by the way they are made. The two most common classifications are compressed tablets and moulded tablets. Compressed tablets are formed by die punch compression of powdered, crystalline or granular substances; however, moulded tablets are made from wet materials placed in moulds.

3.9.5 Compressed Tablets

The most commercially available tablets are primarily prepared by compression, where a measured quantity of powdered or granulated tableting material is compressed under a high pressure (tons). They usually contain a number of pharmaceutical excipients, such as anticaking agents, colourants, flavourants, antioxidants and preservatives (Fig. 3.5).

Multiple-compressed tablets can be considered as multilayered tablets or a tablet within a tablet, which allows the formulation of different and incompatible drugs in one tablet (Fig. 3.6). Each portion of the fill is usually coloured differently for the unique appearance. These multilayered tablets acting as a controlled-release device can provide different drug release profiles.

Chewable tablets are compressed wet granulations that disintegrate rapidly when chewed or allowed to dissolve in the mouth. These are especially useful in tablet

Fig. 3.5 Various shapes and colours of compressed tablets

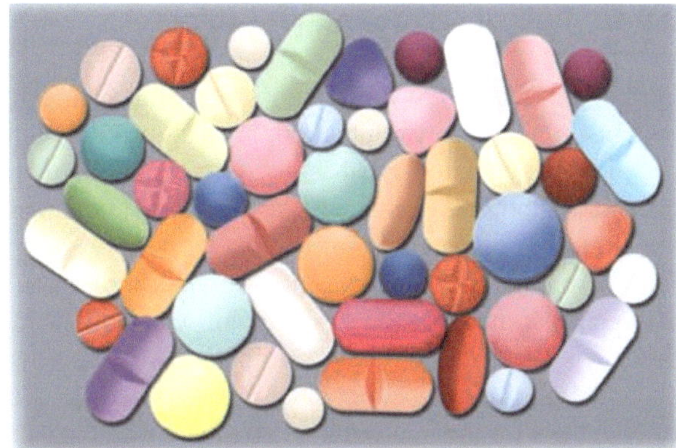

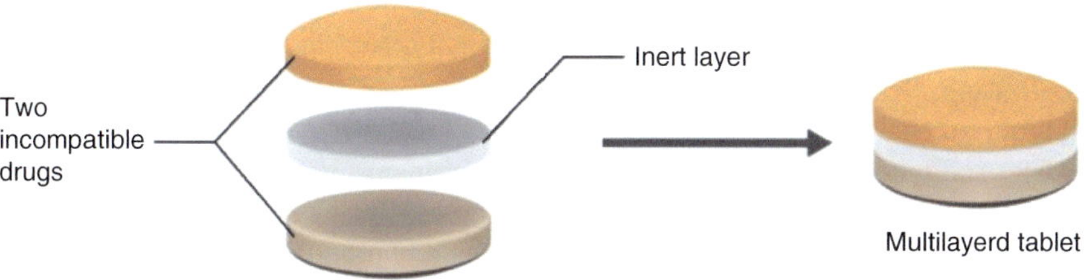

Fig. 3.6 Multilayered tablets

formulations for children and are commonly employed in the preparation of multiple vitamin tablets and also in the formation of antacids and anti-flatulents.

Mannitol (hexahydric alcohol) is a widely used excipient in chewable tablets and may account for 50% or more of the weight of the formulation. Chewable tablets should be chewed, and not swallowed, in order to achieve the desired results.

Sugar-coated tablets are compressed tablets coated with water-soluble coloured or uncoloured sugar layer to mask noxious-tasting or the bad odour of a drug, to add colour to the tablet or to protect the drug from exposure to the environment, for example, air and humidity. Sugar-coated tablets are usually 50% larger and heavier than the original uncoated tablets.

Film-coated tablets are compressed tablets coated with a hard shell of a skinlike film made of a thin layer of a polymer to make the tablet more durable and easier to swallow. The polymer coating is designed to rupture and expose the core tablet at the desired location within the GI tract.

Gelatin-coated tablets are a recent innovation of coated tablets. They are capsule-shaped compressed tablets coated with a gelatin layer and the innovator product is termed gelcaps, for example, Panadol® (acetaminophen). They are easy to swallow, and the coated product is about one-third smaller than a capsule filled with an equivalent amount of powder. Also, gelatin-coated tablets are more tamper evident than an unsealed capsule.

3.9.6   Buccal or Sublingual Tablets

Sublingual tablets are rapidly absorbed and disintegrated, once placed under the patient's tongue, for example, buprenorphine HCl, which is used for the treatment of opioid dependence (used as part of a complete treatment plan that includes psychosocial support). *Buccal* tablets, for example, fentanyl, a potent opioid analgesic, are similar to sublingual tablets, except that they are placed on the gum or on the inner cheek surface; they are disintegrated in the mouth or the lining of the cheek and then absorbed into the bloodstream. Medications may be formulated as either of these types of tablets, if the medications are destroyed by stomach acid, poorly absorbed into the bloodstream or when immediate action is required. This is why some tablets for the treatment of angina pain and general pain are formulated in this manner. Antinausea medicines are particularly suitable for buccal administration as the nausea itself can cause swallowed tablets to be vomited and therefore rendered ineffective.

Dispersible or effervescent tablets are designed to be added to water just prior to swallowing. They are frequently quite large and can contain large amounts of sodium, for example, soluble paracetamol.

The sodium content, however, can cause problems with patients where their sodium intake is restricted. Some dispersible tablets consist of coated granules, and therefore it is not appropriate to crush the dispersible product prior to dispersion.

Enteric-coated tablets have a special coating to prevent the medication from dissolving in the stomach and passing through to the intestine where it is dissolved and absorbed. The term 'enteric' refers to the small intestine and implies that the medication will move from the stomach to the small intestine before it dissolves.

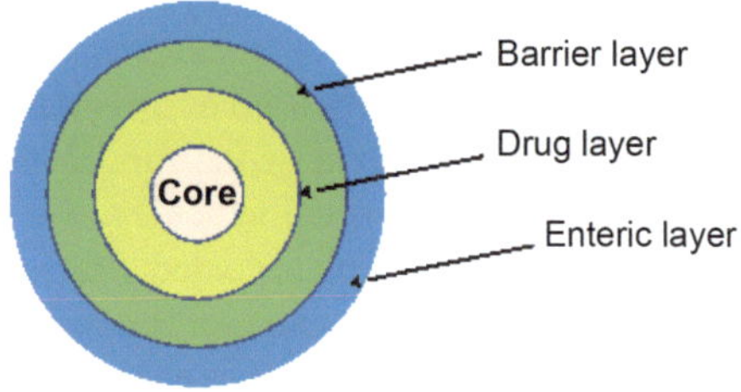

This is intended to prevent irritation of the lining of the stomach from the drug or to prevent the drug from being destroyed by stomach acids. *Tablet triturates* are small, usually cylindrical tablets (prepared by minimal amount of pressure) containing small amounts of potent drugs with a combination of sucrose and lactose as diluents. They must be readily and completely soluble in water and are administered orally or sublingually (e.g. nitroglycerin tablets). They can also be inserted into capsules or dissolved in a small amount of water which can be subsequently mixed with the required volume of the liquid medication.

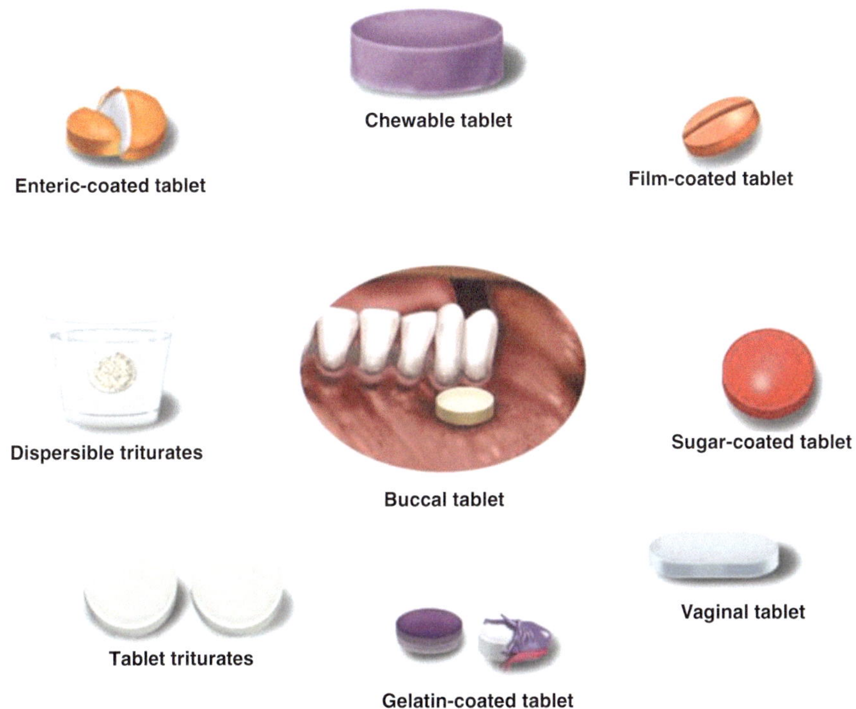

Fig. 3.7 Various solid dosage forms

Vaginal pessaries (vaginal tablets/inserts) are uncoated and bullet or ovoid-shaped tablets which are inserted into the vagina for localised effect. Figure 3.7 shows various commonly used solid dosage forms.

3.9.7 Extended-Release Dosage Forms

These medication dosage forms may be called extended release, sustained-release, long acting, delayed-release or controlled release (Fig. 3.8). While the exact meaning of these terms differs in some respects, each of these terms implies a type of controlled release of medication over a longer period of time than standard dosage forms. Oral tablets and capsules are the most common dosage forms that are formulated as extended release.

There are other dosage forms, such as implants and some intramuscular injections, that are also extended release. In general, several factors must be taken into consideration when manufacturing extended-release dosage forms such as a drug's rate of absorption and excretion, drug solubility, drug potency, therapeutic index (margin of safety) and their intended use (chronic rather than acute conditions). Extended-release dosage forms provide sustained plasma drug levels, which in

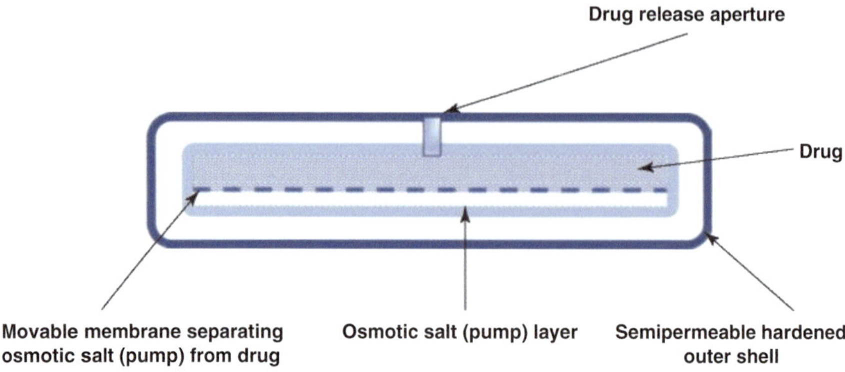

Fig. 3.8 Extended-release dosage form

many cases eliminate the need for night doses, which benefits both the patient and carer. Drug release durations for non-oral rate-controlled delivery systems range from 24 h as in most transdermal patches to 3 months, as with vaginal ring inserts, to 5 years with levonorgestrel subdermal implants. Nevertheless, the main disadvantages of extended-release forms are dose inflexibility and increased risk of sudden and total drug release (dose dumping) due to unexpected failure of the dosage unit technology.

3.9.8 Guidance on Dosage Forms That Cannot Be Altered

Crushing tablets or opening capsules raises a number of issues, amongst them are legal liability and drug licensing, unlicensed medication and product liability, patients' rights and capacity to consent, safety of the person administrating a medication and altered efficacy of treatment and potential adverse effects, even fatality (Schier et al. 2003). It is therefore recommended that the crushing of tablets and/or the opening of capsules should only be carried out where there is not another clear alternative. The nurse or care staff must adhere to local policy and guidelines which should include obtaining written prescriber authorisation and written direction to crush or disperse tablets or to open capsules, and this must be documented in the patient's care plan. Generally, pharmacy advice should always be sought and documented. Medicines that should not be opened and the risk associated are listed in Table 3.4.

3.9.9 Semi-Solid Dosage Forms

In general, semi-solid dosage forms are complex formulations having complex structural elements. Often they are composed of two phases (oil and water), one of which is a continuous (external) phase and the other of which is a dispersed

Table 3.4 Medicines that should not be crushed or opened and the associated risk

Dosage form	Reason for not crushing or opening	Potential risk	Examples
Modified release (name +2 letters, e.g. M/R, LA, SA, CR, XL, SR or retard or slow used in the title[a])	Damage of absorption mechanism and erratic dosing	Increased toxicity/ adverse effects and decreased efficacy	Diclofenac (Voltarol Retard, Diclomax SR) Propranolol (Inderal LA) Nifedipine (Adalat Retard) Felodipine (Plendil) Tramadol (Zydol SR)
Enteric and film coated (name +2 letters, e.g. EN, EC, FC)	Destruction of active pharmaceutical ingredient (API) in the stomach	Decreased stability/ efficacy, unacceptable taste, increased local irritant effect, poor compliance	Diclofenac (Voltarol) Aspirin (Nu-Seals Aspirin) Naproxen (Naprosyn EC) Sulfasalazine (Salazopyrin EN)
Hormonal Cytotoxic steroidal (risk assessment form required if the drug is to be crushed)	Drug may inadvertently affect the administering nurse, contamination	Toxicity, potential hazard to healthcare workers and carers	Tamoxifen Methotrexate Dexamethasone
Nitrate (risk assessment form required if the drug is to be crushed)	Concerns raised over potential explosive nature	Potential harm	Glyceryl trinitrate Isosorbide mononitrate Isosorbide dinitrate

[a]*LA* long acting, *M/R* modified release, *SA* slow acting, *XL* extended release, *SR* slow release

(internal) phase. Topical semi-solid dosage forms are normally presented in the form of creams, gels, ointments or pastes. They contain one or more active ingredients dissolved or uniformly dispersed in a suitable base and any suitable excipients such as emulsifiers, viscosity-increasing agents, antimicrobial agents, antioxidants or stabilising agents.

3.9.9.1 Creams

Creams are homogeneous, semi-solid preparations consisting of opaque emulsion systems, either water-in-oil (w/o) or oil-in-water (o/w) (external phase). Creams are intended for application to the skin or certain mucous membranes for protective, therapeutic or prophylactic purposes, especially where an occlusive effect is not necessary.

3.9.9.2 Hydrophobic Creams (W/O)

Hydrophobic creams are usually anhydrous and absorb only small amounts of water. They contain w/o emulsifying agents such as wool fat, sorbitan esters and monoglycerides.

3.9.9.3 Hydrophilic Creams (O/W)

Hydrophilic creams contain bases that are miscible with water. These creams are essentially miscible with skin secretions.

3.9.9.4 Gels

Gels are usually homogeneous, clear, semi-solid preparations consisting of a liquid phase within a three-dimensional polymeric matrix with physical or sometimes chemical cross-linkage by means of suitable gelling agents. Gels are applied to the skin or certain mucous membranes for protective, therapeutic, or prophylactic purposes.

3.9.9.5 Hydrophobic Gels

Hydrophobic gel bases usually consist of liquid paraffin with polyethylene or fatty oils gelled with colloidal silica or aluminium or zinc soaps.

3.9.9.6 Hydrophilic Gels

Hydrophilic gel (hydrogel) bases usually consist of water, glycerol or propylene glycol gelled with suitable agents such as tragacanth resin, starch, cellulose derivatives, carboxyvinyl polymers and magnesium aluminium silicates.

3.9.9.7 Ointments

Ointments are homogeneous, highly viscous or semi-solid preparations intended for external application to the skin or mucous membranes. They are used as emollients or for the application of active ingredients to the skin for protective, therapeutic or prophylactic purposes and where a degree of occlusion is desired.

3.9.9.8 Hydrophobic Ointments

Hydrophobic (lipophilic) ointments are usually anhydrous and can absorb only small amounts of water. Typical bases used for their formulation are water-insoluble hydrocarbons such as hard, soft and liquid paraffin, vegetable oil, animal fats, waxes, synthetic glycerides and polyalkylsiloxanes.

3.9.9.9 Water-Emulsifying Ointments

Water-emulsifying ointments can absorb large amounts of water. They typically consist of a hydrophobic fatty base in which a w/o agent, such as wool fat, wool alcohols, sorbitan esters, monoglycerides or fatty alcohols, can be incorporated to render them hydrophilic.

3.9.9.10 Hydrophilic Ointments

Hydrophilic ointment bases are miscible with water. The bases are usually mixtures of liquid and solid polyethylene glycols (macrogols).

3.9.9.11 Pastes

Pastes are homogeneous, semi-solid preparations containing high concentrations of insoluble powdered substances (usually not less than 20%), dispersed in a suitable base. The pastes are usually less greasy, more absorptive and stiffer in consistency than ointments because of the large quantity of powdered ingredients present. Some pastes consist of a single phase, such as hydrated pectin, and others consist of a thick, rigid material that does not flow at body temperature. The pastes should adhere well to the skin, in many cases; they form a protective film that controls the evaporation of water.

3.9.10 Guidance for the Use of Semi-Solid Forms

Semi-solid dosage forms should not be diluted. If a dilution is nevertheless necessary, the same type of base should be used in order to obtain a homogeneous mixture. In general, topical semi-solid dosage forms should be of uniform consistency and kept in well-closed containers. When a sample is rubbed on the back of the hand, no solid components should be noticed. The preparation should maintain its pharmaceutical integrity throughout shelf life when stored at the temperature indicated on the label; the temperature should normally not exceed 25 °C. Semi-solid preparations should not be used if they show any evidence of physical instability, for example, a noticeable change in consistency, such as excessive 'bleeding' (separation of excessive amounts of liquid), formation of agglomerates and grittiness, discolouration, emulsion breakdown, crystal growth, shrinking due to evaporation of water, change in odour or evidence of microbial growth. Particular care should be paid to environmental conditions, especially with respect to microbial and cross-contamination.

3.9.11 Liquid Dosage Forms

Liquid dosage forms commonly encountered in pharmaceutical practice are either monophasic or bi−/polyphasic. Monophasic systems are characterised by the presence of a single homogeneous phase, for example, solution, mixtures, elixirs, tinctures, syrups, ear drops, nasal drops, et cetara., whereas bi−/polyphasic liquid dosage forms consist of two or more distinct phases, for example, emulsions and suspensions. Liquid preparations may be administered internally or externally. Figure 3.9 shows a simple classification of liquid dosage forms.

Liquid medication dosage forms usually are faster acting than solid dosage forms, as they are in the dissolved state or are present in small particles, which makes them readily absorbed into the bloodstream. Also, there is more flexibility in liquid forms than solid forms, as it is easier to manipulate liquid volumes than, for example, solid tablets. Table 3.5 shows estimations of the volume/weight commonly used in liquid dosage forms. Moreover, liquid medications are administered where it may not be practical to use solid dosage forms, for example, into the ear. However, liquid dosage forms also have some disadvantages; they often have a shorter expiry time than solid dosage forms, and they sometimes leave an unpleasant taste in the mouth and are more difficult to handle or measure; in

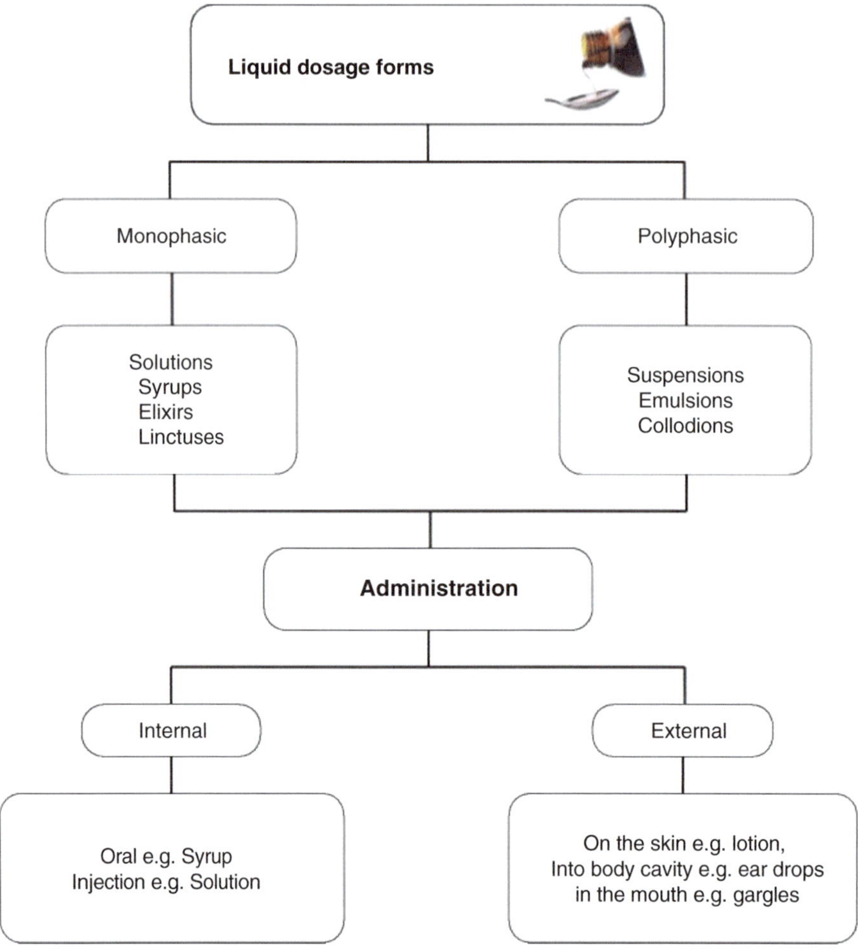

Fig. 3.9 Simple classification of liquid dosage forms

Table 3.5 Estimations for volume/weight of dose of liquid dosage forms

Dose measure	Approx. volume (mL)	Approx. weight (g)
1 drop	0.05	0.05
1 teaspoonful	5.00	5.00
1 tablespoonful	15.0	15.0
20 drops of aqueous solution	1.00	1.00
60 drops of ethanolic solution	1.25	1.00

addition, some liquid forms require special storage and handling, for example, refrigeration and shaking.

3.9.11.1 Solutions

Solutions are evenly distributed, homogeneous mixtures of dissolved medication (solid, liquid or gaseous) in a suitable liquid vehicle. Medications in the solution are absorbed from the stomach, skin or other site of administration. Solutions can be characterised according to the delivery vehicle into aqueous (delivery vehicle is purified water), nonaqueous (delivery vehicle is a solvent other than water) and hydroalcoholic solutions where the delivery vehicle is a mix of alcohol and water.

3.9.11.2 Oral Solutions

Oral liquids are formulated as solutions, suspensions and emulsions depending on the nature of the active ingredient particularly solubility and stability.

3.9.11.3 Mixtures

Simple liquid preparations intended for oral use containing dissolved medicaments may be described as oral solutions or mixtures. For example, rehydration solutions which are used in the mild cases of diarrhoea and dehydration; they are aqueous solutions containing a mixture of Na^+, K^+, $Cl-$, citrate and dextrose in a volume of water.

3.9.11.4 Elixirs

Elixirs are clear, sweet, flavoured hydroalcoholic mixtures intended for oral ingestion. They usually contain either potent or unpleasant-tasting drugs; hence, sweeteners and flavourings are used. In general, nonaqueous solvents (alcohol, glycerine or propylene glycol) form a significant proportion of the vehicle used in elixirs. Although the use of alcohol (3–25%) in elixirs helps to dissolve the drugs, it presents a disadvantage in or contraindication in patients who should not or cannot ingest alcohol. Therefore, children's carers, older people and patients who abuse alcohol should be made aware of the alcohol content of elixirs, because these patients may be especially sensitive to even a small amount of alcohol. Phenobarbital elixir and digoxin paediatric elixir, are two widely prescribed medicated elixirs.

3.9.11.5 Syrups

Syrups are concentrated, viscous aqueous solutions containing one or more sugar components, mainly sucrose. They often contain preservatives against bacterial contamination. Syrups may be flavoured, medicated solutions or without medications (nonmedicated syrups). The high content of sugar in syrups helps to conceal the unpleasant taste of a drug; therefore, syrups are commonly used for paediatric medications. Also, the thick character of syrups has a soothing effect on irritated tissues of the throat; accordingly, syrups are often used for cough formulations. Robitussin® and Benylin® are examples of well-known over-the-counter cough and cold syrups.

3.9.11.6 Linctuses

Linctuses are viscous, liquid oral preparations that are usually prescribed mainly for a demulcent (soothing), expectorant or sedative purpose, for the relief of a cough. They usually contain a high proportion of syrup and glycerol which have a demulcent effect on the membranes of the throat. The dose volume is small (5 mL); however, to prolong the demulcent action, they should be taken undiluted.

3.9.11.7 Spirits

Spirits or essences are alcoholic or hydroalcoholic solutions containing one or more active medicaments dissolved in either absolute or dilute ethanol.

3.9.11.8 Paediatric Drops

These are an oral liquid formulation of potent drugs usually in solution, intended for administration to paediatric patients, for example, amoxil drops, though they may be useful in other patients with swallowing difficulties. The formulation is designed to have very small dose volumes which must be administered with a calibrated dropper.

3.9.11.9 Sprays

Sprays are solutions that are delivered as a mist against the mucous membranes of the nose and throat. Nasal decongestants and antiseptic throat solutions are common spray formulations. The drug may have a local effect, for example, antihistamine, vasoconstrictor or decongestant. Alternatively, the drug may be absorbed through the nasal mucosa to exert a systemic effect, for example, the peptide hormones oxytocin and vasopressin. The use of oily nasal sprays should be avoided because of possible damage to the cilia of the nasal mucosa. Prolonged use of nasal vasoconstrictors may result in rebound vasodilatation and further nasal congestion.

3.9.11.10 Injectable Solutions

Injectable solutions are sterile solutions, suspensions or emulsions in a suitable aqueous or nonaqueous vehicle containing one or more medicaments designed for parenteral administration, and they are usually classified according to their route of administration, for example, intramuscular.

3.9.11.11 Gargles and Mouthwashes

Gargles and mouthwashes are aqueous solutions that are intended for treatment of the throat (gargles) and mouth (mouthwashes) and are generally formulated in a concentrated form. Although gargles and mouthwashes are admitted into the mouth, they should not be swallowed. Gargles are used to treat throat conditions such as a sore throat, while mouthwashes are used to deodorise, refresh or disinfect the mouth, for example, Listerine. A familiar example of a gargle is Chloraseptic® mouth rinse and gargle.

3.9.11.12 Enemas, Douches and Irrigation Solutions

These liquid preparations are often formulated as solutions (though they may be presented as an emulsion or suspension), and are intended for instillation into the rectum (enema) or other orifice, such as the vagina or nasal cavity (douche). Enemas are introduced into the rectum to empty the bowel, for example, osmotic enemas are given to relieve significant constipation or to cleanse the bowel before colonoscopy or surgery. However, douches are used to remove debris from the eyes or to cleanse the nose, throat or vagina. The volumes of these preparations may vary from 5 mL to much larger volumes. Irrigating solutions are sterile, pyrogen-free solutions usually intended for irrigation of body cavities, operation cavities, wounds or the urogenital system. They are similar to douches; however, they usually are used in larger volumes and over larger areas of the body for more general cleansing than douches.

3.9.11.13 Lotions

Lotions are solutions, but may also be suspensions or emulsions, that are intended to be applied to the skin without friction. They contain finely powdered medications, and they cool, soothe, dry or protect the skin. Calamine lotion is a commonplace example of a protective lotion. In some cases, lotions are applied to the scalp, where the vehicle for the medication is alcohol based, allowing for rapid drying of the hair making it more acceptable to the patient, for example, Salicylic Acid Lotion 2%, British Pharmaceutical Codex (BPC). In these cases, problems of flammability are addressed by suitable labelling.

3.9.11.14 Liniments

Liniments are liquid preparation (may be alcoholic, oily solutions or emulsions) intended to be rubbed with friction and massaged onto the skin to obtain analgesic, rubefacient (substance that causes skin redness by vasodilation), or generally stimulating effects. Most are massaged into the skin (counterirritant or stimulating types), but some are applied on a warm dressing or with a brush (analgesic and soothing types). Liniments should not be used on broken skin.

3.9.11.15 Collodions

Collodions are alcoholic solutions of pyroxylin (found in cotton fibres) dissolved in ethyl ether and ethanol. After application to the skin, the ether and ethanol evaporate and leave a pyroxylin film. Collodions that contain medication are useful in the treatment of corns and warts. Nonmedicated collodions, such as liquid adhesive bandages (New-Skin®), may be applied to the skin to protect and seal small wounds. Collodions are highly volatile and highly flammable and care should be taken when used and to label any preparation appropriately.

3.9.11.16 Emulsions

Emulsions are mixtures of two immiscible liquids (usually oil and water). In an emulsion, one liquid is broken into small particles (the internal phase) and evenly scattered throughout the other (the external or continuous). Emulsions may be either water-in-oil (w/o) where droplets of water are dispersed throughout the oil or oil-in-water (o/w) where small oil globules are dispersed throughout water. Most emulsions intended for oral use are of the o/w type; those to be applied to the skin may be of either type. In general, medications that dissolve more readily in oil are applied to the skin as o/w emulsions, in which the oil is the internal phase, while those that dissolve in water are applied as w/o emulsions, in which the water is the internal phase. Some emulsions may also be injected into the bloodstream. For example, fat emulsion Intralipid® and Liposyn® are o/w emulsions which are administered by intravenous infusion.

3.9.11.17 Suspensions

Suspensions are useful for administering a large amount of solid medication that would be inconvenient to take as a tablet or capsule. They are mixtures of fine particles of undissolved solids distributed through gas, liquid or solid. However, most suspensions are solids dispersed in liquids. Largely, suspensions are intended for oral use, where water usually is the vehicle, but some may be administered by other routes such as the rectal, otic and ophthalmic. Moreover, suspensions may be administered via intramuscular route (parenteral route), where oil is used as the vehicle (e.g. testosterone propionate). Generally suspensions need to be shaken before use to redistribute particles that may have risen to the top or settled to the bottom of the container during storage as shown.

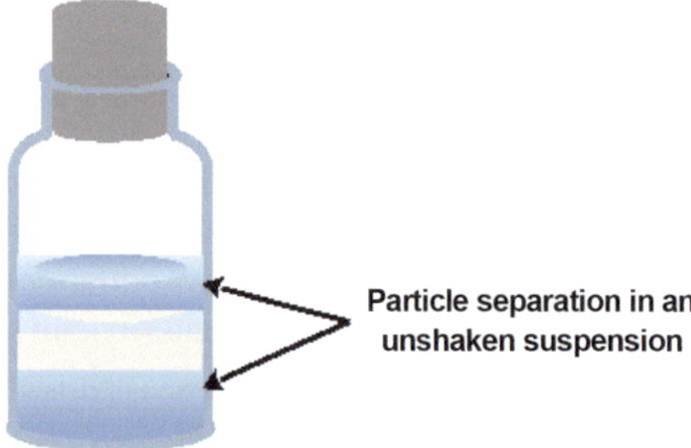

3.9.11.18 Extracts

Extracts are concentrated preparations of active components obtained from plant or animal tissue by extraction methods. In general, the dried plant or the animal tissue is soaked in an appropriate solvent, and the active component is obtained after the solvent is evaporated. With potency as the only difference, tinctures, fluidextracts and extracts are examples of formulations prepared in this manner. Tinctures are alcoholic or hydroalcoholic solutions whose potency equivalent is 100 mg/mL of crude drug. Common examples of tinctures are iodine and paregoric tincture. Fluidextracts are more potent than tinctures (1000 mg/mL of crude drug); however, extracts are the most potent as they are two to six times as potent as the crude drug. *Cascara sagrada* (used to clear the bowel) and vanilla are common examples of fluid extracts and extracts, respectively.

3.9.12 Miscellaneous Forms

3.9.12.1 Aerosols

Pharmaceutical aerosols are pressurised dosage forms containing one or more active ingredients, which upon actuation emit a fine dispersion of liquid and/or solid particles in a gaseous medium. They differ from most dosage forms in their dependence upon the function of the container, its valve assembly and the propellant which may be a liquefied gas or a mixture of liquefied gases that frequently serves dual role of propellant and solvent or vehicle for the active ingredient. Depending on the intended use, aerosol products may be designed to emit their contents as a fine mist, a coarse, wet or dry spray, a steady stream or stable or fast-breaking foams. Inhalants are aerosols that constitute of fine powders or solutions of drugs delivered as a mist through the mouth into the respiratory tract, for example, Primatene mist and Provetil used for the treatment of asthma. Topical aerosols are applied onto the skin, that is, dermatologic sprays such as local anaesthetic (e.g. dibucaine hydrochloride) and ointment-like products. Vaginal aerosol foams containing oestrogenic substances and contraceptive agents and rectal aerosols forms typically containing anti-inflammatory steroids are available. The foams are generally oil-in-water emulsion resembling light creams and are water soluble. Instructions on the use and administration of aerosols should be carefully considered by both healthcare professionals and patients.

3.10 Routes of Administration

In addition to characteristics of the drug substance, the dosage form and a variety of patients factors (e.g. age, body weight, general health conditions, pathologic conditions), routes of administration represent a decisive factor in the process of drug formulation. In clinical medicine, there are several reasons for choosing different routes of administration (Table 3.6). For example, the hepatic first-pass effect can be avoided to a great extent by the use of sublingual tablets, and trans-dermal preparations which provide direct access to systemic (not portal) veins, and to a lesser extent by the use of rectal suppositories which enter the vessels (in the lower rectum) that drain into the inferior vena cava, thus bypassing the liver.

Routes of administration of drugs can be classified into several categories with regard to their effect whether it is systemic as in enteral or parenteral administration or local as in topical administration.

3.10.1 Enteral Administration

Enteral administration involves the oesophagus, stomach and small and large intestines (i.e. the gastrointestinal tract). Methods of administration include oral, sublingual, gastric feeding tube, gastrostomy and rectal. In this route, the drug is

Table 3.6 Characteristics and bioavailability of different routes of administration

Route of administration	Characteristics	Bioavailability %
Oral (PO)	Most convenient, but first-pass effect may be significant	5–<100
Intravenous (IV)	Most rapid onset	100 (by definition)
Intramuscular (IM)	May be painful, but large volumes often feasible	75–≤100
Subcutaneous (SC)	May be painful, smaller volumes than IM	75–≤100
Rectal (PR)	Less first-pass effect than oral	30–<100
Inhalation	Often very rapid onset	5–<100
Transdermal	Used for lack of first-pass effect and prolonged duration of action (very slow absorption)	80–≤100

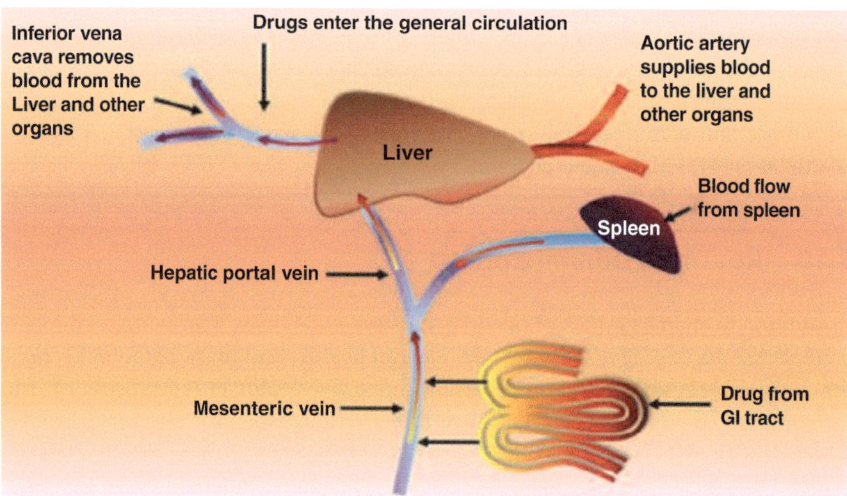

Fig. 3.10 A schematic outline of the route of drugs absorbed from the GI tract

transported to the systemic circulation via absorption into the mesenteric vein through the hepatic portal vein to the liver as shown in Fig. 3.10.

3.10.2 Parenteral Routes of Administration

Parenteral routes may be defined as nonenteral or nonoral; therefore, strictly speaking, the term parenteral includes all products administered other than by the GIT route. The parenteral route is the most popular and viable approach in many cases

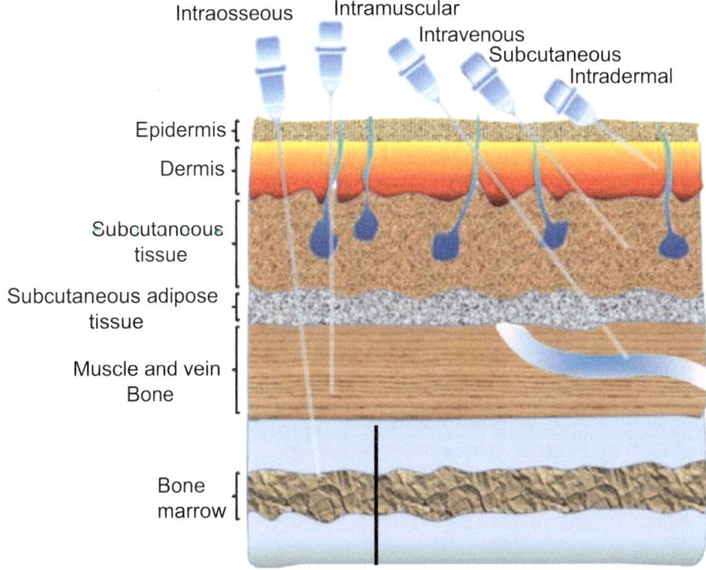

Fig. 3.11 Illustration of the routes of parenteral medication, showing the tissues penetrated by intradermal, subcutaneous, intravenous, intramuscular and intraosseous injections

and remains the primary route for the administration of peptide and protein drugs (Pawer et al. 2004). The most common routes of parenteral administration are intravenous, intramuscular, intraarterial, intracardiac (into the heart), intraosseous infusion (into the bone marrow), intracerebral (into the brain parenchyma), intrathecal (into the spinal canal), intracerebroventricular (into the cerebral ventricular system), epidural (into the epidural space), transdermal (for systemic effect rather than local effect), and subcutaneous (under the skin). Figure 3.11 shows the various routes of parenteral injections.

3.10.3 Topical Administration

Topical administration is the main route of administration to provide a local effect. Topical preparations may be applied to the skin (epicutaneous), mouth (e.g. sublingual), nose, oropharynx (onto the throat), cornea, ear, urethra, vagina or rectum. However, some topical drugs can have systemic effects, especially if given in large doses, in frequent doses or over a long period of time. Table 3.7 shows the various most common routes of administration, their approximate time of action, reasons for choice and example drugs used in each case.

Table 3.7 The most common routes of administration

Route	Approx. time for the onset of drug action	Necessity of choice	Advantage	Disadvantage	Examples
Oral	30–60 min	Whenever possible	Safe, convenient, cost-effective	Slow action, stomach irritation, effect of stomach acid, first-pass effect, not suitable for all patients (with swallowing difficulties or are comatose)	Most medications, for example, analgesics, sedatives, hypnotics, antibiotics
Intramuscular	Several min	For rapid effect, for drugs with poor oral absorption when high blood levels are required	Avoid stomach or GIT effect, rapid effect, accuracy of dosage, irritant drugs can be given to patients with swallowing difficulties or are comatose avoiding first-pass effect	Only small quantities up to 10 mL of the drug can be given at a time, local pain and abscess formation, danger of infection, chances of nerve damage, expensive requires appropriately trained person	Opioid, analgesics, antibiotics
Intravenous	Up to 1 min	Large volumes of drugs, emergency situations	Similar to intramuscular but faster effect, and large volumes can be given, 100% bioavailability	Extravasation of drugs produces irritation and cellulitis, chances of thrombophlebitis, administration difficulties, adverse effects of drugs are difficult to control, danger of infection, expensive and requires an appropriately trained practitioner	IV fluids, nutrient supplements, antibiotics, resuscitative drugs

Intraarterial	Up to 1 min	For local effects within specific target organ, chemotherapy	Diagnostics agents, localised delivery, similar to intravenous	Reserved administration route for clinicians, risk of embolism, similar to intravenous drugs, expensive	Drugs used for treating cancer
Intrathecal	Several min	For local effect within the spinal cord	Localised delivery, minimal adverse effects	Reserved route for medical clinicians, expensive	Subarachnoid/epidural anaesthesia, drugs used for treating cancer
Transdermal	30–60 min	For continuous absorption and systemic effects over extended time (hours, days)	Convenient, no first-pass effect, controlled drug delivery, non-invasive, can be terminated quickly	Require potent drugs, slow action, low bioavailability, can cause irritation, not good for hydrophilic or high-molecular-weight drugs	Nitroglycerin, oestrogen, morphine
Subcutaneous	Several min	For drugs that are inactivated by the stomach	Uniform and sustained drug action, no first-pass effect, can be given to patients with swallowing difficulties or are comatose, avoid GIT effect	Only non-irritant drugs can be given to avoid irritation and necrosis, slower than IM route, danger of infection, only small volumes can be given, expensive	Insulin

(continued)

Table 3.7 (continued)

Route	Approx. time for the onset of drug action	Necessity of choice	Advantage	Disadvantage	Examples
Topical	Up to 60 min	For local effects on skin and mucous membrane of eye, ear, nose, mouth	Effective due to high concentration at the site of action, non-invasive, convenient to some patients, low possibility of systemic effect	Limited contact time, some patients find it messy, might be absorbed due to its lipophilic nature and cause side effects, may cause skin irritation, dosing control	Creams, ointments, sprays, tinctures, lozenges, for example, antibiotics, antiseptics, corticosteroids
Sublingual	Few min	For rapid effect	Rapid effect, avoid first-pass effect, cost-effective	Irritation of oral mucosa, unpleasant taste, only given in small quantities, not suitable for all patients	GTN (nitroglycerin) for angina pectoris
Buccal	Few min	For rapid effect, convenience	Similar to sublingual	Similar to sublingual	Androgenic drugs
Rectal	15–30 min	Local effect, when oral and parenteral routes are not indicated	Higher therapeutic concentrations, used for children and patients with swallowing difficulties or are comatose, little first-pass effect	Inconvenient, drug absorption is slow and erratic, some drugs cause irritation or inflammation of rectal mucosa	Analgesics, antiemetics, laxatives

Vaginal	15–30 min	For local effect	Can be used for local and systemic administration, convenient, controlled delivery, no first-pass effect	Erratic absorption, local administration may be absorbed and cause systemic adverse effects, some irritation, leakage or slipping of formulation	Creams, foams, suppositories
Inhalational	Up to 1 min	For systemic and local effects within respiratory tract	Rapid onset of action, avoid first-pass effects, reduced systemic adverse effects, lower doses are used, high efficacy, non-invasive, wide range of drugs, reproducible absorption kinetics	Only a few drugs can be administered, may cause irritation of pulmonary mucosa, chances of cardiotoxicity, may cause systemic adverse effects, difficult to control doses	Antiasthmatics, bronchodilators

3.11 General Safety Considerations in Handling Hazardous Drugs

Many hazardous drugs including those used for cancer chemotherapy, cytotoxic agents, antiviral drugs, hormones, some bioengineered drugs and other miscellaneous drugs used for the treatment of diseases pose a clear health danger to pharmacists, nurses, physicians and other healthcare workers engaged in the preparation and administration of these agents as well as the disposal of resulting waste products. Since reports of the mutagenic and teratogenic effects of certain cytotoxic agents on healthcare workers first arose (Falck et al. 1979; Hemminki et al. 1985; Rogers and Emmett 1987; Valanis et al. 1999), government agencies have developed increasingly rigorous guidelines for ensuring the safe handling of these hazardous agents. An extensive list of drugs that should be handled as hazardous in addition to drugs that were deleted from previous lists is detailed in the alert published by the National Institute for Occupational Safety and Health (NIOSH 2016). However, this sample list is intended to guide healthcare providers in diverse practice settings and should not be construed as complete representations of all of the hazardous drugs used at the referenced institutions. Some drugs may pose a risk if solid formulations are altered outside a ventilated cabinet (e.g. if tablets are crushed or dissolved or if capsules are pierced or opened). For the protection of healthcare providers using hazardous drugs, national and local policy and guidelines must be followed.

3.11.1 Drug Delivery (DD)

Simply, drug delivery (DD) refers to the processes and technologies involved in transporting a pharmaceutical substance in the body to achieve the desired therapeutic effect. It encompasses the approaches of administering medicinal products in humans and animals to achieve therapeutic efficacy. Drug delivery systems (DDSs) are technological systems that formulate and store drug molecules into suitable forms such as tablets for administration. They accelerate the arrival of drugs to the specific targeted site in the body, thus maximising therapeutic effectiveness and minimising off-target accumulation in the body. However, conventional drug delivery systems can cause systemic adverse effects due to non-specific biodistribution, uncontrolled release, and high doses. Additionally, some major challenges for most drug delivery systems include; intestinal absorption, solubility, poor bioavailability, in vivo stability, prolonged and targeted delivery to site of action, therapeutic efficacy and adverse effects.

Researchers are widely exploring various therapeutic strategies to reduce drug's undesirable adverse effects towards normal cells or tissues. In addition, it should be pointed out that more precise and effective targeted drug delivery systems that have emerged are promising therapeutic strategies for various diseases, especially tumours. Targeted drug delivery (TDD) can achieve the goal of personalised therapy because of low drug dosage used, high efficacy, and few adverse effects.

3.11.2 Targeted Drug Delivery (TDD)

Targeted drug delivery system is considered as a type of novel drug delivery system, by which the drug/medicinal product is specifically targeted to an organ/tissue and release the active therapeutic agent. It specifies the drug moiety directly into its targeted body area (organ, cellular, and subcellular level of specific tissue), to overcome the specific toxic effect adverse effect) of conventional drug delivery, thereby reducing the amount of drug required for therapeutic efficacy. The need for targeted drug delivery over conventional drug delivery systems is pressing to overcome the low efficacy of drugs with conventional delivery systems in terms of pharmaceutical, pharmacokinetic, pharmacodynamic, and pharmacotherapeutic features as shown in Fig. 3.12.

Basic Principles and Applications of Targeted Drug Delivery
The basic principle of targeted drug delivery is to deliver a high concentration of drug to specific organ/tissue (site of action) while minimising its concentration to other normal/ healthy organ/tissue. This principle aids in optimising the drug's therapeutic effects at the site of action while decreasing the adverse effects due to multitarget interactions and higher doses used in conventional drug delivery (Mahajan et al. 2007).

Drug targeting system consists of:

1. Coordinated drug behaviour.
2. Targeting site, which is the specific organ, a cell, or group of cells in chronic or acute condition demanding treatment with which the drug is going to interact.
3. Pharmaceutical carrier, which is a specially engineered molecule or system essential for effective transportation of the loaded drug towards preselected sites.

In order to assure the fulfilment of these characteristics, targeted drug products should be prepared while considering the specific properties of target cells and the nature of transport carriers that express the drug to specific receptors. These

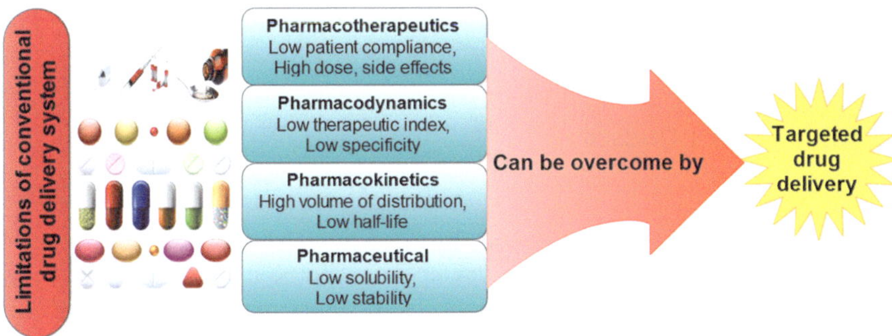

Fig. 3.12 Common problems of conventional drug delivery system (DDS) can be solved by targeted drug delivery

considerable parameters include drug concentration, particulate location and distribution, physicochemical properties, enzymes, physiological environment, nature/concentration of excipients, and surface morphology (shape, charge, size, and density) of carrier system.

Targeted drug delivery systems (TDDSs) has promising applications and purposes which include cancer therapy, vaccine adjuvant, ocular and brain delivery, DNA and oligonucleotide delivery, intracellular and systemic targeting, oral and transdermal delivery, enzyme immunoassays, and radioimaging. TDD can be applied effectively to treat many chronic and infectious diseases; most importantly its application in treating cancerous tumours, due to its better microphage penetration and enhanced concentration at the target site. In general, the reported results of these applications include reduced toxicity, enhanced uptake, prolonged systemic circulation with enhanced bioavailability and drug efficacy, enhanced immunoresponse, improved drug absorption and permeation, and improved drug retention (Bhargav et al. 2013).

3.12 Summary

In this chapter, the various dosage forms and their uses, routes of administration drug delivery and basic principles and applications of targeted drug delivery are discussed:

- Various dosage forms, the necessity for the use of each form, advantages and disadvantages and guidance on their use are discussed. The most common routes of administration, their impact on the choice of dosage forms and their advantages and disadvantages are also discussed.
- General guiding principles for the administration of medicines and the implications it has on patients and healthcare providers are outlined, in addition to precautions and safety consideration in handling hazardous drugs.
- Conventional drug delivery system, its limitations, basic principle and applications of targeted drug delivery system and its advantage over the conventional drug delivery system.

Multiple Choice Questions

1. When discussing drug formulation, drug stability relates to:
   - (a) Stability of the patient who is taking the medication
   - (b) The time it takes to achieve a stable blood serum concentration in a particular patient
   - (c) The stability of the medication against degradation
   - (d) The stability of a drug against drug interactions

2. Commonly, shelf life is defined as:
   (a) The time for the original potency of the active drug to be reduced to 95%
   (b) The time for the original potency of the active drug to be reduced to 90%
   (c) The time for the original potency of the active drug to be reduced to 80%
   (d) The time for the original potency of the active drug to be reduced to 70%
3. Disintegrants and binders are examples of:
   (a) Excipients
   (b) Formulations
   (c) Chelators
   (d) Drug interaction
4. Which population group is generally more likely to experience an excipient-related adverse reaction:
   (a) Older people, as kidney function deteriorates with age
   (b) Preterm babies, because the quantity of excipients may be high relative to body weight
   (c) Preterm babies, because the quantity of excipients may influence physiological processes such as surfactant production
   (d) Older people, because of their higher fat to body water ratio.
5. Capsules should be kept away from:
   (a) Extremes of humidity and dryness
   (b) Extreme humidity
   (c) Extreme dryness
   (d) Extremes of fluctuating temperature
6. Fifty percent of all medications available on the market are in the form of:
   (a) Tablets
   (b) Liquids
   (c) Ointments
   (d) Inhalers
   (e) Intravenous preparations
7. Film coating on tablets is needed to:
   (a) Keep moisture out
   (b) Make tablets easier to swallow
   (c) Ensure they cannot be split
   (d) Ensure they can pass through the stomach without degradation
8. Which form of tablet may contain a large quantity of sodium that may prohibit their use in patients who are sodium restricted?
   (a) Enteric coated
   (b) Multi-compacted
   (c) Effervescent
   (d) Chewable tablets
9. A substance that is usually homogeneous, clear, semi-solid preparations consisting of a liquid phase within a three-dimensional polymeric matrix with physical or sometimes chemical cross-linkage is:
   (a) An ointment
   (b) A cream

    (c) A gel

    (d) A paste

10. Solutions are:

    (a) Evenly distributed, homogeneous mixtures of dissolved medication (solid, liquid or gaseous) in a suitable liquid vehicle

    (b) Clear, sweet, flavoured hydroalcoholic mixtures intended for oral ingestion

    (c) Concentrated, viscous aqueous solutions containing one or more sugar components, mainly sucrose

    (d) Viscous, liquid oral preparations that are usually prescribed mainly for a demulcent (soothing), expectorant or sedative purpose

11. The advantages of developing targeted drug delivery systems over conventional drug delivery systems are:

    (a) TDDS encompasses the approaches of administering medicinal products in humans and animals to achieve therapeutic efficacy

    (b) The delivery of high dosage and non-specific biodistribution of drugs

    (c) The use of low dosage in and limiting the non-specific biodistribution of drugs

    (d) Maximising therapeutic efficacy through the use of high dosage and non-specific biodistribution

Answers

1. (c)
2. (b)
3. (a)
4. (b)
5. (a)
6. (a)
7. (b)
8. (c)
9. (c)
10. (a)
11. (c)

References

Bhargav E, Madhuri N, Ramesh K, Manne A, Ravi V (2013) Targeted drug delivery – a review. J Pharm Pharm Sci 3(1):150–169

Brayfield A (2017) Martindale: the complete drug reference. Pharmaceutical Press, London

British Pharmacopoeia (2019). https://www.pharmacopoeia.com/. Accessed 12 Aug 2019

Cavalla D (2009) APT drug R&D: the right active ingredient in the right presentation for the right therapeutic use. Nat Rev Drug Discov 8(11):849–853

Falck K, Grohn P, Sorsa M, Vainio H, Heinonen E, Holsti LR (1979) Mutagenicity in urine of nurses handling cytostatic drugs. Lancet 1(8128):1250–1251

Gudiksen M, Fleming E, Furstenthal L, Ma P (2008) What drives success for specialty pharmaceuticals. Nat Rev Drug Discov 7:563–567

Hemminki K, Kyyronen P, Lindbohm ML (1985) Spontaneous abortions and malformations in the offspring of nurses exposed to anaesthetic gases, cytostatic drugs, and other potential hazards in hospitals, based on registered information of outcome. J Epidemiol Community Health 39(2):141–147

Lund W (ed) (1994) The pharmaceutical codex. The Pharmaceutical Press, London, pp 277–286. 306–279

Mahajan HS, Patil SB, Gattani S, Kuchekar B (2007) Targeted drug delivery systems. Pharma Times 39:19–21

National Institute for Occupational Safety and Health (NIOSH) (2016) List of antineoplastic and other hazardous drugs in healthcare settings. Centre for Disease Control (CDC), Atlanta. https://www.cdc.gov/niosh/docs/2016-161/pdfs/2016-161.pdf. Accessed 02/02/2019

Pammolli F, Magazzini L, Riccaboni M (2011) The productivity crisis in pharmaceutical R&D. Nat Rev Drug Discov 10(6):428–438

Paul SM, Mytelka DS, Dunwiddie CT, Persinger CC, Munos BH, Lindborg SR, Schacht AL (2010) How to improve R&D productivity: the pharmaceutical industry's grand challenge. Nat Rev Drug Discov 9(3):203–214

Pawer R, BenAri A, Domb AJ (2004) Protein and peptide parenteral controlled delivery. Expert Opin Biol Ther 4(8):1203–1212

Rogers B, Emmett EA (1987) Handling antineoplastic agents: urine mutagenicity in nurses. Image J Nurs Sch 19(3):108–113

Rowe RC, Sheskey PJ, Quinn ME (2009) Handbook of pharmaceutical excipients. Pharmaceutical Press, London

Schier JG, Howland MA, Hoffman RS, Nelson LS (2003) Fatality from administration of labetalol and crushed extended-release nifedipine. Ann Pharmacother 37(10):1420–1423

Selvaag E (1998) Vitiligo caused by chloroquine phototoxicity. J R Army Med Corps 44(3):163–165

US Pharmacopoeia (2019). https://www.usp.org/. Accessed 12 Aug 2019

Valanis B, Vollmer WM, Steele P (1999) Occupational exposure to antineoplastic agents: self-reported miscarriages and stillbirths among nurses and pharmacists. J Occup Environ Med 41(8):632–638

Valeur KS, Holst H, Allegaert K (2018) Excipients in neonatal medicinal products: never prescribed, commonly administered. Pharmaceut Med 32(4):251–258

Nicola Husain

Learning Outcomes

At the end of this chapter, you will be able to:

- Define 'adverse drug reaction' and 'drug interaction'.
- Describe the classification of adverse reactions.
- Understand why adverse drug reactions and drug interactions occur.
- Describe the factors that affect susceptibility to adverse drug reactions and drug interactions.
- Understand that foods and herbal medicines can interact with medicines.
- Discuss how adverse drug reactions and drug interactions can be identified, prevented and managed.
- Understand how you may contribute towards minimising risk of adverse drug reactions and drug interactions.

4.1 Introduction

Adverse drug reactions can be categorised as type A or B: type A reactions are predictable and dose related, whereas type B reactions are idiosyncratic. Type B reactions are rarer than type A but tend to cause greater harm. Some medicines can cause hypersensitivity (allergic) reactions which can be fatal if not treated promptly. Certain factors can affect a patient's susceptibility of experiencing an adverse drug reaction, including extremes of age, co-morbidities, genetic disposition and the characteristics of the medicine.

N. Husain (✉)
Faculty of Life Sciences & Medicine, King's College London, London, UK
e-mail: nicola.husain@kcl.ac.uk

E. Khan, P. Hood (eds.), *Understanding Pharmacology in Nursing Practice*,
https://doi.org/10.1007/978-3-032-03964-4_4

A drug interaction occurs when the effect of one medicine is altered by the presence of another. Interactions that alter the *absorption, distribution, metabolism* or *elimination* of a drug are called 'pharmacokinetic', and interactions that alter the *action* of a drug are called 'pharmacodynamic'. Drug interactions can increase the effect of a drug, resulting in toxicity, or decrease the effects of a drug, resulting in reduced efficacy or treatment failure. Many interacting medicines can be administered safely without causing any harm to the patient through careful monitoring and dose adjustment. However, medicines should only be administered together if the consequences are understood and the risk of harm is outweighed by the therapeutic benefits.

4.2 Adverse Drug Reactions

Adverse drug reactions, commonly referred to as 'side effects', are unwanted effects that occur as a result of taking or using a medicine. An adverse drug reaction can be defined as a response to a drug which is 'noxious and unintended, and which occurs at doses used in man for prophylaxis, diagnosis or therapy' (World Health Organisation 1970: 103). The term 'adverse drug reaction' should not be confused with 'medication error'. Medication errors occur as a result of incorrect prescribing, dispensing or administration of the medicine and are largely considered preventable.

Ideally, medicines would selectively target the site in the body where the therapeutic action is desired. In reality, most medicines lack specificity and as a result cause effects throughout the body. Adverse effects are common and are detrimental to health: they are responsible for significant morbidity and mortality, and evidence suggests they are a contributory causal factor for 6.5% of adult hospital admissions (Pirmohamed et al. 2004). The occurrence of adverse drug reactions is one of the most common reasons patients give for not taking medicines as instructed.

An understanding of how and why adverse drug reactions occur is important for all healthcare professionals. Pharmacological treatment decisions should always be underpinned by consideration of the magnitude and the likelihood of a medicine's anticipated benefits (its desired therapeutic effect) and its potential risk for harm (its adverse effects). There is huge variability in how different people react to the same drug, and although factors have been identified that may predispose certain individuals to experience adverse effects, definitive predictions are difficult. However, acknowledging the potential toxicities of a medicine, and assessing an individual's risk for those toxicities, should lead to appropriate, patient-focused prescribing and patient monitoring.

4.2.1 Identification of Adverse Drug Reactions

Adverse drug reactions are diverse: they can affect single or multiple organs or body systems. They are often non-specific and can bear similarity to symptoms of disease. The severity of an adverse drug reaction can vary from mild to severe or even fatal, the incidence can vary from extremely rare to relatively common and a single medicine may be associated with tens or hundreds of adverse effects. Identifying adverse drug reactions and quantifying the incidence of an adverse effect are consequently extremely complex.

The possibility of an adverse drug reaction should always be considered when assessing a patient's signs and symptoms. Patients sometimes fail to report symptoms of adverse reactions, thinking these are insignificant or unrelated to their medication. Clinicians may also fail to identify the connection between a patient's symptoms and a potential adverse reaction of their medicines. Even when an adverse effect is suspected, it can be difficult, sometimes impossible, to prove a causal relationship between the medicine and the effect. Naranjo et al. (1981) devised an algorithm for determining the likelihood of a patient's symptom being an adverse effect of a medicine. Causality is deemed 'definite', 'probable', 'possible' or 'doubtful', depending on a score calculated from answering ten questions (Table 4.1).

Once an adverse effect is identified, or strongly suspected, it is important that the correct action is taken to minimise further risk to the patient. The management of a patient experiencing an adverse drug reaction is discussed later in this chapter.

Table 4.1 The Naranjo et al. (1981) adverse drug reaction algorithm

		Yes	No	Do not know	Score
1	Are there previous conclusive reports on this reaction?	+1	0	0	
2	Did the adverse event occur after the suspected drug was administered?	+2	−1	0	
3	Did the adverse reaction improve when the drug was discontinued or a specific antagonist was administered?	+1	0	0	
4	Did the adverse reaction reappear when the drug was re-administered?	+2	−1	0	
5	Are there alternative causes (other than the drug) that could have on their own caused the reaction?	−1	+2	0	
6	Did the reaction reappear when a placebo was given?	−1	+1	0	
7	Was the blood detected in the blood (or other fluids) in concentrations known to be toxic?	+1	0	0	
8	Was the reaction more severe when the dose was increased or less severe when the dose was decreased?	+1	0	0	
9	Did the patient have a similar reaction to the same or similar drugs in any previous exposure?	+1	0	0	
10	Was the adverse event confirmed by any objective evidence?	+1	0	0	
	Total score to determine likelihood of causality ≥9, definite; 5–8, probable; 1–4, possible; ≤0, doubtful				Total

Table 4.2 Characteristics and examples of type A and type B adverse drug reactions

	Type A		Type B	
Characteristics	Predictable from known Pharmacological action Dose-related severity High incidence High morbidity and low mortality		Unpredictable from known pharmacological action (and mechanism often not understood) severity not dose related Low incidence Low morbidity and high mortality	
Examples	Reaction	*Drug*	Reaction	*Drug*
	Sedation	*Chlorpheniramine*	Agranulocytosis	*Carbimazole*
	Bradycardia	*Atenolol*	Tinnitus	*Aspirin*
	Constipation	*Morphine*	Anaphylaxis	*Flucloxacillin*
	Headache	*Glyceryl trinitrate*	Aplastic anaemia	*Chloramphenicol*

4.2.2 Classification of Adverse Drug Reactions

Adverse drug reactions can be classified as predictable and dose related (type A) or idiosyncratic (type B) (Rawlins and Thompson 1991). Type A reactions account for approximately 80% of all reported adverse drug reactions, but a type B reaction often results in greater harm. The differentiating features of type A and type B reactions according to the Rawlins and Thompson (1991) classification system and examples of each are listed in Table 4.2.

4.2.3 Mechanisms of Adverse Drug Reactions

Most adverse drug reactions are believed to arise from a pharmacological or immunological action of the active drug or one of its metabolites, although the exact mechanism for many adverse drug reactions has yet to be explained. Some adverse drug reactions occur as a direct, exaggerated effect of the drug's pharmacological action, such as hypotension caused by antihypertensives or hypoglycaemia from insulin. Others are caused by mechanisms that are secondary to the drug's main pharmacological action. For example, tricyclic antidepressants can cause blurred vision by a mechanism that is unrelated to their antidepressant action.

Many adverse drug reactions are known to be dose-dependent, meaning that the extent of the reaction is related to the amount of drug present in the body. Some adverse reactions, however, are related to the *cumulative* dose of a drug received, even when administration has occurred over a long period of time. For example, a well-known adverse effect of the chemotherapeutic agent, doxorubicin, is cardiotoxicity, which is largely associated with lifetime cumulative doses greater than 500 mg/m^2 and may develop months or even years after its use (Chatterjee et al. 2010).

The time at which an adverse reaction occurs in relation to administration of the medicine varies considerably. Some adverse effects occur immediately after the medicine has been administered, whereas others only become apparent months or years later. The harmful effects of medicines that have carcinogenic (causing cancer) or teratogenic (causing foetal malformation) properties are examples of adverse drug reactions that may not present until long after the drug has been eliminated from the body.

The method of drug administration also plays a role in the occurrence of some adverse drug reactions. When administered intravenously, certain drugs, including the antiviral medicine aciclovir, the antiarrhythmic amiodarone, the macrolide antibiotic clarithromycin and some chemotherapeutic agents, can cause phlebitis. The rate at which a medicine is infused can also be a factor: intravenous furosemide, when administered to adults at a rate greater than 4 mg/min, is associated with tinnitus and deafness, and rapid infusion of vancomycin can cause a severe erythematous rash, a condition known as 'red man syndrome' (Sivagnanam and Deleu 2003).

Adverse drug reactions may also be caused by 'excipients', the inactive constituents of a medicine. Excipients are necessary to ensure the safety, stability and efficacy of the active drug. Regular use of sugar-containing liquid medicines can lead to dental caries, and certain preservatives in eye drops can cause local irritation. Some excipients are associated with hypersensitivity reactions, such as arachis (peanut) oil, which is found in some oral and topical medicines, and egg protein, which is present in some vaccines.

4.2.4 Immunological Reactions

The term 'drug allergy' is often incorrectly applied to a multitude of adverse drug reactions or intolerances, but true allergy refers to an immune-mediated reaction. Drug allergies typically present with rash, swelling, bronchoconstriction and hypotension, and symptoms may vary from mild to life-threatening. Allergic reactions are idiosyncratic (type B) adverse effects because they are unrelated to the dose or the pharmacological action of the drug and generally cannot be predicted, although drug allergies may be more common in people with a history of allergy or atopy (a disposition to develop allergies). It is important to be aware that previous exposure to a medicine without any adverse effect does not preclude the development of an allergic reaction following subsequent exposure. Medicines should never be prescribed or administered without finding out the allergy status of the patient.

Anaphylaxis is a severe form of type 1 hypersensitivity characterised by immunoglobulin E (IgE) production. On first exposure to a substance, the immune system of sensitive individuals produces IgE which binds to the surface of basophils and mast cells. When IgE antibodies are exposed to the same allergen on a subsequent occasion, degranulation is triggered and substances such as histamine, prostaglandins and leukotrienes are released. Life-threatening hypotension and bronchoconstriction can develop rapidly, often in combination with cutaneous symptoms such as rash, urticaria and angioedema (oedema and swelling of the skin). Emergency treatment with intramuscular adrenaline must be given promptly because anaphylaxis can be fatal; corticosteroids, antihistamines and intravenous fluids may also be indicated. Whilst penicillins are the most common iatrogenic (drug) cause of

Table 4.3 Some of the most common drug causes of anaphylaxis

Amphotericin
Antibiotics, including penicillins (such as amoxicillin, ampicillin, benzylpenicillin, phenoxymethylpenicillin, flucloxacillin, co-amoxiclav and piperacillin-tazobactam)
Chemotherapy agents
Muscle relaxants (such as suxamethonium, vecuronium and atracurium)
Non-steroidal anti-inflammatory drugs (such as ibuprofen, aspirin and diclofenac)
Radiological contrast agents

anaphylaxis, other drugs are known to be implicated (Table 4.3) (Working Group of the Resuscitation Council 2021). If a drug allergy is suspected, further exposure to the drug must be avoided, which may potentially restrict the patient's future drug choices. For example, if a patient is identified as 'allergic to penicillin', the treatment options available against subsequent infections are limited.

4.2.5 Susceptibility to Adverse Drug Reactions

A number of factors exist that increase the chance of an adverse reaction occurring, some of which relate to the individual and others to the medicine. Factors affecting susceptibility to adverse drug reactions are discussed as follows.

4.2.5.1 Polypharmacy

Patients who require the use of multiple medicines (polypharmacy) are at greater risk of experiencing adverse drug reactions (Leenderte 2008). The combined risk is known to be greater than the summative risk from each medicine, but confounding factors such as multiple disease states, poor organ function and increasing age—which are normally present in people who require multiple medicines—make quantifying this risk difficult. Polypharmacy also increases the risk of a drug–drug interaction, the possibility of non-adherence and the chance of a medication error occurring.

4.2.5.2 Disease States

Disease states, notably renal and hepatic dysfunction, can alter how medicines are processed by the body. The liver is the primary site for drug metabolism, and the kidneys play a key role in excreting drugs and their metabolites. Functional impairment of the liver or kidneys will therefore affect the rate and extent of metabolism and excretion, slowing down drug elimination and resulting in drug or metabolite accumulation and concentration-dependent toxicity. Often, toxicity can be minimised through prudent monitoring of hepatic and renal function, measuring drug plasma levels and reducing the dose or extending the dosage interval when necessary.

Critical illness, immunological disorders, malnutrition, viral infection (including HIV) and cancer may also be associated with a higher incidence of adverse drug reactions from particular medicines, although whether this increased risk arises from other factors, such as polypharmacy or organ failure, is difficult to assess (Joshua et al. 2009; Ulrich 2007).

4.2.5.3 Pregnancy

During pregnancy, changes to body composition, plasma protein concentration and organ function can alter pharmacokinetic parameters, and although most are not thought to be clinically significant, others may cause detrimental effects to the woman. For example, the plasma concentration of several antiepileptic drugs, including phenytoin and carbamazepine, tends to fall during pregnancy, possibly due to a larger vascular volume and greater metabolic clearance, which increases the woman's risk of a seizure (Dawes and Chowienczyk 2001).

The effects of maternal medicines on the development of the foetus must always be considered when administering medicines during pregnancy. Some medicines are known teratogens and should be avoided throughout pregnancy. Isotretinoin, used to treat acne, is an example of a teratogenic medicine. For most medicines, there is a lack of conclusive data surrounding their effects on a foetus when given during pregnancy, primarily because it would be unethical to conduct clinical trials in this patient group. Every pregnancy presents a background risk of congenital malformation, and so even if a medicine is suspected of teratogenicity, a causal effect is hard to prove without epidemiological study.

4.2.5.4 Extremes of Age: Children

Children have additional risk factors for experiencing adverse drug reactions. Pharmacokinetic and pharmacodynamic parameters in neonates (babies up to 4 weeks' old) and children differ to those of adults which can result in variable and unpredictable responses to medicines. Furthermore, children are more likely to require treatment with unlicensed medicines, which may not have undergone the same rigorous safety testing process that licensed medicines have been subjected to.

Drug absorption in a child—be it via the oral, topical or intramuscular route—varies depending on their age. Changes in gastric pH, gastric transit time, skin permeability and muscle mass will affect the rate and extent of absorption. Topical corticosteroids such as hydrocortisone, used in the management of eczema, are more likely to cause systemic effects in children due to greater skin permeation (West et al. 1981).

Neonates have high levels of circulating bilirubin, most of which is bound to albumin. Unbound bilirubin can pass through the blood–brain barrier and enter the central nervous system, where in high levels it can cause a potentially fatal encephalopathy called kernicterus. Drugs that bind strongly to albumin, such as ceftriaxone, can displace bilirubin from its protein binding site, allowing it to penetrate the blood–brain barrier (Martin et al. 1993). Kernicterus can cause permanent neurological damage, which may result in hearing loss, seizures and death.

The tetracycline class of antibiotic, including minocycline, tetracycline and doxycycline, distributes into calcifying tissue, such as the bones and teeth of children (Sanchez et al. 2004). Tetracycline administration to children under the age of 12 may result in permanent discolouration of teeth, and usage is therefore avoided.

Metabolic pathways that convert drugs to inactive compounds, such as the cytochrome P450 (CYP450) enzyme system, are not fully functional in early childhood (Johnson 2003). The rate at which hepatic enzymatic pathways develop during childhood varies between individuals, which can lead to variability in drug disposition and metabolism and the occurrence of adverse reactions that are not apparent in the adult population.

Reye's syndrome is a rare but serious condition that causes damage to the liver and brain. The aetiology of Reye's syndrome is complex, but it is believed to be an idiosyncratic (type B) adverse drug reaction associated with the use of aspirin in children with a concurrent viral illness (Ulrich 2007). The belief that aspirin is linked to the development of Reye's syndrome is supported by the dramatic fall in cases since the avoidance of aspirin in children was recommended in the 1980s (Belay et al. 1999).

Children are also exposed to a greater risk of adverse effects from excipients. The preparation of phenobarbital elixir that is licensed in the United Kingdom contains 38% alcohol, ingestion of which could result in significant alcohol toxicity in a child. Propylene glycol is a solvent contained in many medicines, including injectable forms of phenobarbital, phenytoin and diazepam, which in sufficient quantities can cause seizures or respiratory arrest in neonates. Caution is required to ensure that the cumulative dose of excipients does not reach toxic levels.

4.2.5.5 Extremes of Age: Older People

As age increases, the percentage of total body water content decreases, total body fat content increases, compensatory and homeostatic mechanisms become less efficient and renal and hepatic function tend to decline. In fact, it should be assumed that all older people—although most significantly in patients over the age of 75—have a degree of renal impairment, even if plasma creatinine is not raised (Rowe et al. 1976). These physiological changes can affect pharmacokinetic and pharmacodynamic parameters, resulting in a patient's susceptibility to certain adverse drug reactions increasing with age. Older people are also more likely to suffer from multiple illnesses, so require multiple medicines, which increase their risk of adverse drug reactions.

Digoxin is a water-soluble, renally excreted cardiac glycoside that is prescribed for heart failure and arrhythmias. As age increases, the volume of distribution of digoxin decreases and its elimination via the kidneys is reduced (Currie et al. 2011). The resulting increase in digoxin plasma concentration dramatically increases the risk of dose-related toxicities, such as nausea, dizziness and blurred vision. This example highlights the necessity of caution when dosing renally excreted medicines for older patients. Older people are also more sensitive to nephrotoxic effects of drugs, as is frequently observed with non-steroidal anti-inflammatory drugs (NSAIDs), especially when renal function is already impaired. Often prescribed to older people for arthritis, NSAIDs can impair renal function by reducing renal blood flow and glomerular filtration rate (Weinblatt 1991).

Plasma protein concentrations tend to be lower in older people, possibly as a result of the ageing process, although malnutrition and concurrent disease states may also contribute. Lowered protein concentration affects the distribution of highly protein-bound drugs, such as warfarin and phenytoin. As the amount of protein available for drug binding is reduced, the proportion of unbound drug, which is the component available for receptor interaction, is increased, enhancing its effects and increasing the risk of toxicity. This is particularly important for drugs that have a small margin between their therapeutic and toxic plasma level (high-risk drugs).

Hepatic blood flow and the liver's capacity for drug metabolism are also affected by older age. Propranolol is a lipid-soluble beta-blocker that is extensively hepatically metabolised during its first pass through the portal circulation. However, in older people, portal blood flow is reduced, and so a greater proportion of propranolol reaches the systemic circulation, resulting in raised propranolol plasma levels (Castleden et al. 1975). The half-life of drugs which are predominantly metabolised by the liver can be significantly increased in older age due to reduced metabolic enzyme activity. The half-life of diazepam increases substantially with age due to a reduction of its metabolism by the liver (Greenblatt et al. 1991). Unless doses are adjusted, the patient may be exposed to significant risk of diazepam toxicity.

Although the majority of adverse drug reactions that affect older people have a pharmacokinetic basis, pharmacodynamic changes also occur with ageing. Postural hypotension occurs commonly in older people receiving antihypertensives such as diuretics or calcium channel blockers. Baroreceptors, which are located within the blood vessels, detect changes in blood pressure and provide constant feedback to regulate and maintain normal blood pressure. With increasing age, the sensitivity of this reflex mechanism declines: postural hypotension may occur, which can lead to a fall. Adverse drug reactions affecting cognition, sedation or motor function may also increase an older person's risk of falls. Antidepressants, opioids and benzodiazepines are all implicated, especially as older people tend to have greater sensitivity to the effects of medicines on the central nervous system.

Osteoporosis is primarily a condition of old age, particularly affecting postmenopausal women for whom a decline in oestrogen levels is associated with a fall in bone density. Glucocorticoids such as prednisolone reduce bone mineral density and impair bone formation, and so their use presents the older person—especially postmenopausal women—with a significant risk of fracture (Mazziotti et al. 2006).

As a general rule, medicines for older people should be initiated at low doses and increased gradually to minimise the risk of adverse effects occurring.

4.2.5.6 Pharmacogenomics

Increasingly, variation in an individual's genetic profile, particularly within genes that code for drug-metabolising enzymes and drug transporters, is known to play a role in determining an individual's risk of adverse drug effects. 'Pharmacogenomics' is the study of how a person's genomic profile affects their response to medicines. Pharmacogenomic testing enables clinicians to select drugs and doses that optimise effectiveness and minimise the risk of adverse effects for a specific patient (Swen et al. 2023).

An estimated 400 million people worldwide express a genetic variant that results in a deficiency of the enzyme glucose-6-phosphate dehydrogenase (G6PD)

Table 4.4 Drugs with risk of haemolysis in individuals who are G6PD deficient

Drugs with definite risk of haemolysis in most G6PD-deficient individuals	Drugs with definite risk of haemolysis in most G6PD-deficient individuals
Dapsone and other sulfones	Aspirin
Fluoroquinolones (including ciprofloxacin, moxifloxacin, norfloxacin and ofloxacin)	Chloroquine
Methylthioninium chloride (methylene blue)	Menadiol sodium phosphate
Niridazole [not on UK market]	Quinine
Nitrofurantoin	Sulfonylureas
Pamaquin [not on UK market]	
Primaquine	
Quinolones	
Rasburicase	
Sulfonamides such as co-trimoxazole	

(Youngster et al. 2010). The major complication of G6PD deficiency is haemolytic anaemia precipitated by exposure to certain drugs. The drugs that are most commonly associated with drug-induced haemolysis are listed in Table 4.4 (Joint Formulary Committee 2025), although it should be noted that individual susceptibility and severity of haemolysis varies considerably between patients.

Hypersensitivity reactions following initiation of the antiretroviral abacavir occur in approximately 4% of patients, although studies have shown that prevalence varies across ancestral groups (Symonds et al. 2002; Hetherington et al. 2002). Abacavir hypersensitivity is strongly associated with the presence of the *HLA-B*5701* allele, a genetic marker that is more common in White European than Black sub-Saharan African people, highlighting the variation in pharmacogene allele frequency across populations (Orkin et al. 2009). Patients should be tested for *HLA-B*5701* prior to commencing antiretroviral treatment, and abacavir should be avoided in those who are *HLA-B*5701* positive.

Variants in the mitochondrial *MT-RNR1* gene are associated with ototoxicity (hearing loss) following exposure to aminoglycoside antibiotics, which are active against Gram-negative bacteria (McDermott et al. 2022). People who are predisposed to Gram-negative infections, such as those with cystic fibrosis, can be tested for the associated genetic variants and prescribed alternative antibiotics if a risk of ototoxicity is identified.

Azathioprine is an immunosuppressive agent that is indicated for inflammatory conditions including inflammatory bowel disease and rheumatoid arthritis. A subset of the population produce only low levels of the enzyme thiopurine methyltransferase (TPMT) which catalyses the S-methylation reaction that metabolises azathioprine, necessitating a much lower dose to avoid toxicity (Weinshilboum 2001). Testing for TPMT prior to starting therapy allows for lower dose selection for patients with low levels of enzyme.

A greater understanding of pharmacogenomics will allow therapy to be tailored for a specific patient, leading to individualised dosing and minimisation of adverse effects.

4.2.6 High-Risk Drugs

Drugs which have a small margin separating their subtherapeutic and toxic level are described as having a narrow therapeutic index. Examples include digoxin, carbamazepine, phenytoin, sodium valproate, phenobarbital, ciclosporin, lithium, gentamicin, vancomycin, warfarin and theophylline. Extensive patient variability exists in what dose will produce a therapeutic response, and so toxic adverse effects can easily occur.

For most drugs with a narrow therapeutic index, therapeutic drug monitoring—monitoring of plasma levels or therapeutic efficacy—can be utilised to ensure plasma levels within the therapeutic window are maintained. The typical adult therapeutic plasma range for some narrow therapeutic index drugs is shown in Table 4.5 (Brayfield and Cadart 2025), although clinical circumstance may necessitate different target levels.

In addition to possessing a narrow therapeutic index, some drugs exhibit nonlinear pharmacokinetics, which means that plasma concentration is not directly proportional to the dose. In the case of phenytoin, this occurs when hepatic metabolic pathways become saturated, and large increases in plasma level may result from small changes to the dose (Ludden 1991).

Despite the common perception that they are 'safe', serious adverse reactions can also occur with alternative or herbal remedies and medicines that can be bought over-the-counter without a prescription. It is therefore important when asking about a patient's medication history to always enquire about medicines and remedies that have been purchased as well as those that have been prescribed.

4.2.7 Pharmacovigilance: Reporting and Monitoring of Adverse Drug Reaction Data

In response to the thalidomide tragedy in the 1960s, when thousands of mothers gave birth to babies with disabilities and birth defects as a result of taking thalidomide to alleviate morning sickness, the Medicines Act (1968) was passed which required all new medicines to undergo clinical trials to assess safety, quality and efficacy prior to market authorisation. Common adverse effects are usually revealed during this process, but rarer effects may not become apparent until after the

Table 4.5 Typical adult therapeutic plasma range for narrow therapeutic index drugs

Drug	Plasma range
Carbamazepine	4–12 mg/L
Digoxin	0.5–2 µg/L
Phenytoin	10–20 mg/L
Phenobarbital	15–40 mg/L
Theophylline	10–20 mg/L
Vancomycin	10–15 mg/L

medicine is licensed when usage has expanded to a wider patient population. For this reason, it is critical that information is collected about the type and incidence of adverse effects that occur with medicines.

In the United Kingdom, a national reporting system, the Yellow Card Scheme, is provided by the Medicines and Healthcare products Regulatory Agency (MHRA) to collate and monitor data about suspected adverse reactions to medicines, vaccines, medical devices, blood products and electronic cigarettes (Medicines and Healthcare products Regulatory Agency 2025). Yellow Card data is continually evaluated to help improve understanding of adverse reactions and to identify previously unreported reactions. Reports can be submitted by healthcare professionals or members of the public, even if causality is not proven. The following adverse effects should always be reported:

- Adverse effects that are severe or result in harm.
- Adverse effects that occur in children or the patients over 65.
- Suspected delayed drug effects or congenital abnormalities.
- Suspected adverse effects from biological medicines or vaccines.
- Suspected adverse effects from complementary remedies such as homeopathic and herbal products.
- Adverse effects that occur with medicines that are intensively monitored by the MHRA (indicated in the *British National Formulary* and recognised throughout Europe by a black triangular symbol ▼).

Similar pharmacovigilance reporting systems exist in countries across Europe and beyond. As new data emerges the safety profile of a medicine may be revised and additional warnings or precautions introduced. Occasionally, a medicine may be withdrawn from the market if new information indicates that the medicine's therapeutic benefits no longer outweigh its risks.

4.2.8 Managing Adverse Drug Reactions

Patients should be educated about the possible adverse effects that might occur with their medicines, and every dispensed medicine in the United Kingdom must be accompanied by the manufacturer's patient information leaflet, which provides detailed information about the medicine, including undesirable effects. All healthcare professionals should play a role in patient education, and nurses are particularly well-placed to talk to patients about their medicine's adverse effects and to ensure they know what to do should an adverse reaction occur, especially if the medicine is associated with serious or harmful effects. For example, carbimazole, a medicine that is used to treat hyperthyroidism, can cause life-threatening agranulocytosis, and so patients should be warned to report immediately any signs of infection, such as a sore throat or fever.

When an adverse drug reaction is suspected, there are several factors that will affect the course of action that should follow. For adverse reactions that are dose related, a reduction in the dose may be enough to alleviate the symptoms of the reaction without losing the therapeutic benefits of the medicine. For example, the hypoglycaemic effects of insulin therapy can be minimised by dose adjustment. For adverse effects that are known to usually be mild and transient, such as gastrointestinal disturbance following the initiation of metformin therapy for type 2 diabetes, simply continuing therapy and providing reassurance that the effects are self-limiting may be sufficient management. For more serious or troublesome reactions, switching to an alternative drug within the same pharmacological class may be appropriate, assuming the same effects are not anticipated with the second drug. In the case of adverse reactions that are known to be class effects, such as angioedema induced by ACE inhibitors, avoidance of all medicines within the therapeutic class is necessary, and an alternative class of drug should be selected. In some cases, the best course of action may be to use an additional drug to treat the adverse effect, such as a laxative to treat constipation caused by morphine.

4.3   Drug Interactions

When two or more medicines are taken together, there is a chance that the drugs will interact. A 'drug–drug interaction' occurs when the effect of one drug is altered by the presence of another. Drug interactions can also occur when medicines are taken with certain foods, chemicals, herbal remedies or illicit drugs. The consequences of drug interactions can range from trivial to life-threatening and the symptoms they present are highly variable. Most drug interactions can be classed as 'pharmacokinetic' or 'pharmacodynamic', and the characteristics of each are described below.

4.3.1   Pharmacokinetic Interactions

Pharmacokinetic drug interactions are due to the effect one drug has on the pharmacokinetic characteristics—absorption, distribution, metabolism or elimination—of another. Pharmacokinetic interactions usually result in a change in the plasma concentration of a drug: a concentration increase may result in drug toxicity whereas a concentration decrease may cause therapeutic failure.

4.3.1.1 Absorption
The rate or extent that a medicine is absorbed can be enhanced or inhibited by the concurrent administration of another medicine. Drug absorption via the gastrointestinal tract may be affected by agents that alter gut pH or gastric transit time (Baxter and Preston 2025). Proton pump inhibitors (such as omeprazole) and H2-receptor antagonists (such as ranitidine) exert their therapeutic effect by suppressing gastric acid secretion. The rise in pH that follows their administration can inhibit the absorption of the HIV drug atazanavir because its solubility is reduced in an alkaline environment (Klein et al. 2008). Metoclopramide is an antiemetic which accelerates gastrointestinal transit time and gastric emptying. When administered with

digoxin, intestinal motility is accelerated to such an extent that absorption of digoxin is reduced (Manninen et al. 1973).

Drug absorption can also be impaired by the presence of substances that chemically bind with drugs in the gastrointestinal tract. For example, calcium salts—commonly administered to patients at risk of osteoporosis—form insoluble, poorly absorbed chelate complexes with ciprofloxacin, tetracycline and levothyroxine in the gut. Iron compounds and indigestion remedies comprising aluminium-containing and magnesium-containing salts exert similar effects to calcium (D'Arcy and McElnay 1987; Garty and Hurwitz 1980; Kara et al. 1991). Ensuring a window of several hours between administration of the salt and the interacting drug can minimise the effect of this interaction.

4.3.1.2 Distribution

Drugs that are highly protein-bound may compete with other protein-bound drugs for binding sites. For example, if Drug A is bound to albumin within plasma, the addition of Drug B, which has greater affinity for albumin than Drug A, will displace Drug A from its binding sites leading to greater levels of 'free' or unbound Drug A. Often, the rise in circulating free drug is countered by an increase in its breakdown, because only unbound drug is free to be metabolised. For most drugs, the temporary rise in plasma levels is not considered of clinical importance, and protein displacement alone is rarely the cause of a significant drug interaction (Rolan 1994).

Some drugs can inhibit or enhance the function of efflux transporter proteins, such as P-glycoprotein, which remove drugs from cells or organs including the brain. Ritonavir is an antiretroviral drug that is removed from the brain by P-glycoprotein. When administered together with ketoconazole, a triazole antifungal that inhibits P-glycoprotein, the concentration of ritonavir within the brain is increased (Khaliq et al. 2000). In some cases, this interaction can be beneficial but the risk of toxicity also increases.

4.3.1.3 Metabolism

Some of the most important and frequently encountered drug interactions involve drugs that inhibit or induce hepatic enzymes that are responsible for drug metabolism. Drugs that are enzyme inhibitors will reduce the enzymatic metabolism of other drugs, resulting in higher drug plasma levels, whereas drugs that are enzyme inducers will speed up the metabolism of drugs via that pathway, resulting in lower drug plasma levels. Some common enzyme inducers and inhibitors are listed in Table 4.6.

Rifampicin, an antimicrobial used to treat tuberculosis, is known to increase the expression of the 3A family of CYP450 enzymes and the efflux transporter, P-glycoprotein. As a result, rifampicin considerably increases the metabolism (and therefore lowers the plasma concentration) of a multitude of drugs including oral contraceptives, phenytoin and members of the protease inhibitor class of antiretrovirals (including atazanavir, darunavir and lopinavir).

Table 4.6 Common enzyme inducers and inhibitors

Enzyme inducers	Enzyme inhibitors		
Alcohol (chronic use)	Alcohol (acute use)	Fluconazole	Omeprazole
Barbiturates	Allopurinol	Fluoxetine	Oral contraceptives
Carbamazepine	Amiodarone	Gemfibrozil	Protease inhibitors
Griseofulvin	Cimetidine	Grapefruit juice	Sulphonamides
Phenytoin	Ciprofloxacin	Isoniazid	Terbinafine
Rifampicin	Clarithromycin	Itraconazole	Verapamil
St John's wort	Diltiazem	Ketoconazole	Voriconazole
Tobacco smoke	Erythromycin	Metronidazole	

Some enzyme inducers augment the effects of the enzyme that is responsible for their own metabolism. Carbamazepine is an example of a drug that causes 'autoinduction'; a fall in plasma levels is often seen a few days after initiation or following a dose increase (Kudriakova et al. 1992).

The cholesterol-lowering agent simvastatin is metabolised in the liver by the isoenzyme 3A4, and co-administration of a 3A4 inhibitor can increase drug levels which can subsequently increase the patient's risk of adverse effects, including rhabdomyolysis (muscle breakdown, a recognised serious adverse effect of statins) (Jacobson 2004). Simvastatin should be withheld in patients taking potent inhibitors of 3A4, such as the antibiotics erythromycin and clarithromycin, due to the significance of this interaction. Of note is that erythromycin and clarithromycin bind irreversibly to the enzyme, rendering it inactive until further enzyme has been synthesised. Most other enzyme inhibitors bind reversibly, so they can be displaced by other drugs with greater affinity.

Amiodarone, an antiarrhythmic, is one of numerous medicines that interact with the anticoagulant, warfarin. Amiodarone inhibits the enzymes 3A4, 2C9 and 1A2, all of which are involved in the metabolism of warfarin. Amiodarone has an extremely long half-life, and so the full effects of the interaction may not be evident for up to 7 weeks after its introduction (Sanoski and Bauman 2002).

Although most drug metabolism involves the CYP450 system, drug interactions also occur with other metabolic enzymes. For example, allopurinol inhibits xanthine oxidase, the enzyme that metabolises the anticancer drug, 6-mercaptopurine. When administered with allopurinol, the activity of 6-mercaptopurine is prolonged, and to prevent significant drug toxicity, its dose should be reduced by 75% (Zimm et al. 1983).

4.3.1.4 Elimination

Drug elimination via the kidney can be altered by drugs that affect renal blood flow, glomerular filtration rate, active tubular secretion or urinary pH. Some of these mechanisms are illustrated by the interaction between NSAIDs and methotrexate, a cytotoxic agent that is excreted almost exclusively unmetabolised via the urine. NSAIDs inhibit the synthesis of prostaglandins which are involved in regulating blood flow through the kidney and are believed to reduce methotrexate elimination by reducing renal blood flow. In addition, NSAIDs compete with methotrexate for the active transport system that secretes both drugs into the renal tubular lumen (Frenia and Long 1992). Toxic levels of methotrexate can cause bone marrow suppression, hepatotoxicity and death.

Excretion of drugs in bile via the enterohepatic circulation may be affected by other drugs that alter normal gut flora or affect the function of drug transporter proteins. Mycophenolic acid, the active form of the immunosuppressant mycophenolate mofetil, is metabolised in the liver to an inactive glucuronide conjugate, which is secreted into bile by multidrug resistance protein 2 (MRP-2). In the gut, a proportion of the glucuronide conjugate is converted back to mycophenolic acid by a beta-glucuronidase enzyme produced by gut bacteria, allowing it to be reabsorbed into the circulation. Several drugs can disrupt this process if administered concurrently: ciclosporin inhibits MRP-2 which prevents excretion of the glucuronide conjugate into bile (Hesselink et al. 2005), and broad-spectrum antibiotics can reduce beta-glucuronidase activity by destroying gut flora (Naderer et al. 2005). Both interactions reduce the efficacy of mycophenolate mofetil. Mycophenolate is commonly used to prevent rejection following organ transplant, and so loss of efficacy could result in organ rejection unless careful dose adjustments are made to counteract the interaction.

4.3.2 Pharmacodynamic Interactions

In contrast to pharmacokinetic interactions which affect the plasma level of a drug, pharmacodynamic interactions occur when the action of a drug is altered by the presence of another. Pharmacodynamic interactions are described as 'additive' if they involve two drugs causing similar effects; such interactions are often predictable. The co-administration of a benzodiazepine and an opioid can cause profound sedation due to the combined adverse effects of both drugs. Sometimes additive pharmacodynamic interactions are used positively: a patient whose hypertension is not controlled with a calcium channel blocker alone may benefit from the addition of another antihypertensive agent, such as an ACE inhibitor.

Antagonistic pharmacodynamic drug interactions also occur, an example of which is the co-administration of NSAIDs and diuretics. NSAIDs cause renal sodium and water retention which can limit the clinical response to diuretics—which reduce blood pressure by increasing sodium and water excretion—by up to 20% (Brater 1999). Another example involves warfarin, an anticoagulant used to treat or prevent thromboemboli in susceptible patients. Warfarin inhibits the enzyme vitamin K epoxide reductase to suppress the synthesis of vitamin K-dependent clotting factors and its therapeutic action can be reversed by the administration of vitamin K.

4.3.3 Food–Drug Interactions

The presence of food in the gastrointestinal tract may help or hinder the absorption of some medicines administered by the oral route. The difference that food makes can be profound, sometimes increasing the bioavailability of the drug up to four-fold, as is the case for the antiarrhythmic drug dronedarone when administered with food (Dorian 2010).

Table 4.7 lists some frequently encountered medicines for which oral absorption is affected by the concurrent ingestion of food. The British National Formulary (BNF) lists cautionary and advisory warning labels that pharmacists should ensure are printed on the dispensing label when issuing prescribed medicines to patients (Joint Formulary Committee 2025). If a medicine should be taken with or after food or a meal, the patient should be advised that a small quantity of food is usually sufficient. It should be noted that many other medicines should be given with food but for the purpose of preventing gastrointestinal irritation rather than reasons related to drug absorption.

For some drugs, the correct timing of administration in relation to food differs depending on the formulation. The absorption of oral standard-release clarithromycin tablets is not significantly affected by the presence or absence of food; however, absorption of the modified-release tablets is impaired if taken on an empty stomach. Itraconazole capsules should be taken immediately after a meal to ensure maximum absorption (peak concentration is doubled) but the liquid should be taken on an empty stomach. It has even been found that co-administration of itraconazole capsules and cola may enhance absorption further because the cola creates an acidic environment that favours itraconazole absorption (Lange et al. 1997).

Table 4.7 Medicines for which oral absorption is affected by the presence of food and the BNF advice that applies to its administration

Absorption increased by food	Absorption decreased by food	
BNF advice: *take with or just after food or a meal*	BNF advice: *take 30–60 min before food*	BNF advice: *take when your stomach is empty. This means an hour before food or 2 h after food*
Acitretin	Capecitabine	Ampicillin
Alfuzosin (modified-release tablets)	Deferasirox	Azithromycin (capsules)
	Dipyridamole	Flucloxacillin
Clarithromycin (modified-release tablets)	Domperidone	Itraconazole (liquid)
	Hydrocortisone (modified-release tablets)	Montelukast (chewable tablets)
Dronedarone		Norfloxacin
Exemestane	Isoniazid	Oxytetracycline
Fenofibrate	Lansoprazole	Phenoxymethylpenicillin
Griseofulvin	Penicillamine	Tacrolimus
Isotretinoin	Peppermint oil	Tetracycline
Itraconazole (capsules)	Perindopril	Voriconazole
Ribavirin	Rifampicin	Zafirlukast

The role that calcium-containing salts play in pharmacokinetic drug interactions has already been discussed. The same interactions that occur with pharmaceutical preparations of calcium can be observed with dietary calcium. For example, administration of milk can reduce the oral absorption of ciprofloxacin (Hoogkamer and Kleinbloesem 1995).

It may seem an unlikely culprit, but grapefruit is responsible for a number of important drug–food interactions. Certain compounds in grapefruit juice are potent inhibitors of 3A4, the enzyme responsible for metabolising numerous drugs. Drugs for which concurrent administration of grapefruit can lead to serious drug toxicity include simvastatin, atorvastatin, ciclosporin, tacrolimus, sirolimus, verapamil, amiodarone and carbamazepine (Seden et al. 2010). Patients should be advised to avoid or minimise their intake of grapefruit and grapefruit juice whilst taking these medicines.

Alcohol can enhance the effects of sedative drugs such as benzodiazepines, opioids and certain antihistamines. Co-administration can lead to drowsiness and impairment of skilled tasks, and so patients should be alerted to the risks of drinking even small quantities of alcohol whilst taking such medicines.

4.3.4 Herbal Medicine–Drug Interactions

Both pharmacokinetic and pharmacodynamic interactions can occur between medicinal drugs and herbal remedies. Although widely assumed by the general public to be free from adverse effects, some herbal products have the potential to cause serious harm when combined with conventional medicines.

St John's wort is an herbal remedy that claims antidepressant properties. Its mechanism of action is not well understood but it is believed to enhance the effects of neurotransmitters, including serotonin, within the brain. When St John's wort is administered concurrently with selective serotonin reuptake inhibitor (SSRI) antidepressants, serotonin toxicity can occur (Lantz et al. 1999). Excess serotonin can cause 'serotonin syndrome' which can present with confusion, tachycardia, agitation and in extreme cases seizures, arrhythmias or coma.

Constituents of St John's wort may also induce P-glycoprotein (Hennessy et al. 2002) and the isoenzyme 3A4 (Roby et al. 2000), which can result in increased metabolism and therefore reduced effectiveness of many drugs including antiepileptics, antiretrovirals, oral contraceptives, warfarin and digoxin.

4.3.5 Physicochemical Interactions

Interaction between medicines before they have entered the body can have adverse consequences for the patient. Drugs that are administered intravenously should not be mixed unless it is known with certainty that they are physically and chemically compatible. When an infusion of the diuretic furosemide is mixed with an infusion of the beta-blocker labetalol, a white, insoluble precipitate immediately appears

(Trissel 2012), which would be extremely harmful if infused into a vein. Many intravenous drugs can be safely diluted with either sodium chloride 0.9% or glucose 5%, but this is not the case for all: amiodarone and liposomal amphotericin B are incompatible with sodium chloride solutions, whereas caspofungin and phenytoin are incompatible with glucose solutions, so care must always be taken to ensure that the correct diluent is chosen for every drug.

4.3.6 The Risk of Harm from Drug Interactions

Most drug interactions do not result in significant injury to the patient and many are of no clinical consequence at all. However, there are particular factors that can increase the risk of harm. For certain groups of medicines, a small reduction in therapeutic efficacy can have catastrophic consequences for the patient. For example, a reduction in the level of an antiepileptic could cause a patient to experience a seizure, and an interaction that increases the metabolism of an antiretroviral drug could lead to HIV viral resistance. Interactions involving drugs with a narrow therapeutic index have the potential to cause harm because a small change in plasma level can result in toxicity or a loss of efficacy. Conversely, other medicines tolerate wide variability in plasma levels without any apparent detrimental effects.

As with adverse drug reactions, there are certain patient characteristics that place some individuals at greater risk of experiencing harm from drug interactions than others, although predicting a patient's risk of experiencing a drug interaction is difficult: there is huge variation in how individuals respond to combinations of drugs and a drug interaction that occurs in one person may not be evident in another. The wide patient variability that has been observed for many drug interactions suggests that genetic polymorphisms play a role. Age, polypharmacy and organ dysfunction may also affect an individual's risk of experiencing harm from a drug interaction.

4.3.7 Prediction, Prevention and Management of Drug Interactions

Some interactions can be predicted from what is known of the pharmacology and pharmacokinetics of the drugs in question. For example, if Drug A, which is a known inhibitor of Enzyme E, is administered to a patient taking Drug B, which is metabolised by Enzyme E, it can be predicted that the plasma level of Drug B will increase. However, many interactions that are predicted theoretically are not borne out in practice and others are not predictable at all.

Prior to prescribing or administering a new medicine, a full and complete history of the medications that a patient takes, including herbal, illicit (where possible) and over-the-counter medicines, must be obtained. Without this information, it is impossible for the healthcare professional to know whether the newly prescribed medicine is indeed safe for the patient. Several reference sources exist for checking whether medicines are known or likely to interact (refer to the recommended reading), and pharmacists can provide advice about the likelihood and consequence of two or more drugs interacting. If an interaction is identified, the course of action that is taken will likely depend on the following:

- The necessity of each drug.
- The availability of an alternative agent.
- The severity of the interaction.
- Whether the effects of the interaction can be minimised, for example, using therapeutic drug monitoring and/or adjusting doses or timing of doses.

The simplest way to prevent drug interactions is to minimise polypharmacy and avoid prescribing combinations of medicines that have the potential to interact.

If an alternative, non-interacting drug is available that has equivalent safety and efficacy, it may be sensible to choose it in preference to the interacting drug. An example would be selecting azithromycin rather than clarithromycin for the treatment of pneumonia in an epileptic patient already taking carbamazepine. Azithromycin and clarithromycin are both macrolide antibiotics with similar antibacterial activity. However, clarithromycin increases levels of carbamazepine by inhibiting its metabolism, whereas azithromycin does not cause the same interaction (Pauwels 2002).

Sometimes both drugs in question are deemed essential, and no therapeutic alternatives exist. Consider a female patient who requires treatment with tamoxifen for breast cancer but is already taking warfarin following the insertion of a metallic replacement heart valve. Tamoxifen can increase the anticoagulant effect of warfarin and therefore increase the patient's risk of bleeding (Tenni et al. 1989). This interaction can be overcome by closely monitoring the patient's international normalised ratio (INR) and reducing the dose of warfarin if the INR starts to rise. Of course, when tamoxifen therapy is no longer required, a decrease in INR must be anticipated. The patient should also be advised to promptly report any unexplained bruising or bleeding that could indicate a raised INR.

Some interactions can be minimised by changing the timing of drug administration. For example, iron supplementation with oral ferrous sulphate can inhibit the oral absorption of bisphosphonates (such as alendronic acid), which are prescribed for osteoporosis. The effects can be minimised by delaying the administration of ferrous sulphate until several hours after the bisphosphonate has been taken.

4.4 Summary

Adverse drug reactions and drug interactions occur commonly and contribute to significant morbidity and mortality. The mechanisms of adverse drug reactions and drug interactions are complex and many are not well understood. Multiple factors including age, genetic make-up and co-morbidities play a role in increasing a patient's susceptibility to experiencing an adverse drug reaction or harm from a drug interaction. Although their occurrence cannot always be predicted, an understanding of how and why adverse drug reactions and drug interactions occur can help healthcare professionals to choose appropriate medicines, at optimum doses, that are least likely to cause a patient harm. Nurses have a responsibility to educate patients by alerting them to what signs or symptoms can be expected from a particular medicine or combination of medicines, alongside monitoring, documenting and reporting to the prescriber any adverse effects that occur. Nurses must also take particular care to ensure patients with drug allergies do not receive medicines that would be expected to cause a hypersensitivity reaction.

In the United Kingdom, data concerning adverse drug reactions is collated by the MHRA, and nurses are encouraged to report suspected adverse reactions via the Yellow Card Scheme. The data will improve understanding of the adverse effects of medicines and lead to greater patient safety.

Multiple Choice Questions

1. Which of the following adverse drug reactions could be characterised as a type B reaction according to the Rawlins and Thompson classification system?
   (a) Drowsiness in a patient taking the antihistamine chlorphenamine
   (b) Toxic epidermal necrolysis in a patient taking the antimalarial drug chloroquine
   (c) Hypokalaemia in a patient taking the loop diuretic furosemide
   (d) Cold extremities in a patient taking the beta-blocker atenolol
2. Which of the following adverse reactions does not need to be reported to the MHRA via the Yellow Card Scheme?
   (a) A minor reaction in an adult following administration of a 'Black Triangle' medicine
   (b) A minor reaction in a child following administration of an established medicine
   (c) A minor reaction in an adult following administration of an established medicine
   (d) A minor reaction in an adult following administration of an herbal medicine
3. Which of the following is not a common symptom of anaphylaxis?
   (a) Hypertension
   (b) Urticaria
   (c) Rash
   (d) Angioedema
4. Which of the following drugs could be safely considered for a patient who has previously experienced a severe hypersensitivity reaction with amoxicillin?
   (a) Co-amoxiclav
   (b) Phenoxymethylpenicillin
   (c) Erythromycin
   (d) Piperacillin-tazobactam

5. Which of the following patients with a urinary tract infection can safely receive the oral antibiotic ciprofloxacin?
   (a) A patient who is allergic to penicillin
   (b) A patient who is G6PD deficient
   (c) A patient who is epileptic
   (d) A patient taking oral calcium supplements for osteoporosis
6. Which of the following drugs is not known to induce cytochrome P450 enzymes?
   (a) Rifampicin
   (b) Carbamazepine
   (c) Phenobarbital
   (d) Simvastatin
7. Why is a patient taking warfarin at particular risk of harmful drug interactions?
   (a) Warfarin is a substrate of cytochrome P450 enzymes and has a narrow therapeutic index
   (b) Warfarin is an enzyme inducer
   (c) Only a small fraction of warfarin is protein-bound
   (d) Warfarin is renally excreted and many other medicines affect a person's renal function
8. Which of the following statements about adverse drug reaction and drug interactions is incorrect?
   (a) Age is a factor that can affect a patient's risk of experiencing an adverse drug reaction
   (b) Drug interactions do not occur between conventional and herbal medicines
   (c) Adverse drug reactions sometimes arise from excipients in the medicine
   (d) Drug interactions may not become apparent until several weeks after the combination of medicines is initiated
9. Which of the following is not a known drug–food interaction?
   a. Grapefruit and simvastatin
   b. Milk and ciprofloxacin
   c. Vodka and lorazepam
   d. Potatoes and amlodipine
10. Methadone is a long-acting opioid that is often prescribed to patients with opioid dependence. It is metabolised by the cytochrome P450 enzyme 3A4. Fluconazole is an antifungal drug that inhibits 3A4. What effects would you expect if methadone and fluconazole were administered together?
    (a) A decrease in methadone plasma levels
    (b) An increase in methadone plasma levels
    (c) A decrease in fluconazole plasma levels
    (d) An increase in fluconazole plasma levels

Answers

1. (b)

    Toxic epidermal necrolysis is a rare and severe cutaneous adverse drug reaction that cannot be predicted from the known pharmacology of chloroquine. It is a type B reaction according to the Rawlins and Thompson classification system. Drowsiness from chlorphenamine, hypokalaemia from furosemide and cold extremities from atenolol are all commonly occurring, dose-related adverse reactions that can be predicted from the pharmacology of the drug and are therefore type A reactions.

2. (c)

    Serious adverse drug reactions, reactions that occur in children and reactions following administration with herbal remedies or medicines that are intensively monitored by the MHRA (indicated by a black triangle symbol) should always be reported, even if causality is not proven. Minor reactions that occur in adults following the administration of an established medicine that no longer requires additional monitoring do not need to be reported.

3. (a)

    Anaphylaxis is a severe form of type 1 hypersensitivity characterised by immunoglobulin E (IgE) production following the administration of an allergen, such as a medicine. Anaphylaxis commonly causes rash, urticaria, angio-edema and hypotension (not hypertension).

4. (c)

    The patient has previously experienced a severe hypersensitivity reaction to amoxicillin, which is a penicillin, and so should avoid further exposure to amoxicillin and all other penicillins. Co-amoxiclav, phenoxymethylpenicillin and piperacillin-tazobactam are all penicillin-containing drugs and so must be avoided. Erythromycin is a macrolide antibiotic and so can be safely considered for this patient.

5. (a)

    Ciprofloxacin belongs to the 'quinolone' class of antibiotics and so can safely be administered to patients who have an allergy to penicillin. Exposure to ciprofloxacin can precipitate haemolytic anaemia in patients who are G6PD deficient, and ciprofloxacin is known to reduce the seizure threshold in susceptible individuals, so it should not be administered to patients who are G6PD deficient or epileptic. Oral calcium supplements reduce the oral absorption of ciprofloxacin, which may result in inadequate treatment of the urinary tract infection.

6. (d)

    Simvastatin is a known enzyme inhibitor of cytochrome P450 enzymes, not an inducer. Rifampicin, carbamazepine and phenobarbital are all known inducers of cytochrome P450 enzymes.

7. (a)

Warfarin is a substrate of cytochrome P450 enzymes, and therefore its metabolism can be impaired or enhanced by a multitude of drugs that induce or inhibit the enzyme system. The margin between its subtherapeutic and toxic concentration—the therapeutic index—is narrow, and therefore even a small increase or decrease in plasma level can cause the patient harm.

8. (b)

Drug interactions can and do occur between conventional medicines and herbal medicine; an example is the interaction between St John's wort and digoxin. St John's wort is an enzyme inducer and can reduce the plasma levels of digoxin.

9. (d)

Grapefruit juice contains compounds that inhibit cytochrome P450 3A4, the enzyme responsible for metabolising simvastatin. Calcium-containing products such as milk can impair the absorption of ciprofloxacin by forming insoluble complexes in the gastrointestinal tract. The combination of alcohol and a benzodiazepine such as lorazepam can cause marked sedation. There is no known interaction between potatoes and the calcium channel blocker amlodipine.

10. (b)

Methadone is broken down by the enzyme 3A4. Fluconazole inhibits this enzyme, so if it is administered with methadone, there will be less enzyme available to metabolise the methadone which will cause a rise in the amount of methadone circulating in plasma. Patients receiving methadone together with inhibitors of 3A4, such as fluconazole, should be monitored for signs of opioid toxicity, which include drowsiness and respiratory depression.

References

Baxter K, Preston CL (eds) (2025) Stockley's drug interactions. [online] Pharmaceutical Press, London http://medicinescomplete.com/. Accessed 29.01.25

Belay ED, Bresee JS, Holman RC, Khan AS, Shahriari A, Schonberger LB (1999) Reye's syndrome in the United States from 1981 through 1997. N Engl J Med 340(18):1377–1382

Brater DC (1999) Effects of nonsteroidal anti-inflammatory drugs on renal function: focus on cyclooxygenase-2—selective inhibition. Am J Med 107(6):65–70

Brayfield A, Cadart C (eds) (2025) Martindale: the complete drug reference. [online]. Pharmaceutical Press, London http://www.medicinescomplete.com/. Accessed on 29.01.25

Castleden CM, Kaye CM, Parsons RL (1975) The effect of age on plasma levels of propranolol and practolol in man. Br J Clin Pharmacol 2(4):303–306

Chatterjee K, Zhang J, Honbo N, Karliner JS (2010) Doxorubicin cardiomyopathy. Cardiology 115(2):155–162

Currie GM, Wheat JM, Kiat H (2011) Pharmacokinetic considerations for digoxin in older people. Open Cardiovasc Med J 5:130–135

D'Arcy PF, McElnay JC (1987) Drug-antacid interactions: assessment of clinical importance. Drug Intell Clin Pharm 21(7–8):607–617

Dawes M, Chowienczyk PJ (2001) Pharmacokinetics in pregnancy. Best Pract Res Clin Obstet Gynaecol 15(6):819–826

Dorian P (2010) Clinical pharmacology of dronedarone: implications for the therapy of atrial fibrillation. J Cardiovasc Pharmacol Ther 15(S4):15S–18S

Frenia ML, Long KS (1992) Methotrexate and nonsteroidal antiinflammatory drug interactions. Ann Pharmacother 26(2):234–237

Garty M, Hurwitz A (1980) Effect of cimetidine and antacids on gastrointestinal absorption of tetracycline. Clin Pharmacol Ther 28(2):203–207

Greenblatt DJ, Harmatz JS, Shader RI (1991) Clinical pharmacokinetics of anxiolytics and hypnotics in the elderly. Therapeutic considerations (part I). Clin Pharmacokinet 21(3):165–177

Hennessy M, Kelleher D, Spiers JP, Barry M, Kavanagh P, Back D, Mulcahy F, Feely J (2002) St Johns wort increases expression of P-glycoprotein: implications for drug interactions. Br J Clin Pharmacol 53(1):75–82

Hesselink DA, Van Hest RM, Mathot RAA, Bonthuis F, Weimar W, De Bruin RWF, Van Gelder T (2005) Cyclosporine interacts with mycophenolic acid by inhibiting the multidrug resistance-associated protein 2. Am J Transplant 5(5):987–994

Hetherington S, Hughes AR, Mosteller M, Shortino D, Baker KL, Spreen W, Lai E, Davies K, Handley A, Dow DJ, Fling ME, Stocum M, Bowman C, Thurmond LM, Roses AD (2002) Genetic variations in HLA-B region and hypersensitivity reactions to abacavir. Lancet 359:1121–1122

Hoogkamer JF, Kleinbloesem CH (1995) The effect of milk consumption on the pharmacokinetics of fleroxacin and ciprofloxacin in healthy volunteers. Drugs 49(S2):346–348

Jacobson TA (2004) Comparative pharmacokinetic interaction profiles of pravastatin, simvastatin, and atorvastatin when coadministered with cytochrome P450 inhibitors. Am J Cardiol 94(9):1140–1146

Johnson TN (2003) The development of drug metabolising enzymes and their influence on the susceptibility to adverse drug reactions in children. Toxicology 192(1):37–48

Joint Formulary Committee. British National Formulary (online). Available at: https://bnf.nice.org.uk [Accessed: 29.01.25].

Joshua L, Devi P, Guido S (2009) Adverse drug reactions in medical intensive care unit of a tertiary care hospital. Pharmacoepidemiol Drug Saf 18(7):639–645

Kara M, Hasinoff BB, McKay DW, Campbell NR (1991) Clinical and chemical interactions between iron preparations and ciprofloxacin. Br J Clin Pharmacol 31(3):257–261

Khaliq Y, Gallicano K, Venance S, Kravcik S, Cameron DW (2000) Effect of ketoconazole on ritonavir and saquinavir concentrations in plasma and cerebrospinal fluid from patients infected with human immunodeficiency virus. Clin Pharmacol Ther 68(6):637–646

Klein CE, Chiu YL, Cai Y, Beck K, King KR, Causemaker SJ, Doan T, Esslinger HU, Podsadecki TJ, Hanna GJ (2008) Effects of acid-reducing agents on the pharmacokinetics of lopinavir/ritonavir and ritonavir-boosted atazanavir. J Clin Pharmacol 48(5):553–562

Kudriakova TB, Sirota LA, Rozova GI, Gorkov VA (1992) Autoinduction and steady-state pharmacokinetics of carbamazepine and its major metabolites. Br J Clin Pharmacol 33(6):611–615

Lange D, Pavao JH, Wu J, Klausner M (1997) Effect of a cola beverage on the bioavailability of itraconazole in the presence of H2 blockers. J Clin Pharmacol 37(6):535–540

Lantz MS, Buchalter E, Giambanco V (1999) St. John's wort and antidepressant drug interactions in the elderly. J Geriatr Psychiatry Neurol 12(1):7–10

Leenderte A (2008) Frequency of and risk factors for preventable medication-related hospital admissions in The Netherlands. Arch Intern Med 168(17):1890–1896

Ludden TM (1991) Nonlinear pharmacokinetics: clinical implications. Clin Pharmacokinet 20(6):429–446

Manninen V, Melin J, Apajalahti A, Karesoja M (1973) Altered absorption of digoxin in patients given propantheline and metoclopramide. Lancet 301(7800):398–400

Martin E, Fanconi A, Kälin P, Zwingelstein C, Crevoisier C, Ruch W, Brodersen R (1993) Ceftriaxone-bilirubin-albumin interactions in the neonate: an in vivo study. Eur J Pediatr 152(6):530–534

Mazziotti G, Angeli A, Bilezikian JP, Canalis E, Giustina A (2006) Glucocorticoid-induced osteoporosis: an update. Trends Endocrinol Metab 17(4):144–149

McDermott JH, Wolf J, Hoshitsuki K, Huddart R, Caudle KE, Whirl-Carrillo M, Steyger PS, Smith RJH, Cody N, Rodriguez-Antona C, Klein TE, Newman WG (2022) Clinical Pharmacogenetics Implementation Consortium guideline for the use of aminoglycosides based on MT-RNR1 genotype. Clin Pharmacol Ther 111(2):366–373

Medicines Act (1968) Chapter 67. HMSO, London. https://www.legislation.gov.uk/ukpga/1968/67. Accessed 27.01.25

Medicines and Healthcare Products Regulatory Agency (2025) Online reporting site for the Yellow Card Scheme [online]. https://yellowcard.mhra.gov.uk/. Accessed 28.01.25

Naderer OJ, Dupuis RE, Heinzen EL, Wiwattanawongsa K, Johnson MW, Smith PC (2005) The influence of norfloxacin and metronidazole on the disposition of mycophenolate mofetil. J Clin Pharmacol 45(2):219–226

Naranjo CA, Busto U, Sellers EM, Sandor P, Ruiz I, Roberts EA, Janecek E, Domecq C, Greenblatt DJ (1981) A method for estimating the probability of adverse drug reactions. Clin Pharmacol Ther 30(2):239–245

Orkin C, Sadiq ST, Rice L, Jackson F, UK EPI Team (2009) Prospective epidemiological study of the prevalence of human leukocyte antigen (HLA)-B*5701 in HIV-1-infected UK subjects. HIV Med 11(3):187–192

Pauwels O (2002) Factors contributing to carbamazepine-macrolide interactions. Pharmacol Res 45(4):291–298

Pirmohamed M, James S, Meakin S, Green C, Scott AK, Walley TJ, Farrar K, Park BK, Breckenridge AM (2004) Adverse drug reactions as cause of admission to hospital: prospective analysis of 18 820 patients. Br Med J 329(7456):15–19

Rawlins MD, Thompson JW (1991) Mechanisms of adverse drug reactions. In: Davies DM (ed) Textbook of adverse drug reactions, 4th edn. Oxford Medical Publications, Oxford

Roby CA, Anderson GD, Kantor E, Dryer DA, Burstein AH (2000) St John's Wort: effect on CYP3A4 activity. Clin Pharmacol Ther 67(5):451–457

Rolan PE (1994) Plasma protein binding displacement interactions—why are they still regarded as clinically important? Br J Clin Pharmacol 37(2):125–128

Rowe JW, Andres R, Tobin JD, Norris AH, Shock NW (1976) The effect of age on creatinine clearance in men: a cross-sectional and longitudinal study. J Gerontol 31(2):155–163

Sanchez AR, Rogers RS, Sheridan PJ (2004) Tetracycline and other tetracycline-derivative staining of the teeth and oral cavity. Int J Dermatol 43(10):709–715

Sanoski CA, Bauman JL (2002) Clinical observations with the amiodarone/warfarin interaction: dosing relationships with long-term therapy. Chest 121(1):19–23

Seden K, Dickinson L, Khoo S, Back D (2010) Grapefruit-drug interactions. Drugs 70(18):2373–2407

Sivagnanam S, Deleu D (2003) Red man syndrome. Crit Care 7(2):119–120

Swen JJ, van der Wouden CH, Manson LEN, Abdullah-Koolmees H, Blagec K, Blagus T et al (2023) A 12-gene pharmacogenetic panel to prevent adverse drug reactions: an open-label, multicentre, controlled, cluster-randomised crossover implementation study. Lancet 401(10374):347–356

Symonds W, Cutrell A, Edwards M, Steel H, Spreen B, Powell G, McGuirk S, Hetherington S (2002) Risk factor analysis of hypersensitivity reactions to abacavir. Clin Ther 24(4):565–573

Tenni P, Lalich DL, Byrne MJ (1989) Life threatening interaction between tamoxifen and warfarin. Br Med J 298(6666):93

Trissel LA (ed) (2012) Handbook on injectable drugs, 17th edn. American Society of Health-System Pharmacists, Bethesda

Ulrich RG (2007) Idiosyncratic toxicity: a convergence of risk factors. Annu Rev Med 58:17–34

Weinblatt ME (1991) Nonsteroidal anti-inflammatory drug toxicity: increased risk in the elderly. Scand J Rheumatol 20(S91):9–17

Weinshilboum R (2001) Thiopurine pharmacogenetics: clinical and molecular studies of thiopurine methyltransferase. Drug Metab Dispos 29(4):601–605

West DP, Worobec S, Solomon LM (1981) Pharmacology and toxicology of infant skin. J Invest Dermatol 76:147–150

Working Group of Resuscitation Council UK (2021) Emergency treatment of anaphylaxis. Guidelines for healthcare providers. Resuscitation Council (UK), London

World Health Organisation (1970) International drug monitoring: the role of the hospital—a WHO report. Ann Pharmacother 4(4):101–110

Youngster I, Arcavi L, Schechmaster R, Akayzen Y, Popliski H, Shimonov J, Beig S, Berkovitch M (2010) Medications and glucose-6-phosphate dehydrogenase deficiency: an evidence-based review. Drug Saf 33(9):713–726

Zimm S, Collins JM, O'Neill D, Chabner BA, Poplack DG (1983) Inhibition of first-pass metabolism in cancer chemotherapy: interaction of 6-mercaptopurine and allopurinol. Clin Pharmacol Ther 34(6):810–817

Further Reading

Aronson JK (ed) (2016) Meyler's side effects of drugs: the international encyclopedia of adverse drug reactions and interactions, 16th edn. Elsevier, Oxford

Baxter K, Preston CL (eds) (2025) Stockley's drug interactions. [online] Pharmaceutical Press, London. http://medicinescomplete.com/ Accessed 29.01.25

Brayfield A, Cadart C (eds) (2025) Martindale: the complete drug reference. [online] Pharmaceutical Press, London. http://www.medicinescomplete.com/. Accessed on 29.01.25

Karalliedde L, Clarke SFJ, Gotel U, Karalliedde J (2016) Adverse drug interactions: a handbook for prescribers, 2nd edn. CRC Press, Taylor & Francis Group, FL

Lee A, Cuthbert M (2023) Adverse drug reactions, 3rd edn. Pharmaceutical Press, London

Williamson EM, Driver S, Baxter K (eds) (2009) Stockley's herbal medicines interactions: a guide to the interactions of herbal medicines, dietary supplements and nutraceuticals with conventional medicines, 2nd edn. Pharmaceutical Press, London

Pharmacology of Pain

5

Sheila Turner

Learning Outcomes
At the end of this chapter, you will be able to:

- Appreciate the biopsychosocial complexity of pain
- Have an awareness of the variety of analgesic drugs available
- Understand the key features of the medications discussed
- Recognise in which circumstances certain analgesic medications might not be prescribed
- Consider the need to adopt a multimodal approach incorporating pharmacologic and non-pharmacologic methods to achieve effective analgesia

5.1 Introduction

The evolutionary purpose of pain is that it is a protective measure. With the wide range of approaches both pharmacologic and non-pharmacologic currently available, there is no reason for anyone to endure pain unnecessarily. Because the experience of pain is subjective and influenced by psychology and even culture, it is very difficult to define, but McCaffery proposes pain is 'whatever the experiencing person says it is, existing whenever he/she says it does' (McCaffery and Pasero 1999: 17). Therefore, the nurse must appreciate and understand all the possible influences upon the experience of pain to determine the best approaches to achieve analgesia (Royal College of Nursing 2015).

S. Turner (✉)
Florence Nightingale Faulty of Nursing, Midwifery & Palliative Care, King's College London, London, UK

E. Khan, P. Hood (eds.), *Understanding Pharmacology in Nursing Practice*,
https://doi.org/10.1007/978-3-032-03964-4_5

109

5.2   Definition of Terms

Acute pain is of sudden onset and usually has a recognisable cause, its duration is said by some authors to be no more than 30 days (Thienhaus and Cole 2002) and others, no longer than 3 months (McCaffery and Beebe 1994; Green 2013). Healthcare professionals frequently encounter patients in pain because of injury, disease, investigations and/or surgery. Pain may subside as healing occurs; however, persistent (possibly poorly treated) acute pain may become chronic pain; this is frequently difficult to manage and will have a major impact on a person. Persistent or *chronic* (from the Greek *chronos* time) *pain* is where pain persists beyond an expected repair and recovery time (Turk and Okifuji 2010).

'Pain' is a word which evokes an emotional response. The International Association for the Study of Pain [IASP] defines pain as an 'an unpleasant sensory and emotional experience associated with, or resembling that associated with, actual or potential tissue damage' (Srinivas et al. 2020). So, pain is much more than a simple physiological response necessary for survival. Anxiety and the fear of pain can amplify the experience of pain. Much more than an automatic response, pain involves many aspects of the central nervous system (CNS) and is influenced by areas such as the limbic system, the seat of emotions. There are also social and cultural influences which effect how pain is expressed. The nurse's role is to alleviate suffering, so complaints of pain must not be ignored but must be promptly attended to; poorly controlled pain can delay patient recovery, for example, a patient in pain might not be able to breathe deeply or want to cough, posing the risk of respiratory infection: similarly patients in pain tend to move less, so the risk of thrombo-embolism and pressure ulcers increase. The nurse must ensure that the patient is as comfortable as possible.

5.3   What Is the Nurse's Role in Pain Management?

The difficulty for nurses caring for patients experiencing pain is how to achieve analgesia. If pain is a complex phenomenon, how can it be effectively assessed and managed?

It could be argued that the nurse cannot 'assess' patient pain; only the person experiencing it can determine the extent of their pain. Since the publication of McCaffery's aforementioned statement that pain is 'whatever the experiencing person says it is, existing whenever he/she says it does' (McCaffery and Pasero 1999: 17), research indicates that when nurses do attempt to assess a patient's pain it seems they do not always believe or respond to reports of pain and, as a result, fail to effectively treat the patient in pain (Sloman et al. 2005; Ene et al. 2008). Research has identified that when the nurse has some discretion as to how much prescribed analgesia to administer, he/she does not always make the correct choice (McCaffery and Ferrell 1994; Gordon et al. 2008). For example, Tanabe et al. (2010) report nurses' reluctance to administer the maximum dose of opioid analgesia prescribed to those with sickle cell disease [SCD] because, they assert, the patient might become 'addicted' to the drugs: such attitudes are worrying because they reflect ignorance about analgesia, opioid tolerance and sickle cell disease.

To be effective care providers, nurses must understand pain physiology. The experience of pain can be compounded by the patient's emotional response. Colloca and Benedetti (2007) describe the 'nocebo effect', when anxiety and anticipation of pain lead to an experience of pain greater than might be expected given the clinical situation; in appreciating the complexity of pain nurses should be able to empathise with and offer patients in pain the care and support they require.

5.4 How Does Pain Arise?

The nerve endings which relay pain 'signals' to the central nervous system are widely located throughout the body. Cutaneous pain is often described as 'sharp' or 'burning'. Pain from the viscera (the internal organs) might initially be difficult to locate, for example, in appendicitis the patient often reports a generalised abdominal pain before it can be localised to the right iliac fossa.

Somatic pain arises in deep tissues: tendons, muscles joints, periosteum and blood vessels. Pain initiates the 'fight-or-flight' response, increasing the heart rate, blood pressure and respiratory rate, delaying gastric emptying (with the risk of nausea and vomiting), decreasing urinary output and mobilising resources to elevate blood glucose levels (Fig. 5.1).

5.4.1 What Is Pain?

Pain is frequently categorised as 'neuropathic' or 'nociceptive'.

Neuropathic pain arises as a result of compromise of or damage to the nervous system, for example, post-herpetic neuralgia—the persistent pain that may be experienced by some people having had herpes zoster ('shingles'). Neuropathic pain can also arise as a result of poorly treated acute pain and is, therefore, pain which is often very difficult to treat.

Nociceptive pain normally arises as the result of an injury. For example, the wound made to facilitate surgery is, as would be expected, a source of pain and tissue injury is associated with the inflammatory response. When cells are damaged, processes begin to clean away the debris; this involves the mobilisation of non-specific defence mechanisms, making local blood vessels 'leaky' so that white blood cells (monocytes) can escape the circulation to move into the tissues where they become macrophages to engulf and destroy damaged cells. If cell damage persists, this inflammatory response is increased by the degranulation of mast cells to release the chemical histamine, which dilates blood vessels (increasing blood flow to the area), opening pores in blood vessel walls and signalling to monocytes that they are needed in the tissues. When the monocytes become macrophages, they release pyrogens, chemicals such as interleukin 1, which cause an uprating of the thalamic temperature set point allowing the body temperature to rise and making the

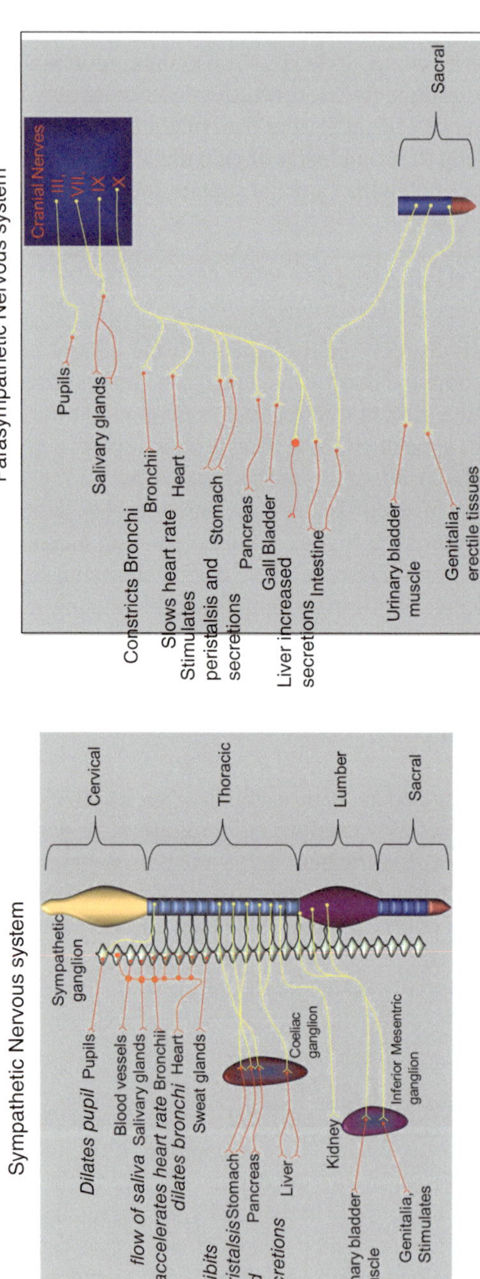

Fig. 5.1 The fight and flight response (sympathetic) and opposing parasympathetic effects on the body

site of damage less hospitable to microorganisms which might otherwise invade and establish a site of infection. The pain experienced by the patient who has undergone surgery arises from the stimulation of specific receptors—nociceptors, which respond to what are termed 'noxious stimuli', generated as a result of tissue damage (Fig. 5.2). The extent of a person's pain might be influenced by the extent of tissue damage and/or the continued presence of the chemical mediators of the inflammatory response.

The four pain message relay processes are transduction, transmission, perception and modulation (McCaffery and Pasero 1999). Transduction arises from the stimulation of nociceptors. The resultant pain 'message' is transmitted from the site of provocation (usually where damage occurred) to the central nervous system. Pain perception occurs because sufficient messages have been received by a number of areas in the brain, including the somatosensory cortex, the reticular and limbic systems. Pain modulation involves approaches to reduce or, in some circumstances, increase the overall experience of pain.

5.4.2 Transduction

Transduction involves nociceptor response to noxious stimuli. The nociceptors can be 'free nerve endings' within tissue, nerve endings which respond to specific stimuli, for example, pressure, temperature or chemical changes, or 'polymodal receptors' which respond to more than one stimulus (Fig. 5.2).

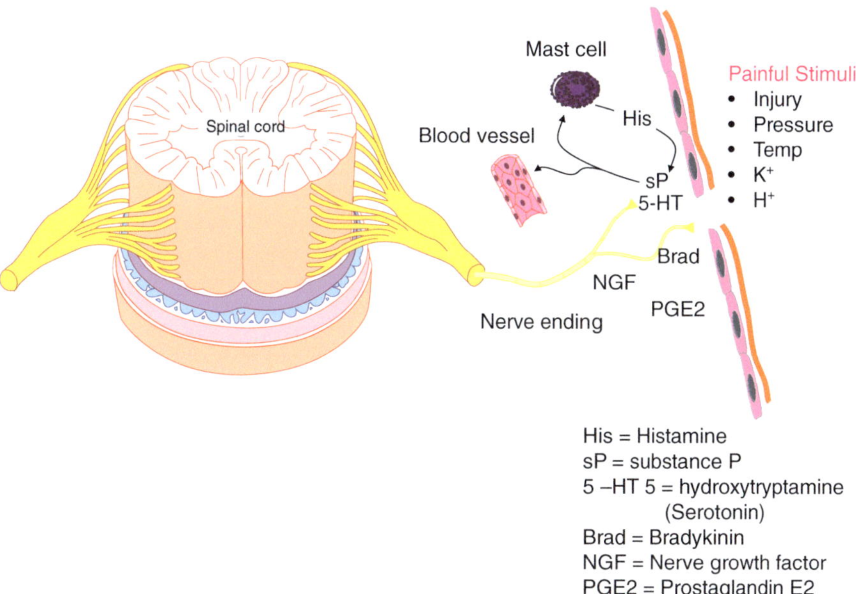

Fig. 5.2 Mechanisms associated with the peripheral sensitisation to pain

Nociceptors are widely distributed throughout the body, but lacking in solid organs. The pain associated with disease in solid organs might be experienced as 'referred pain' because there is a deficiency of established sensory pathways directly connecting the injured tissue with the sensory cortex of the brain, for example, victims of acute coronary syndrome (a 'heart attack') do not locate pain in the heart; what they frequently describe is a central crushing chest pain which radiates to the jaw and arm. Another example is in the renal system where the solid kidney has few nociceptors so a large calculus forming in the organ causes little pain; such a calculus is often diagnosed when the patient has an acute episode of haematuria. But the hollow ureter is supplied with multiple nociceptors so the passage of a very small fragment of calculus through that ureter can be extremely painful, a condition called 'renal colic'.

5.4.3 Transmission

Transmission involves the relay of pain impulses (or signals) to the central nervous system where the location and intensity of pain might be determined.

Like many nerve cells, nociceptors are highly excitable; before activation, they have a resting potential which reflects a slight imbalance of positively charged particles between the nerve cell interior and the environment outside the nerve. When a nociceptor is stimulated sodium channels in the nerve axon open, the resultant influx of sodium ions result in a potential (voltage) change within the nerve to the point where a threshold (potential) is exceeded leading to depolarisation, this depolarisation is conducted along the nerve towards the central nervous system.

The two nerve fibre types recognised as nociceptors differ in diameter and, therefore, speed; the myelinated, insulated, thicker conducting fibres relay signals more rapidly than the unmyelinated thinner fibres. Both types of fibre terminate in the dorsal horn of the spinal cord.

$A\delta$ (delta) fibres are myelinated having a conduction speed of 5–30 m/s; they are mechanoreceptors, commonly associated with touch.

C fibres are non-myelinated with a conduction speed of 1 m/s; they are the polymodal nociceptors which can respond to temperature, pressure and chemical changes in the tissues, for example, substances (K^+) generated by cell damage or even neurotransmitters.

Any noxious event, for example, the swelling and increased pressure associated with tumour growth or abscess development, can result in the release of chemicals (Fig. 5.2):

- Peptides, for example, Bradykinin
- Amides, for example, Serotonin and Histamine
- Arachidonic acid derivative, for example, Prostaglandin

The presence of these chemicals contributes to the persistence of pain and in some circumstances acts as a 'wind-up' mechanism increasing the pain experienced. The cytokines (cell mover chemicals), such as prostaglandin, bradykinin and serotonin, promote non-specific immune defence activity, causing inflammation at the injured site, further sensitising the polymodal nociceptors.

'First pain' is transmitted via Aδ (A-Delta) fast fibres, mechanoreceptors responding to just one stimulus, frequently expressed by the person experiencing it as 'sharp and stabbing' and represents superficial damage. The 'second pain' transmitted via C (slow) fibres, from polymodal nociceptors, is more diffuse and is expressed as 'throbbing and aching' and represents significant damage because the receptors involved respond to more than one stimulus. It is the combination of the messages received from the two fibres which contribute to both the ability to locate the site from which pain originates and the extent of patient suffering.

5.4.4 Reflex Arc

When appropriate, even before nociceptive impulses are relayed towards the brain, the 'first pain', transmitted via A-Delta fibres, results in reflex activity to move away from the cause of pain; this spinal cord response initiates an immediate withdrawal of the affected part, away from a harmful situation, to minimise damage and (therefore) pain (Fig. 5.3).

Transmission involves the relay of nociceptive impulses to the spinal cord, then upwards to the brain. There is a synapse between the 'first-order neurons' which relay peripheral signals towards the spinal cord and the 'second-order neurons' which continue the relay in the cord. Neurotransmitter chemicals like adenosine triphosphate (ATP), calcitonin gene-related peptide (CGRP), bradykinin, nitric oxide and substance P facilitate impulse relay across synapses. The nociceptive impulses are relayed in the spinothalamic tracts of the dorsal horn of the spinal cord.

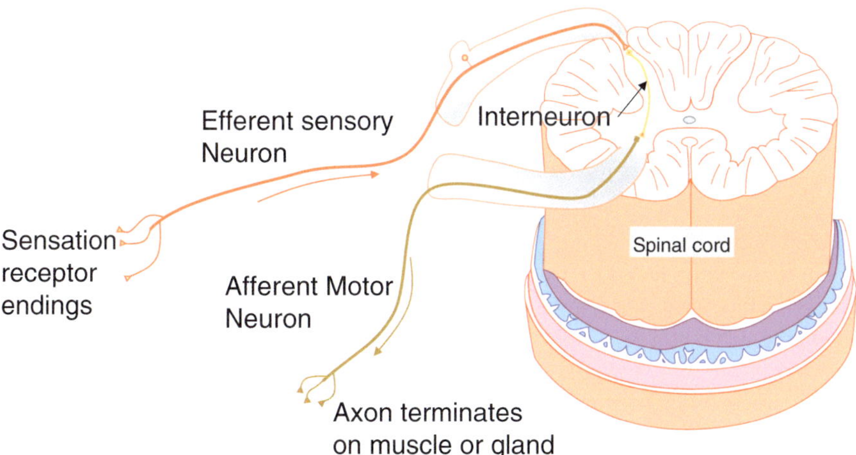

Fig. 5.3 Reflex arc

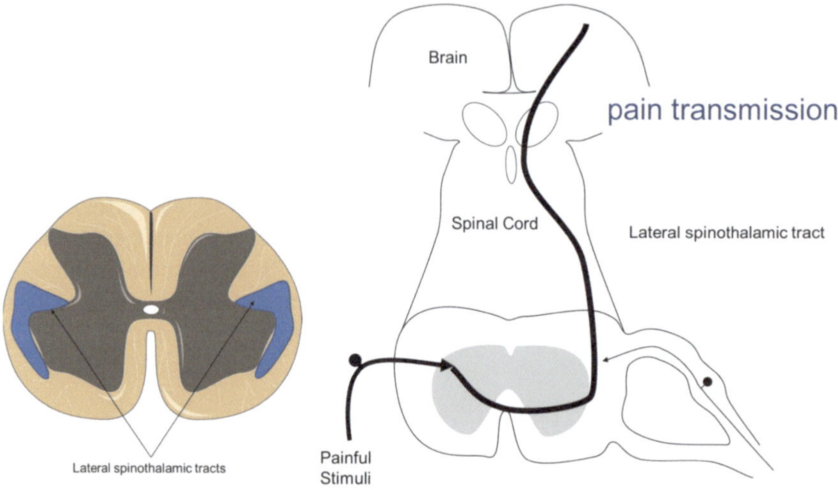

Fig. 5.4 Spinothalamic tracts

Messages relayed from Aδ fibres synapse at the spinal cord and are immediately relayed to the thalamus (Fig. 5.4). Messages from C fibres synapse at the spinal cord and are relayed to the brain stem and the thalamus. Once nociceptor input has reached the brain stem and hypothalamus a number of regions of the cortex become activated to allow discrimination of the 'messages', to determine the location of their source and the possible extent of injury (damage).

The somatosensory cortex interprets input from the nociceptors to determine the site of injury (source of pain); influenced by the memory of previous painful events, this results in the quality and quantity of pain experienced before any pain responses, other than a reflex, can be initiated (Fig. 5.4).

5.4.5 Modulation

Modulation of the transmission of pain occurs because the physiological response is to protect, as a result it involves processes to inhibit or change nociceptive impulse relay in the spinal cord.

5.4.5.1 Inhibition

Some inhibitory processes have been identified as the basis of the 'gate control theory', which suggests that there is mechanism much like a gate in an area of tissue called the substantia gelatinosa in the dorsal horn of the spinal cord regulating nociceptor impulse relay towards the brain (and therefore sensation). That 'gate' is not merely an open-close mechanism, but it can distinguish between impulses, for example, non-pain impulses can close the gate to nociceptor impulses. The 'gate' mechanism is influenced by large diameter fibres (Aδ) which tend to inhibit transmission and small diameter fibres (C) which facilitate transmission increasing the spread of the pain impulses to specific areas of the brain.

One process contributing to modulation involves the stimulation of Aβ fibres, very similar to Aδ fibres, resulting in 'gate closure' with a reduction in pain. For example, an instinctive human response to a minor injury is to rub the affected area. Such mechanical stimulation of Aβ fibres results in less pain being experienced.

When Melzack and Wall (1965) proposed the 'gate control theory', they recognised that there must be modulatory mechanisms influencing nociceptive input to the higher centres of the brain, and they suggested that there is downward regulation by the brain upon the nociceptive inputs from the periphery. Such downward regulation via 'descending modulatory pain pathways' [DMPP] can lead to inhibition, suppressing the experience of pain, or excitation, increasing pain; both processes being protective.

Descending inhibition involves the release of chemicals acting as neurotransmitters to block nociceptive impulse relay into the CNS, for example, neuropeptides or endogenous (internal) opioids (β-endorphins, enkephalin and dynorphin), serotonin (5-HT), norepinephrine and gamma amino butyric acid (GABA); which partially block the transmission of nociceptive impulses.

Most endogenous processes attempt to minimise the experience of pain. But endogenous pain relief activity is not limited to the spinal cord; it has been identified at the site of injury, disrupting pain impulse relays from the site of injury towards the central nervous system. Greater understanding about how endogenous processes contribute to the pain experience has led to the development of contemporary approaches to analgesia.

5.5   Pain Assessment

Heikkinen et al. (2005: 596) noted that, certainly upon initial assessment, 'nurses are inclined to underestimate severe pain and to overestimate mild pain', poor assessment of pain can lead to poor outcomes for patients. Pain assessment tools allow nurses to employ simple techniques to document what is happening to the patient as well as how they respond to nursing intervention. So pain assessment should be the first stage in achieving effective pain management; this is particularly important because poorly managed acute pain could lead to a chronic pain scenario, which might be even more challenging to manage effectively. The principles of pain assessment involve talking with the patient, evaluating both the physical signs (vital signs measurements) and non-verbal indicators. The National Institute for Healthcare Excellence (NICE) produces up-to-date evidence to support healthcare practice and the 'Clinical Knowledge Summary Scenario about the assessment of pain', was last reviewed in 2023.

Townsend and Cox (2007: 342) advocate the following approach when assessing the patient reporting pain:

- *Location* (where is it?)
- *Nature* (does it radiate?)
- *Pattern* (is it brief, intermittent or constant?)
- *Description* (is it dull, heavy, aching, sharp, stabbing, burning or pricking?)
- *Intensity* (how strong is it?)
- *What makes it worse?* (e.g. coughing, deep breathing, walking).
- *What makes it better?* (rest, heat pack, analgesia, rubbing).

5.5.1 Pain Assessment Tools

Simple tools are available to facilitate accurate pain assessment, for example, the pain score which is the simplest *numeric rating scale*, popular in the post-anaesthetic care unit, involves asking the patient to rate the pain they are experiencing where 0 is no pain, 1 mild pain, 2 moderate pain and 3 worst pain imaginable. Other versions of this tool use a scale of 0 to 10, but patients recovering from anaesthesia and surgery and in other situations find it difficult to process the information required to rate their pain against a range greater than 0–3. Similarly, recovering patients are often unable to answer Townsend and Cox (2007) more detailed questions.

A *verbal descriptor scale* apportions a statement about the pain experience in a numeric value:

Excruciating	10
	9
	8
	7
Moderate	6
	5
	4
Slight	3
	2
	1
No pain	0

A *visual analogue scale* requires the patient to indicate where their pain sits against a scale similar to that on a graph or thermometer (Fig. 5.5).

The Wong-Baker faces pain score (Wong-Baker 2018) allows a patient to rate their pain using pictorial representation, at one end a very smiley emoji (representing minimal pain/feeling good) through a number of emojis representative of worsening pain (or feelings) to the most miserable emoji (representing the worst pain imaginable/feeling bad); this tool is suitable for use with children and patients for whom English or even language might be difficult, for example, aphasia following a neurovascular event.

Fig. 5.5 Example of visual analogue scale

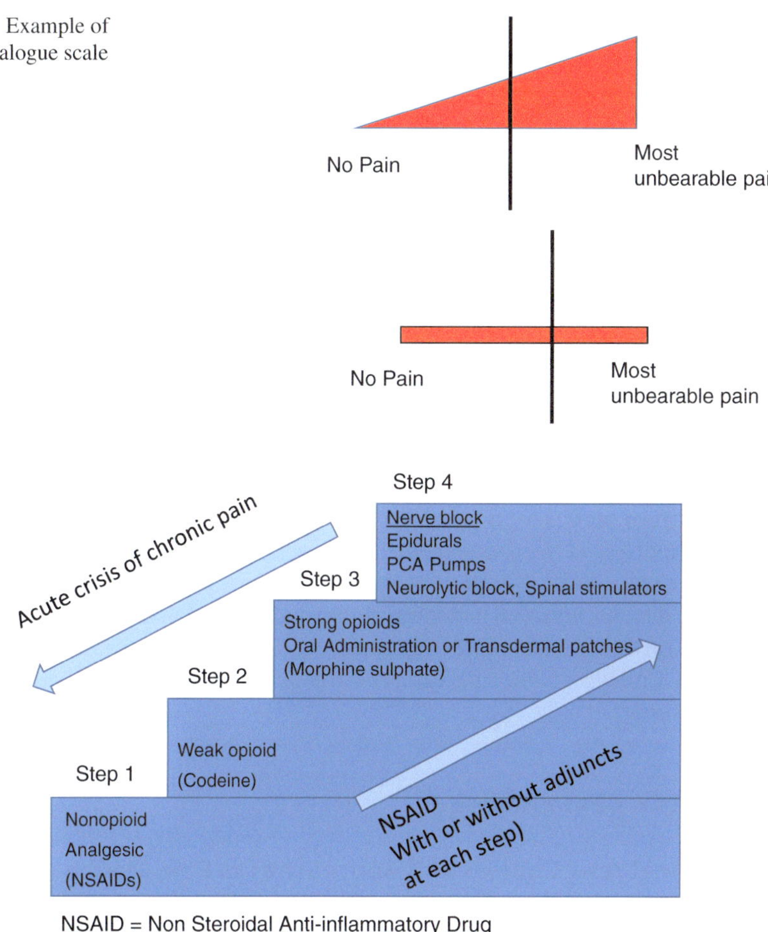

NSAID = Non Steroidal Anti-inflammatory Drug
PCA = Patient controlled analgesia

Fig. 5.6 Pain control ladder

The analgesic ladder has undergone many adaptations since 1986, as more complex clinical scenarios have emerged and new analgesic drugs/methods have been introduced (Fig. 5.6).

5.5.2 Behavioural Pain Assessment

It is designed for use with paediatric or cognitively impaired patients; it is a useful tool for the immediate assessment of a patient who is recovering from anaesthesia.

The CALMS scale

	0	1	2
C Comfort	Responds quietly when touched	Reassured when hand is held or brow stroked	Difficult to comfort
A Activity	Breathes deeply and coughs and moves freely	Reluctant to take deep breaths or cough	Moves only minimally when asked
L Looks	Relaxed or sleeping	Grimaces only when moved	Screwed up face and clenched jaw
M Moves	Relaxed	Tense muscles when moved	Continuous clenched grasp, or rigid, may writhe around
S Speaks	Quiet	Moans only when moved	Continually grunts or whimpers

Score out of 10
From: Craig and Hatfield (2020)

There are a wide variety of tools available for the assessment of acute pain. Different tools have been designed for use with people who experience chronic pain. Whichever tool has been identified for a clinical environment must be used diligently, data documented and intervention and evaluation undertaken.

Where medication has been prescribed, the Royal Pharmaceutical Society and the Royal College of Nursing (2019) have published guidance about medicine administration.

5.6 Pain pharmacology

5.6.1 Analgesic Choices and Approaches to Pain Management

Effective pain relief and the perception of pain are influenced by many individual factors, for example, age, previous experience and psychosocial status. Any analgesic approaches might use or mimic the endogenous processes. Drug choice depends on many things, for example, the results of pain assessment and patient reporting, the duration of pain and patient response to pain-relieving interventions including drugs.

Frequently Used Medications
- Local anaesthetics
- Non-opioid analgesics
  - Paracetamol
  - Non-steroidal anti-inflammatory drugs (NSAIDs)
  - Gamma aminobutyic acid (GABA) analogues
  - Tricyclic antidepressants
  - Antispasmodic, for example, Hyoscine or Baclofen (a GABA derivative)
- Opioid analgesics (including synthetic opioids)

5.6.2 Local Anaesthesia

On the basis that the surgical wound is a major source of post-operative pain, one approach employed to minimise the experience of post-operative pain is the injection of local anaesthetic into the wound edges as surgery is completed; this approach can be very successful but is not effective for every patient. However, with the advent of enhanced recovery programmes, surgery without the deposition of local anaesthesia around the wound at the end of a procedure is considered unacceptable (Whiteman et al. 2011).

Local anaesthetics cause a reversible blockade of conduction along nerve fibres. As has been identified, nociceptor impulses are relayed along nerves by an action potential generated by the opening of sodium channels and the movement of sodium into the nerve axon (associated latterly with an outward movement of potassium). Local anaesthetic drugs penetrate a nerve in a non-ionised lipophilic form, and once inside the nerve axon ionised molecules (Chaps. 2 and 7) are formed which block sodium channels preventing the influx of sodium necessary to generate action potentials. All nerve fibres are sensitive to local anaesthetics; smaller diameter sensory fibres are more sensitive than large diameter motor fibres so the medium into which a local anaesthetic drug is injected can be significant—the most effective block, whereby all impulses (both motor and sensory) are intercepted, is achieved by drug deposition into a fluid, rather than a solid tissue. A differential block can be achieved where the smaller diameter pain and autonomic fibres are blocked, while the larger diameter coarse touch and movement fibres are spared; before any local anaesthetic for a surgical procedure where they expect to be totally pain-free, patients must be advised that not every sensation is eliminated with local anaesthesia.

Local anaesthetic drugs vary widely in potency, duration of action, toxicity and ability to penetrate mucous membranes, for example, Lidocaine causes loss of sensation in the skin rapidly upon injection, whereas Bupivacaine or Ropivacaine does not. So the drug selected by the anaesthetist/surgeon must be the most appropriate for the technique as well as suitable for the site of drug administration. This is because any drug which can disrupt impulses travelling through 'excitable' tissues such as sensory nerves can also disrupt similar processes in other excitable tissues such as the myocardium leading to abnormal heart rhythms or arrhythmias this may happen when sufficient quantities of the local anaesthetic enters the systemic circulation.

Lidocaine can cause abnormalities of cardiac rhythm, even cardiac arrest and death. The myocardium is much less sensitive to Bupivacaine or Ropivacaine, which are most effective when injected into the tissue in the epidural space or into the fluid (CSF) in the subarachnoid space. Therefore, Bupivacaine and Ropivacaine become the drugs of choice when large doses, which might gradually enter the circulation before elimination, are required as in regional (epidural and spinal) anaesthesia. Intravenous regional anaesthesia involves the deliberate injection of a local anaesthetic drug intravenously (under very specific and carefully controlled circumstances), and Prilocaine is the most stable from the cardiovascular perspective (least likely to cause abnormalities of cardiac rhythm) of all the local anaesthetic drugs.

The more lipid-soluble, the more potent the local anaesthetic agent; Bupivacaine is four times more potent than Lidocaine. Drug potency influences the concentrations of the drugs available for clinical use: Bupivacaine is presented in 0.25–0.5% solutions, while Lidocaine 0.5–2% solutions. Lidocaine and Bupivacaine are metabolised in the liver by amidases, a relatively slow process, so repeated doses of these local anaesthetics can accumulate in the patient's bloodstream. The metabolites are excreted renally.

Topical application of local anaesthesia can be very effective for small cutaneous procedures and to minimise the pain of injection in children and needle phobic patients. The drug is applied to the skin and then covered with an occlusive dressing for the requisite time. When the dressing is removed, the product is wiped off; while a local anaesthetic makes procedures less painful, the anaesthetic gel softens the skin making it more difficult to insert needles/devices. The two products used topically are EMLA and Ametop®. EMLA (Eutectic Mixture of Local Anaesthetic—Lidocaine and Prilocaine) is applied 60 min before a procedure, while Ametop (Tetracaine) is applied 30 min before a procedure.

For more information about the local anaesthetics refer to Taylor and McLeod (2020).

5.6.2.1 Medication Choices and Pharmacology

If a medicine is to be effective, it must prevent the pain impulses entering the CNS. If administered orally, sufficient drug following first-pass metabolism in the liver must enter the circulation. Administered by intravenous injection, analgesic drugs do not undergo first-pass metabolism; such a route of administration is a very efficient method for delivering a high percentage of a medication directly into the circulation. Successful analgesia depends upon the speed with which drugs target their site of action. Moore (2009: 134) identifies the 'ideal analgesic' as characterised by the following:

1. Rapid onset of action
2. Prolonged duration of action
3. Minimisation of interruption by pain
4. Production of analgesia over a wide variety of pain types
5. Effectiveness in different patient populations
6. Good tolerability profile.

The National Institute for Health and Care Excellence Clinical Knowledge Summary: mild to moderate pain (NICE 2023) advocates the use of single analgesic drugs before resorting to combinations of analgesic drugs; the initial use of drugs in combination can make it difficult to determine the most effective drug/drug combination for the individual patient.

5.6.3 Non-opioid Analgesics

5.6.3.1 Paracetamol (Acetaminophen)

This drug remains the most popular 'over-the-counter' analgesic. Paracetamol is considered a 'weak' analgesic and it is often administered in combination with opioid or NSAID analgesics (Jóźwiak-Bebenista and Nowak 2014).

The comprehensive mode of action of paracetamol has yet to be identified, but what is known is that the drug demonstrates very limited anti-inflammatory properties so it cannot be described a 'non-steroidal' analgesic; it therefore occupies a group of its own.

Well absorbed from oral administration, paracetamol can also be administered very effectively per rectum and intravenously. Because it has no impact upon level of consciousness, Paracetamol is often administered intravenously during the immediate post-operative period.

15–20% plasma protein bound, Paracetamol is uniformly distributed in the body tissues and fluids (but not in body fat, which is why it has a relatively short half-life). Peak plasma concentration of paracetamol occurs within 1 h of administration.

Paracetamol metabolism occurs in the liver by conjugation with glucuronic acid and sulphate; the conjugate is excreted in the urine (85–95% within 24 h).

An overdose can irreversibly damage the liver because of an accumulation of one toxic metabolite (N-acetyl-p-benzoquinone imine) within liver cells.

With a half-life of 3–4 h, no more than 4 g of paracetamol can be administered in any 24 h period, so it is prescribed to be administered every 6 h.

So, while local anaesthetics disrupt message relay from nerves at the site of injury and paracetamol has both a local and central action, drugs which act differently might prove useful. A multimodal approach to pain management, tackling different aspects of the physiology of pain, should offer more chance of blocking pain impulses to provide the most effective analgesia.

5.6.3.2 Non-steroidal Anti-inflammatory Drugs (NSAIDs) Analgesics
Examples:

- Aspirin
- Ibuprofen
- Naproxen
- Diclofenac
- Celecoxib

The acute pain from surgery or a traumatic injury involving damage to skin, tissues (including bone) and hollow organs is largely provoked by the inflammatory response. Drugs specifically targeted at reducing inflammation should therefore provide effective analgesia. Because the inflammatory response leads to an elevation in body temperature, anti-inflammatory drugs are also very effective anti-pyretics. The steroid hormones are the best naturally occurring anti-inflammatory chemicals, but the anti-inflammatory drugs which are used to achieve analgesia are not steroids; hence, their name 'non-steroidal anti-inflammatory drugs' is abbreviated as NSAIDs. The NSAIDs are prostaglandin inhibitors; prostaglandin is a key contributor to mechanisms increasing the experience of pain; blocking these processes should result in analgesia. Dependent upon cyclooxygenase (enzyme mediated) pathways, the prostaglandins are manufactured from arachidonic acid. The pathway most closely associated with pain is COX-2. Very few NSAIDs are COX-2-specific. Most NSAIDs disrupt both COX-1 and COX-2 (Fig. 5.7).

COX-1 is an inflammatory prostaglandin pathway, initiated in the gastrointestinal (GI) tract when the mucus membrane lining the GI tract is damaged. The resultant inflammatory response mobilises protective resources to reduce gastric acid secretion and prevent further damage. So there is a risk that long-term NSAID use, while providing good analgesia, can block the protective prostaglandin pathway in the GI tract leading to erosion and bleeding.

Prostaglandins are also involved in renal blood flow and the maintenance of glomerular filtration rate (GFR); the use of NSAIDs can reduce GFR causing sodium and water retention, which can lead to hypertension and renal failure. Many NSAIDs are acidic and can irritate the gastric mucosa on ingestion. NSAIDs can also induce allergic reactions, and caution is advised in asthmatics; they may develop an acute bronchospasm when given NSAID preparations. NSAIDs can also delay clotting.

In patients requiring long-term NSAID treatment, or when patients have experienced symptoms of gastric disturbance or ulceration, a proton pump inhibitor drug might be administered daily to reduce gastric acid secretion and protect the delicate gastric mucosa. Omeprazole 20 mg daily is an example of a proton pump inhibitor. It must be noted that, when a drug is introduced to off-set the possible adverse

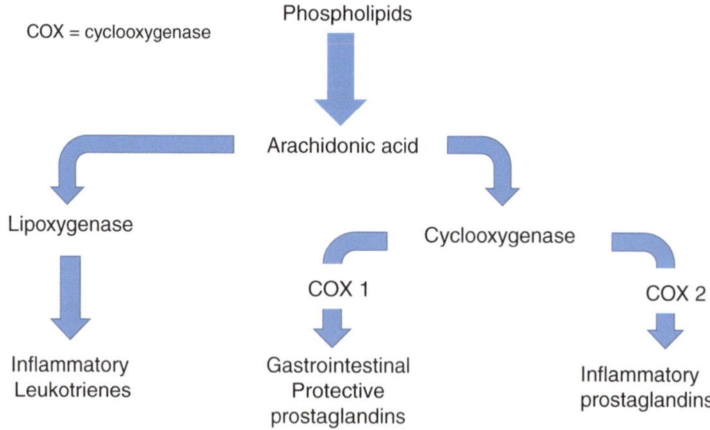

Fig. 5.7 Simplified inflammatory mediator pathway showing location of cyclooxygenase enzymes

actions of another drug, it might be more difficult to determine the cause of adverse drug response/reaction/interaction.

Aspirin

Acetylsalicylic acid, derived from willow bark, has been used as an analgesic for two millennia. Pharmacologically aspirin was identified in the late nineteenth century, but its mode of action was only recognised in the 1970s. Unlike the other NSAIDs, which have a reversible effect on cyclooxygenase, Aspirin has an irreversible effect. Aspirin also inhibits inflammatory mediator chemicals.

Aspirin has antiplatelet activity through inhibition of Thromboxane, the chemical which causes platelets to aggregate (stick together) when a clot forms (see Chap. 15).

Rather than through prostaglandin inhibition, Aspirin has a direct negative action upon the gastric mucosa.

Aspirin is not licensed for use in children because of the risk of Reye's syndrome which can result in fatal liver and neurological damage.

Aspirin is most frequently administered orally; it can also be administered per rectum and is well absorbed from the GI tract.

Protein binding is dose-dependent; at low doses, the drug is 90% protein bound, at higher doses 75%.

Aspirin is hydrolysed in the plasma to its active form, salicylic acid; peak plasma concentration of salicylic acid occurs within 1–2 h of administration.

Salicylic acid is widely distributed to all tissues of the body, highest concentrations in plasma, liver and renal cortex.

Aspirin (Acetylsalicylic acid) is conjugated in the liver to form salicylic acid and other metabolites, excreted by the kidneys.

Salicylic acid has a plasma half-life of 6 h.

Dose

- Because of the risk of GI disturbance, oral Aspirin should always be taken with food.
- Mild to moderate pain and fever 325–650 mg, repeated every 4–6 h. Maximum daily dose 4 g.
- As an anti-inflammatory (for arthritis pain), 3000–5000 mg daily in equally divided doses 4–6 h.
- As an antiembolic (in cardiovascular disease), 75 mg (enteric coated) once daily.

Ibuprofen

Ibuprofen has become a very popular over-the-counter medication for the treatment of mild to moderate pain; it is analgesic, anti-inflammatory and anti-pyretic. Initially introduced as a prescription-only medicine in the 1970s, Ibuprofen became a popular choice with prescribers because it exhibited fewer serious side effects than drugs like aspirin. Ibuprofen causes a reversible disruption to the anti-inflammatory cyclo-oxygenase-mediated pathways.

Pharmacokinetically ibuprofen is:

- Rapidly absorbed from the GI tract following oral administration, peak plasma concentration occurs within 1–2 h of administration.
- 90–99% of Ibuprofen is plasma protein bound.
- Metabolised via cytochrome P450 in the liver, the metabolites are renally excreted.
- Serum half-life of 2 h.
- Within 24 h of the last dose, the drug will have been completely eliminated.

Dose (Adult)
- For mild to moderate pain, 200–400 mg every 4–6 h.
- As an anti-inflammatory, 400–800 mg 3–4 times daily.

Naproxen
Is a prescription only medicine (POM) with an action similar to that of Ibuprofen, it is used for the relief of pain in musculoskeletal conditions, it has a history of a higher incidence of gastro-intestinal disturbance than Ibuprofen and NHS guidance advocates that the smallest therapeutically beneficial dose be administered across the shortest period of time.

Pharmacokinetically naproxen is:

- Rapidly absorbed from the GI tract following oral administration, peak plasma concentration occurs within 1–2 h of administration.
- 99% of Naproxen is plasma protein bound.
- Undergoing phase I and phase II metabolism in the liver, the metabolites are renally excreted.
- Serum half-life of 2 h.
- Within 17 h of the last dose, the drug will have been completely eliminated.

Dose (Adult)
- For pain in rheumatic disease 0.5–1 g daily in divided doses.
- For pain and inflammation in musculo-skeletal disorders and dysmenorrhoea 500 mg as an initial does, the 250 mg every 6–8 h, as required.

Diclofenac
Introduced in the UK in 1979, initially as a prescription-only medicine, diclofenac has been available as an over-the-counter preparation since 2008.

An anti-inflammatory, anti-pyretic analgesic, Diclofenac causes a reversible disruption of the anti-inflammatory cyclooxygenase-mediated pathways; it also inhibits monocyte migration during the inflammatory response.

Diclofenac can be administered orally, rectally, intravenously or topically.

Completely absorbed following oral administration, first-pass metabolism results in only 50–60% of the original dose reaching the systemic circulation. Peak plasma concentration occurs within 2–3 h of administration. A significant proportion of Diclofenac is distributed into the synovial fluid; 3–6 h after administration, there is more drug detectable in the synovial fluid than in the plasma. It also appears that Diclofenac is relatively slow to return to the systemic circulation from the synovial fluid.

Pharmacokinetically diclofenac is:

- 99% plasma protein bound.
- Extensively metabolised in the liver, 65% of an oral dose is renally excreted, while 35% is excreted in the bile.
- Relatively short-lived with a half-life of 2 h. However drug action is much longer, and this might be because the drug persists within synovial joints far longer than in the plasma.

Dose
- Oral 75–150 mg/day in 2–3 divided doses.

Intravenous Administration
- Intravenous infusion 75 mg repeated, when necessary after 4–6 h, for a maximum of 2 days.
- Post-operatively, immediately after surgery: 25–50 mg over 15–60 min, then 5 mg for a maximum of 2 days.
- For acute pain, for example, post-operative pain; deep i.m. (gluteal) injection 75 mg once daily for a maximum of 2 days.
- For ureteric colic, deep i.m. (gluteal) injection 75 mg, then a second dose after 30 min, if necessary.
- *Per rectum* suppositories 75–150 mg daily in divided doses.

The maximum total daily dose by any route is 150 mg.

Diclofenac is contraindicated in patients with congestive cardiac failure, neuro-vascular, cardiovascular or peripheral vascular disease.

Topical Preparations
- 1% cream
- 3% gel
- Eye drops

5.6.3.3 COX-2-Specific NSAIDs

The long-term use of NSAIDs presents significant risks, mainly associated with GI erosion and bleeding. A COX-2-specific inhibitor drug which would only target the production of prostaglandins associated with pain was initially welcomed. Subsequently, however, ongoing research indicates the use of a number of these medications is associated with potentially fatal adverse cardio-vascular effects (De Vecchis et al. 2014).

Celecoxib
One of the most recent NSAIDs, Celecoxib, is a COX-2-specific anti-inflammatory, anti-pyretic analgesic.

Oral Administration
- Relatively slowly absorbed from the GI tract following oral administration, peak plasma concentration occurs within 2–4 h of administration.
- 95–99% of Celecoxib is plasma protein bound.
- Metabolised in the liver, the metabolites are excreted renally and in the bile.
- Serum half-life of 11 h indicates why the drug only needs to be administered twice daily.

Dose
- Osteoarthritis: 100 mg twice daily or a single dose of 200 mg daily.
- Rheumatoid arthritis: 200–400 mg daily in two divided doses.
- Like Diclofenac, Celecoxib is contraindicated in patients with congestive cardiac failure, neurovascular, cardiovascular or peripheral vascular disease (British National Formulary 2024), and guidance about all NSAIDs recommends that the lowest possible drug dose is prescribed for the shortest length of time to achieve analgesia and that patients are regularly monitored, for example, blood pressure is measured and documented before and during treatment (Scottish Executive 2006).

5.6.4 Opioids

Opioids are identified as 'weak' (Rodriguez et al. 2007) or 'strong' (National Institute for Health and Care Excellence 2016a); the 'strong' opioids include a number of synthetic, as well as naturally occurring, drugs. The synthetic drugs have been developed with the aim of eliminating some of the unpleasant adverse effects of the naturally occurring opioids, but with limited success. The naturally occurring opioids, which include codeine, morphine and papaverine, are still derived from opium extracts. Diamorphine hydrochloride is manufactured by heating morphine with acetic anhydride. Diamorphine is more potent than morphine and more lipid soluble so it penetrates the CNS more rapidly, causing effective analgesia, but it has a shorter half-life.

Three important opioid receptors, Mu, Delta and Kappa, have been identified. The endogenous opioids, for example, β-endorphin (which has 80 times the analgesic potency of morphine), enkephalin and dynorphin, have a preference for and stimulate the Mu receptor. When combined with the Mu receptor, opioid drugs provide very good analgesia but, in an area of the brainstem called the locus coeruleus opioids can also give rise to respiratory depression by reducing respiratory centre sensitivity to CO2, they also cause a fall in systemic blood pressure, drowsiness, and a reduced cough reflex.

Opioids also act upon the GI tract, inhibiting enteric nerves, leading to reduced gut motility and constipation. Nurses must ensure patient comfort, and in certain circumstances where the patient must not strain to defecate, for example, following neurosurgery the patient may be prescribed stool softeners. The opioid drugs do not just stimulate Mu receptors, the binding of opioid drugs with other opioid receptors results in analgesia that is far less effective than the endogenous processes, for example, drug combination with the Delta receptor causes nausea and vomiting and combination with Kappa receptors in the limbic system can cause euphoria which can contribute to opioid addiction. Opioid binding with Kappa receptors can also cause miosis (pin-point pupils) although this occurs less frequently with synthetic opioids. Most opioid drugs contract the biliary muscles and should not be used to treat biliary colic; they relax the detrusor muscle, which can lead to retention of urine. Similar problems are exhibited by synthetic opioids, as yet nothing has been manufactured which can compare in potency and efficacy with endogenous substances.

When opioid drugs are prescribed, patients must be closely monitored for both effective (analgesia) and adverse effects (respiratory depression, drowsiness). When strong opioid side effects become a problem, the competitive opioid antagonist naloxone might be used to reverse (by blocking the opioid receptors normally occupied by opioid drugs) the unwanted effects of the strong opioids, but naloxone does not simply reverse the unwanted effects of the drugs, it also stops the analgesic effects. As naloxone might have other systemic effects, for example, it can cause tachycardia and dysrhythmias, hypotension, nausea and vomiting and pulmonary oedema; it is only used in potentially life-threatening situations.

All opioid use is strictly regulated in accordance with the NICE clinical guideline NG46 (National Institute for Health and Care Excellence 2016b).

The Medicines and Healthcare products Regulatory Agency [MHRA] published Opioid-specific guidance in March (2020a) cautioning against the prescription of Benzodiazepines with opioids because of the risk of 'potentially fatal respiratory depression'. In September (2020b) the MHRA also published guidance about the risk of 'opioid dependence and addiction' cautioning healthcare professionals about the risk of 'long-term opioid use (greater than three months) in patients suffering non-malignant pain'.

5.6.4.1 Weak Opioids
Codeine

A relatively weak opioid, Codeine needs to be metabolised to form a morphine metabolite which binds with spinal opioid receptors to cause analgesia and narcosis (the drowsiness specifically associated with narcotic (opioid) analgesics). Codeine forms a popular over-the-counter purchase in combination with paracetamol.

Codeine is well absorbed from oral, intramuscular and intravenous administration.

Pharmacokinetically codeine is metabolised in the liver which results in the production of conjugates of codeine, norcodeine and morphine.

Codeine has rapid urinary excretion, 67% is eliminated within 6 h, 10% is unchanged codeine, 40% conjugates of codeine, 10% norcodeine and 10% morphine. Its half-life is 3 h.

Codeine is often used as an analgesic for patients following traumatic injury because it is less likely to cause drowsiness, respiratory depression and nausea, and vomiting associated with morphine and its effects are, therefore, less likely to mask any cerebral events associated with the trauma.

Codeine offers little to the patient suffering acute pain in the hospital setting, but some patients find it very useful to manage acute episodes of pain (e.g. headache, earache) at home. Codeine is a very effective cough suppressant. Prolonged use can result in constipation because codeine slows gastrointestinal motility.

5.6.4.2 Strong Opioids

Naturally Occurring
Morphine
Opium was first identified in the early nineteenth century and by the mid-nineteenth century, following the development of the hypodermic needle, widely marketed. Morphine can relieve most types of pain, having an impact upon both sensory and emotional components. Analgesia is produced by morphine binding with Mu opioid receptors in the dorsal horn of the spinal cord, inhibiting the relay of pain impulses to the brain; it also activates descending modulatory pain pathways and has an inhibitory action on pain impulses arising in the tissues, all mediated through combination with Mu opioid receptors. Morphine is the opioid most likely to cause urinary retention. As many as 40% of morphine recipients experience nausea and vomiting because morphine stimulates the chemoreceptor trigger zone (CTZ) in the brain; a combined morphine and antiemetic preparation (Cyclimorph) is available for sub-cutaneous/intramuscular/intravenous administration.

Morphine can be administered orally, rectally, subcutaneously (as bolus doses or by infusion), intramuscularly, intravenously (as bolus doses or via a patient-controlled analgesia device [PCA]), intrathecally or epidurally and inhaled via a nebulizer. In clinical use, it is most frequently administered intravenously. Nurses tend to be cautious when administering morphine because of the risk of adverse effects. There is no doubt that respiratory depression can be frightening, but the patient in pain deserves sufficient analgesia. One adverse effect nurses should be concerned about is the risk of hypotension, but in a normotensive/normovolaemic patient there is minimal risk of hypotension, it seems that this risk is used as an 'excuse' to delay the administration of analgesia; but this can inappropriately prolong patient distress.

When taken orally, Morphine is rapidly metabolised in the liver, so that only 40–50% of the original drug escapes first pass metabolism. Plasma concentration of Morphine peaks 30 min after oral administration. Oral preparations included sustained released products for prolonged analgesia.

Plasma concentration of Morphine peaks 20 min after s/c or i.m. administration. Following hepatic metabolism 87% of a dose of Morphine is excreted in the urine within 72 h of drug administration.

Of the two main metabolites of Morphine metabolism, 60% morphine-3-glucuronide (M3G) and 10% morphine-6-glucuronide (M6G), M3G has no analgesic effect, while M6G is half as potent as Morphine.

Morphine half-life is 2 h.

Dose
- *Acute Pain*
- Subcutaneous or intramuscular injection 10 mg 4 hourly as necessary.
- Intravenous injection 25–50% corresponding subcutaneous/i.m. dose.
- PCA Trust policies dictate the concentration and dosing of Morphine via PCA pumps.

5.6.4.3 Synthetic Opioids

Pethidine

The first synthetic opioid manufactured in 1932 was very popular in the late twentieth century because of the belief that Pethidine exhibited fewer adverse effects than Morphine. Nevertheless, Pethidine can cause all the known opioid adverse effects and can cause convulsions in overdose.

Pethidine has greater lipid solubility than morphine, so enters the CNS and acts more rapidly.

Pethidine can be administered by intramuscular and intravenous injection.

Pethidine is metabolised in the liver to pethidinic acid and the toxic metabolite norpethidine, which has none of the beneficial properties of an opioid, only the unwanted ones. Because of this toxic metabolite, which has a longer half-life than Pethidine and cannot be blocked with antagonists like Naloxone, Pethidine it is only administered for short periods of time.

Pethidine has a half-life of 3–5 h and provides analgesia for 2–4 h.

One additional use of Pethidine is that, in low doses, it is very effective in treating normothermic post-anaesthetic shivering.

Fentanyl

A potent synthetic opioid, described as 50–100× more potent than Morphine, was once described as the most frequently prescribed opioid worldwide.

Because it can cause significant respiratory depression upon intravenous administration, intravenous Fentanyl is only administered in critical care clinical areas. Used in combination with sedative drugs to support mechanical ventilation, Fentanyl is also used as preemptive analgesia during the induction of anaesthesia. Outside the critical care environment Fentanyl is most frequently used in transdermal patches for the relief of acute and chronic pain. Fentanyl administered buccally/sublingually as a 'rapid onset opioid' is a novel approach to the management of chronic and 'breakthrough' pain (Stanley 2014). However, like many opioids Fentanyl is a potential drug of abuse: in overdose, it can cause fatal respiratory depression.

Oxycodone

Described as a 'semi-synthetic' opioid (Ordóñez Gallego et al. 2007), Oxycodone is very effective when compared with morphine. Oxycodone can be administered orally, subcutaneously (by bolus and infusion) and intravenously (by bolus and PCA). When taken orally, Oxycodone undergoes less first-pass metabolism than morphine, 60–85% of the drug does not undergo first-pass metabolism. Oxycodone is 45% plasma protein bound.

Following hepatic metabolism, Oxycodone and its metabolites are renally excreted. Oxycodone half-life is 3–5 h.

Dose

- Oral 5 mg every 4–6 h. Dose can be increased to a maximum 400 mg daily.
- Slow intravenous injection 1–10 mg every 4 h as necessary.
- Subcutaneous injection 5 mg every 4 h as necessary.
- Subcutaneous infusion initially 7.5 mg every 24 h.
- PCA Trust policies dictate the concentration and dosing of Oxycodone via PCA pumps.

5.6.5 Other Approaches to Achieve Analgesia

GABA Analogues

Gamma-amino butyric acid (GABA) is an inhibitory neurotransmitter in the CNS, regulating neuronal activity; without it there might be excessive neuronal activity resulting in seizures or anxiety. A GABA analogue mimics the action of GABA. Drugs which increase the effects of GABA include the benzodiazepines and alcohol.

Gabapentin, an antiepileptic medication, has been found to be an effective analgesic, particularly for neuropathic pain, but its precise mode of action is unknown. Gabapentin has very low plasma protein binding. Gabapentin undergoes no metabolism and is excreted unchanged by the kidneys. Initial dose 300 mg orally, rising to 300 mg three times a day to a maximum of 3.6 g per day.

Large doses of Gabapentin cause drowsiness, MHRA (2017) guidance cautioned against the use of high doses because of the risk of severe respiratory depression. In 2019 the MHRA changed the status of Gabapentin, recognising the potential for addiction, the drug became a Class C-controlled substance and a Schedule 3 drug.

Similar in action to Gabapentin:

Pregabalin is prescribed as an anxiolytic, anti-convulsant and in chronic neuropathic pain as an analgesic. A recent Cochrane review suggests that dosing with

300–600 mg daily Pregabalin can achieve good analgesia (Derry et al. 2019). Pregabalin is also a Class C-controlled substance and Schedule 3 drug (MHRA 2019), in 2021 the MHRA warned about the risk of respiratory depression with high doses of Pregabalin.

Because serotonin and noradrenaline are neurotransmitters involved in pain modulation, they can be pharmacologically manipulated. Selective serotonin reuptake inhibitors (SSRIs) and tricyclic antidepressants (e.g. amitriptyline) therefore have analgesic properties and may prove useful in treating chronic and neuropathic pain.

5.6.5.1 Antispasmodics

Hyoscine is an alkaloid anticholinergic, acting on the parasympathetic nervous system; it reduces the incidence of nausea and vomiting associated with travel sickness and is a powerful antispasmodic. It used to treat the pain of irritable bowel syndrome and sold in over-the-counter (OTC) preparations for menstrual pain; it also causes a dry mouth and tachycardia. It is administered by injecting 200–600 µg subcutaneously or intramuscularly, orally 10 mg tablets and by transdermal patch (to treat nausea and vomiting).

Baclofen is a GABA analogue which has powerful antispasmodic properties; it also causes a decreased release of substance P. Baclofen can be administered orally in doses beginning at 15 mg and rising to a maximum 100 mg; it can also be administered via an implanted pump device which delivers the drug directly into the cerebrospinal fluid to control severe muscular spasticity (in cerebral palsy and after CVA).

5.6.5.2 Ketamine

A drug used to induce anaesthesia, Ketamine has powerful analgesic properties, acting directly on the substantia gelatinosa (the 'gate') in the spinal cord blocking the upwards relay of pain messages. Ketamine also has a direct effect on the thalamus preventing it from relaying messages from the limbic system to the sensory cortex, where pain impulses become a conscious experience of pain. Ketamine can be used to good effect in combination with opioid analgesia, particularly when treating intractable pain. Ketamine is currently used in the chronic rather than the acute pain scenario. As it can cause hallucinations, Ketamine is a drug of abuse; it is stored, handled and its use documented in the same way as the opioids.

Dosing for analgesia: intravenous 0.5 mg/kg, intramuscular 2–4 mg/kg; Ketamine can also be administered by controlled intravenous infusion; in combination with ketoprofen and lidocaine, it can also be administered topically to treat neurogenic pain.

5.6.6 Molecular Targets: The Future of Analgesia in Chronic Pain?

One approach to pain management involves targeting cytokines using anti-tumour necrosis factor (TNF) to reduce inflammation, for example, Adalimumab® is used in inflammatory bowel disease; the drug reduces the unpleasant symptoms associated with Crohn's disease and ulcerative colitis including the acute pain experienced by disease sufferers (Bouhnik et al. 2018). Another drug Tanezumab® is an anti-nerve growth factor, as yet unproven, which might be effective in disease processes involving less inflammation, for example, osteoarthritis (Chen et al. 2017).

5.6.7 Psychologic Approaches

This chapter acknowledges the biopsychosocial nature of pain; therefore, it must be acknowledged that the psychological aspects cannot be ignored (Royal College of Nursing 2015) and the nurse must offer an empathic and appropriate response to patient reports of pain. It is beyond the remit of this chapter to consider the non-pharmacologic approaches which might be employed, it is recommended to review sources related to this aspect of care for example, Johnson and Bjordal (2009).

5.7 Summary

When attempting to assess the extent and severity of pain, nurses must acknowledge the patient's own assessment of their pain. As has been outlined, pain can vary, and no two individuals' experiences are the same. Each patient must be nursed according to their reported pain and the emotional contribution to the experience of pain acknowledged. All patients reporting pain deserve a prompt and appropriate response.

- Analgesia choices are limited by the medical prescription; the nurse must recognise when it is appropriate to employ non-pharmacologic approaches.
- A multi-modal approach involving different analgesics which target the pain impulses in more than one way, for example, in the periphery at the site of damage as well as at the level of the spinal cord, should be more effective at preventing the pain impulses reaching the patient's consciousness than simply targeting one aspect of the pain impulse relay.
- The strong analgesics (opioids) cause adverse effects which might pose a risk causing, for example, respiratory depression and somnolence.

Craig and Hatfield (2020) Advocate the Mnemonic CARER
C—Cause of pain
A—Assess the amount of pain
R—Reassure and comfort the patient

E—Effective and appropriate analgesia
R—Reassess

Working collaboratively with the patient, the nurse must assess and document pain; the nurse must then make the correct decision about how to manage that pain.

When giving analgesia, the nurse must regularly reassess the patient to determine both the effects and adverse effects of the chosen approach. When the patient reports no benefit from the analgesia, the nurse must recognise when it is appropriate to summon clinical assistance to identify and prescribe suitable alternative analgesia.

Rosa (2018) opines that 'through the skillful integration of theory, practice, and the ability to build respectful and responsible patient-client partnerships, pain management nurses can deliver contextually relevant care that promotes safety, quality, and healing'.

Multiple Choice Questions

1. Acute pain becomes chronic pain when:
   - (a) It persists for more than 30 days.
   - (b) It becomes difficult to treat.
   - (c) It persists after healing.
   - (d) It becomes more intense.
2. Pain does not indicate:
   - (a) A threat
   - (b) Healing
   - (c) Cell death
   - (d) Anxiety
3. An optimal approach to acute pain management requires:
   - (a) Minimal side effects
   - (b) Minimal cost
   - (c) Minimal nursing activity
   - (d) Minimal monitoring
4. The drug most commonly prescribed for pain management in the immediate post-operative period is:
   - (a) IV Paracetamol
   - (b) Morphine
   - (c) Codeine
   - (d) Ibuprofen
5. The benefits of using paracetamol for treating acute pain include:
   - (a) It combines with opioid receptors.
   - (b) It is safe to exceed the maximum dose.
   - (c) It causes moderate sedation.
   - (d) There is no effect on level of consciousness.

6. Non-steroidal anti-inflammatory drugs do not result in:
   (a) Bronchospasm
   (b) Gastric irritation
   (c) Hypercoagulability
   (d) Reduced renal blood flow
7. Opioids administered in the immediate post-operative period are unlikely to cause:
   (a) Somnolence
   (b) Respiratory depression
   (c) Itch
   (d) Anxiety
8. Identify the main benefit of patient-controlled analgesia:
   (a) Reduced nurse workload
   (b) Reduced cost of analgesia
   (c) Reduced pain
   (d) Reduced monitoring requirements

Answers

1. (b)

   Acute pain becoming a chronic scenario is not a simple time issue; it is more than the experience of pain can overwhelm a patient, even in the absence of obvious wound/tissue damage and the situation becomes more and more complex and difficult to manage.

2. (b)

   Pain can indicate a threat to tissues and, eventually, cell death. An anxious patient is going to have a very different pain experience to a patient who has been well-prepared; for example, the anxious patient might suffer more pain because of the anticipation of a painful event. If a wound is healing, then pain should subside; it should not persist; if pain remains an issue, the underlying cause must be identified and managed; it is not good enough to simply treat (medicate) the pain.

3. (a)

   Most drugs exhibit some adverse effects, a humanitarian approach advocates the use of the drugs which cause minimal adverse effects and the nurse needs to be aware about and observe for any potential issues when administering drugs to the patient. Cost should not be the determining issue when a prescriber is deciding how to treat a patient. Whatever the treatment prescribed, the nurse is obliged to regularly assess the patient and determine the effectiveness (or otherwise) of the intervention employed; so reducing nursing activity and patient monitoring cannot be issues when analgesia is the goal.

4. (a)

   Paracetamol has none of the adverse effects, for example, the depression and somnolence associated with the potent opioids like morphine. Weak opioids are analgesic and have less effect on level of consciousness; but codeine would not be the first choice for post-operative pain management because it is a less effective analgesic, it can be a stimulant at low doses and with frequent use it can cause uncomfortable constipation (in some circumstances, constipation and straining at stool must be avoided post-operatively). Non-steroidal anti-inflammatory drugs like ibuprofen are effective analgesics, but their adverse effects, for example, bronchospasm, gastric irritation and decreased renal perfusion, are more numerous and potentially more hazardous than the adverse effects of paracetamol.

5. (d)

   While the mechanism of action of the drug has yet to be properly defined, what is known is that Paracetamol does not combine with opioid receptors, because of the risk of hepatic damage during drug metabolism for elimination the maximum does of 4 g daily must not be exceeded and the drug does not cause sedation.

6. (c)

   Non-steroidal drugs like aspirin reduce platelet aggregation, reducing coagulability of blood. To a greater or lesser extent the non-steroidal medication may cause the other factors listed.

7. (d)

   Opioid analgesics cause somnolence, respiratory depression and itch. Without sufficient analgesia the patient may become anxious, but the opioids are not, themselves, the cause of anxiety. Endogenous opioids form effective anxiolytics, an adaptive mechanism to ward off negative situational responses (taken from: https://journals.sagepub.com/doi/abs/10.1177/0269881110367726;   last accessed 1st December 2024).

8. (c)

   Patient-controlled analgesia should optimise pain control physiologically and psychologically.

References

Bouhnik Y, Carbonnel F, Laharie D, Stefanescu C, Hébuterne X, Abitbol V, Nachury M, Brixi H, Bourreille A, Picon L, Bourrier A, Allez M, Peyrin-Biroulet L, Moreau J, Savoye G, Fumery M, Nancey S, Roblin X, Altwegg R, Bouguen G, Bommelaer G, Danese S, Louis E, Zappa M, Mary J-Y (2018) Efficacy of adalimumab in patients with Crohn's disease and symptomatic small bowel stricture: a multicentre, prospective, observational cohort (CREOLE) study. Gut 67(1):53–60

British National Formulary (2024) Celecoxib. https://bnf.nice.org.uk/drug/celecoxib.html. Accessed 1 Dec 2024

Chen J, Li J, Li R, Wang H, Yang J, Xu J, Zha Z (2017) Efficacy and safety of Tanezumab on osteoarthritis knee and hip pains: a meta-analysis of randomized controlled trials. Pain Med 18(2):374–385

Colloca L, Benedetti F (2007) Nocebo hyperalgesia: how anxiety is turned into pain. Curr Opin Anaesthesiol 20(5):435–439

Craig A, Hatfield A (2020) The complete recovery room book, 6th edn. OUP Oxford

De Vecchis R, Baldi C, Di Biase G, Ariano C, Cioppa C, Giasi A, Valente L, Cantatrione S (2014) Cardiovascular risk associated with celecoxib or etoricoxib: a meta-analysis of randomized controlled trials which adopted comparison with placebo or naproxen. Minerva Cardioangiol 62(6):437–448

Derry S, Bell R, Straube S, Wiffen PJ, Aldington D, Moore R (2019) Pregabalin for chronic neuropathic pain in adults. From the Cochrane library: Accessed 1 Dec 2024

Ene KW, Nordberg G, Bergh I, Johansson FJ, Sjöström B (2008) Postoperative pain management-the influence of surgical ward nurses. J Clin Nurs 17(15):2042–2050. https://www.cochrane.org/CD007076/SYMPT_pregabalin-chronic-neuropathic-pain-adults

Gordon DB, Pellino TA, Higgins GA, Pasero C, Murphy-Ende K (2008) Nurses' opinions on appropriate administration of PRN range opioid analgesic orders for acute pain. Pain Mgmt Nurs 9(3):131–140

Green L (2013) Assessment of acute and chronic pain. Anaesthesia Intens Care Med 14(11):488–490

Heikkinen K, Salanterä S, Kettu M, Taittonen M (2005) Prostatectomy patients' postoperative pain assessment in the recovery room. J Adv Nurs 52(6):592–600

Johnson MI, Bjordal JM (2009) Chapter 9: Non-pharmacologic approaches to pain management. In: Dickman A, Simpson KH (eds) Chronic pain. Oxford University Press, Oxford

Jóźwiak-Bebenista M, Nowak JZ (2014) Paracetamol: mechanism of action, applications and safety concern. Acta Pol Pharm 1(1):11–23

McCaffery M, Beebe A (1994) Pain clinical manual for nursing practice. Mosby, London

McCaffery M, Ferrell BR (1994) Understanding opioids and addiction. Nursing 28(4):56–59

McCaffery M, Pasero C (1999) Pain: clinical manual. Mosby, Michigan

Medicines and Healthcare products Regulatory Agency (2017) Gabapentin (Neurontin) risk of severe respiratory depression. Drug Saf Update (2017) 11(3):2

Medicines and Healthcare products Regulatory Agency (2019) Pregabalin (Lyrica), Gabapentin (Neurontin) and risk of abuse and dependence: new scheduling requirements from 1 April. Drug Saf Update (2019) 12(9):4

Medicines and Healthcare products Regulatory Agency (2020a) Benzodiazepines and opioids: reminder of risk of potentially fatal respiratory depression. Drug Saf Update 2020 13(8):5

Medicines and Healthcare products Regulatory Agency (2020b) Opioids: risk of dependence and addiction. Drug Saf Update (2020) 14(2):1

Medicines and Healthcare products Regulatory Agency (2021) Pregabalin (Lyrica): reports of severe respiratory depression. Drug Saf Update 14(7):2

Melzack R, Wall PD (1965) Pain mechanisms: a new theory. Science 150(3699):971–979

Moore ND (2009) In search of an ideal analgesic for common acute pain. Acute Pain 11:129–137

National Institute for Health and Care Excellence (2016a) CG 140, palliative care for adults: strong opioids for pain relief NICE London.

National Institute for Health and Care Excellence (2016b) NG46 controlled drugs: safe use and management. https://www.nice.org.uk/guidance/ng46. Accessed 5 Dec 2024

National Institute for Health and Care Excellence (2021) Clinical Knowledge Summary Scenario Analgesia for mild to moderate pain. https://cks.nice.org.uk/topics/analgesia-mild-to-moderate-pain/#:~:text=The%20analgesics%20used%20to%20relieve,Aspirin%20(a%20salicylate%20NSAID). Accessed 5 Dec 2024

National Institute for Health and Care Excellence (2023) Clinical knowledge summary scenario: pain assessment. https://cks.nice.org.uk/topics/palliative-cancer-care-pain/management/assessment-of-pain/. Accessed 5 Dec 2024

Ordóñez Gallego A, González Barón M, Espinosa Arranz E (2007) Oxycodone: a pharmacological and clinical review. Clin Transl Oncol 9(5):298–357

Rodriguez RF, Bravo LE, Castro F, Montoya O, Castillo JM, Castillo MP, Daza P, Restrepo JM, Rodriguez MF (2007) Incidence of weak opioids adverse events in the Management of Cancer Pain: a double-blind comparative trial. J Palliat Med 10(1):56–60

Rosa WE (2018) Transcultural pain management: theory, practice, and nurse-client partnership. Pain Manag Nurs 19(1):23–33

Royal College of Nursing (2015) Pain knowledge and skills framework for the nursing team. RCN, London

Royal Pharmaceutical Society and the Royal College of Nursing (2019) Professional Guidance on the Administration of Medicines in Healthcare Settings. https://www.rpharms.com/Portals/0/RPS%20document%20library/Open%20access/Professional%20standards/SSHM%20and%20Admin/Admin%20of%20Meds%20prof%20guidance.pdf?ver=2019-01-23-145026-567. Accessed 1 Dec 2024

Scottish Executive (2006) Safety of selective and non-selective NSAIDs. https://www.publications.scot.nhs.uk/files_legacy/sehd/publications/DC20061024nsaids.pdf. Accessed 1 Dec 2024

Sloman R, Rosen G, Rom M, Shir Y (2005) Nurses' assessment of pain in surgical patients. J Adv Nurs 52(2):125–132

Srinivas NR, Carr DB, Cohen M, Finnerup NB, Flor H, Gibson S, Keefe F, Mogil JS, Ringkamp M, Sluka KA, Song X-J, Stevens B, Sullivan M, Tutleman P, Ushida T, Vader K (2020) The revised IASP definition of pain: concepts, challenges and compromises. Pain 161(9):1976–1982

Stanley TH (2014) The fentanyl story. J Pain 15(12):1215–1226

Tanabe P, Reddin C, Thornton VL, Todd KH, Wun T, Lyons JS (2010) Emergency department sickle cell assessment of needs and strengths (ED-SCANS), a focus group and decision support tool development project. Acad Emerg Med 17(8):848–858

Taylor A, McLeod G (2020) Basic pharmacology of local anaesthetics. Br J Anaesthesia 20(2):34–41

Thienhaus O, Cole BE (2002) Classification of pain. In: Weiner RS (ed) Pain management: a practical guide for clinicians, 6th edn. American Academy of Pain Management

Townsend R, Cox F (2007) Standardised analgesia packs after day case orthopaedic surgery. J Perioperat Pract 17(7):340–346

Turk DC, Okifuji A (2010) Chapter 2: Pain terms and taxonomies. In: Fishman SM, Ballantyne JC, Rathmell JP (eds) Bonica's management of pain, 4th edn. Lippincott Williams & Wilkins, Philadelphia, pp 13–23

Whiteman A, Bajaj S, Hasan N (2011) Novel techniques of wound infiltration. Continuing education in anaesthesia. Crit Care Pain 11(5):167–171. http://ceaccp.oxfordjournals.org/content/11/5/167.full.pdf. Accessed 1 Dec 2024

Wong-Baker (2018) Wong-Baker Faces Foundation. https://wongbakerfaces.org/. Accessed 1 Dec 2024

Additional Activity

The Royal College of Anaesthetists Faculty of Pain Medicine have produced e-PAIN described as "The resource for NHS workers who want to better understand and manage pain". https://fpm.ac.uk/e-pain. Accessed 1 Dec 2024

Additional Resources

International Association for the Study of Pain (2014) IASP Taxonomy, offers a detailed explanation about the formal definition of pain. https://www.iasp-pain.org/resources/terminology/?ItemNumber=169. Accessed 1 Dec 2024

National Institute for Health and Care Excellence Chronic pain (primary and secondary) in the over 16s: assessment of all chronic pain and management of chronic primary pain NG193. https://www.nice.org.uk/guidance/ng193. Accessed 5 Dec 2024

The Faculty of Pain Medicine of the Royal College of Anaesthetists have an excellent web-based resource: opioids aware, which provides up-to-date information on many drugs used to achieve analgesia, including Ketamine at https://www.fpm.ac.uk/opioids-aware. Accessed 5 Dec 2024

The Royal College of Nursing Pain Subject Guide. https://www.rcn.org.uk/library/Subject-Guides/pain. Accessed 1 Dec 2024

Edward Purssell

Learning Outcomes

At the end of this chapter, you will be able to:

- Discuss pharmacologically important differences of different types of microorganism.
- Provide an understanding of different drug targets in microorganisms.
- Provide an understanding of factors that govern the choice of antimicrobial agents.

6.1 Introduction

This chapter will consider the role that antimicrobial medications have in the treatment of infection and healthcare more generally. This will be realised by considering infection from an ecological perspective; that is, the world is a changing and dynamic community of organisms, of which humans are only a very small part. It is this aspect that makes treating infectious diseases so challenging, because infections are the result of an interaction between two organisms, both of which are evolving to exploit or reject the other. Consequently, the relationship is ever changing and dynamic; in the case of humans, this is most notably being seen in the development of immunity throughout the lifespan.

Although some microorganisms can cause disease, most do not, and seeing all microorganisms as dangerous is to misunderstand our relationship with them and reliance upon them. As will be explained, most microorganisms on the planet live in the soil and in the sea and will never encounter a human, let alone cause infection.

E. Purssell (✉)
Faculty of Health, Medicine and Social Care, Anglia Ruskin University, Chelmsford, UK
e-mail: edward.purssell@aru.ac.uk

E. Khan, P. Hood (eds.), *Understanding Pharmacology in Nursing Practice*,
https://doi.org/10.1007/978-3-032-03964-4_6

For those that do, and in terms of understanding how infections are treated, the focus throughout is on a concept known as selective toxicity: how can we damage or inhibit the infecting microorganism without damaging the host?

Because there are general principles that apply across the different groups of microorganism, each group will be considered in turn, starting with bacteria and viruses which cause most infections. These are followed by fungi, and finally protozoa and helminths, which are only briefly referred to because severe diseases caused by these are rare in most developed countries, although globally protozoa such as those that cause malaria are a major problem. Throughout this chapter, the reader is asked to consider the vital question above; how can we damage or inhibit the infecting microorganism without damaging the host?

6.2 Microbial Ecology

The world in which we live is a complex and diverse one containing many different species and communities of different organisms. It is estimated that there are around 4–6×10^{30} prokaryotes in the world (these are non-nucleated organsisms and comprise bacteria and archea), in contrast to the approximately 8.2×10^9 (8.2 billion) humans (Whitman et al. 1998). Fortunately, very few microorganisms cause disease; it has been estimated that there are in the region 1407 pathogenic species of organism, of which bacteria comprise 538, fungi 307, helminths 287, viruses 208, and protozoa 57 (Woolhouse and Gowtage-Sequeria 2005). Although this estimate is somewhat elderly and probably underestimates this number, even doubling this would still represent a small proportion of the total number of organisms. Some of these, around 816, are shared with animals, known as zoonoses; and around 13% are new or re-emerging pathogens. Recently, emerged diseases include human immunodeficiency virus (HIV) and severe acute respiratory syndrome (SARS), and more recently severe acute respiratory syndrome coronavirus 2 (SARS-CoV-2) the virus that causes coronavirus disease (COVID-19), while other infections such as tuberculosis (TB) and influenza continue to circulate and in the case of influenza to evolve and change at a rapid rate.

The human body is similarly diverse, providing a home for many different types and species of microorganism. In most cases, these organisms receive benefit from the relationship without causing any harm to the host, the technical term for this being that they are commensal. This is in contrast with mutual relationships where both benefit, or parasitic ones where one benefits but damages the other. Some parts of the body have a large number of organisms, while others are normally sterile, examples of the latter being most internal organs, bones and the blood and central nervous system. If microorganisms do infect these normally sterile sites, the resulting infection is known as an invasive infection. Because this means that microorganisms have gained access to a normally sterile site, such infections are often associated with injury or serious disease. Many of the most serious infections such as meningitis, septicaemia and osteomyelitis are invasive infections.

The normal range of microorganisms found in a particular part of the body is known as the flora or microbiome, and sometimes these play an important part in host defence, for example, the normal microbiome of the gastrointestinal tract is important in preventing pathogens from colonising and growing in the gastrointestinal tract, and one of the main risk factors for Clostridioides (*Clostridium*) *difficile* infection is the use of broad spectrum antimicrobials that damage this flora. Maintenance of a healthy and balanced flora is important for this and other reasons, for example, it is thought that it helps to regulate the immune system and reduce the risk of allergy (Belkaid and Hand 2014). In addition to not using antimicrobials unnecessarily, other factors such as diet may be important, this being the rationale for the use of pre- and probiotics; prebiotics being non-digestible substances that encourage a healthy flora, while probiotics are the organisms themselves (sometimes referred to in advertising as 'friendly' or 'good' bacteria).

6.3   Treating Infections: Selective Toxicity

The aim of antimicrobial therapy is to kill or inhibit the infecting organism without damaging the host; this is known as selective toxicity. This is commonly accomplished through the use of antimicrobial drugs. The terminology surrounding the drugs used to treat infections is complex; a strict definition of the term antibiotic, for example, is that it is a substance produced by one living organism that kills or inhibits the growth of another. This definition excludes completely synthetic products which are antimicrobials, a broader term referring to any substance that has this effect.

Many of the antimicrobials in common use are true antibiotics, being isolated from bacteria and fungi, but some are not. For example, penicillin is made by a number of fungi in the genus *Penicillium* and vancomycin by a bacterium known as *Amycolatopsis orientalis*, and both are therefore true antibiotics, while ciprofloxacin and linezolid are synthetic products and so are technically antimicrobials. Some drugs, such as the newer penicillins, are semi-synthetic, which means that they have a natural base that has been altered synthetically. In practice this makes very little difference, but it does have implications for the development of resistance, as it means that some resistance genes are found in the producing organism or the environment; for example, a bacterium producing an antibacterial substance must itself be resistant to the substance it is producing if it is not to kill itself. From a resistance perspective, this becomes problematic if these resistance genes spread into medically significant bacteria (Davies and Davies 2010).

The aim of selective toxicity means that those developing antimicrobials have to identify structures or metabolic processes in the microorganism that is different to or absent from the host. In the case of bacteria, our evolutionary relationship is distant, meaning we have had a lot of time to evolve to be different and there are many selective targets; however, this is not the case with fungi to which we are more closely related and so relatively similar on a cellular basis. Viruses present a more difficult problem again, as they do not have their own metabolic or growth capabilities, instead, they use those of the host cell. This means that they are obligate intracellular organisms (they have to be inside cells to reproduce). Therefore, damaging viruses or preventing their growth usually means damaging the infected host cells, and while the immune system is able to differentiate infected from non-infected cells, it is more difficult to find drugs that are able to do this. This explains why drug formularies contain many antibacterial drugs and far fewer antifungal and antiviral drugs and why some of the latter are associated with the toxicities and adverse effects resulting from poor selective toxicity; that is they damage the microorganism but also the host. Protozoa are even more problematic because they often have a complex life cycle, are relatively similar to human cells in many respects, and are often found in developing countries with limited healthcare budgets.

6.4   Bacteria

Many serious infections are caused by bacteria, and the first task in their treatment is their identification. There are many ways of identifying bacteria, for example, by shape; by their ability to take up and retain certain stains (e.g. Gram's stain); by their susceptibility to antimicrobials (antibiogram); or, increasingly, by molecular methods. The first three of these are known as phenotypic traits, that is, they are observable characteristics; the latter are genotypic, being based on bacterial genetics. Although most tests used in everyday practice identify phenotypic characteristics, molecular and genetic methods such as the polymerase chain reaction (PCR) are becoming increasingly important.

Bacteria are prokaryotes, that is, they do not have a nucleus and, consequently, are relatively simple organisms. Because they are only distantly related to humans, there are a lot of selective targets, some of the more important of which are shown in Table 6.1. The bacterial cell wall is an important target because it is a structure that is lacking from human cells and is made of a substance known as peptidoglycan, which again human cells do not have; thus, it is a very good selective target. Bacterial ribosomes are a target not because these are lacking in humans, but because they are of different sizes, so most drugs that bind to bacterial ribosomes do not bind to the human equivalents. Similarly, some of the enzymes involved in the reproduction of bacterial nucleic acid are different to their equivalents in humans. Folic acid synthesis is an example of a metabolic process that differs between bacteria and humans; while bacteria synthesise their own folic acid, humans gain theirs from the diet. Hence, blocking the synthesis of folic acid production is selective against bacteria.

The evolutionarily distant relationship of bacteria to humans means that there are lots of differences between human and bacterial cells and so lots of selective targets. However, the clinician still needs to identify the infecting organism, establish the best treatment and deliver that treatment in a way that can resolve the infection. Although the details differ, many of these principles are common to most infections and are considered later in this chapter.

Table 6.1 Common targets in bacteria (Tenover 2006)

Target and mode of action	Examples of drug groups	Examples of drugs
Damage cell wall	*β-lactams*	
	Penicillins	Penicillin
	Cephalosporins	Cefuroxime
	Monobactams	Aztreonam
	Carbapenems	Meropenen
	β-lactam with β-lactamase inhibitor	Amoxicillin/clavulanic acid (co-amoxiclav)
	Glycopeptides	Vancomycin
Prevent protein synthesis by binding to ribosome	Macrolides	Erythromycin
	Chloramphenicol	Chloramphenicol
	Lincosamides	Clindamycin
	Streptogramins	Quinupristin-dalfopristin
	Oxazolidanones	Linezolid
	Aminoglycosides	Gentamycin
	Tetracyclines	Doxycycline
Prevent nucleic acid synthesis	Flouroquinolones	Ciprofloxacin
	Rifampicin	Rifampicin
	Nitroimidazoles	Metronidazole
Inhibit metabolic pathway	Sulfonamides	Sulfamethoxazole
	Folic acid analogues	Trimethoprim
Disrupt membrane structure	Polymixins	Colistin
	Lipopeptides	Daptomycin
Inhibit adenosine triphosphate (ATP) synthase	Diarylquinolines	Bedaquiline
Inhibit mycobacterial cell wall synthesis	Dihydro-nitroimidazooxazoles	Delamanid Pretomanid

Some bacteria are inherently difficult to treat. For example, those which have resistance mechanisms which will be considered later. Others are difficult to treat because they grow or reproduce slowly, or have 'resting' stages where they form spores. Most antimicrobials work by inhibiting or preventing growth or reproduction, so slowly growing or spore-forming organsisms are often difficult to treat.

Mycobacterium tuberculosis which causes tuberculosis is one such organism which can be both slow-growing and has a dormant state (Connolly et al. 2007). This requires complex and long-term treatments which can be difficult for people to take. The result of this is often partially treated infection and the development and spread of antimicrobial resistance. The general treatments for tuberculosis have not change very much for many years; however, there have been recent developments with novel anti-mycobacterial agents, most notably bedaquiline which targets mycobacterial adenosine triphosphate (ATP) synthase. As ATP synthesis is a key part of energy production needed for replicating and non-replicating cells alike, targeting this key process leads to cell death and so is bactericidal (Goulooze et al. 2015). Its selective toxicity comes from human ATP synthase having a 20,000-fold lower sensitivity to the drug than the mycobacterial equivalent (Haagsma et al.

2009). Delamanid is another relatively recent anti-tuberculosis drug. This works by inhibiting the synthesis of the mycobacterial cell wall components methoxymycolic acid and ketomycolic acid (Matsumoto et al. 2006). Both drugs are generally recommended for resistant TB where other drugs are not suitable.

Clostridioides difficile (formerly known as *Clostridium difficile*) is another challenging organism. Its acquisition and spread is associated with the use of broad spectrum antibiotics, older age, and hospitalization. This combination of risk factors means that those likely to have it are already likely to be ill and in a position to transmit it to others. It also forms spores which are like 'resting' stages, and are hard to treat and may survive in the environment for long periods. The traditional mainstay of treatment has been oral vancomycin. A newer alternative is fidxomicin, which is a macrocyclic drug with a relatively narrow Gram-positive spectrum of activity. It also has little effect against the normal colonic microbiotica (Czepiel et al. 2019). Although fidoxomicin has been shown to be more effective in some circumstances, it is substantially more expensive making it a second-line drug in most cases (National Institute for Health and Care Excellence n.d.).

A less positive recent development concerns the flouroquinolones, a very important group of drugs which includes imipenem and meropenem. Although these are highly effective broad-spectrum antibacterials their use has been associated with an increase in the risk of tendon, muscular joint, nerve, and mental health problems. As a result of this guidance now recommends that systemic fluoroquinolones should only be prescribed when other recommended antimicrobials are inappropriate (Medicines and Healthcare Products Regulatory Agency n.d.).

Priority Areas in Antibacterial Research

Based on their assessment of the need for research and development and the public health importance of each, the World Health Organization regularly prioritises a number of bacterial pathogens. The critical group have been identified as *Acinetobacter baumannii* (carbapenem-resistant), Enterobacterales (third-generation cephalosporin-resistant), Enterobacterales (carbapenem-resistant), *Mycobacterium tuberculosis* (rifampicin-resistant); those which are considered of high importance are *Salmonella Typhi* (fluoroquinolone-resistant), *Shigella* spp. (Fluoroquinolone-resistant), *Enterococcus faecium* (vancomycin-resistant), *Pseudomonas aeruginosa* (carbapenem-resistant), Non-typhoidal *Salmonella* (fluoroquinolone-resistant), *Neisseria gonorrhoeae* (third-generation cephalosporin, and/or fluoroquinolone-resistant), *Staphylococcus aureus* (methicillin-resistant); while the medium group are Group A Streptococci (macrolide-resistant), Streptococcus pneumoniae (macrolide-resistant), Haemophilus influenzae (ampicillin-resistant), Group B Streptococci (penicillin-resistant). This list is interesting both as an indication of significant pathogens, and resistance patterns that are of particular concern (World Health Organization 2024).

6.5 Fungi

Because fungi are relatively closely related to humans, compared to bacteria, they have had less time to evolve differences, and so fewer selective targets exist (Table 6.2). This means that there are far fewer drugs to treat fungal infections than there are to treat bacterial infections, and many of those which do exist, particularly older antifungal drugs, have toxicities associated with them. A further complication is that many people who have severe systemic fungal diseases also have comorbidities, in particular, immunodeficiencies, further compromising the ability to treat the infection. Fungi can take two main forms: a yeast-like form that usually grows on surfaces and a hyphal form where it grows as finger-like projections that can force their way between cells and so become invasive; this is sometimes referred to as being a 'mould' (one may see these growing on bread). *Candida* species are examples of the former, and *Aspergillus* the latter. In addition, some fungi can take both forms, these are known as dimorphic fungi.

Most antifungal agents work by inhibiting the cell wall or membrane which is the main difference between fungal and human cells. Human cells do not have a cell wall, and the fungal cell wall which contains glucan and chitin, is the target for a range of drugs. The other main target is ergosterol which is a component of the fungal cell membrane, a structure that humans do have but in fungi the membrane sterol is ergosterol, in humans the equivalent is cholesterol. Although there is a difference between these two sterols, the difference is not great, reducing the selective toxicity and explaining some of the toxicities associated with the main drugs that bind to this the polyene drugs amphotericin B and nystatin. Amphotericin, which has historically been the most important drug for treatment of severe fungal disease, has a range of toxicities including nausea, vomiting, rigours, fever and hypotension or hypertension. However, of most concern is its effect upon the renal system, where it can cause nephrotoxicity, particularly in those individuals with existing renal problems, on high doses, who are dehydrated or on other nephrotoxic drugs (Laniado-Laborín and Cabrales-Vargas 2009). These can partly be overcome through the use of liposomal preparations, where the drug is contained within a lipid bilayer. The liposome is formulated to maximize the anti-fungal activity of the drug while minimizing drug-related toxicity (Stone et al. 2016).

These adverse effects are reduced in those drugs that inhibit its production rather than bind to it and in liposomal preparations where the amphotericin molecules are enclosed in a lipid membrane. Additionally, polyenes are not absorbed through the

Table 6.2 Main antifungal targets

Target	Drugs
Cell wall—Glucan inhibitors	Echinocandins (caspofungin, micafungin)
Cell membrane—Ergosterol binders	Polyenes (amphotericin B, nystatin)
Cell membrane—Ergosterol inhibitors	Azoles (ketoconazole, itraconazole, fluconazole, voriconazole, posaconazole, ravuconazole)

gastrointestinal tract, making nystatin a safe drug for the topical treatment of superficial fungal infections. Less commonly used drugs include flucytosine which inhibits fungal nucleic acid synthesis, griseofulvin which has the same effect upon microtubules and the polyoxins and nikkomycin which inhibit chitin in the fungal cell wall (Kathiravan et al. 2012).

One major drug has been approved recently, that is Rezafungin, a long-acting echinocandin (Garcia-Effron 2020). Primarily indicated for the treatment of invasive candidiasis, it can be given as a loading dose, then once a week. Other antifungals in development include Olorofim from a novel class of drugs known as orotomides which inhibit pyrimidine synthesis, damaging the cell wall and resulting in cell lysis (Wiederhold 2020); and Fosmanogepix which interrupts the trafficking and anchoring of mannoproteins to the cell membrane and cell wall (Shaw and Ibrahim 2020). Because both are novel drugs, they may eventually be used to treat fungal isolates that are resistant to existing classes of drugs.

Priority Areas in Antifungal Research

Based on their assessment of the need for research and development and the public health importance of each, the World Health Organization regularly prioritises a number of fungal pathogens. The critical group have been identified as *Cryptococcus neoformans*, *Candida auris*, *Aspergillus fumigatus* and *Candida albicans*; those which are considered of high importance are *Nakaseomyces glabrata* (Candida glabrata), *Histoplasma* spp., eumycetoma causative agents, *Mucorales*, *Fusarium* spp., *Candida tropicalis* and *Candida parapsilosis*; while the medium group are *Scedosporium* spp., *Lomentospora prolificans*, *Coccidioides* spp., *Pichia kudriavzeveii* (Candida krusei), *Cryptococcus gattii*, *Talaromyces marneffei*, *Pneumocystis jirovecii* and *Paracoccidioides* spp. This list is interesting both as an indication of significant pathogens, and because some of the names may be different to those in common use. Renaming organisms usually happens when new information suggests that different evolutionary lineages (World Health Organization 2022).

6.6 Viruses

Viruses are simple organisms that have no metabolism of their own. Consequently, they have to use the metabolism of host cells to replicate, making them obligate intracellular pathogens. This is problematic for treating viral infections because it means there are few selective targets, and while the immune system is able to differentiate infected from non-infected cells, it is hard to produce drugs that can damage or inhibit infected cells while leaving uninfected cells alone; and targeting all cells would lead to severe toxicity or even death. Consequently, most therapies in this area have tended to maximise immunity through immunisation rather than treat established infections.

Viruses that can most successfully be treated are usually those which have something in their structure or replication cycle which is different to or not found in human cells. The first viruses to be successfully treated were the herpes viruses, in particular, cytomegalovirus (CMV), varicella-zoster virus (VZV) and herpes simplex virus type 1 (HSV1) and type 2 (HSV2). These can be treated using drugs such as acyclovir that inhibit viral DNA polymerase, which is the enzyme that copies viral DNA during replication. Its selective toxicity stems from its specificity for the viral polymerase rather than the human equivalent, and because the drugs are inactive in the form given needing to be activated by phosphorylation which is preferentially done by a viral enzyme known as thymidine kinase. Although humans also have this enzyme, the drug is specific for the viral version, hence its selective toxicity.

The human immunodeficiency virus (HIV) is among the most significant human pathogens in history. HIV is a retrovirus, meaning that it uses a viral-specific enzyme known as reverse transcriptase (RNA-dependent DNA polymerase) to turn the viral RNA genome into DNA. This DNA copy is then integrated into the DNA genome of the infected cell using another viral enzyme known as integrase. Although human cells make DNA copies of DNA when cells replicate and mRNA copies of DNA for protein production, they never produce DNA copies of RNA. Because of this, the reverse transcriptase enzyme has to be produced from the viral genome and so is a highly selective and important target for anti-HIV drugs. There are two groups of drugs that target this enzyme, the nucleoside reverse transcriptase inhibitors (NRTI) which mimic the normal nucleotides and nuclosides in the DNA genome. They are then incorporated into the newly formed viral DNA by reverse transcriptase, but as they lack a 3′-hydroxyl group reverse transcriptase is unable to add the next nucleotide, bringing the process to an end. This is quite a common strategy for anti-viral drugs, and is similar to that used by acyclovir. Non-nucleoside reverse transcriptase inhibitors (NNRTI) generally bind to the active site of reverse transcriptase.

Another viral enzyme, protease, is the third major target as it is required for viral assembly and maturation. Although the human body does contain proteases, these are different to the viral enzyme, again making this a good selective target. Drugs that target this enzyme are known as protease inhibitors (PIs). Another important target for the treatment of HIV is the integration of the newly formed HIV DNA into that of the host cell. Integrase strand transfer inhibitors (INSTI) that prevent the incorporation of the viral genome into that of the host cell have become increasingly important within many HIV treatment regimens due to their lower toxicity compared to NNRTI and PI options and equal to slightly superior levels of viral suppression. Other drugs target the process of viral binding and entry into the cell. These drugs have the potential to prevent cells becoming infected in the first place, not merely preventing or reducing viral replication after infection.

In order to maximise the effectiveness of these drugs and to reduce the risk of resistance developing, they are given in combinations of drugs from at least two of the groups. This is often referred to as ART which is short for anti-retroviral therapy. A new approach to treating HIV is the long-acting injectable combination of cabotegravir (INSTI) and rilpivirine (NNRTI) (sometimes shortened to CAB-RPV) which can be given every 2 months. This may be particularly useful for people who are not able to take oral drugs consistently (Sax et al. 2024). Because the risk of transmission is related to the viral load, effective treatment raises the prospect of eradicating HIV (Joint United Nations Programme on HIV/AIDS (UNAIDS) 2023).

The Role of Antimicrobials in COVID-19

Coronaviruses are viruses with a single-stranded RNA genome. They have been responsible for a number of epidemics, most notably SARS (Severe acute respiratory syndrome) and MeRS (Middle East respiratory syndrome), and more recently the COVID-19 pandemic. The impact of this virus on individuals and society demonstrates the complexity of the management and treatment of infectious diseases, and the need to adapt these as the organism evolves and knowledge develops. Non-pharmacological interventions formed an important part of the COVID-19 prevention and control strategies. Pharmacological approaches take three main forms:

- Vaccination
- Immunotherapy and immunomodulation
- Treatments for infection

Vaccines

Over the course of the COVID-19 pandemic a number of different vaccines were produced. Vaccines have two mechanisms of action: the direct protection of those receiving the vaccine, the individual-level effect; and providing herd immunity by leaving too few unprotected people for the disease to circulate widely in the community, this is the population-level effect. Vaccines may prevent the organism colonising a person sometimes referred to as sterilising immunity; or allow colonisation but prevent severe disease.

Currently there are two main vaccine technologies used for COVID-19. The first are mRNA (messenger RNA) vaccines. mRNA is used by cells to produce proteins. RNA polymerases make mRNA copies of genes which are then translated into proteins. Cells in the vicinity of the injection site take up the injected mRNA and subsequently produce the peptides that make up the spike protein which forms part of the structure of the virus. This is similar to the process of protein production in viral infection, resulting in a strong immune response. It is important to understand that mRNA is translated into proteins in the cytoplasm of the cell, it does not enter the nucleus, and it is quickly broken down (Han et al. 2021).

Other vaccines administer a small part of the virus to which it is hoped immunity will develop. The manufacturing process involves using recombinant DNA technology to make laboratory cells produce viral spike proteins which can then be injected. This is referred to as a recombinant form of the SARS-CoV-2 spike protein, allowing immunity to the spike protein to develop without exposure to the virus. Because this approach does not mimic the viral lifecycle in the same way as the mRNA vaccine, another substance referred to as an adjuvant is added to improve the immune response (Moderna 2024; Novavax 2024; Pfizer-BioNTech 2024).

One vaccine that was widely used, but is no longer available made use of a viral vector. These use a harmless virus (the vector) to deliver the spike protein genes which are then taken up and processed by cells just as any virus would be. One extensively administered vaccine used single recombinant, replication-deficient chimpanzee adenovirus vector encoding the spike glycoprotein of SARS-CoV-2 (AstraZeneca 2022). Other possible approaches include live attenuated vaccines which use a virus which is able to replicate but not cause severe disease (these are widely used for influenzas vaccines), killed or inactive vaccines (for example, the injected polio vaccine), and non-replicating viruses and virus-like particles.

Immunotherapy and Immunomodulation
The aim of this approach to treatment is to prevent the excessive immune response and the 'cytokine storm' associated with severe COVID-19 disease (Al-Hajeri et al. 2022). Clearly there is a balance to be struck here, as an appropriate immune response is important.

Corticosteroids regulate and reduce the immune response through a variety of actions on the innate (non-specific) and acquired (specific) immune systems (Cain and Cidlowski 2017).

IL-6 receptor blockers inhibit the production of interleukin-6, a pro-inflammatory and pyrectic cytokine produced by macrophages as part of the innate immune system.

Baricitinib is a drug that was originally developed for the treatment of more severe cases of conditions such as rheumatoid arthritis and atopic dermatitis. This is a Janus kinase (JAK) 1 and 2 inhibitor, which interferes with the JAK-STAT signalling pathway and so inhibits the production of inflammatory cytokines (Shawky et al. 2022).

Treatments for COVID-19 Infection
There are many candidate drugs for the treatment of COVID-19, yet few have proven efficacy or effectiveness. This is partly due to the complexity of producing drugs that can interrupt the viral lifecycle without causing significant damage to the host. Currently, the two main targets are the viral RNA-dependent RNA-polymerase (RdRp) and protease.

Drugs targeting the viral RNA polymerase using nucleoside or nucleotide analogues. These drugs mimic natural nucleotides or nucleosides and so can be incorporated into the viral genome in their place. The result of this is either termination of nucleic acid synthesis (known as chain termination), or the accumulation of mutations that leads to non-functional RNA (error catastrophe or lethal mutagenesis) or damages its chemical structure (chemical corruption) (Shannon and Canard 2023). Monlupavir is a prodrug that is converted in the body to the active form N-hydroxycytidine (NHC). Its incorporation in the viral genome by the viral RdRp is thought to cause genetic corruption leading to eventual error catastrophe (Maas et al. 2024; Shannon and Canard 2023). Remdesivir is also a prodrug, that is converted into remdesivir-triphosphate, an analogue of the normal adenosine tri-phosphate which can be incorporated into new viral RNA by RdRp leading to delayed chain termination and chemical corruption of the structure of the RNA molecule (Eastman et al. 2020; Shannon and Canard 2023).

Nirmatrelvir/Ritonavir is a combination of two drugs, the main active component is nirmatrelvir which major inhibits the major protease (Mpro) responsible for turning the long polyprotein produced during viral replication into the individual proteins needed to build the virus. Although ritonavir is also a protease inhibitor its main purpose is to inhibit the cytochrome P450 3A enzyme that metabolises nirmatrelvir so increasing its half-life in the body (Hashemian et al. 2023).

Different approaches to treating viruses are shown in the treatment of hepatitis B and C viruses. Because hepatitis B has both RNA and DNA polymerases, some of the reverse transcriptase inhibitors used for the treatment of HIV also have activity against it. Other approaches to the treatment of this virus and hepatitis C virus include therapies aimed at improving the immune response, known as immunomodulators; these include drugs such as interferons, which are antiviral substances produced by the body in response to viral infections (Antonelli and Turriziani 2012; Littler and Oberg 2005).

6.7 Parasites—The Protozoa and Helminths

The term parasitology is normally applied to the study and treatment of protozoa, helminths or worms, and ectoparasites.

Protozoa: Theses single celled-organisms include some important human pathogens. There are a number of distinct groups of protozoa:

- Mastigophora which are flagellated, for example *Giardia, Leishmania*
- Sarcodina which are amoeboid, for example *Entamoeba*
- Sporozoa/Apicomplexa which includes *Babesia, Plasmodium* spp., *Cryptosporidium parvum*, and *Toxoplasma gondii*. This group includes some of the most important human pathogens, most notably those that cause malaria *Plasmodium falciparum, Plasmodium vivax, Plasmodium ovale, Plasmodium malariae* and *Plasmodium knowlesi*.
- Ciliated protozoa or ciliates such as *Balantidium coli*

Helminths are worms, which can be sub-divided into the following:

- Flatworms (also known as platyhelminths) which include trematodes (flukes) and cestodes (tapeworms). Trematodes are often grouped according to the area of the body in which they cause disease. These include intestinal trematodes/flukes, lung trematodes/flukes, and liver trematodes/flukes.
- Nematodes (roundworms). The most common nematodes are the roundworm (*Ascaris lumbricoides*), the whipworm (*Trichuris trichiura*) and hookworms (*Necator americanus* and *Ancylostoma duodenale*).

Ectoparasites live on or externally to the host, including fleas, ticks and lice.

The treatment of some of these organisms, particularly those such as the *Plasmodium* spp. which have different intra-cellular, extra-cellular, or dormant stages can be complex. Some of the more important drugs are now discussed:

Praziquantel is used to treat cestodes (tapeworms) and trematodes such as schistosomes. It does this by increasing membrane Ca^{2+} permeability, leading to paralysis in the contracted state and disrupting the exterior surface of the worm (Chan et al. 2013).

Albendazole and mebendazole can be used to treat a wide variety of nematodes, trematodes, cestodes, and some protozoans. The work by inhibiting the polymerization of ß-tubulin into microtubules and reducing glucose uptake leading to glycogen depletion. They also inhibit cell division because these prevent spindle fibre formation (Chai et al. 2021).

Ivermectin has activity against a variety of gastrointestinal nematodes, lungworms, lice and mange. Its main effect is to open inhibitory glutamate-gated chloride ion channels allowing an influx of negatively charged Cl, leading to hyperpolarisation of cell membranes (Martin et al. 2021).

Artemisinin has a complex and not completely understood mechanism of action against *Plasmodium* spp. It seems to damage the mitochondria of the malarial parasite, causing damage to lipids and proteins, and by acting on hemin within the parasite to form toxic oxygenated products (Khanal 2021).

Primaquine is used for patients with P. vivax or P. ovale to prevent relapse from dormant liver-stage hypnozoites.

Metranidazole is active against a variety of anaerobic bacteria and protozoal organisms where it causes damage to DNA. In order to have this action, it needs to be converted into its active form through reduction by reduced ferredoxin to form nitroso radicals. This electron transfer from can only take place in the presence of pyruvate:ferredoxin oxidoreductase (PFOR) which is absent in eukaryotes and other bacteria. Additionally, oxygen competes with metronidazole for these electrons in oxygenated environments (Samuelson 1999).

6.7.1 Choosing an Antimicrobial

It is important when treating infections that the most appropriate antimicrobial is used. Choosing an antimicrobial regimen is complex and involves clinical experience and interpreting test results, but at the same time being careful not to overuse drugs that might ultimately result in resistance and reduced effectiveness in the future. There are four questions that a clinician needs to ask in this respect (Leibovici et al. 1999):

1. Based on the prescriber's understanding and results of tests, is this the right drug for the known or likely infection?
2. Is the balance of likely benefit against harm appropriate in this case?
3. Given the cost of the drug, is its use appropriate?
4. Is there an equally good option which would be less likely to promote resistant organisms?

Recent guidance from National Institute for Health and Care Excellence (NICE) in the United Kingdom (National Institute for Health and Care Excellence 2015) states that when prescribing antimicrobials the prescriber should follow any local or national guidance on:

- Prescribing the shortest effective course.
- At the most appropriate dose.
- Using the best route of administration.

Unlike any other treatments though, the antimicrobial prescriber has an additional consideration, which is the likelihood of antimicrobial resistance developing at either the individual or population levels.

In some cases treatment can be delayed until test results are known (remembering that false-negative results, or contamination resulting in a false-positive may occur); but in others such as febrile neutropenia, this is not possible and empirical therapy may be needed while awaiting test results.

There are a variety of tests that are used in informing antimicrobial use, but they all aim to help the clinician find the best drug for the infecting organism. Depending upon the results, each drug-microorganism combination can be put into one of three categories (Rodloff et al. 2008):

1. Susceptible: The bacterium is inhibited in vitro by a concentration of the drug that is associated with a high likelihood of therapeutic success.
2. Intermediately resistant: The bacterium is inhibited in vitro by a concentration of the drug that is associated with an uncertain therapeutic effect.
3. Resistant: The bacterium is inhibited in vitro by a concentration of the drug that is associated with a high likelihood of therapeutic failure.

These are usually calculated using breakpoints and the drug-bacterium minimum inhibitory concentration. A breakpoint is a specified concentration of an antimicrobial which is used to define susceptibility or resistance of a bacteria to it. The susceptibility of a particular organism is based on this and the minimum inhibitory concentration or MIC of the specific organism, which is the lowest (or minimum) concentration of the antimicrobial which inhibits the growth of the organism. If the MIC is equal to or less than the breakpoint that defines susceptibility, the bacteria is categorised as being susceptible to that antibiotic; if it is more, it is either resistant or intermediately resistant (British Society for Antimicrobial Chemotherapy 2018).

For example, the current breakpoint between susceptibility and resistance for vancomycin for the treatment of *Staphylococcus aureus* is defined by the minimum concentration of the drug that will stop the bacterium from growing, currently set at a level of 2 mg/L. If it is less than or equal to this, it is sensitive; if above this, it is resistant. This is based on the minimum concentration that inhibits growth; it is not necessarily the same as the concentration that kills the bacterium (the minimum bactericidal concentration). For practical reasons, most tests are based on inhibition rather than killing the bacteria. There is no intermediate category between these two outcomes as vancomycin is a toxic drug and higher doses cannot usually be given to account for this. This is in contrast to drugs such as penicillin, where higher doses can usually be safely given.

The most common tests used are those using phenotypic traits (these are things that are measureable or observable); for example, microscopy, culture and sensitivity (MC&S), but genotypic tests looking for specific microbial genes and molecular tests are increasingly being used. These have the benefit of not requiring the laboratory to be able to grow the organism, as it does for tests such as MC&S. Such techniques include polymerase chain reaction (PCR), high-throughput genome sequencing and matrix-assisted laser desorption/ionization–time-of-flight mass spectrometry (MALDI-TOF MS).

When interpreting any test result, one must be aware of the possibilities of false-positive, or in this case the more likely scenario of false-negative results, where the test fails to identify an infecting organism. While there are many reasons why this may occur, an important consideration is that laboratory conditions do not replicate those found in the human body, and in particular the attempt to culture individual species does not reflect the polymicrobial nature of the body where multiple species and subspecies interact.

6.8 Delivering the Drug

Choosing the best drug to treat a particular infection is only part of the answer. The next part is to deliver the drug to the site of the infection in sufficient quantities or concentrations to achieve the desired outcome. The science of how drugs move from the site of administration to site of activity and their subsequent elimination is known as pharmacokinetics, while the concentration of the drug as it relates to its clinical effect is known as pharmacodynamics.

As most drugs are taken orally or given intravenously, getting a drug into the bloodstream is relatively straightforward. However, most infections occur in the tissues, and so the drug needs to be able to leave the bloodstream and get to the site of the infection. In some cases, where the blood supply is poor or absent, this can be particularly problematic. For example, the cornea has a limited blood supply, which is why many eye medications are given as eye drops. More problematic can be infections of implantable devices, such as orthopaedic implants, necrotic tissue or abscesses, all of which have limited or no blood supply. Therefore, the serum concentration of a drug is unlikely to be representative of the actual concentration at the site of infection, unless this is the bloodstream. One way of remembering this is that whatever the blood results are saying about serum concentrations of antimicrobials, 'it is the tissue that is the issue'.

Another problematic type of infection is that which occurs on hard surfaces, such as orthopaedic implants. Layers of bacteria and other microorganisms can form, known as biofilms. While those on the top of the film can be treated, those in the deeper layers of the biofilm are more difficult to treat, partly because of the physical protection of those above, but also because they are often metabolically less active. Biofilms that form on implantable devices, such as orthopaedic implants, also benefit from the lack of blood supply making it difficult to deliver sufficient concentrations of the drug to the site of the infection, making them even more difficult to treat successfully. Biofilms can be extremely complicated, and in some cases a number of different organisms can form a stable and difficult to treat community of organisms.

6.9 Antimicrobial Dosing

Most antimicrobial drugs express their effect either through being static (e.g. bacteriostatic) or cidal (bactericidal). Static drugs stop the organism from growing but do not necessarily kill it; cidal drugs generally kill the microorganism at concentrations that can be achieved clinically.

Antimicrobials may also be concentration or time-dependent. Concentration-dependent drugs usually have a longer action, and many are taken up by the target organism. In these cases, the important issue with regard to dosing is not how many doses a patient has, but what concentration of the drug can be achieved, so these are generally given in fewer but larger doses. With time-dependent drugs on the other hand, the important parameter is not the maximum dose, but the length of time that the drug persists above the MIC at the site of infection. These drugs tend to be given in smaller but more frequent doses. Gentamicin is an example of a concentration-dependent drug; hence, it is usually given in one large dose, while penicillin which is time-dependent is normally given a multiple daily doses to maximise its time over the MIC.

In general, the best approach to treatment is to give a single highly targeted antimicrobial. However, there are many exceptions to this rule, for example, in those who are immunosuppressed and for whom waiting for test results is not an option or who might be at an increased risk of polymicrobial infection with more than one organism. In these cases, the treatment approach might be to give combination empirical therapy (empirical meaning treatment based not on test results, but on knowledge and experience of what they are most likely to have). As there is limited information available, such therapies are often less targeted and broad spectrum antimicrobial medications are prescribed (the spectrum referring to the range of organisms targeted by the drug). In addition to broadening the spectrum of the therapy, combinations might also show synergy, that is, the drugs work better together than on their own. However, by increasing the spectrum of the therapy the risk of drug interactions and adverse reactions is increased, as is the cost of the treatment, and more damage is likely to be done to the normal flora of the body, increasing the risk of opportunistic infections such as *C. difficile*.

6.10 Resistance

Antimicrobial resistance has become a matter of increasing concern in recent years. It is important to be clear about the difference between intrinsic and acquired resistance. Intrinsic resistance occurs where some feature of an organism means that it is inherently undamaged by an antimicrobial. For example, Gram-negative bacteria have an outer membrane that prevents glycopeptides such as vancomycin from accessing the cell wall where the drug is active, making the bacteria intrinsically resistant to these drugs (Cox and Wright 2013). This being a feature of this group of bacteria, there is nothing that can be done to prevent this. A more serious problem is that of acquired resistance, where a previously susceptible organism develops a new resistance to one or more groups of antibiotics. The latter is known as multiple resistance and is often seen in methicillin-resistant Staphylococcus aureus (MRSA). One particularly concerning development is the acquisition of vancomycin resistance by MRSA, which may already be resistant to a range of antimicrobials including all β-lactams apart from perhaps the new fifth generation cephalosprins which are active against MRSA, macrolides, aminoglycosides, fluoroquinolones and tetraclines; and for which vancomycin would normally be the treatment of choice (Appelbaum 2007; Foster 2017).

Bacteria can become resistant in two main ways: the first is that they undergo a genetic mutation that changes an antimicrobial target in some way (Hughes and Andersson 2017) and the second is that they acquire resistance genes from another bacterium or the environment. While the first of these are chance events, the sheer number of bacteria means that such mutations probably occur quite frequently. Most of these will not cause resistance, and may actually be damaging to the bacterium, but a small number may confer resistance allowing that bacterium to survive or grow in the presence of the antimicrobial.

Probably more problematic than this is the acquisition of resistance genes, either from other bacteria or the environment (Sultan et al. 2018). This most commonly occurs in one of three ways (Gillings and Stokes 2012):

1. Acquisition of resistance genes from the environment, a process known as transformation (remember that many antimicrobials are produced by organisms which therefore need resistance genes to survive their own antibiotic).
2. Transfer of resistance genes from one bacterium to another by viruses, a process known as transduction.
3. The direct physical transfer of resistance genes from one bacterium to another, through a process known as conjugation.

Conjugation usually involves larger genetic elements that may contain a number of different resistance genes, or possible genes for toxins or other traits that aid bacterial survival. There are a number of different types of such genetic elements, the most complex being plasmids which may contain many different genes, and acquisition of such a plasmid by a bacterium might confer multiple resistances upon that bacterium. Plasmids may also contain genes encoding for toxins, in which case the bacterium may be capable of causing severe disease.

The development of resistance is almost inevitable when antimicrobials are used. This is because populations of microorganisms are heterogenous, that is to say all are a little different; for example, some will be very susceptible to an antimicrobial, while others may be a less susceptible. This is sometimes referred to as heteroresistance. Often a resistance mechanism reduces growth rates of organisms that have it, meaning that they are less likely to predominate than their susceptible equivalents.

For example, a thickened cell-wall might reduce susceptibility but it might also take longer to grow. However, the use of that antimicrobial, particularly if the dose is not sufficient or it is not given for sufficient time may result in it killing the susceptible organisms but not the less susceptible ones, turning the disadvantage of resistance into an advantage and allowing them to 'take over'. Over time this leads to selection of resistant organism, the use of the antimicrobial resulting in 'selection pressure' for resistance. Although this may seem complicated, it is a simple Darwinian selection occurring as a result of antimicrobial use. This is the reason why antimicrobials are fundamentally different to all other medicines; they have both an individual effect (curing the infection) and a population effect (selection for resistance), and sometimes these conflict (Sandoval-Motta and Aldana 2016). The main mechanisms of resistance are shown in Table 6.3.

The World Health Organization adopted a global action plan on antimicrobial resistance in 2015 (World Health Organization 2015), which contained five objectives:

1. To improve awareness and understanding of antimicrobial resistance
2. To strengthen the knowledge and evidence base through surveillance and research
3. To reduce the incidence of infection through effective sanitation, hygiene and infection prevention measures
4. To optimize the use of antimicrobial medicines in human and animal health
5. To increase investment in new medicines, diagnostic tools, vaccines and other interventions

The last point, although perhaps the most obvious, is not without its difficulties, in particular the long development period required for human medicines and the

Table 6.3 Mechanisms of resistance in bacteria (Giedraitienė et al. 2011; Kapoor et al. 2017)

Category of resistance	Example of resistance	Examples of organisms
Altered target prevents the drug from binding	Altered penicillin binding proteins in cell wall	Methicillin resistant *S. aureus*
	Change in cell wall structure	Glycopeptide resistant *S. aureus*
Decreased permeability or uptake prevents the drug from entering the cell	Change in outer membrane permeability	Multiple resistances in *Pseudomonas aeruginosa*
Efflux mechanisms pump the drug out of the cell	Acquired and chromosomally encoded efflux pumps	*Acinetobacter baumannii* multiple resistance
Enzymatic degradation breaks the drug down or changes its structure	β-lactamase enzymes that degrade β-lactam drugs	*Klebsiella peumoniae* that produce extended spectrum β-lactamases
Target overproduction overwhelms the drug	Overproduction of cell wall components targeted by glycopeptides	Vancomycin intermediately resistant *S. Aureus*

relatively poor financial return that drug companies receive from antimicrobials compared to other drug groups.

Current Issues in Antimicrobial Resistance

There are many current issues in the treatment of resistant infections. These include bacteria that are inherently hard to treat, such as *P. aeruginosa which is resistant to many drugs due to a relatively impermeable* outer membrane, efflux pumps, and the enzymatic deactivation of some antibacterial drugs. Two other major issues are the development and spread of β-lactamases and methicillin resistance, which are discussed below.

Extended-Spectrum β-Lactamases

β-lactamases are enzymes that are able to hydrolyze (break down) the active part of β-lactam drugs. This very large and important group of drugs includes the penicillins, cephalosporins, carbapenems, and monobactams. There are a number of different β-lactamase enzymes which have different effects, with not all affecting all drugs. One group, the extended spectrum β-lactamases (ESBLs) are able to confer bacterial resistance to a broad range of β-lactams, including the penicillins, the first (cefalexin, cefadroxil), second (cefuroxime, cefaclor), and third (ceftazidime, ceftriaxone, and cefotaxime) generation cephalosporins, and aztreonam. They do not however affect the cephamycins or carbapenems (ertapenem, meropenem, imipenem) and are inhibited by β-lactamase inhibitors such as clavulanic acid and avibactam (Paterson and Bonomo 2005).

Organisms that most commonly produce ESBLs include members of the Enterobacterales, including *Escherichia coli*, *Klebsiella pneumoniae*, *Klebsiella oxytoca*, and *Proteus mirabilis*. You may hear these collectively referred to as ESBL-E (extended spectrum β-lactamases producing Enterobacterales). Carbapenems are often considered to be the first-line treatment for ESBL-E infections outside of the urinary tract (Tamma et al. 2022). Different treatments are usually needed for treating urinary infections because of the range of causative organisms, and the need for renal elimination and its concentration of the drug in the urine (Abbott et al. 2023).

The role of the carbapenems for the treatment of ESBL-E infections is notable because these are β-lactams with a very broad spectrum of activity including many Gram-negative and Gram-positive bacteria making their use superficially attractive (Papp-Wallace et al. 2011). However, their increased use has led to the development and spread of another group of β-lactamases, the carbapenemases.

Carbapenemases are β-lactamases that can hydrolyze a broader range of drugs including the cephalosporins, carbapenems and monobactams. This means that bacteria that carry this resistance mechanism are resistant to most β-lactam drugs including the carbapenems. As discussed previously, the carbapenems are among the recommended treatments for ESBL-E infections. This resistance can be transferred between bacterial strains, and often co-exists alongside resistance to other antimicrobials leading to multiple resistance.

The recommended treatment for carbapenem-resistant Enterobacterales (CRE) infections outside of the urinary tract are β-lactam/ β-lactamase inhibitor combinations, including ceftazidime-avibactam, meropenem-vaborbactam, and imipenem-cilastatin-relebactam, with tigecycline and eravacycline from the broad tetracycline-class being alternative options (Tamma et al. 2022). Again, different treatments are generally required for urinary infections.

Methicillin Resistant *Staphylococcus aureus* (MRSA)

Staphylococcus aureus is a bacterium that provides a good lesson in microbial adaptability and evolution. Even before its introduction into clinical practice in the early 1940s it was known that some isolates were not susceptible because they produced enzymes known as penicillinases. In 1959 a penicillinase resistant drug, methicillin was introduced into practice. By 1961 the first cases of what became known as MRSA were reported (Jevons 1961). By 2002, resistance to vancomycin which is the primary treatment for MRSA was reported in *S. aureus* (Centers for Disease Control and Prevention (CDC) 2002). Although this has not spread as quickly and as far as many had feared, it is a salutary lesson on microbial evolution in the face of antimicrobial pressure.

Methicillin-sensitive and resistant *Staphylococcus aureus* (MSSA/MRSA) cause a wide variety of infections. Additionally, some isolates produce toxins that can lead to very severe disease. These include pore-forming toxins (PFTs), exfoliative toxins (ETs) and superantigens (SAgs) (Oliveira et al. 2018). Although traditionally associated with healthcare institutions, community strains of MRSA also exist some of which produce a toxin known as Panton Valentine Leukocidin. For most MRSA infections recent UK guidance suggests first line treatments using vancomycin or teichoplanin, with linezolid as an alternative. Older American guidance puts greater emphasis upon daptomycin although this should never be used for pneumonia as it is inactivated by surfactant (Liu et al. 2011). Newer anti-staphylococcal drugs include the fifth generation cephalosporins ceftobiprole and ceftaroline; the fluoroquinolone delafloxacin, an oxazolidinone tedizolid, and the lipoglycopeptides telavancin and oritavancin. Some antimicrobials have particular characteristics that can be used, for example clindamycin and rifampicin have toxin-inhibiting effects as well as their direct antimicrobial action, which may be beneficial for the treatment of necrotizing infections (Brown et al. 2021). However, overall there remains a lack of high-quality evidence on which to base practice (Mahjabeen et al. 2022).

6.10.1 Antimicrobial Policies

All healthcare organisations should have an antimicrobial policy, which aims to guide clinicians as to the best and most rational use of these drugs. Such policies have a number of aims, specifically to:

1. Ensure that a sufficient range of antimicrobials remain available
2. Guide prescribing
3. Avoid their unnecessary use
4. Reduce the emergence and spread of resistance
5. Promote good practice
6. Contain costs (Mayon-White and Wiffen 2005)

Although the exact content will differ between institutions as the type of patient treated and local resistance patterns might vary, they should include guidance as to the treatment of common infections, including dosages and special considerations or cautions, details of who to contact for advice in the treatment of infection and details of restricted drugs, for example, new or expensive drugs, or those which for other reasons such as resistance are restricted. Some of this information is available on a national basis from the British National Formulary or other national formularies, although this needs to be read and interpreted in light of local conditions.

6.11 Opportunistic Infections

Some groups are at particularly high risk of infection, for example, newborn infants because of their immature immune system and reliance upon others for their hygiene and daily care, and those who are immune suppressed either due to an immunosuppressive disease or because they are having immunosuppressive therapy. The range of microorganisms that can cause infections in these groups is often very wide and may include microorganisms that would not normally cause disease; these are referred to as opportunistic infections (they literally take the opportunity of immune suppression to cause disease). One example of this is the first cases of acquired immune deficiency syndrome (AIDS) that were reported in the United States; they were noted because apparently otherwise healthy young men were becoming infected with *Pneumocystis carinii* (now known as *Pneumocystis jirovecii*), a fungus that does not normally cause disease in healthy people (Centres for Disease Control and Prevention 1981). Of course, it is now known that they were not healthy, as the opportunistic infection occurred because of immunosuppression due to AIDS.

Because the range of microorganisms that can cause infections is wider than that normally encountered, and because they often have other risk factors such as recurrent hospitalisations, the treatment of infection in these groups poses a particular challenge. Furthermore, because of the rarity of some of the infections that they have, treatment options and experience may be limited. A general approach may be to give broad spectrum antimicrobials, the exact regimen being adjusted according to specific risk factors, with frequent reassessment and the switching of antimicrobials and consideration of the introduction of antifungals if there is no improvement after 48 hours.

6.12 New Therapies

Although the development of new antimicrobial drugs would seem one answer to the development of resistance, there are problems with relying on this. Firstly, the new therapeutics need to be available. However, secondly there are specific issues related to antimicrobials, in particular: the limited time which people will take, typically no more than 7–10 days for most people; many infections occur in people or places with limited financial resources making pricing important; and in order to reduce the risk of resistance, developing new drugs is likely to be restricted whatever the cost may be. Some new drugs have been developed, and a selection is shown in Table 6.4. Other possible treatments include those aimed at boosting the immune response such as vaccines and pre-formed antibody products, and bacteriophage therapies, these being viruses that infect bacteria.

Despite this, new drugs are being developed. Examples of drugs at earlier stages of development include Teixobactin, a drug that targets lipid II, which is a precursor of the peptidoglycan that makes up the bacterial cell wall (Shukla et al. 2022). This has activity against Gram-positive bacteria such as *S. aureus* and mycobacteria including *M. tuberculosis*, and being a novel product there does not appear to be existing resistance (Piddock 2015). The producing organism has been tentatively named *Eleftheria terrae*. Other novel antimicrobials target Gram-negative bacteria by inhibiting lipopolysaccharide transport in *Acinetobacter* sp., which are particularly troublesome (Pahil et al. 2024). However, the road from discovery to clinical use is a long one.

Nanomaterials and Nanoparticles
One potentially promising area of research into the treatment of infections is that of nanoparticles. These are very small particles, ranging in size from 10 to 1000 nm which can be used either as a vector to deliver antimicrobial agents or used for their own antimicrobial properties. Depending upon the size, shape and chemistry of the particle, they may be able to interact with and penetrate cells, causing direct damage or carrying antimicrobials into the cell. Damage may also result from electrostatic interactions between the particle and the cell membrane, particles binding to intracellular components or organelles, the induction or increase in reactive oxygen species. It has been hypothesised that the novelty of these approaches, and the multiple targets that they could have makes the development of resistance less likely (Ndayishimiye et al. 2022). A number of clinical trials are being undertaken to investigate various nanoparticle formulations (Mondal et al. 2024) including those involving the delivery of amphotericin B which often results in significant side effects.

Table 6.4 New drugs approved in Europe and the United States, or at an advanced stage of development (Leone et al. 2019; Rai et al. 2013; Topouzis et al. 2025)

Drug	Notes
Aztreonam-avibactam	Monobactam/β-lactamase inhibitor against Gram-negative including *Pseudomonas aeruginosa*
Berdazimer	Treatment of *Molluscum contagiosum*
Cefiderocol	Carbapenem active against Gram-negative including *Pseudomonas aeruginosa*
Ceftobiprole medocaril	*Cephalosporin, S. aureus bacteremia, bacterial skin and soft tissue infections, community acquired pneumonia*
Ceftaroline-fosamil	Cephalosporin, active against Gram-positive including MRSA and VISA
Ceftazidime-avibactam	Cephalosporin/β-lactamase inhibitor active against Gram-negative
Cefepime-enmetazobactam	*Cephalosporin/β-lactamase used for complex UTI*
Ceftobiprole-medocaril	Cephalosporin active against Gram-positive including MRSA
Ceftolozane-tazobactam	Cephalosporin/β-lactamase inhibitor active against Gram-negative including *Pseudomonas aeruginosa*
Dalbavancin	Lipoglycopeptide active against Gram-positive
Daptomycin	Lipopeptide active against Gram-positive bacteria
Delafloxacin	Fluoroquinolone active against broad spectrum
Eravacycline	Tetracycline active against broad spectrum
Imipenem-relebactam-cilastatin	Carbapenem/β-lactamase inhibitor active against broad spectrum
Meropenem-vaborbactam	Carbapenem/β-lactamase inhibitor active against broad spectrum
Omadacycline	Tetracycline active against broad spectrum
Oritavancin	Lipoglycopeptide active against Gram-positive
Plazomicin	Aminoglycoside active against broad spectrum
Sulopenem etzadroxil-probenecid	*Carbapenem used for UTI*
Tedizolid	Oxazolidinone active against Gram-positive including MRSA and VRE
Telithromycin	Ketolide active against broad spectrum
Tigecycline	Glycylcycline active against broad spectrum

6.13 Preventing Infections

Although most attention is placed upon treating infections, prevention is a better strategy, and relatively simple public health interventions can have significant results. With regard to medicines, the most common way of preventing infections is through prophylaxis; this is a treatment not to cure an existing infection but to prevent infection.

There are a number of different groups who might benefit from antimicrobial prophylaxis, for example:

- Patients undergoing some types of surgery where there is a high risk of contamination, such as surgery involving the placement of a prosthesis or implant, clean surgery or clean-contaminated surgery or contaminated surgery (National Institute for Health and Care Excellence 2019).
- Those who are severely immunosuppressed: the exact details of what prophylaxis they require will depend upon the nature, extent and length of their immunosuppression, but may include antibacterials, antifungals and antivirals.
- People who are functionally or anatomically asplenic should be considered for lifelong pneumococcal prophylaxis with penicillins or macrolides (Davies et al. 2011).

The use of prophylaxis for long periods of time is not without its risks however, as it might hasten the development of resistance, increase the risk of secondary infections if the prophylaxis damages the normal flora and may be expensive.

Another approach to prophylaxis is passive immunisation, where pre-formed antibodies are given. This may be specific for an organism, for example, V-ZIg (varicella-zoster immunoglobulin antibodies), or be pooled antibodies from a large number of people, in which case it will provide antibodies against a large number of organisms, but at a lower level. It is important to note that as with antimicrobial prophylaxis and unlike active immunisation this does not provide long-term protection (Berger 2018).

6.14   Summary

- Microorganisms are ubiquitous and outnumber other forms of life many times, but most are not harmful to humans.
- The key to treating infections is selective toxicity, that is, the ability to damage the infecting organism without damaging the host.
- Bacteria have many selective targets because of their distant evolutionary relationship with humans Fungi and protozoa have fewer selective targets, and viruses fewer still because they use host metabolism to reproduce.
- Antimicrobial resistance is an increasing problem and is driven by the selective effect of antimicrobial use.

Multiple Choice Questions

1. The real meaning of the term antibiotic is:
   - (a) Any substance used to treat an infection
   - (b) A substance produced by one living organism that kills or inhibits the growth of another
   - (c) An antibacterial drug only
   - (d) An antiviral drug only

2. Viruses are difficult to treat because:
   (a) They replicate rapidly.
   (b) They are very small.
   (c) They use host cell metabolism to replicate.
   (d) They are often resistant to commonly used antimicrobials.
3. Antimicrobial resistance usually occurs because:
   (a) Of the common use of older, cheaper drugs.
   (b) The use of the wrong drugs.
   (c) The use of the wrong doses.
   (d) Their use selects for resistant organisms through natural selection.
4. In terms of the number and range of drugs available:
   (a) Bacterial infections are easier to treat than fungal infections.
   (b) Fungal infections are easier to treat than bacterial infections.
   (c) Both are equally easy to treat.
   (d) Most infections cannot be treated.
5. Selective toxicity refers to:
   (a) Antimicrobials that are toxic to both human and microbial cells
   (b) Antimicrobials that are toxic to neither human or microbial cells
   (c) Antimicrobials that are more toxic to human than microbial cells
   (d) Antimicrobials that are more toxic to microbial than human cells
6. When treating a patient with an infection:
   (a) You should always wait for the culture results before starting treatment.
   (b) Never wait for the culture results—always treat straight away.
   (c) Asses if the severity of infection permits receipt of culture results before starting treatment.
   (d) Always treat with broad spectrum antimicrobials, so it does not matter.
7. A negative blood culture result in a patient with a fever:
   (a) Proves that the patient does not have an infection, the fever is due to something else.
   (b) Suggests it but does not prove it, it may be a false-negative result.
   (c) Needs more time to become positive as the patient has a fever.
   (d) Is of no clinical significance and should be ignored.
8. The main measure of susceptibility of a microorganism to a drug is:
   (a) The maximum dose that can be given
   (b) The minimum inhibitory concentration
   (c) The minimum toxic concentration
   (d) The minimum cidal concentration

Answers

1. (b)
2. (c)
3. (d)
4. (a)

5. (d)
6. (c)
7. (b)
8. (b)

References

Abbott IJ, Peel TN, Cairns KA, Stewardson AJ (2023) Antibiotic management of urinary tract infections in the post-antibiotic era: a narrative review highlighting diagnostic and antimicrobial stewardship. Clin Microbiol Infect 29:1254–1266. https://doi.org/10.1016/j.cmi.2022.05.016

Al-Hajeri H, Baroun F, Abutiban F, Al-Mutairi M, Ali Y, Alawadhi A, Albasri A, Aldei A, AlEnizi A, Alhadhood N, Al-Herz A, Alkadi A, Alkanderi W, Almathkoori A, Almutairi N, Alsayegh S, Alturki A, Bahbahani H, Dehrab A, Ghanem A, Haji Hasan E, Hayat S, Saleh K, Tarakmeh H, by the Kuwait Association of Rheumatology (2022) Therapeutic role of immunomodulators during the COVID-19 pandemic- a narrative review. Postgrad Med 134:160–179. https://doi.org/10.1080/00325481.2022.2033563

Antonelli G, Turriziani O (2012) Antiviral therapy: old and current issues. Int J Antimicrob Agents 40:95–102. https://doi.org/10.1016/j.ijantimicag.2012.04.005

Appelbaum PC (2007) Reduced glycopeptide susceptibility in methicillin-resistant Staphylococcus aureus (MRSA). Int J Antimicrob Agents 30:398–408. https://doi.org/10.1016/j.ijantimicag.2007.07.011

AstraZeneca (2022) VAXZEVRIA (COVID-19 Vaccine AstraZeneca). Doc ID-004459550 V18.0

Belkaid Y, Hand TW (2014) Role of the microbiota in immunity and inflammation. Cell 157:121–141. https://doi.org/10.1016/j.cell.2014.03.011

Berger M (2018) Antibodies to vaccine antigens in pooled polyclonal human IgG products. Transfusion 58:3096–3105. https://doi.org/10.1111/trf.15017

British Society for Antimicrobial Chemotherapy (2018) Definitions | BSAC. http://www.bsacsurv.org/science/mics/. Accessed 24 Feb 2019

Brown NM, Goodman AL, Horner C, Jenkins A, Brown EM (2021) Treatment of methicillin-resistant *Staphylococcus aureus* (MRSA): updated guidelines from the UK. JAC-Antimicrob Resist 3:dlaa114. https://doi.org/10.1093/jacamr/dlaa114

Cain DW, Cidlowski JA (2017) Immune regulation by glucocorticoids. Nat Rev Immunol 17:233–247. https://doi.org/10.1038/nri.2017.1

Centers for Disease Control and Prevention (CDC) (2002) Staphylococcus aureus resistant to vancomycin–United States, 2002. MMWR Morb Mortal Wkly Rep 51:565–567

Centres for Disease Control and Prevention (1981) Pneumocystis pneumonia—Los Angeles. MMWR 30:250–252

Chai J-Y, Jung B-K, Hong S-J (2021) Albendazole and mebendazole as anti-parasitic and anti-cancer agents: an update. Korean J Parasitol 59:189–225. https://doi.org/10.3347/kjp.2021.59.3.189

Chan JD, Zarowiecki M, Marchant JS (2013) Ca2+ channels and praziquantel: a view from the free world. Parasitol Int 62:619–628. https://doi.org/10.1016/j.parint.2012.12.001

Connolly LE, Edelstein PH, Ramakrishnan L (2007) Why is long-term therapy required to cure tuberculosis? PLoS Med 4:e120. https://doi.org/10.1371/journal.pmed.0040120

Cox G, Wright GD (2013) Intrinsic antibiotic resistance: mechanisms, origins, challenges and solutions. Int J Med Microbiol 303:287–292. https://doi.org/10.1016/j.ijmm.2013.02.009

Czepiel J, Dróżdż M, Pituch H, Kuijper EJ, Perucki W, Mielimonka A, Goldman S, Wultańska D, Garlicki A, Biesiada G (2019) Clostridium difficile infection: review. Eur J Clin Microbiol Infect Dis 38:1211–1221. https://doi.org/10.1007/s10096-019-03539-6

Davies J, Davies D (2010) Origins and evolution of antibiotic resistance. Microbiol Mol Biol Rev 74:417–433. https://doi.org/10.1128/MMBR.00016-10

Davies JM, Lewis MPN, Wimperis J, Rafi I, Ladhani S, Bolton-Maggs PHB, British Committee for Standards in Haematology (2011) Review of guidelines for the prevention and treatment of infection in patients with an absent or dysfunctional spleen: prepared on behalf of the British Committee for Standards in Haematology by a working party of the haemato-oncology task force. Br J Haematol 155:308–317. https://doi.org/10.1111/j.1365-2141.2011.08843.x

Eastman RT, Roth JS, Brimacombe KR, Simeonov A, Shen M, Patnaik S, Hall MD (2020) Remdesivir: a review of its discovery and development leading to emergency use authorization for treatment of COVID-19. ACS Cent Sci 6:672–683. https://doi.org/10.1021/acscentsci.0c00489

Foster TJ (2017) Antibiotic resistance in Staphylococcus aureus. Current status and future prospects. FEMS Microbiol Rev 41:430–449. https://doi.org/10.1093/femsre/fux007

Garcia-Effron G (2020) Rezafungin-mechanisms of action, susceptibility and resistance: similarities and differences with the other echinocandins. J Fungi Basel Switz 6:262. https://doi.org/10.3390/jof6040262

Giedraitienė A, Vitkauskienė A, Naginienė R, Pavilonis A (2011) Antibiotic resistance mechanisms of clinically important bacteria. Medicina (Kaunas) 47:137–146

Gillings MR, Stokes HW (2012) Are humans increasing bacterial evolvability? Trends Ecol Evol (Amst) 27:346–352. https://doi.org/10.1016/j.tree.2012.02.006

Goulooze SC, Cohen AF, Rissmann R (2015) Bedaquiline. Br J Clin Pharmacol 80:182–184. https://doi.org/10.1111/bcp.12613

Haagsma AC, Abdillahi-Ibrahim R, Wagner MJ, Krab K, Vergauwen K, Guillemont J, Andries K, Lill H, Koul A, Bald D (2009) Selectivity of TMC207 towards mycobacterial ATP synthase compared with that towards the eukaryotic homologue. Antimicrob Agents Chemother 53:1290–1292. https://doi.org/10.1128/AAC.01393-08

Han X, Xu P, Ye Q (2021) Analysis of COVID-19 vaccines: types, thoughts, and application. J Clin Lab Anal 35:e23937. https://doi.org/10.1002/jcla.23937

Hashemian SMR, Sheida A, Taghizadieh M, Memar MY, Hamblin MR, Bannazadeh Baghi H, Sadri Nahand J, Asemi Z, Mirzaei H (2023) Paxlovid (Nirmatrelvir/Ritonavir): a new approach to Covid-19 therapy? Biomed Pharmacother 162:114367. https://doi.org/10.1016/j.biopha.2023.114367

Hughes D, Andersson DI (2017) Evolutionary trajectories to antibiotic resistance. Ann Rev Microbiol 71:579–596. https://doi.org/10.1146/annurev-micro-090816-093813

Jevons MP (1961) "Celbenin" – resistant Staphylococci. BMJ 1:124–125. https://doi.org/10.1136/bmj.1.5219.124-a

Joint United Nations Programme on HIV/AIDS (UNAIDS) (2023) The path that ends AIDS. 2023 UNAIDS global aids update. UNAIDS, Geneva

Kapoor G, Saigal S, Elongavan A (2017) Action and resistance mechanisms of antibiotics: a guide for clinicians. J Anaesthesiol Clin Pharmacol 33:300–305. https://doi.org/10.4103/joacp.JOACP_349_15

Kathiravan MK, Salake AB, Chothe AS, Dudhe PB, Watode RP, Mukta MS, Gadhwe S (2012) The biology and chemistry of antifungal agents: a review. Bioorg Med Chem 20:5678–5698. https://doi.org/10.1016/j.bmc.2012.04.045

Khanal P (2021) Antimalarial and anticancer properties of artesunate and other artemisinins: current development. Monatshefte Für Chem Chem Mon 152:387–400. https://doi.org/10.1007/s00706-021-02759-x

Laniado-Laborín R, Cabrales-Vargas MN (2009) Amphotericin B: side effects and toxicity. Rev Iberoam Micol 26:223–227. https://doi.org/10.1016/j.riam.2009.06.003

Leibovici L, Shraga I, Andreassen S (1999) How do you choose antibiotic treatment? BMJ 318:1614–1616

Leone S, Cascella M, Pezone I, Fiore M (2019) New antibiotics for the treatment of serious infections in intensive care unit patients. Curr Med Res Opin 35(8):1331–1334. https://doi.org/10.1080/03007995.2019.1583025

Littler E, Oberg B (2005) Achievements and challenges in antiviral drug discovery. Antivir Chem Chemother 16:155–168. https://doi.org/10.1177/095632020501600302

Liu C, Bayer A, Cosgrove SE, Daum RS, Fridkin SK, Gorwitz RJ, Kaplan SL, Karchmer AW, Levine DP, Murray BE, Rybak MJ, Talan DA, Chambers HF (2011) Clinical practice guidelines by the Infectious Diseases Society of America for the treatment of methicillin-resistant Staphylococcus aureus infections in adults and children. Clin Infect Dis 52:e18–e55. https://doi.org/10.1093/cid/ciq146

Maas BM, Strizki J, Miller RR, Kumar S, Brown M, Johnson MG, Cheng M, De Anda C, Rizk ML, Stone JA (2024) Molnupiravir: mechanism of action, clinical, and translational science. Clin Transl Sci 17:e13732. https://doi.org/10.1111/cts.13732

Mahjabeen F, Saha U, Mostafa MN, Siddique F, Ahsan E, Fathma S, Tasnim A, Rahman T, Faruq R, Sakibuzzaman M, Dilnaz F, Ashraf A (2022) An update on treatment options for methicillin-resistant Staphylococcus aureus (MRSA) bacteremia: a systematic review. Cureus 14:e31486. https://doi.org/10.7759/cureus.31486

Martin RJ, Robertson AP, Choudhary S (2021) Ivermectin: an anthelmintic, an insecticide, and much more. Trends Parasitol 37:48–64. https://doi.org/10.1016/j.pt.2020.10.005

Matsumoto M, Hashizume H, Tomishige T, Kawasaki M, Tsubouchi H, Sasaki H, Shimokawa Y, Komatsu M (2006) OPC-67683, a nitro-dihydro-imidazooxazole derivative with promising action against tuberculosis in vitro and in mice. PLoS Med 3:e466. https://doi.org/10.1371/journal.pmed.0030466

Mayon-White RT, Wiffen P (2005) Audit of antibiotic policies in the south east of England, 2004. J Antimicrob Chemother 56:204–207. https://doi.org/10.1093/jac/dki152

Medicines and Healthcare Products Regulatory Agency (n.d.) Fluoroquinolone antibiotics: must now only be prescribed when other commonly recommended antibiotics are inappropriate [WWW document]. GOV.UK. https://www.gov.uk/drug-safety-update/fluoroquinolone-antibiotics-must-now-only-be-prescribed-when-other-commonly-recommended-antibiotics-are-inappropriate. Accessed 26 Feb 25

Moderna (2024) Fact sheet for healthcare providers administering vaccine: emergency use authorization of moderna COVID-19 vaccine (2024–2025 formula), for individuals 6 months through 11 years of age

Mondal SK, Chakraborty S, Manna S, Mandal SM (2024) Antimicrobial nanoparticles: current landscape and future challenges. RSC Pharm 1:388–402. https://doi.org/10.1039/D4PM00032C

National Institute for Health and Care Excellence (n.d.) Clostridioides difficile infection: antimicrobial prescribing NICE guideline [NG199]. Published: 23 July 2021

National Institute for Health and Care Excellence (2015) Antimicrobial stewardship: systems and processes for effective antimicrobial medicine use [NG15] [WWW document]. https://www.nice.org.uk/guidance/ng15. Accessed 24 Feb 2019

National Institute for Health and Care Excellence (2019) Surgical site infections: prevention and treatment, clinical guideline [NG125]. https://www.nice.org.uk/guidance/ng125/chapter/Recommendations#preoperative-phase

Ndayishimiye J, Kumeria T, Popat A, Falconer JR, Blaskovich MAT (2022) Nanomaterials: the new antimicrobial magic bullet. ACS Infect Dis 8:693–712. https://doi.org/10.1021/acsinfecdis.1c00660

Novavax (2024) Fact sheet for healthcare providers administering vaccine: emergency use authorization of Novavax COVID-19 vaccine, adjuvanted (2024–2025 formula), for individuals 12 years of age and older

Oliveira D, Borges A, Simões M (2018) Staphylococcus aureus toxins and their molecular activity in infectious diseases. Toxins 10:252. https://doi.org/10.3390/toxins10060252

Pahil KS, Gilman MSA, Baidin V, Clairfeuille T, Mattei P, Bieniossek C, Dey F, Muri D, Baettig R, Lobritz M, Bradley K, Kruse AC, Kahne D (2024) A new antibiotic traps lipopolysaccharide in its intermembrane transporter. Nature 625:572–577. https://doi.org/10.1038/s41586-023-06799-7

Papp-Wallace KM, Endimiani A, Taracila MA, Bonomo RA (2011) Carbapenems: past, present, and future. Antimicrob Agents Chemother 55:4943–4960. https://doi.org/10.1128/AAC.00296-11

Paterson DL, Bonomo RA (2005) Extended-spectrum beta-lactamases: a clinical update. Clin Microbiol Rev 18:657–686. https://doi.org/10.1128/CMR.18.4.657-686.2005

Pfizer-BioNTech (2024) Fact sheet for healthcare providers administering vaccine: emergency use authorization of Pfizer-BioNTech COVID-19 vaccine (2024–2025 formula), for 6 months through 11 years of age

Piddock LJV (2015) Teixobactin, the first of a new class of antibiotics discovered by iChip technology? J Antimicrob Chemother 70:2679–2680. https://doi.org/10.1093/jac/dkv175

Rai J, Randhawa GK, Kaur M (2013) Recent advances in antibacterial drugs. Int J Appl Basic Med Res 3:3–10. https://doi.org/10.4103/2229-516X.112229

Rodloff A, Bauer T, Ewig S, Kujath P, Müller E (2008) Susceptible, intermediate, and resistant – the intensity of antibiotic action. Dtsch Arztebl Int 105:657–662. https://doi.org/10.3238/arztebl.2008.0657

Samuelson J (1999) Why metronidazole is active against both bacteria and parasites. Antimicrob Agents Chemother 43:1533–1541. https://doi.org/10.1128/AAC.43.7.1533

Sandoval-Motta S, Aldana M (2016) Adaptive resistance to antibiotics in bacteria: a systems biology perspective: adaptive resistance to antibiotics in bacteria. Wiley Interdiscip Rev Syst Biol Med 8:253–267. https://doi.org/10.1002/wsbm.1335

Sax PE, Thompson MA, Saag MS, IAS-USA Treatment Guidelines Panel (2024) Updated treatment recommendation on use of cabotegravir and rilpivirine for people with HIV from the IAS-USA guidelines panel. JAMA 331:1060. https://doi.org/10.1001/jama.2024.2985

Shannon A, Canard B (2023) Kill or corrupt: mechanisms of action and drug-resistance of nucleotide analogues against SARS-CoV-2. Antivir Res 210:105501. https://doi.org/10.1016/j.antiviral.2022.105501

Shaw KJ, Ibrahim AS (2020) Fosmanogepix: a review of the first-in-class broad spectrum agent for the treatment of invasive fungal infections. J Fungi Basel Switz 6:239. https://doi.org/10.3390/jof6040239

Shawky AM, Almalki FA, Abdalla AN, Abdelazeem AH, Gouda AM (2022) A comprehensive overview of globally approved JAK inhibitors. Pharmaceutics 14:1001. https://doi.org/10.3390/pharmaceutics14051001

Shukla R, Lavore F, Maity S, Derks MGN, Jones CR, Vermeulen BJA, Melcrová A, Morris MA, Becker LM, Wang X, Kumar R, Medeiros-Silva J, Van Beekveld RAM, Bonvin AMJJ, Lorent JH, Lelli M, Nowick JS, MacGillavry HD, Peoples AJ, Spoering AL, Ling LL, Hughes DE, Roos WH, Breukink E, Lewis K, Weingarth M (2022) Teixobactin kills bacteria by a two-pronged attack on the cell envelope. Nature 608:390–396. https://doi.org/10.1038/s41586-022-05019-y

Stone NRH, Bicanic T, Salim R, Hope W (2016) Liposomal amphotericin B (AmBisome(®)): a review of the pharmacokinetics, pharmacodynamics, clinical experience and future directions. Drugs 76:485–500. https://doi.org/10.1007/s40265-016-0538-7

Sultan I, Rahman S, Jan AT, Siddiqui MT, Mondal AH, Haq QMR (2018) Antibiotics, resistome and resistance mechanisms: a bacterial perspective. Front Microbiol 9:2066. https://doi.org/10.3389/fmicb.2018.02066

Tamma PD, Aitken SL, Bonomo RA, Mathers AJ, van Duin D, Clancy CJ (2022) Infectious Diseases Society of America 2022 guidance on the treatment of extended-spectrum β-lactamase producing enterobacterales (ESBL-E), carbapenem-resistant enterobacterales (CRE), and Pseudomonas aeruginosa with difficult-to-treat resistance (DTR-P. aeruginosa). Clin Infect Dis 75:187–212. https://doi.org/10.1093/cid/ciac268

Tenover FC (2006) Mechanisms of antimicrobial resistance in bacteria. Am J Med 119:S3–S10; discussion S62-70. https://doi.org/10.1016/j.amjmed.2006.03.011

Topouzis S, Papapetropoulos A, Alexander SPH, Cortese-Krott M, Kendall DA, Martemyanov K, Mauro C, Nagercoil N, Panettieri RA, Patel HH, Schulz R, Stefanska B, Stephens GJ, Teixeira MM, Vergnolle N, Wang X, Ferdinandy P (2025) Novel drugs approved by the EMA, the FDA and the MHRA in 2024: a year in review. Br J Pharmacol:bph.17458. https://doi.org/10.1111/bph.17458

Whitman WB, Coleman DC, Wiebe WJ (1998) Prokaryotes: the unseen majority. Proc Natl Acad Sci 95:6578–6583. https://doi.org/10.1073/pnas.95.12.6578

Wiederhold NP (2020) Review of the novel investigational antifungal olorofim. J Fungi Basel Switz 6:122. https://doi.org/10.3390/jof6030122

Woolhouse MEJ, Gowtage-Sequeria S (2005) Host range and emerging and reemerging pathogens. Emerg Infect Dis 11:1842–1847. https://doi.org/10.3201/eid1112.050997

World Health Organization (2015) WHO | Global action plan on antimicrobial resistance [WWW document]. WHO, New York. http://www.who.int/antimicrobial-resistance/publications/global-action-plan/en/. Accessed 24 Feb 2019

World Health Organization (2022) WHO fungal priority pathogens list to guide research, development and public health action, 1st ed. World Health Organization, Geneva

World Health Organization (2024) WHO bacterial priority pathogens list 2024: bacterial pathogens of public health importance, to guide research, development, and strategies to prevent and control antimicrobial resistance, 1st ed. World Health Organization, Geneva

Medications Used for the Cardiovascular System

7

Joan Adams and Ehsan Khan

Learning Outcomes
At the end of this chapter, you will be able to:

- Explore the mechanism of drug action, clinical indications, pharmacokinetics and contraindications associated with prescribed organic nitrates, angiotensin-converting enzyme inhibitors, angiotensin II receptor antagonists, calcium-channel blockers and beta-adrenoceptor blocking drugs, antiarrhythmic drugs and statins.
- Identify the common adverse effects and important drug–drug interactions associated with organic nitrates, angiotensin-converting enzyme inhibitors, angiotensin II receptor antagonists, calcium-channel blockers and beta-adrenoceptor blocking drugs.
- List the routes of administering organic nitrates and the information patients would require when taking these medications.
- Review the similarities and differences between amlodipine, verapamil and diltiazem, enalapril and candesartan cilexetil.
- Identify the IV classes of antiarrhythmic drugs and state the differences between them listing the common adverse effects.
- Review the common adverse effects and drug–drug interactions associated with statins.
- Outline the nursing considerations and the information patients require when prescribed angiotensin-converting enzyme inhibitors, calcium-channel blockers, beta-adrenoceptor blocking drugs, antiarrhythmic drugs and statins.

J. Adams (Retired) (✉)
Florence Nightingale Faculty of Nursing, Midwifery and Palliative Care,
King's College London, London, UK

E. Khan
Faculty of Nursing Midwifery and Palliative Care, King's College London, London, UK
e-mail: eu.khan@kcl.ac.uk

171

E. Khan, P. Hood (eds.), *Understanding Pharmacology in Nursing Practice*,
https://doi.org/10.1007/978-3-032-03964-4_7

7.1 Introduction

This chapter focuses on the pharmacology of medication that influences cardiac function by reviewing the underlying physiology of the cardiovascular system, the pharmacokinetics and pharmacodynamics of such medication and the adverse effects of cardiac drugs, alongside the clinical indications, contraindications and possible drug–drug interactions.

The classes of drugs that affect cardiac function through their action on the vascular system are organic nitrates, angiotensin-converting enzyme inhibitors and angiotensin II receptor antagonists. Calcium-channel blockers and beta-blockers act on myocardial cells with the former also acting on vascular smooth muscle resulting in vasodilation. Antiarrhythmic drugs act by either blocking or modulating the ion channels in the heart, thereby influencing the action potential and the conduction mechanism by direct action (ion channel blockers) or via receptor modulation (beta-adrenoceptor blocking drugs). Statins have an inhibitory action on hepatic cholesterol synthesis and are effective in lowering plasma low-density lipoprotein (LDL) cholesterol.

Healthcare practitioners are ideally placed to facilitate and enhance a service user's understanding of their prescribed medication; therefore, an understanding of the mechanisms of drug action and applying this knowledge to clinical practice is an essential element of the nurse's role.

7.2 Organic Nitrates

These medications are primarily used in the management of angina pectoris and for acute coronary syndrome.

7.2.1 Angina Pectoris

The heart is a pump that distributes oxygen and nutrients to the organs and tissues of the body by way of the systemic circulation. A constant supply of oxygen is required by the myocardium to maintain contraction. Oxygenated blood is supplied to the myocardium through the coronary arteries which subdivide into smaller branches feeding the myocardial muscle cells. Blood flow to the myocardium can be adjusted by the sympathetic nervous system controlling vasodilation and vasoconstriction. Blood flow is also adjusted by autoregulation mechanisms. When blood flow is unable to meet tissue demands, oxygen levels fall, and metabolic waste products, such as hydrogen ions, potassium and adenosine, accumulate stimulating autoregulation. This can result in dilatation of vascular smooth muscle and the release of nitric oxide from vascular endothelial cells leading to vasodilation (Marieb and Hoehn 2013).

Narrowing of the arteries due to atheromatous plaque reduces the radius of the vessels, impairing the blood supply and depriving the muscle of adequate oxygen and nutrients; this is known as myocardial ischaemia. Angina pectoris is a symptom of ischaemic heart disease where there is insufficient oxygen (O_2) supplying the myocardium. In normal cardiac function, oxygen balance is maintained between supply and demand. When experiencing the symptom of angina, myocardial demand for oxygen exceeds supply. The poor blood supply is typically a result of atherosclerotic narrowing, but may also be due to thickened (hypertrophied muscle) or non-atherosclerotic abnormalities of the coronary artery structure.

Ischaemia of the myocardium causes coronary vessels to dilate through autoregulation adjusting blood flow. When demand increases, such as in exercise, cold weather, after a substantial meal, emotional stress or anxiety, greater dilatory capacity may be inadequate, and central chest pain radiating to the arm and neck may be experienced. Such transient episodes of ischaemia are known as *stable angina*. This type of pain may be relieved with rest or with pharmacological intervention as detailed in Box 7.1.

> **Box 7.1 Major Groups of Drugs Used in the Management of Stable Angina**
> - Organic nitrates: vasodilators—drug, e.g. isosorbide mononitrate
> - Calcium-channel blockers: vasodilators—drug, e.g. amlodipine
> - Beta-adrenoceptor blocking drugs: slows heart rate and reduces metabolic demand—drug, e.g. atenolol

7.2.2 Acute Coronary Syndrome

It is a syndrome that includes unstable angina; when there is a rupture of atheromatous plaque, the vessels are not completely occluded. Pain occurs at rest or when sleeping. Plaque rupture may also occlude a vessel and lead to death of heart muscle (myocardial infarction). Acute coronary syndrome includes cardiac chest pain resulting from unstable angina and chest pain that occurs in the initial stages of a myocardial infarction.

Variant angina is caused by a sudden spasm of the coronary artery decreasing myocardial blood flow and results in ischaemia (Moini 2012).

7.2.2.1 Organic Nitrates: Vasodilators
The mechanisms of preload and afterload are important concepts in understanding. the action of organic nitrates (Box 7.2).

Box 7.2 Preload and Afterload

Preload can be defined as the degree to which cardiac muscle cells are stretched at the end of diastole (Fig. 7.1a). The volume of blood in the ventricles before they contract determines preload. The greater the stretch, the larger the preload, with oxygen requirement of the myocardial muscle cells being greater. Venous return is an important factor influencing the volume and the degree of stretch. Preload can be reduced by venous dilation.

Afterload is the resistance that has to be overcome for the ventricles of the heart to eject blood into the circulation (Fig. 7.1b). This is determined by two factors: the distensibility of large arteries and total peripheral resistance. Vasodilation of arterial vessels will reduce vascular resistance and therefore afterload. Oxygen demand and cardiac workload will be reduced (Montague et al. 2005; Marieb and Hoehn 2013).

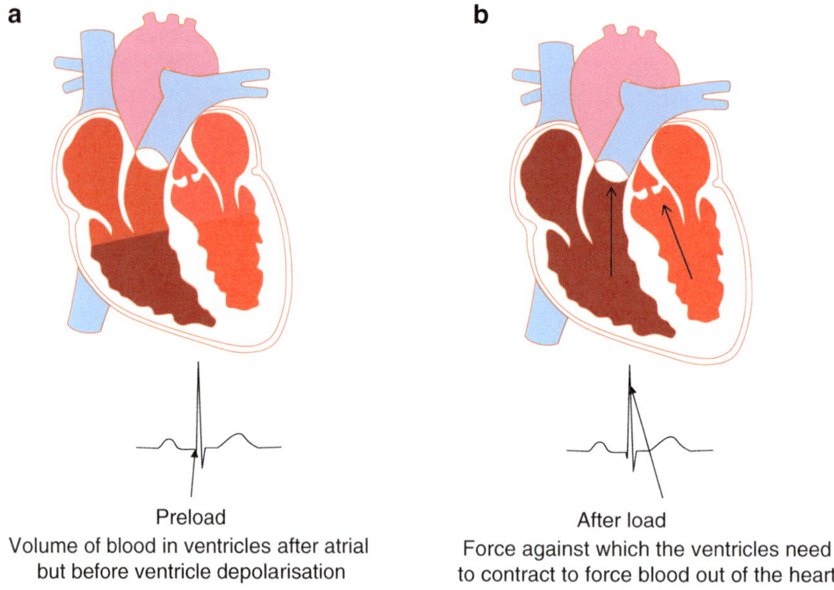

Fig. 7.1 (**a**) Preload: Volume of blood in ventricles after atrial but before ventricle depolarisation. (**b**) Afterload: Force against which the ventricles need to contract to force blood out of the heart

Fig. 7.2 Effect of nitrates on preload

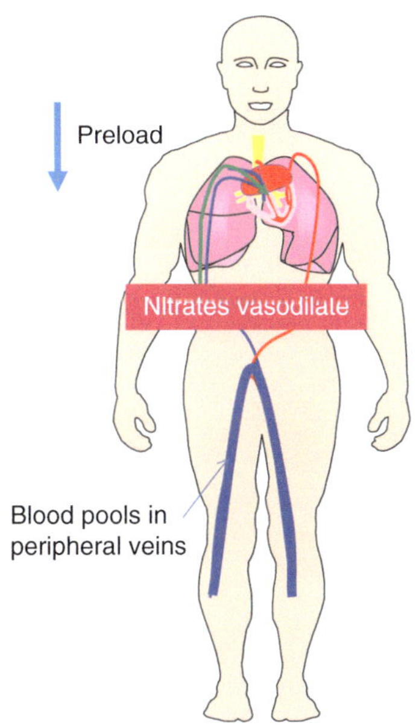

Mechanism of Action of Organic Nitrates

Organic nitrates form nitric oxide the sequence of events culminates in relaxation of venous and arteriolar smooth muscle, resulting in dilation. The vasodilatory effects of these drugs reduce preload through venous dilation and afterload through arterial dilation (Fig. 7.2), while improving coronary blood flow through dilation of the coronary vasculature.

Veins Veins are known as capacitance vessels or capacity vessels (Marieb and Hoehn 2008). Peripheral venodilation increases their capacity, reducing venous return, and central venous pressure, reducing preload. Reducing preload decreases the ventricular end diastolic volume, oxygen demand and oxygen consumption by the myocardial muscle cells. With less blood to be ejected by the ventricles, there is less mechanical stress, reducing myocardial workload and oxygen consumption.

Arteries Organic nitrates dilate larger muscular elastic arterial vessels and have a lesser effect on smaller resistance arteries. Reducing arterial resistance will reduce cardiac afterload (Rang et al. 2011).

Action on coronary arteries Organic nitrates have been shown to dilate the coronary vasculature increasing blood flow. The diameter of the vessel determines the vasodilatory response with a greater response seen in those vessels larger than 100 μm in diameter (Harrison and Bates 1993). Blood is redistributed through dilated collateral vessels from the unaffected vessels to ischaemic areas (Rang et al. 2011).

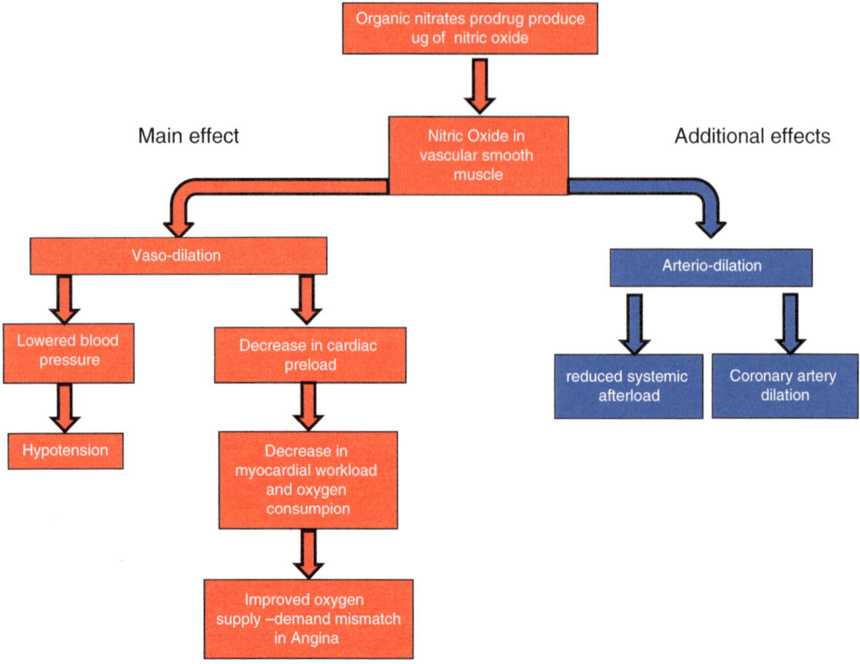

Fig. 7.3 The cardiovascular action of organic nitrates

The cardiovascular actions of organic nitrates are detailed in Fig. 7.3.

Additional Effects of Organic Nitrate Medication

Organic nitrates relax most smooth muscle tissue, for example, in the biliary and gastrointestinal system and in bronchial smooth muscle.

Pharmacokinetics

The action of nitrates induces vasodilation in both intact and dysfunctional blood vessel endothelium (the inner layer of the blood vessel). Organic nitrates are pro-drugs[1]; they are absorbed from the mucous membrane of the mouth, skin and gastrointestinal tract and undergo chemical reduction to liberate nitric oxide. *Glyceryl trinitrate (GTN)* is absorbed rapidly when given sublingually in spray or tablet form. The onset of action is within 1–3 min of administration, and the effect lasts for approximately 30 min. The half-life $(T1/2)$[2] of GTN is 1–3 min.

With oral administration, GTN undergoes extensive first-pass metabolism in the liver, resulting in low bioavailability, limiting the clinical use of this route. GTN is

---

[1] A prodrug is one that is administered in the inactive form and becomes active after metabolism.

[2] $T1/2$ half-life is the time taken for plasma concentration of the drug to fall to half of its original value.

also absorbed through the skin and can be administered as transdermal patches; this mode of administration avoids first-pass metabolism.

Isosorbide mononitrates are longer-acting nitrate drugs taken twice a day, namely, in the morning and early afternoon to reduce the problem of tolerance (a reduction in the antianginal effect). They are available as a sustained release preparation and given daily as the drug is not released over the whole of a 24-h period; this provides nitrogen-free periods, thereby reducing the risk of tolerance.

Isosorbide dinitrates are converted in the liver to activate mononitrates and excreted by the kidneys (Page et al. 2006; Rang et al. 2011).

Table 7.1 illustrates speed and duration of action.

Adverse Reactions of Organic Nitrate Medication

The adverse effects are mainly due to excessive vasodilation and can include the following:

- Flushing of the face and neck is caused by arteriolar vasodilation and headaches by vasodilation of the cerebral vessels.
- High doses may increase venous pooling reducing venous return and arteriolar resistance, leading to hypotension. Pallor, dizziness and syncope[3] may be experienced; alcohol intake can accentuate these effects.
- Excessive dilation may result in reflex tachycardia caused by lowering of blood pressure and a compensatory sympathetic response.[4]
- Postural hypotension may be associated with standing, caused by venous pooling and vasodilation. This may increase the risk of falling especially in older people.
- Rashes have been reported especially with transdermal patches, and hypersensitivity can be experienced.
- Nausea and vomiting have been reported.

Precautions

Organic nitrates should be withdrawn slowly as abrupt discontinuation may lead to vasospasm. They should be used with caution for individuals with liver and renal impairment (Table 7.2).

---

[3] Syncope: a transient loss of consciousness.

[4] A hypotensive state leads to an increase in baroreceptor activity. This compensatory response triggers the sympathetic nervous system, which is coordinated in the cardiovascular centre in the medulla oblongata. Vasomotor tone increases, causing vasoconstriction increasing peripheral resistance. Sympathetic activity increases heart rate, contractility and stroke volume resulting in an increase in cardiac output increasing blood pressure. This compensatory system provides some evidence to support why organic nitrates have a lesser effect on resistance arteries. In patients who have autonomic dysfunction, this compensatory activity would be impaired.

Table 7.1 Speed and duration of action of some organic nitrates

Drug	Speed of action	Duration of action
Glyceryl trinitrate		
Sublingual tablets	1–3 min	<30 min
Spray	1–4 min	<30 min
Transdermal patch	30 min	24 h with continuous application
Sustained release tablets and capsule	Slow	8–12 h
Intravenous route	Immediate	Once the infusion is finished
Isosorbide dinitrate		
Sustained release tablets	Slow	
Intravenous route	Immediate	
Isosorbide mononitrate		
Oral tablets	30–40 min	6–12 h
Sustained release tablets	Slow	12–24 h

Adapted from Opie and Gersh (2009), Brunton et al. (2011), and Electronic Medicine Compendium (eMC) accessed (2025)

Note: These figures are examples as individual preparations will vary

Table 7.2 Specific cautions

	Pregnancy	Breastfeeding	Renal and hepatic impairment
Glyceryl trinitrate (GTN)	No harmful effects observed in animal studies but safety especially in first trimester of pregnancy[a] not known	Manufacturers state use if the benefits outweigh the risks	Manufacturers advise caution if used in those with severe impairment
Isosorbide dinitrate (ISDN)	There is no data to suggest it is harmful to the foetus. It has been suggested that it may cross the placenta. Not prescribed unless the benefits outweigh the risks to foetus	No information available	Manufacturers advise caution in those with severe impairment
Isosorbide mononitrate (ISMN)	It is suggested that they are avoided unless there is potential benefit	Unknown as to whether nitrates are in breast milk	Manufacturers advise caution in those with severe impairment

Joint Formulary Committee (2024) and Electronic Medicines Compendium (eMC) accessed (2025)

[a]The first trimester begins with fertilisation of an ovum and finishes at week 12 of pregnancy

Contraindications

- Hypotension and hypovolaemia
- Increased intracranial pressure due to cerebral haemorrhage as vasodilation of the cerebral arteries could enhance intracranial bleeding
- Hypersensitivity to nitrates, hypertrophy cardiomyopathy, pulmonary oedema and aortic stenosis (Joint Formulary Committee 2024).

Examples of Interactions with Other Drugs

Sildenafil, tadalafil and vardenafil are phosphodiesterase 5 inhibitors and used for the treatment of erectile dysfunction. If prescribed with nitrates, extreme hypotension will result (Joint Formulary Committee 2024).

Tolerance

Tolerance (a reduction in the therapeutic effect) to the antianginal effect may be observed in organic nitrates such as isosorbide mononitrates, transdermal patches and those administered by the intravenous route. Tolerance tends to be dose dependent but improves with nitrogen-free periods. This is achieved by administrating organic nitrates intermittently (Joint Formulary Committee 2024), for example, transdermal patches may be removed at night, or giving modified release formulations of isosorbide mononitrate once a day, leaving nitrate-free intervals when the patient is at their lowest risk and generally at rest.

Clinical Considerations

The patient's blood pressure should be measured prior to administration of organic nitrates to identify possible hypotension and any other contraindications. After administration, assess for adverse effects such as hypotension, reflex tachycardia, headaches, dizziness and skin reactions. Safety is important as postural hypotension may increase the potential risk of falls, especially in older people. Patients should be advised to get up from a sitting or lying position slowly. When administering short-acting GTN, individuals should be advised to sit down rather than lie down or stand, as they may feel dizzy. GTN produces a therapeutic effect within 1–3 min and is prescribed for acute angina pain. Organic nitrates such as isosorbide mononitrate and transdermal patches are prescribed prophylactically. The patient's skin should be assessed for hypersensitivity if transdermal patches are used and any adverse effects documented and reported to a medical prescriber. When sustained released preparations are prescribed, these should not be chewed or crushed as this will alter the pharmacological action. Tolerance is also an important consideration requiring the need for nitrogen-free periods.

Intravenous glyceryl trinitrate may be used in the management of acute heart failure which reduces blood pressure.

Table 7.3 outlines the use of sublingual sprays, transdermal patches and sublingual tablets.

Table 7.3 The use of sublingual spray, transdermal patches and sublingual tablets

Organic nitrate preparation	Comments
Sublingual spray	Breath held, sprayed under the tongue or on the buccal mucosa; then the mouth is closed; do not inhale. In an acute episode of angina pain, pain levels are evaluated using a pain tool
Transdermal patches	Transdermal patches are applied to the trunk or upper arm, upper abdomen and chest and are not suitable for relieving acute angina attacks; they should be applied to unbroken, clean, dry and hair-free areas, and the position changed when reapplying the patch to prevent soreness (Electronic Medicine Compendium accessed 2025)
Sublingual tablets (GTN)	Sublingual tablets (GTN) have an 8-week expiry from package opening; after this date they will have no pharmacological action. GTN tablets are placed under the tongue and can be removed or swallowed when pain is relieved. Stopping its action reduces the risk of a headache occurring; if the mouth is dry, moisten prior to administration. This preparation is infrequently prescribed.

7.3 Calcium-Channel Blockers

7.3.1 Mechanism for Action and Indications for Use

The concentration of intracellular calcium ions is an important trigger for contraction of muscle. Extracellular calcium ions enter into the cell triggering the release of stored intracellular calcium ions (Marieb and Hoehn 2013). Calcium-channel blockers (CCB) bind to L-type calcium channels (voltage-sensitive calcium channels that span the membrane of the myocyte, particularly found in smooth muscle and cardiac muscle) interfering with the inward movement of calcium into the myocardium, the cells of the conducting system and vascular smooth muscle cells. They depress myocardial contractility, slow the formation and propagation of electrical impulses in conducting tissue and reduce the tone in both the systemic and coronary arterial vessels. This results in vasodilation of vascular smooth muscle decreasing peripheral resistance, reducing afterload and lowering blood pressure and dilating coronary arteries. They are used in the management of hypertension and angina pectoris (Rang et al. 2011). Their action on the conducting system can slow the rate of the propagation of impulses from the sinoatrial node to the atrial ventricular nodal cells, which can lead to a negative dromotropic effect (decrease in conduction) in the AV node. Verapamil is licensed and used in the treatment of some cardiac arrhythmias.

They are a diverse group of drugs consisting of three chemically distinct classes:

- Dihydropyridines, i.e. amlodipine.
- Phenylalklamines, i.e. verapamil hydrochloride.
- Benzothiazepines, i.e. diltiazem hydrochloride.
- Verapamil and diltiazem are known as non-dihydropyridines. This class of drug binds to different sites on the L-type calcium channel.

7.3.2   Dihydropyridines

This medication acts on arterial smooth muscle, resulting in peripheral vasodilation. This action reduces peripheral resistance, decreases afterload and reduces blood pressure (Opie and Gersh 2009). Many of the drugs in this class dilate the coronary arteries increasing blood flow.

The National Institute for Health and Care Excellence (NICE) publication 'Hypertension: The clinical management of primary hypertension in adults guide lines' (NICE 2013, 2019) suggests these are the first choice of drug for those who do not have type 2 diabetes and; are over 55 years, or are people of black African and Caribbean family origin (of any age).

Figure 7.4 presents an algorithm of drugs prescribed for the management of hypertension.

Dihydropyridines have a limited effect on depressing myocardial contractility and only a minimal effect on the conducting cells as the vasodilatory effect of peripheral dilation can cause a sympathetic reflex in an attempt to maintaining cardiac output when the blood pressure drops following their administration.

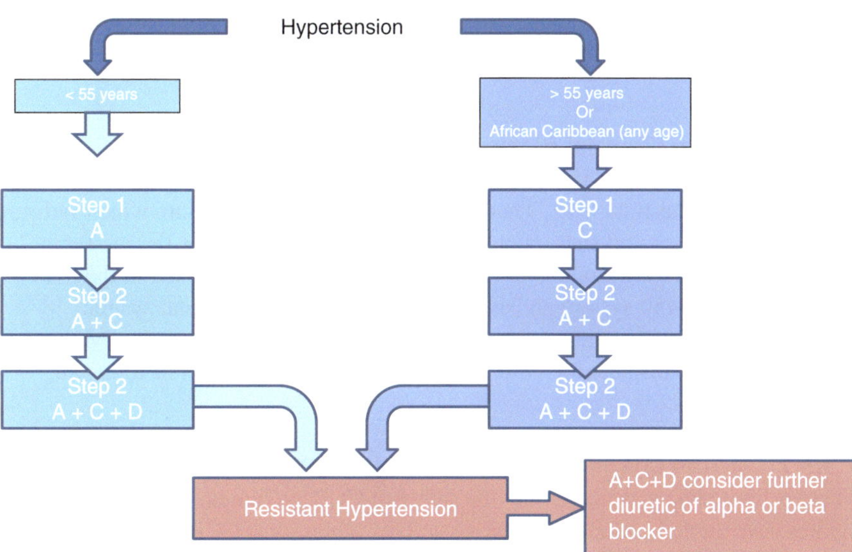

A = ACE inhibitor or Angiotensin II receptor antagonist
C = Calcium channel blocker
D = Diuretics

Fig. 7.4   Drug choice in hypertension. **A** ACE inhibitor or angiotensin II receptor antagonist, **C** calcium channel blocker, **D** diuretics. The National Institute for Health and Care Excellence (2019). Note: Calcium channel blockers will only be first choice if the patient does not have type 2 diabetes

7.3.3   Non-dihydropyridines

Verapamil and diltiazem are similar in action to dihydropyridines in that they reduce vascular tone in both peripheral and coronary vessels, thereby reducing blood pressure and preventing angina pain; however, they are more cardioselective. The action of these drugs interferes with calcium entry into the myocardial cells reducing the force of contraction and having an inhibitory effect on the sinoatrial node and atrioventricular nodal cells of the conducting system of the heart. Both tend to decrease heart rate and reduce contraction. They slow conduction and prolong the refractory period. For this reason, verapamil is known as a class IV antiarrhythmic drug. Verapamil has similar actions to beta-adrenergic blocking drugs, reducing automaticity of the sinoatrial node and slowing the propagation of electrical impulses to the atrio-ventricular nodal cells. Contractility is reduced (negative inotropic effect), as is heart rate and cardiac output. Atrio-ventricular conduction may be affected and therefore these medications should not be used with beta-adrenoceptor blocking drugs. Both verapamil and diltiazem may precipitate heart failure due to their negative inotropic effects. Diltiazem is licensed for the management of hypertension and angina pectoris.

Table 7.4 outlines the site of action, clinical indications and contraindications of some calcium-channel blockers. Table 7.5 presents dihydropyridine amlodipine and non-dihydropyridines diltiazem and verapamil and the effects on the cardiovascular system.

7.3.3.1 Calcium Channel Blocker Pharmacokinetics

Following oral administration, calcium-channel blockers (CCB) are well absorbed from the gastrointestinal tract. They undergo first-pass metabolism, which reduces their bioavailability and the amount of drug reaching the target tissue. Table 7.6 identifies the pharmacokinetics of four CCBs. They are metabolised in the liver by the cytochrome P450 system and excreted mainly through the renal system.

Calcium-channel blockers are highly protein bound, and those such as verapamil could potentially displace or be displaced by other protein bound drugs such as anticoagulants.

7.3.3.2 Calcium Channel Blocker Contraindications

There is limited data available into the safety of CCBs in human pregnancy. Animal studies have demonstrated reproductive toxicity when some CCBs were used in rats and mice. Trials have demonstrated that CCBs such as verapamil can cause foetal hypoxia due to reduced blood flow to the uterus (Joint Formulary Committee 2024). Recommendations state that verapamil should be avoided in the first trimester and CCBs not used during pregnancy unless there is a greater benefit for the mother. Most calcium-channel blockers cross the placenta barrier. Calcium-channel blocker properties are found in breast milk (Miller et al. 1986) and should not be used when breast feeding, unless there are significant benefits for the mother (Joint Formulary Committee 2024).

Table 7.4 Site of action, clinical indications and contraindications of some calcium-channel blockers

Drug	Specific cardiovascular sites of action	Clinical indications	Contraindication
Dihydropyridines			
Amlodipine	Vascular smooth muscle Limited effect on myocardium	Hypertension and chronic stable angina	Shock including cardiogenic shock, unstable angina, severe aortic stenosis, unstable heart failure
Felodipine	Vascular smooth muscle Limited effect on myocardium	Hypertension and chronic stable angina	Unstable angina, uncontrolled decompensated heart failure, severe aortic stenosis; within 1 month after a myocardial infarction, pregnancy
Nicardipine hydrochloride	See under amlodipine	Mild to moderate hypertension and chronic stable angina	Cardiogenic shock, unstable angina and acute angina pain; within 1 month after a myocardial infarction, acute porphyria, severe aortic stenosis, pregnancy and lactation
Nifedipine	Vascular smooth muscle Limited effect on myocardium	Hypertension, chronic stable angina, Raynaud's phenomenon	Cardiogenic shock, unstable angina, acute pain; within 1 month after a myocardial infarction, severe aortic stenosis
Nimodipine	Vascular smooth muscle Limited effect on myocardium	Prevention and treatment of ischaemic neurological deficits following subarachnoid haemorrhage	Unstable angina; within 1 month after a myocardial infarction, acute porphyria, contraindicated if prescribed, e.g. antiepileptic drugs or rifampicin
Non-dihydropyridines			
Diltiazem hydrochloride	Vascular smooth muscle, myocardium and conducting tissue	Angina and mild to moderate hypertension	Severe bradycardia, second- or third-degree heart block, sick sinus syndrome, decompensated heart failure, pregnancy
Verapamil hydrochloride	Vascular smooth muscle, myocardium and conducting tissue	Superventricular arrhythmias hypertension and angina	Hypotension, bradycardia, second- or third-degree heart block, AV block, uncompensated heart failure, atrial flutter or fibrillation which is associated with pathways of conduction. Not given in the first trimester of pregnancy

Adapted from McGavock (2005), Brunton et al. (2011), Joint Formulary Committee (2024), and Electronic Medicines Compendium (eMC) accessed (2025)

Table 7.5 Effects of calcium-channel blockers on the cardiovascular system

Drug	Amlodipine	Diltiazem	Verapamil
Peripheral smooth muscle	Hypotensive effect +++	Hypotensive effect ++	Hypotensive effect ++
Coronary smooth muscle	Anti-angina effect ++	Anti-angina effect ++	Anti-angina effect ++
Myocardium cardiac muscle	Reduces contractility +	Reduces contractility ++	Reduces contractility ++
Sino atrial node and atrial ventricular nodal cells	Effect on conduction +	Effect on conduction ++	Effect on conduction +++
Heart rate	Minimal changes, hypotension resulting from action of drug induces reflex tachycardia	Minimal effect	Reduces
Reduction in afterload	Decreases peripheral resistance +++	++	++

Adapted from McGavock (2005)

+ Limited effect, ++ Good effect, +++ Significant effect

7.3.3.3 Calcium Channel Blocker Adverse Reactions

Many of the adverse effects of calcium-channel blockers are due to their pharmacological actions (type A adverse effects) and include facial flushing, headache and dizziness caused by the vasodilatory action (it is not a cardiac effect but due to vasodilation) and are more common with dihydropyridines especially short-acting nifedipine and less common with verapamil and long-acting preparations. Ankle swelling results from an increase in precapillary hydrostatic pressure, pushing fluid into the interstitial spaces. Ankle swelling is, however, less common with verapamil. Calcium-channel blockers may cause bradycardia and heart block due their inhibiting action on calcium influx into atrio-ventricular nodal cells. This is less common in the dihydropyridine group. They may exacerbate heart failure due to their action on contractility; this is more marked with verapamil.

Non-cardiac effects Calcium-channel blockers act on smooth muscle and cause relaxation in the gastrointestinal tract leading to nausea and vomiting and gastro-oesophageal reflux. Constipation is a commonly reported adverse effect of verapamil due to reduced peristalsis.

Interaction with other drugs

These vary according to the different classes of calcium-channel blockers. Some examples are as follows:

- Verapamil increases serum digoxin levels displacing it from its binding sites, decreasing elimination and increasing the risk of bradycardia and toxicity (Joint Formulary Committee 2024).
- Beta-adrenoceptor blocking drugs have a negative effect on contractility of the myocardium, heart rate and conduction, which may increase the incidence of

Table 7.6 Pharmacokinetic profile of oral calcium-channel blockers

Drug	Oral absorption (%)	Bioavailability (%)	Protein binding (%)	Metabolism $T1/2$	Elimination	Elimination in %
Dihydropyridines						
Amlodipine	90	64–80	97.5	Hepatic	35–50 h	Renal 60% excreted in urine
Nifedipine	90	45–75	92–98	Hepatic	2 h	Renal 60% excreted in urine 15% via gastrointestinal tract
Non-dihydropyridines						
Diltiazem	90	45	80–86	Hepatic	6–8 h	Renal 35% excretion in urine, 65% via gastrointestinal tract
Verapamil	90	10–20	87–93	Hepatic	3–7 h	Renal 75% excretion in urine, 25% via gastrointestinal tract

Adapted from Opie and Gersh (2009), Brunton et al. (2011), and Electronic Medicines Compendium (eMC) accessed (2025)
Note: These figures are examples as individual preparations will vary

heart failure hypotension and arrhythmias when prescribed with verapamil and diltiazem.

- There is an enhanced hypotensive effect when calcium-channel blockers are administered with alpha-blockers and general anaesthesia.
- Diltiazem increases the plasma levels of statins: atorvastatin and simvastatin.
- Cimetidine increases the plasma levels of most dihydropyridines (Schwartz et al. 1988) but not amlodipine.
- St John's Wort reduces the concentration in plasma of verapamil and nifedipine.

It is suggested that the components of grapefruit juice increase the bioavailability of some calcium-channel blockers by increasing plasma concentration (Joint Formulary Committee 2024). The possible rationale for this is that grapefruit juice components inhibit the cytochrome P450 enzyme system, namely, isoenzyme CYP3A found in the walls of the intestine, reducing first-pass metabolism and increasing bioavailability (Bailey et al. 2000). Amlodipine and diltiazem are minimally affected. Some studies have indicated that fresh grapefruit has the same effect (Bailey et al. 2000; Baxter and Stockley 2010).

Clinical Considerations
- The prescriber must take a careful medical history and assess the patient to determine any known allergies, prescribed medication that could interact with the prescription, the possibility of pregnancy and/or renal and liver impairment that could influence treatment.
- Measurement of blood pressure and heart rate, rhythm and amplitude should be undertaken to identify a baseline and to indicate the possibility of adverse effects such as hypotension and tachycardia with dihydropyridines and bradycardia with non-dihydropyridines. Assess for ankle swelling.
- Abrupt withdrawal can cause rebound hypertension.
- Establish with the patient whether any other medicines are used or herbal remedies such as St John's Wort as this can interact with the effectiveness of the drug.

The patient should be advised about food that could cause interactions, such as grapefruit juice.

7.4 Angiotensin-Converting Enzyme Inhibitors

7.4.1 Introduction to Renin–Angiotensin–Aldosterone System

The renin–angiotensin–aldosterone system is an important mechanism for controlling blood pressure and fluid volume. Angiotensin II is a vasoconstrictor hormone and, by its action on the cortex of the adrenal glands, stimulates the secretion of mineral corticoid aldosterone, which increases sodium ion reabsorption. This action results in an increase in blood pressure and blood volume and a decrease in urine output.

7.4.2 Angiotensin-Converting Enzyme Inhibitors (ACE Inhibitors)

These are an important group of drugs that are used in treating and reducing the risk of cardiovascular disease. They block the conversion of angiotensin I to angiotensin II. This class of drug is used in the treatment of hypertension, heart failure, acute coronary syndrome and diabetic nephropathy.

7.4.3 Renin–Angiotensin–Aldosterone System (RAAS)

7.4.3.1 Formation of Angiotensin II

The formation of angiotensin II is initiated by renin, an enzyme secreted into the circulation by cells of the juxtaglomerular apparatus of the kidney. It is released in response to various physiological phenomena as follows:

1. A fall in sodium concentration in part of the distal convoluted tubule in the nephron of the kidneys.
2. A hypotensive state where blood volume is reduced or cardiac pumping is ineffective.
3. Stimulation of renal sympathetic nerves by $\beta1$ adrenoceptor agonists (Rang et al. 2011).

Angiotensinogen is a circulating plasma alpha 2 globulin, synthesised in the liver. Figure 7.5 represents the physiological cascade of events that occurs when renin is released.

The enzyme renin cleaves decapeptide angiotensin I from angiotensinogen (Marieb and Hoehn 2013). Angiotensin-converting enzyme (ACE) catalyses the conversion of angiotensin I to angiotensin II and is a membrane-bound enzyme located on the surface of vascular endothelial cells. High levels are found in the lungs; different forms of the same protein (isoforms) are located in other vascular tissue including the brain, heart and kidneys (Rang et al. 2011). Bradykinin has vasodilator abilities and increases vascular permeability. Angiotensin-converting enzyme (ACE) deactivates bradykinin. This increases vasoconstriction (Levick 2000).

7.4.3.2 Main Action of Angiotensin II

The main action of angiotensin II is mediated through the angiotensin II subtype I receptor (AT1) found in blood vessels and the cortex of the adrenal gland, heart, brain, kidneys and lungs (Fig. 7.6).

The effects include the following:

1. Vasoconstriction through its action on vascular smooth muscle increases vascular tone in the blood vessels. Constriction of the efferent arterioles of the renal glomerulus increases perfusion pressure (Rang et al. 2011). Vasoconstriction

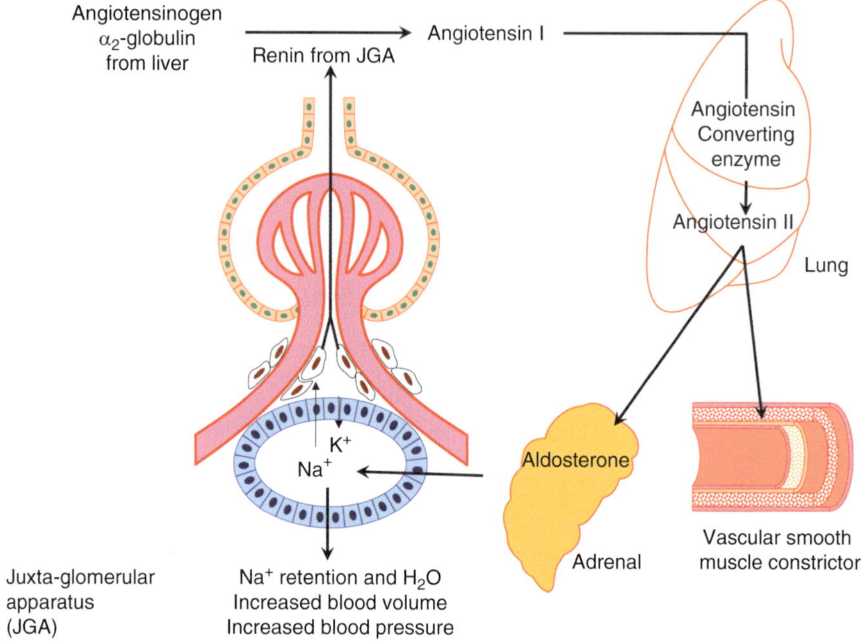

Fig. 7.5 Renin–angiotensin–aldosterone system

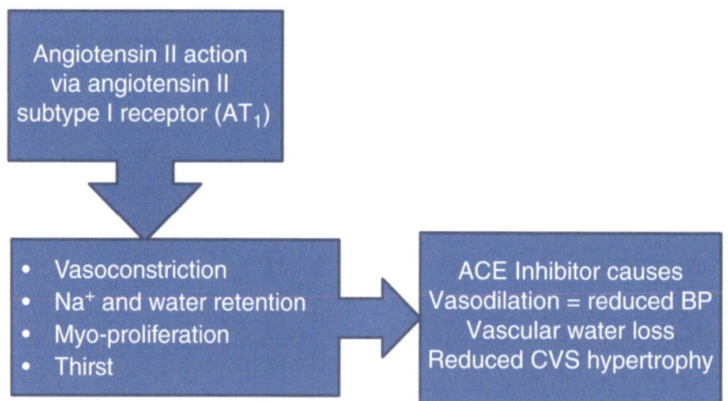

Fig. 7.6 Effects of angiotensin II and its pharmacological inhibition

increases peripheral vascular resistance, i.e. afterload, and increases venous return, i.e. preload, resulting in an increase in blood pressure.

2. Increased levels of noradrenaline (due to stimulation of the sympathetic nerve fibres) and increased levels of catecholamines from the adrenal medulla cause vasoconstriction.

3. Angiotensin II stimulates aldosterone secreted from the cortex of the adrenal gland. This increases the permeability of the distal convoluting tubule membrane and the collecting duct to both sodium and chloride ions and the reabsorption and excretion of potassium. Furthermore, stimulation of the posterior lobe of the pituitary gland releases antidiuretic hormone, resulting in water reabsorption in the distal convoluted tubules and collecting duct of the kidney increasing blood volume (Marieb and Hoehn 2013).
4. Stimulates proliferation of vascular and cardiac muscles cells that are implicated in ventricular hypertrophy (Brunton et al. 2011).

7.4.4 Angiotensin-Converting Enzyme Inhibitor (ACE Inhibitor)

7.4.4.1 Mechanism of Action

ACE inhibitors block the conversion of angiotensin I to angiotensin II, reducing the vasoconstrictory effect on vascular smooth muscle and lowering peripheral resistance. They enhance excretion of sodium and chloride ions in the urine and water loss due to reduced aldosterone secretion and prevent the breakdown of bradykinin, a vasodilator that contributes to a reduction in peripheral resistance.

Specific ACE inhibitors, and their clinical indications, are listed in Table 7.7.

In the management of hypertension, the National Institute for Health and Care Excellence (2019) recommend their use in those under 55, although not for

Table 7.7 Angiotensin-converting enzyme inhibitor

Drug	Comments	Clinical uses
Captopril	Take 1 h prior to food	Hypertension, heart failure with left ventricular dysfunction, after a myocardial infarction, diabetic nephropathy
Enalapril maleate	Prodrug	Hypertension, heart failure
Fosinopril sodium	Prodrug	Hypertension, heart failure
Imidapril hydrochloride	Prodrug take before food	Hypertension
Lisinopril		Hypertension, heart failure, after a myocardial infarction, in diabetic patients who have renal complications
Moexipril hydrochloride	Prodrug	Hypertension
Quinapril	Prodrug Absorption may be reduced by food	Hypertension, heart failure
Ramipril	Prodrug	Hypertension, heart failure, following a myocardial infarction, prevention of further cardiovascular problems in those with diabetes
Trandolapril	Prodrug	Hypertension, after a myocardial infarction

Adapted from Opie and Gersh (2009), Brunton et al. (2011), and Joint Formulary Committee (2024)

Table 7.8 Pharmacokinetics of ACE inhibitors

Drug	Pharmacokinetics	Comments
Oral captopril	Absorbed rapidly Bioavailability 75%[a] Peak plasma concentration within 60–90 min $T1/2$ 2 h Most excreted by the kidneys	Should be taken on an empty stomach absorption is reduced by 30–40% when food is in the gastrointestinal tract dose reduced in renal dysfunction may cause skin rashes and impair taste
Oral enalapril maleate	Absorbed rapidly A prodrug hydrolysed in the liver to active drug enalaprilat Bioavailability 60% Peak plasma concentration within 3–4 h $T1/2$ of enalaprilat 11 h Excreted mainly by the kidneys	Absorption not affected by food dose reduced in renal dysfunction
Lisinopril	Absorbed slowly and based on urinary recovery the average extent of absorption is between 25–30%, although there is considerable variability over the dose range Peak concentration in plasma after 7 h $T1/2$ (plasma) 12 h Excreted unchanged by the kidneys	Food does not affect absorption dose reduced in renal dysfunction

Adapted from Opie and Gersh (2009), Brunton et al. (2011), Joint Formulary Committee (2024), and Electronic Medicine Compendium (eMC) accessed (2025)

Note: These figures are examples as individual preparations will vary

[a]The bioavailability takes into account both absorption and metabolism and describes the proportion of the drug that passes into the systemic circulation

individuals of black African and Caribbean family origin. The rationale for this is that people 55 years and under with hypertension tend to have higher levels of renin, whereas those over 55 years and black people of African Caribbean family origin tend to have lower renin levels and respond less effectively.

7.4.4.2 Pharmacokinetics

Angiotensin-converting enzyme inhibitors are well absorbed from the gastrointestinal tract and are excreted mainly via the kidneys, with the exception of fosinopril sodium. The pharmacokinetics of three ACE inhibitors are presented in Table 7.8.

The hypotensive effect is greater in those with high plasma renin levels. An exaggerated hypotensive state can be observed in those with prescribed diuretics (loop diuretics), who have salt-depleted diets, who are dehydrated or in heart failure.

Careful monitoring is required for those with liver impairment, especially if prescribed prodrugs. They tend not to affect cardiac contractility.

ACE inhibitors are known to cross the placenta and are associated with foetal abnormalities. ACE inhibitors can also be detected in breast milk.

7.4.4.3 Contraindications

Contraindications for ACE inhibitors are given in Tables 7.9 and 7.10.

7.4.4.4 Common Adverse Effects

Cough A cough has been reported in 5–35% of those prescribed ACE inhibitors (Dicpinigaitis 2006). It is proposed that a dry cough results from the accumulation of bradykinin and there is an increased sensitivity of the cough reflex. This is not observed in those prescribe angiotensin II receptor antagonists, as angiotensin II is still available to inactivate bradykinin.

Hypotension Individuals most at risk include those who have high renin levels (those who have a low sodium diet, prescribed loop diuretics and heart failure and those who are dehydrated or having dialysis) as the hypotensive effect is more exag-

Table 7.9 Pregnancy and breastfeeding

Drugs	Comments
All ACE inhibitors	Not to be used in pregnancy unless essential. Can affect foetal and neonatal blood pressure control and renal function
Fosinopril sodium, imidapril hydrochloride, lisinopril, moexipril hydrochloride, perindopril erbumine, ramipril and trandolapril	Not recommended if breastfeeding

Joint Formulary Committee (2024)
If these drugs are prescribed to mothers with older infants (4 weeks to 1 year), the baby's blood pressure should be monitored (Joint Formulary Committee 2024)

Table 7.10 General contraindications

Contraindications	Comments
Hypersensitivity to ACE inhibitors	This includes angioedema: a vascular reaction characterised by swelling involving the deep dermis, submucosa or subcutaneous tissue. It can involve the lips, eyes, face and airway
Pregnancy	In addition to blood pressure and renal function mentioned in Table 7.9. It may also cause skull defects and oligohydramnios (amniotic fluid deficiency)
Bilateral renal artery stenosis Renovascular disease	Glomerular filtrate is either diminished or abolished and can lead to progressive renal failure Drugs prescribed for chronic kidney disease can cause progressive severe impairment of renal function, especially in older people there is a greater risk of hyperkalaemia and other side effects in those with renal impairment
Hepatic dysfunction	The patients liver function should be monitored when prescribed a prodrug

Adapted from Joint Formulary Committee (2024)

gerated. Hypotension following a first dose of medication may be experienced, and to reduce this risk, the first dose may be taken just before retiring.

Hyperkalaemia This is associated with decreased levels of aldosterone leading to a reduction in potassium ion secretion. The co-administration of potassium-sparing diuretics, such as spironolactone, increases the risk of hyperkalaemia as does salt supplements which contain potassium.

Hypersensitivity A rash and angioedema due to immune interactions may be observed. There is an increased incidence in those of African and Caribbean decent (Brown et al. 1996).

Renal impairment Angiotensin II acts by constricting the efferent arteriole to maintain glomerular filtration when there is low perfusion. Inhibition of this can cause acute renal insufficiency.

7.4.4.5 Drug Interactions

Patients prescribed ACE inhibitors often have other long-term conditions and are on a combination of drugs. Potential interactions can occur when co-administered with diuretics, lithium or nonsteroidal anti-inflammatory drugs (NSAIDs). Further details are found in Table 7.11.

7.4.5 Angiotensin II Receptor Antagonists

7.4.5.1 Pharmacology

The biological effects of angiotensin II receptor antagonists are similar to that of ACE inhibitors in that they decrease vasoconstrictor activity and inhibit aldosterone release. Unlike ACE inhibitors, angiotensin II receptor antagonists selectively bind to the angiotensin II receptor AT_1, blocking angiotensin II from binding. This blocks the action of angiotensin II. They do not inhibit the breakdown of bradykinin so are

Table 7.11 Examples of potential serous drug interactions with ACE inhibitors and angiotensin II receptor antagonists

Drug	Comment
Diuretics	Enhanced hypotensive effect
Potassium-sparing diuretic such as spironolactone Potassium salts Ciclosporin	Increased risk of hyperkalaemia
Lithium	Increased lithium concentrations due to reduced excretion
Nonsteroidal anti-inflammatory drugs	Increased risk of renal impairment, hypotensive effect of ACEI antagonised

Joint Formulary Committee (2024)

less likely to cause a cough. Table 7.12 lists some of the angiotensin II receptor antagonists licensed in the United Kingdom, and the pharmacokinetics of two angiotensin II receptor antagonists are presented in Table 7.13.

7.4.5.2 Adverse Reactions

These are similar to ACE inhibitors; however, angiotensin II receptor antagonists do not cause cough as circulating angiotensin deactivates bradykinin.

7.4.6   Clinical Considerations of ACE Inhibitors and Angiotensin Receptor Antagonists

7.4.6.1 Assessment for Adverse Effects

Hyperkalaemia Assess serum potassium levels and report if the individual presents with the signs and symptoms of hyperkalaemia such as an irregular heart rate, numbness and tingling of limbs, fatigue and muscle weakness. Patients should be advised not to take salt substitutes containing potassium, for example, products such as 'low sodium salt' which could cause hyperkalaemia. If the patient is taking drugs that contain potassium or are potassium sparing, they may need to be discontinued.

Table 7.12 Angiotensin II receptor antagonists

Drug	Comments
Candesartan cilexetil, irbesartan, losartan potassium, olmesartan medoxomil	Bioavailability not affected by food
Eprosartan	Food may affect the absorption
Valsartan	Food decreases absorption

Adapted from Electronic Medicines Compendium (eMC) accessed (2025)

Table 7.13 Pharmacokinetics of two angiotensin II receptor antagonists

Drug	Pharmacokinetics
Candesartan cilexetil	A prodrug, converted to the active form during the absorption process from the gastrointestinal tract Plasma peak levels in 3–4 h Plasma $T1/2$ 9 h 40% excreted unchanged via biliary system and faeces and (60%) excreted in urine No effect if taken with food
Losartan potassium	A prodrug activated in the liver to an active metabolite Peak plasma level achieved in 1–3 h For oral administration $T1/2$ is variable depending upon preparation 6–9 h Excreted mainly via the biliary system in faeces and excreted in urine Consuming with food has minimal effect

Adapted from Opie and Gersh (2009), Brunton et al. (2011), Joint Formulary Committee (2024), and Electronic Medicines Compendium (eMC) accessed (2025)

Hypotension The first dose of an ACE inhibitor may cause severe hypotension, fainting or dizziness. The most at risk include those prescribed a loop diuretic or who are dehydrated and have high renin levels. Diuretics may be discontinued prior to starting treatment. If the service user is being treated outside a hospital or care facility, i.e. in the community, they should be advised to administer the first dose when retiring for the night to avoid the possible outcome of a hypotensive episode.

Older people have a greater risk of falls and hypotension may increase this risk. The blood pressure and pulse rate should be monitored to assess for changes and the individual advised to get up slowly. If prescribed with captopril, the individual's blood pressure may decrease after a few hours (short-acting drug), whereas with enalapril maleate, a longer-acting preparation, a fall in blood pressure can last longer.

Fluid Balance Ensure appropriate hydration.

Blood biochemistry Renal function test (including estimated glomerular filtrate rate) and electrolytes and urea should be taken prior to starting either ACEI or angiotensin II receptor antagonists and then after 1–2 weeks and monitored during treatment to assess for changes in renal function. Food may affect absorption of some ACE inhibitors or ARBs.

7.5 Neprilysin Inhibitors

7.5.1 Mechanism of Action

Natriuretic peptides such as atrial natriuretic peptide (ANP) and brain natriuretic peptide (BNP) are released from the heart when the atria and ventricles are over stretched due to increased blood volume. These peptides initiate a central nervous system, renal and vascular response that leads to natriuresis (sodium rich renal fluid loss), and a reduction in sympathetic nerve tone and arterio and veno dilation (Fig. 7.7). Together these influences reduce cardiac workload and ventricular dilatation.

Neprilysin is a neutral endopeptidase that breaks down a number of peptides in the body including ANP and BNP. Inhibition of these hormones by neprilysin results in termination of their effect of reducing cardiac stretch and workload. Sacubitril is the first clinically available medication that inhibits neprilysin, prolonging the affects of ANP and BNP on the heart.

Clinically sacubitril is available in combination with the angiotensin II receptor blocker valsartan in the form of the medication Entresto. This combination amplifies the pharmacological effect of these two medications. This includes vasodilation, reduced blood pressure, reduction in aldosterone levels and a reduction in sympathetic nerve tone. In addition, the presence of an ARB reduces the effect of an increase in angiotensin II caused by sacubitril-related fluid loss.

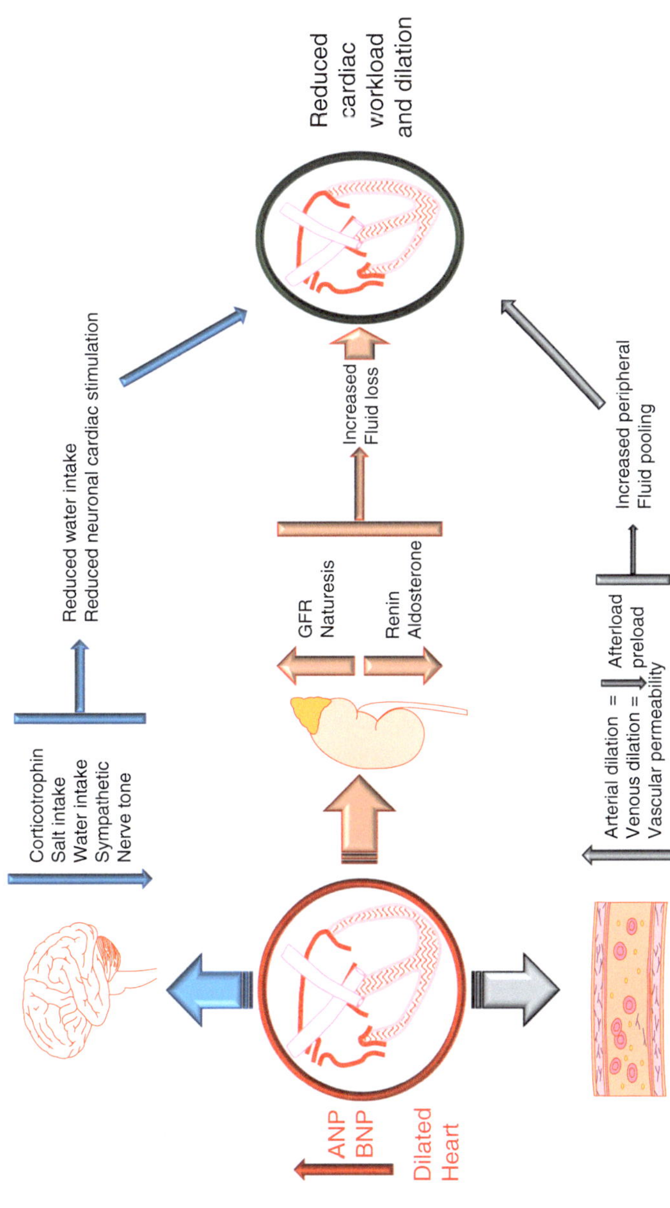

Fig 7.7   The effect of natriuretic peptides on the heart

7.5.2 Pharmacokinetics

Sacubitril is a prodrug and is converted to its active metabolite LBQ657 by carboxylesterases found in different parts of the body including the liver, kidneys and intestine.

Sacubitril, LBQ657 and valsartan are highly plasma protein bound 94–97%. In relation to metabolism neither valsartan, sacubitril or LBQ657 significantly interact with CYP450 isoenzymes therefore there is limited potential for Entresto to cause drug interactions.

Just over 50% of sacubitril, primarily as LBQ657, is excreted by the kidney with the remaining being excreted in faeces. Approximately 86% of Valsartan is excreted in faeces, Owing to these excretion patterns circulating sacubitril and LBQ657 levels are elevated by approximately 1.5–2-fold in moderate to severe renal failure respectively (Electronic Medicines Compendium (eMC) accessed 2025).

7.5.3 Indications for Use

Entresto is recommended by NICE (TA388 2016) to be used in control of symptoms in chronic heart failure in patients who have a New York Heart Association (NYHA) classification of II–IV, with an ejection fraction $\leq 35\%$ and have been on a stable dose of ACE or ARB inhibitor.

7.5.4 Adverse Effects

Similar to ARB and ACE inhibitors Entresto may cause hypotension, hyperkalaemia, angioedema and cough. The risk of angioedema may increase with previous use of ace inhibitors. It has been recommended that ace inhibitors be discontinued at least 36 h prior to starting Entresto (Hubers and Brown 2016).

7.6 Beta-Adrenoceptor Blocking Drugs

7.6.1 Classification of Adrenoceptors

The autonomic nervous system consists of two branches: the parasympathetic and the sympathetic division. Regulation of the heart originates in the cardiovascular centre of the medulla oblongata, receiving stimuli from both sensory receptors and higher centres. The cardiovascular centre coordinates the response by increasing or decreasing the frequency of nerve impulses in both the sympathetic and parasympathetic nervous system. The major neurotransmitter released at the postganglionic nerve ending of the sympathetic division is noradrenaline, and stimulation of the sympathetic nervous system (SNS) increases the release of the catecholamines, mostly adrenaline with small amounts of noradrenaline. These are synthesised in the medulla of the adrenal glands.

There are two main classes of adrenergic receptors: alpha- and beta-adrenoceptors which are subdivided into the following:

- Alpha (α) 1 and 2.
- Beta (β) 1, 2 and 3.

The different receptors have different preferences for adrenaline and noradrenaline. Table 7.14 identifies the adrenergic receptor these ligands preferentially bind to.

The sympathetic nervous system has an important and diverse regulatory function in organs and peripheral vessels, achieved by the binding of noradrenaline or adrenaline to specific α and β receptor subtypes. Pharmacological manipulation of these receptors therefore leads to widespread effects, depending upon the receptor and its location in the body. The location of these subtypes and physiological effect of binding to either α and β subtypes are presented (Table 7.15).

7.6.2 β1 Adrenoceptors: Mechanism of Action

β1 adrenoceptors are located in the heart, kidneys and smooth muscle in the gastrointestinal tract.

7.6.2.1 Cardiac Effects

The sympathetic nervous system increases heart rate and force of contraction through the activation of β1 adrenoceptors located in the myocardium and the cells of the sinoatrial node and conducting tissue. The binding of noradrenaline and adrenaline results in an increase in heart rate (and an increase in the strength of ventricular contraction). These events increase cardiac output and myocardial oxygen consumption and can lead to increases in blood pressure. Increased levels of catecholamines can cause arrhythmias (Rang et al. 2011).

7.6.2.2 Kidney

β1 adrenoceptors are located in the juxtaglomerular granular cells in the kidney, and stimulation of these by the SNS results in the release of the enzyme renin into the renal blood vessels leading to the formation of angiotensin II. Peripheral resistance is increased due to the action of angiotensin II, a known vasoconstrictor, and aldosterone release increases sodium ion reabsorption, resulting in increased blood volume.

Table 7.14 Adrenoceptor ligand preference in the sympathetic nervous system

Ligand	Receptor
Adrenaline	Beta 1, beta 2 and beta 3
Noradrenaline	Alpha 1, alpha 2 and beta 1

Table 7.15 The major location and physiological effects of binding to α and β adrenoceptors

Location: organ and peripheral vessels	Receptor subtype	Physiological effects of the sympathetic nervous system when binding
Heart	β1	Increased heart rate and force of contraction
Kidney		Stimulates release of renin
Smooth muscle	β2	
Bronchial		Dilates the bronchial in response to adrenaline released from the adrenal medulla
Blood vessels		Dilates
Gastrointestinal tract		Decreases motility
Uterus		Relaxation
Bladder sphincter		Relaxation
Ciliary muscles		Relaxation
Skeletal muscle		Tremor and increase in speed of contraction
Liver		Glycogenolysis/glyconeogenesis
Mast cells		Inhibits histamine release
Adipose tissue	β3	Stimulates lipolysis and thermogenesis
Smooth muscle	α1	Increases rate and force of contraction
Bronchial		Constriction
Blood vessels		Constriction
Gastrointestinal tract		Relaxation
Gastrointestinal sphincters		Constriction
Bladder sphincters and uterus		Contraction
Liver		Glucogenolysis
Ciliary muscle		Contraction of ciliary muscles
Smooth muscle	α2	Increases rate and force of contraction
Blood vessels		Dilate/constrict
Gastrointestinal tract		Relaxes
Pancreas		Decreases insulin secretion

Adapted from Bennett and Brown (2008), Brunton et al. (2011), Rang et al. (2011), and Walker and Whittlesea (2011)

7.6.2.3 Gastrointestinal Tract

Relaxation of smooth muscle is achieved through β2 adrenoceptors; however, in the gastrointestinal tract, it is not clear whether it is β1 or β2 (Rang et al. 2011).

7.6.3 Beta-Adrenoceptor Blocking Drugs: Mechanism of Action and Indications for Use

These drugs prevent the ligand noradrenaline and adrenaline from binding to the adrenoceptor by competing for its binding site. They are competitive antagonists. Their action reduces heart rate, cardiac contractility and excitability; they reduce blood pressure in hypertension and have a stabilising effect on the membrane being classified as class II and class III antiarrhythmic drugs. Due to their blocking effect on the granular cells in the juxtaglomerular in the kidney, renin secretion is reduced, hence resulting in reduced formation of angiotensin II. Their indications for use are listed in Box 7.3.

Box 7.3 Indications for Use
- Ischaemic heart disease
- Selected tachycardia arrhythmias
- Heart failure
- Hypertension

The administration of beta-adrenoceptor blocking drugs (beta-blockers) in stable heart failure has been shown to improve patients' survival. The proposed reason being reduced sympathetic activity. These drugs are not prescribed in acute heart failure as they reduce myocardial contractility, which worsen heart failure. Nebivolol, bisoprolol fumarate and carvedilol are licensed for treating heart failure.

Beta-blockers have different actions according to their affinity to the receptor subtype; they vary in their lipid solubility and their selectivity.

7.6.4   Action of Specific Classes of Beta-Blockers

7.6.4.1 Selective Agents for β1 Sites

Beta-blockers such as atenolol and bisoprolol fumarate are known as cardioselective agents. They have a greater affinity for the β1 site than β2; however, selectivity diminishes with increasing doses, and no beta-blocking agent is fully cardiac specific. These agents may cause bronchospasm through their potential blocking action on β2 sites.

7.6.4.2 Nonselective Agents Block Both β1 and β2 Adrenoceptors

Drugs such as propranolol hydrochloride and oxprenolol hydrochloride block both β1 and β2 adrenoceptors equally and are a pure antagonist. Their action on β2 adrenoceptors may induce bronchospasm especially in those with asthma by blocking β2 adrenoceptors in airway smooth muscle affecting the sympathetic reflex (Chap. 10). The Asthma Guidelines state that beta-blockers are contraindicated in asthma unless clinically important (BTS, NICE, SIGN 2024, NG245) and caution when prescribed for those with chronic obstructive pulmonary disease (COPD). Their action may also result in vasoconstriction due to their blocking action on vascular smooth muscle.

7.6.4.3 Nonselective Mixed Agents

Drugs such as labetalol hydrochloride and carvedilol have a pharmacological effect on β1, β2 and α adrenoceptors. The advantage is that vasoconstriction is minimised, due to the enhanced vasodilation due to interaction with α adrenoceptors. Nebivolol although β1 selective has a mixed effect as it vasodilates via a nitric oxide pathway.

7.6.4.4 Intrinsic Sympathomimetic Activity (ISA)

Drugs such as oxprenolol hydrochloride, pindolol and celiprolol hydrochloride both block the adrenoceptor and have the capacity to stimulate (partial agonist); therefore, they do not have the same maximum effect as a full antagonists. These may reduce the risk of bradycardia and cold hands (Joint Formulary Committee 2024).

7.6.5   Other Differences Between Beta-Blockers

Lipid solubility determines the degree of penetration of the beta-blocker into the central nervous system (CNS). Lipophilic beta-adrenoceptor blocking drugs such as propranolol hydrochloride and carvedilol have a greater tendency to cause sleep disturbances, nightmares, hallucinations and depression than those that are more hydrophilic (water soluble) such as atenolol, celiprolol hydrochloride and sotalol hydrochloride. They undergo hepatic metabolism to make them more water soluble for excretion. Water-soluble drugs such as atenolol, celiprolol hydrochloride and sotalol hydrochloride are partially absorbed and are not subject to significant first-pass metabolism in the liver. They are marginally protein bound and do not cross the blood–brain barrier. They are filtered unchanged in the kidney without reabsorption (McGavock 2005). The kidneys mainly excrete these drugs, and therefore, their dose may be reduced in those with renal dysfunction. They have less effect on the central nervous system (CNS) resulting in less risk of sleep disturbances, nightmares and depression.

7.6.6   Pharmacokinetics of Selected Beta-Blockers

7.6.6.1 Atenolol

This drug when administered orally is incompletely absorbed and reaches the systemic circulation. When taken with food, the bioavailability is reduced by 20%. It is hydrophilic (water soluble) and excreted unchanged via the kidneys; therefore, accumulation in those with renal dysfunction may be seen. As it is water soluble, its penetration of the CNS is limited. Its elimination half-life is 6–9 h.

7.6.6.2 Propranolol Hydrochloride

This drug is 90% absorbed after oral administration and metabolised in the liver with high first-pass metabolism. There are individual variations in the clearance of the drug in the liver, and approximately 25% reaches the circulation. It is lipophilic and penetrates the CNS and has a large volume of distribution. It is approximately 90% bound to plasma proteins.

7.6.6.3 Pindolol

A nonselective beta-adrenoceptor blocking drug with intrinsic sympathomimetic activity (ISA) has low lipid solubility. This drug has partial agonist properties resulting in a smaller reduction of heart rate and blood pressure. 90% of the drug is absorbed after oral administration. Approximately 50% is metabolised in the liver and then excreted in the urine (Brunton et al. 2011; Walker and Whittlesea 2011; Electronic Medicines Compendium (eMC) accessed 2025).

Table 7.16 presents the pharmacokinetics of beta-adrenoceptor blocking drugs.

7.6.7   Common Adverse Effects

Bronchospasm β2 adrenoceptors are located in the bronchial smooth muscle, and circulating catecholamines such as adrenaline cause a dilatory effect resulting in bronchial dilation. Beta-blockers may block this physiological effect causing bronchospasm leading to breathlessness and wheezing. This is important in those with respiratory conditions such as asthma and COPD. The asthma guidelines (BTS, NICE, SIGN 2024,

Table 7.16   Pharmacokinetics of some beta-blockers

Drug	Antagonist effect on receptor	Water soluble	Lipid soluble	Oral absorption	$T1/2$ in hours	Elimination
Atenolol[a]	β1 greater than β2	Yes	–	40–60%	6–9	Mainly renal
Bisoprolol fumerate[a]	β1 low β2	–	–	Nearly completely absorbed in the intestine	10–12	Renal and hepatic
Carvedilol[b]	β1, β2, α1	–	Yes	80%	4–10	Hepatic via bile excreted in faeces and renal
Celiprolol hydrochloride[b]	β1, α2	Yes	–	30–70%	5–6	Hepatic via bile excreted in faeces and renal
Labetalol hydrochloride[b]	β1, β2, α1 α2		Low	Completely absorbed	4–8 h	Hepatic via bile excreted in faeces and renal
Nadolol[c]	β1, β2	Yes	–	30%	16–24	Renal
Pindolol[c, d]	β1, β2	–	Yes	90%	3–4	Hepatic via bile excreted in faeces and renal
Propranolol hydrochloride[c]	β1, β2	–	Yes	90%	3–6	Hepatic liver removes 90% of oral dose
Sotalol hydrochloride[c]	β1, β2	Yes	–	70%	10–20	Renal

Adapted from Bennett and Brown (2008), Brunton et al. (2011), Rang et al. (2011), Walker and Whittlesea (2011), and Electronic Medicines Compendium (eMC) accessed (2025)
[a]β1 selective
[b]Nonselective mixed
[c]Nonselective
[d]Intrinsic sympathomimetic activity (ISA)

NG245) state that these drugs should states that non-selective betablockers are not recomended for use in patuents with asthma, however cardioselective betablockers may be used with caution when clinically needed. Cardiac selective drugs have a lessening effect on β2 adrenoceptors, so a lesser effect on airway resistance.

Cold peripheries β2 adrenoceptors are located in the vascular smooth muscle, and circulating catecholamines such as adrenaline causes a dilatory effect resulting in vasodilation. Beta-blockers may block this physiological effect causing vasoconstriction resulting in cold peripheries, and they are contraindicated in peripheral vascular disease should be used with caution in Raynaud's phenomenon.

Cardiac effect This may cause excessive bradycardia and hypotension, exacerbation of conduction disorders, a decrease exercise capacity and exacerbation of acute heart failure (Joint Formulary Committee 2024).

Sleep disturbances, nightmares, hallucinations and depression Lipophilic drugs such as propranolol hydrochloride and carvedilol may cause sleeplessness, nightmares, hallucination and depression compared to hydrophilic drugs such as atenolol and celiprolol hydrochloride and sotalol hydrochloride.

Fatigue Sympathetic activity at rest is minimal; beta-blockers have a greater effect in exercise and situations of stress. Fatigue may result because of reduced muscle perfusion due to a decreased cardiac output.

Hypoglycaemia The liver releases glucose in response to adrenaline, and the sympathetic response to hypoglycaemia is tachycardia; beta-blockers reduce this response and hypoglycaemia may not be recognised.

Gastrointestinal disturbances Due to sympathetic adrenergic receptors being blocked, there is a potential increase in parasympathetic activity.

The common adverse effects are listed in Box 7.4.

Box 7.4 Common Adverse Reactions
Effects on smooth muscle

- Peripheral vasoconstriction—cold hands and feet
- Bronchospasm dyspnoea

Exaggerated cardiac effect

- Bradycardia
- Hypotension
- Conduction disorders

(continued)

Box 7.4 (continued)

CNS

- Fatigue
- Sleep disturbances
- Nightmares
- Psychosis
- Sexual dysfunction
- Gastrointestinal disturbances
- Metabolic effects
- Causes hypo/hyperglycaemia
- Masks tachycardia in hypoglycaemia

7.6.8   Contraindications

Beta-blocker drugs are contraindicated in asthma and caution in those with chronic obstructive pulmonary disease (COPD) due to their blocking action of β2 adrenoceptors in airway smooth muscle.

They are contraindicated in acute heart failure, bradycardia, cardiogenic shock and different forms of AV conduction block, especially in the presence of heart failure, due to the negative effect on pacemakers and conduction and a depressive effect on myocardium.

In pregnancy, beta-blockers may cause intrauterine growth restriction, hypoglycaemia and bradycardia in neonates. The level of many beta-blockers in breast milk is low but with celiprolol hydrochloride, esmolol hydrochloride and nebivolol manufacturers would advise avoidance if breastfeeding (Joint Formulary Committee 2024; Electronic Medicine Compendium (eMC) accessed 2025).

7.6.9   Clinical Considerations

- Assess and be aware of the contraindications, any known allergies and other prescribed medication and over-the-counter medication that could influence treatment.
- Clinical assessment: measurement of blood pressure and pulse rate, rhythm and amplitude to identify a baseline measurement and to indicate adverse effects such as hypotension, postural hypotension and bradycardia. Observe for breathlessness.
- Monitor glucose level in patients with type I and type II diabetes.
- Be aware of the adverse effects associated with the specific beta-blockers, for example, liver damage associated with labetalol hydrochloride. Liver function tests may be included in the patient's management plan.
- Some beta-blockers can cause nightmares and hallucination.

- Specific protocols are used when beta-blockers are administered via the intravenous route.
- Beta-blockers are not prescribed for the initial treatment of hypertension.
- Beta-blockers should not be discontinued suddenly but gradually withdrawn over several weeks especially after long-term treatment as beta-adrenergic receptors become more sensitive to catecholamines. This could exacerbate angina and precipitate sudden death (Brunton et al. 2011).

7.6.10 Summary

Organic nitrates relax both venous and arteriolar smooth muscle resulting in vasodilation improving myocardial perfusion and reducing cardiac workload. Many of the adverse effects are a result of the vasodilatory action and include facial flushing headaches and hypotension. They are used in the management of angina pectoris and acute coronary syndrome and may be used in acute heart failure.

Calcium-channel blockers (CCB) consist of two distinct classes, dihydropyridines and non dihydropyridines, and bind to L-type channels interfering with the movement of calcium into the myocardium and vascular smooth muscle cells. This reduces peripheral vascular resistance and dilates coronary blood vessels lowering blood pressure and improving myocardial perfusion. Non-dihydropyridines have a greater propensity on the conducting system of the heart and are used in the treatment of some arrhythmias. Many adverse effects are a result of their action such as facial flushing. Bradycardia and heart block are a result of inhibition of myocardium calcium reflux.

Angiotensin-converting enzyme inhibitors block the conversion of angiotensin I to angiotensin II and breaks down bradykinin. ARBs block the action of angiotensin II by selectively binding to angiotensin II receptor AT1. They do not inhibit the breakdown of bradykinin and, therefore, are less likely to cause a cough as an adverse effect. These drugs reduce peripheral vascular resistance and increase sodium ions and water excretion and are used in the treatment of hypertension and heart failure. Their adverse effects result from their action and include hypotension, hyperkalaemia and cough.

Beta-adrenergic blocking drugs block the normal sympathetic response of noradrenaline and adrenaline by binding to beta-adrenoceptors in the heart and kidneys. Their pharmacological action and adverse effects are associated with this action. They reduce heart rate, contractility and excitability reducing cardiac workload, and their blocking effect in the kidneys decreases renin secretion, hence reducing the formation of angiotensin II. They are prescribed in the management of angina, arrhythmias, hypertension and heart failure. Cardio-specific agents have a greater affinity for beta I receptors, whereas nonselective agents can block beta I beta 2 and alpha 1 sites. They may cause bronchospasm which limits their use in those with respiratory disorder and are contraindicated in those with asthma and cautioned in those with COPD. Their adverse effects are associated with their actions and may cause bradycardia, hypotension, cold peripheries, sleep disturbances and hypotension.

7.7 Antiarrhythmics

Antiarrhythmic drugs mainly modulate ion channels in the heart to change contractility or conduction. The change in ion channel may be direct on the ion channel itself (ion channel blockers) or be indirect via receptor modulation, for example, beta-adrenergic receptor blockade. Antiarrhythmic medications are currently categorised according to a modification of the original Vaughan Williams classification, which categorises medications according to their antiarrhythmic effect rather than the drug target (Lau et al. 2000) (Table 7.17).

As many antiarrhythmic medications have an effect on action potentials in the heart, a brief and simplified review of the action potential pertinent to antiarrhythmic pharmacology will be provided.

7.7.1 The Action Potential

The action potential represents voltage change during the activation and relaxation of cells in the heart and applies to muscle cells (myocardium) and conduction tissues, including the sinoatrial node (SAN) and atrioventricular node (AVN).

The voltage change in the action potential describes the two electrical states found in muscles and conductive tissue cells in the heart, namely, a polarised state,

Table 7.17 Modified Vaughan Williams classification

Class number	Function	Example
I	Sodium channel blocker	
Ia		Quinidine, procainamide, disopyramide
Ib		Lidocaine, mexiletine, tocainide, phenytoin
Ic		Encainide, flecainide, Propafenone
		Quinidine, procainamide, disopyramide
II	Beta blocker	Propranolol, esmolol, acebutolol, l-sotalol
III	Potassium channel blocker	Amiodarone, bretylium, D,l-sotalol, ibutilide
IVa	Calcium channel blocker	Verapamil, diltiazem
IVb	Potassium channel opener	Adenosine, ATP
Miscellaneous		Digoxin

where the cells are at rest, and a depolarised state, where the cells are activated or working, i.e. myocardium is contracting and conduction tissue is conducting.

The action potential is divided into different phases, numbered 0–4.

The action potential mainly depends upon passive ion movement across ion channels. The beginning of the action potential (phases 0–1) precedes the systolic period of the cardiac cycle and then continues through it (phases 2–3). The diastolic period is mainly associated with phase 4 of the action potential or the resting phase.

The aim of the action potential is to take the cell from a resting phase during which the cell is negative inside (polarised state) to an activated state, during which the cell becomes positive inside (depolarised state). Depolarisation of the cell leads to calcium entry that initiates myocardial contraction or conductive tissue conduction.

7.7.1.1 Phase 0

The action potential (Fig. 7.8) begins when the pacemaker voltage opens sodium ion channels. Sodium moves passively into the cell down its concentration gradient. If the pacemaker voltage is strong enough, then sufficient sodium ions enter the myocardial cell to change the resting negative polarised state of the cell to a more positive state (Fig. 7.8, phase 0); this signifies the beginning of the action potential or phase 0.

7.7.1.2 Phase 1

As more and more sodium ions enter the cell, the inside of the cell becomes more positive. The increased positive charge opens up calcium ion channels that allow calcium to enter the cell passively, maximising the positive charge in the cell. At this time, potassium ion channels also open up. As the concentration gradient of potassium is outwards, potassium begins to flow out of the cell. This causes a sudden drop in the membrane voltage leading to the notch descriptive of phase 1 of the myocardial action potential.

7.7.1.3 Phase 2

During phase 2 of the action, potential calcium ions enter the cell and initiate and perpetuate the myocardial contraction. Calcium ion entry is balanced by potassium ions leaving the cell, resulting in no net change in cell voltage. This keeps the cell voltage constant which is seen as a plateau on the action potential during phase 2 (Fig. 7.8, phase 2). The duration of phase 2 is determined by potassium leaving the cell. Eventually, calcium ion channels begin to close and additional potassium ion channels open. This results in a net loss of positive ion from inside the myocardial cell and causes the cell voltage to drop. This signifies the end of phase 2 and the beginning of phase 3.

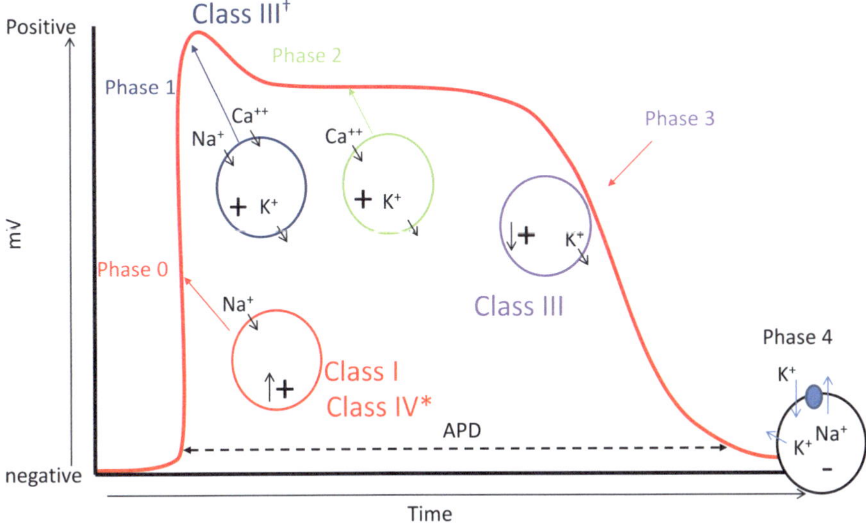

Fig. 7.8 Simplified myocardial action potential, showing site of action of antiarrhythmic drug groups (*Class IV drugs act on nodal action potentials that have different action potentials; †Some class III drugs are only effective on atrial myocardium). APD action potential duration

7.7.1.4 Phase 3

Phase 3 of the action potential is of significant pharmacological importance. During this phase, a number of potassium ion channels open (Fig. 7.8, phase 3) (for detail, see Khan et al. 2012). Movement of potassium ions down their concentration gradient out of the cell causes a net loss of positive ion from the cell, bringing the membrane voltage eventually back to the resting negative (polarised) voltage. Therefore, potassium ion loss during phase 3 of the action potential repolarises the myocardial cell. Once the cell is repolarised, phase 3 finishes, and the resting phase, phase 4, begins. The duration of phase 3 determines the duration of the action potential in ventricular myocardium.

7.7.1.5 Phase 4

Phase 4 coincides broadly with the diastolic period. During this time, active transport mechanisms remove calcium and sodium ions from the cell. During this period, lost cellular potassium is also actively replenished. However, there is a very small potassium 'leak' out of the cell; together with the removal of sodium, the potassium leak keeps the myocardial cell negatively changed, i.e. polarised during phase 4 (Fig. 7.8, phase 4).

7.7.2 Antiarrhythmic Class

7.7.2.1 Class I Sodium Channel Blockers

Sodium channel blockers exert an effect by inhibiting sodium ion entry into the myocardium during phase 0 of the action potential (Fig. 7.9). This inhibition delays the upstroke of the action potential, which may help terminate a number of arrhythmias that are formed because of abnormal depolarisation of the heart cells.

Sodium channel blockers are further subdivided into subclasses (Table 7.17). This subdivision is based upon the drugs' interaction with potassium ion channels.

Class 1a

Class 1a drugs have a moderate sodium ion channel blockade effect and also cause a small amount of blockage on potassium ion channels. This results in a class 1 effect (sodium channel blockage) but also a delayed potassium efflux from the cell resulting in a prolongation of the action potential.

Class 1b

Class 1b drugs are weak sodium channel blockers and have an additional potassium channel opening effect that leads to an enhanced potassium efflux. This results in shortening of the action potential duration.

Class 1c

Class 1c drugs are strong sodium channel blockers and have no effect on potassium ion channels and have no effect on the action potential duration. Consequently, class 1c medications are pure sodium channel blockers.

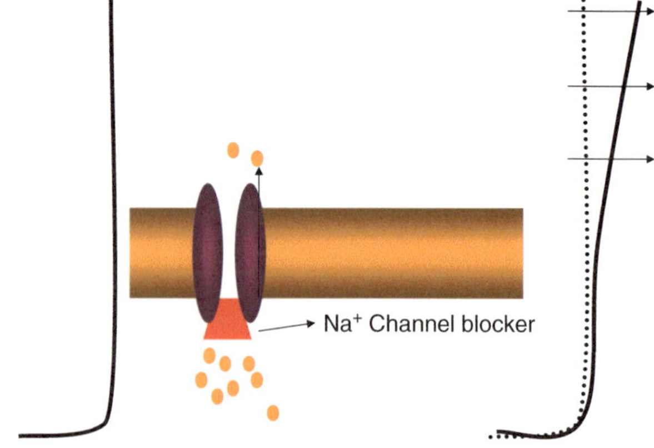

Fig. 7.9 Sodium channel blockers inhibiting the passage of sodium ions (Na⁺) into the cell during the excitation of myocardial action potentials

Table 7.18 Main adverse effects of the four main classes of drugs

Class I	Class II	Class III	Class IV
Proarrhythmic effects:	Sinus bradycardia	Sinus bradycardia	Sinus bradycardia
IA—Torsades de pointes	AV block	Torsades de pointes	AV block
IB—negative inotropic effect	Depression of LV function (adrenergic-dependent)		Negative inotropic effect
IC—proarrhythmic			

Adverse reactions of these class 1 drugs are influenced by the drug's effect on potassium ion channels (Table 7.18).

7.7.2.2 Class II

Class II inhibits the sympathetic adrenergic pathways. Beta-blockers are designed to act primarily on the beta 1 (β1) receptor found in the heart; inhibition of this receptor results in reducing the effects of adrenaline and noradrenaline on the heart:

- S/A node increased firing rate.
- A/V node increased conduction velocity.
- Myocardium increased force of contraction.

Refer to preceding section on beta-receptor antagonists in this chapter for further detail.

7.7.2.3 Class III

Class III medications block potassium ion channels (Fig. 7.10a). Potassium ion channel opening occurs during two phases in the action potential: during phase 1, which is prominent in atrial myocardium, and during phase 3, which is important for both atrial and ventricular myocardium. Potassium ion movement out of the cell governs the action potential duration (APD). This is important because during the action potential, the cell is relatively resistant or refractive to electrical stimuli that may initiate an arrhythmia (Fig. 7.10a). Refractivity of the cell is divided into two forms: absolutely refractive, during which time the cell cannot be stimulated, and relatively refractive, during which time the cell may be stimulated if the stimuli is strong enough (Fig. 7.10a). By prolonging potassium efflux from the cell, potassium channel blockers prolong the action potential duration and consequently the refractivity of the cell, making it more resistant to arrhythmia formation.

QT Prolongation

As with many situations in nature, too much of a good thing is detrimental. This is the case with prolongation of the APD. If the APD prolongs too much, there is risk of generating a specific form of ventricular tachycardia known as torsade de pointes (TdP). Prolongation of the APD is clinically measured on the electrocardiograph (ECG) as the QT interval (Fig. 7.10b). Accurate measurement of the QT interval requires correct heart rate. The QT interval varies slightly with gender, but generally the normal QT interval is 0.43 s or 430 ms.

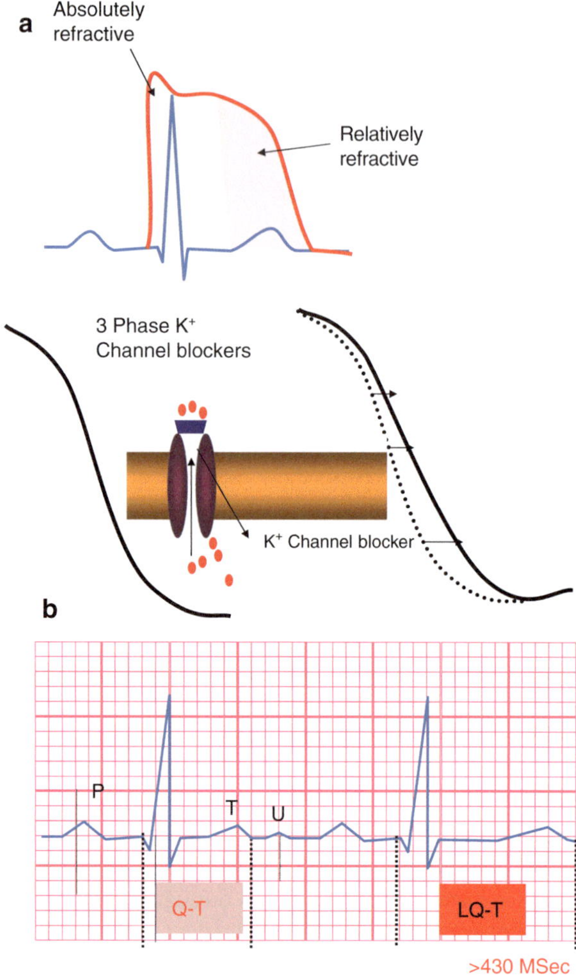

Fig. 7.10 Effect of class III antiarrhythmics: inhibition of potassium efflux from the myocardial cell delays repolarisation (solid line) (**a**). Within limits this reduces the possibility of the muscle eliciting an abnormal depolarisation or contraction. Too much potassium channel blockade may however lead to an abnormally long delay in repolarisation seen on the electrocardiograph (ECG) as a prolonged QT interval (**b**). QT interval prolongation may lead to a potentially fatal ventricular arrhythmia known as torsade de pointes

As the main effect of class III drugs is potassium channel blockade, most if not all drugs in this class carry the potential to prolong the QT interval and subsequently are associated with a risk of causing TdP.

Amiodrone is the most popular drug in this class. Its frequent use is derived from its ability to terminate a wide number of arrhythmias. This is due to the mixed nature of its mechanism of action. Although it is a class III agent (potassium channel blocker), it has powerful class I and class II characteristics. Due to its effectiveness, it tends to become a drug of convenience, despite the time it takes to load in the blood stream. There are, however, many adverse effects associated with its short- and long-term administration. Recent studies have now demonstrated that procainamide is comparable to amiodarone in terms of efficacy in cardiovert ventricular tachycardia and has fewer adverse effects (Kelson and deSouza 2019).

Adverse Reactions of Amiodarone

Adverse reactions are common (occur in more than 75% of patients receiving drug) and increases after a year of treatment; some toxicities may be fatal. The half-life of amiodarone is 25–110 days which may prolong toxicity. Specific adverse effects of amiodarone include the following:

- Pulmonary toxicity and fibrosis (10–15%) can cause death in 10% of those affected); as this effect is associated with tissue fibrosis, this may be irreversible.
- Constipation may occur in 20% of patients.
- Corneal deposits may occur; these may effect vision and are normally reversible when the medication is discontinued.
- Neuronal effects include peripheral neuropathy, dizziness, depression, nightmares and hallucinations.
- As the amiodarone molecule contains two atoms of iodine, they may disturb thyroid function resulting in changes in plasma thyroxine level.
- Amiodarone accumulates in the subcutaneous tissues where the iodine fluoresces as the iodine reacts to sunlight. This causes cutaneous photosensitivity and blue-grey skin discolorations.
- Amiodarone may increase LDL-cholesterol plasma concentrations.
- Amiodarone and its metabolites interact with a number of metabolic enzymes including cytochrome P450 (2D6, 1A2 and 3A4 McDonald et al. 2015). This may enhance the effect of warfarin and increases the serum concentrations of digoxin, quinidine, procainamide, flecainide, theophylline and other medications.
- Adapted from Anon (1991).

To help reduce the occurrence of these adverse effects, a low maintenance dose of amiodarone (200 mg/day) is now suggested (Joint formulary committee 2024).

It is important to reiterate that amiodarone needs to be administered via a wide bore cannula appropriately diluted, as IV administration is associated with considerable risk of phlebitis (Norton et al. 2013).

General adverse effects of class III medications are shown in Table 7.18.

Novel Class III Medications

A number of new medications have recently been developed that specifically block potassium ion channels in phase 1 of the action potential (Fig. 7.8). These ion channels play a significant role in atrial repolarisation. Therefore, blockade of phase 1 potassium ion channels has potential to inhibit/terminate atrial fibrillation (AF). One such drug, vernakalant, has been licensed for use in Europe. This drug has been demonstrated to be effective in converting acute-onset AF back to sinus rhythm; however, there are safety concerns with this medication that caution its wider clinical use and licence for use in the USA (Akel and Lafferty 2018). NICE, have not provided any guidance regarding the use of this drug owing to a lack of provided evidence (TA675, 2021). However there is a small body of evidence that continues to demonstrate clinical benefits of the drug, for example, a systematic review exploring the use of vernakalant in cardioversion of rapid onset AF including 12 studies (2365 patients, 887 events) demonstrated a significantly great rate of cardioversion compared to placebo and other active comparators (risk ratio = 5.60; 95% CI, 2.83–11.09; I2 test for heterogeneity, 92%) (Yu et al. 2023).

7.7.2.4 Class IV

Class IV antiarrhythmics are the main area where the original Vaughan Williams classification and the later Sicilian Gambit differ. Class IV antiarrhythmics are now subdivided into subgroups IVa and IVb. Although they both inhibit calcium ion channels from conducting (class IV effect), this effect is achieved by different mechanisms.

Class IVa calcium-channel blockers such as verapamil and diltiazem have a relatively localised inhibitory effect on nodal (SA and AV node) calcium ion channels; these have great therapeutic importance. This is because the upstroke (phase 0) of the AV-node and SA-node action potential is Ca^{++} dependent (Fig. 7.11) rather than Na^+ dependent, as in myocardial tissue (Fig. 7.8). By inhibiting the upstroke of the AV node, these drugs have the ability to slow down nodal depolarisation (Fig. 7.11). This effect is important as it reduces AV node conduction, an effect that helps disrupt a number of tachycardic arrhythmias involving the AV node, collectively known as re-entry arrhythmias. Other calcium-channel blockers such as nifedipine and amlodipine do not possess this effect because their effect is primarily on vascular smooth muscle calcium channels.

Antiarrhythmic calcium-blocking drugs are almost exclusively used to terminate AV node implicated tachycardia, although they do have some use in treatment of fast atrial arrhythmias.

Class IV b

These drugs are classified as such because their net effect is calcium ion channel inhibition (class IV effect). However, this effect is achieved indirectly. Class IVb antiarrhythmics are potassium channel openers by action.

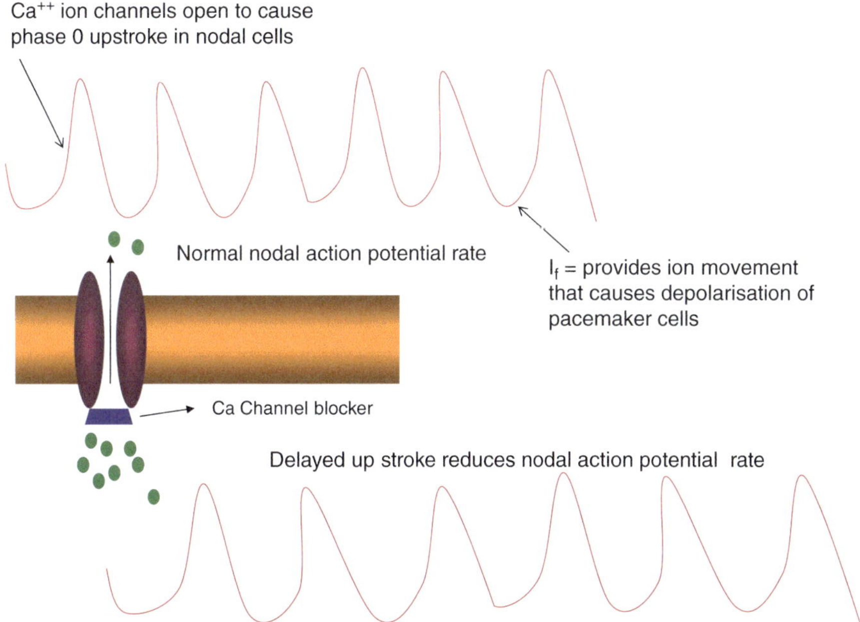

Fig. 7.11 Effect of antiarrhythmic calcium ion channel blockers on nodal action potentials

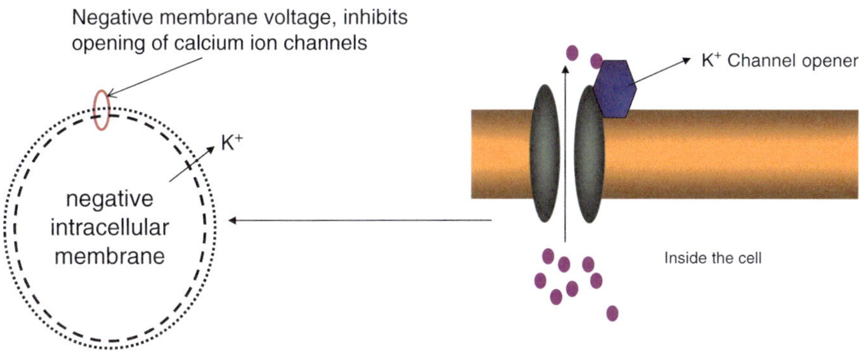

Fig. 7.12 Mechanism of action of potassium channel openers

Potassium moves passively out of the cell when its ion channel opens. Potassium loss from the cell reduces the membrane potential to a more negative voltage (Fig. 7.12); this affects how the cell depolarises. Sodium ion channels open when the membrane is electrically stimulated (by the pacemaker) at very low voltages. This is why sodium ion channels and not calcium ion channels initiate the action potential. Calcium channels open once the membrane potential is more positive (or less negative). Potassium ion channel openers increase the efflux of positively charged potassium ions from the cell, rendering the membrane potential (voltage) very negative (hyperpolarise). Medications such as adenosine act as potassium ion channel openers and hyperpolarise nodal membranes making it difficult for the cells to depolarise and open calcium ion channels. When these medications are administered to patients with re-entry of tachycardia involving the AV node, these drugs disrupt the synchrony of the re-entry mechanism by slowing done AV node firing rates and terminate the arrhythmia.

Although not found in the classic antiarrhythmic classification, digoxin is a widely prescribed antiarrhythmic drug that is indicated for use for atrial fibrillation.

7.7.2.5 Digoxin

Digoxin as a therapeutic medication has been used for over 200 years. It has a two-fold effect on the heart: one is directly on the myocardium itself and the second is believed to be via a modification of sympathetic nerve tone on the heart.

Digoxin inhibits the Na/K ATP-dependent ion exchange pump found in the myocardial membrane. Normally, this pump removes Na^+ from and loads K^+ into the cell, in a ratio of 3:2, i.e. 3 Na^+ ions are removed from inside of the cell for each 2 K^+ ions loaded into the cell (Fig. 7.13a). This low intracellular Na^+ concentration drives another ion exchange mechanism, called the Na^+/Ca^{++} exchanger, to load Na^+ into the cell at the expense of unloading Ca^{++} ions (Fig. 7.13a).

When digoxin inhibits the Na/K pump, Na^+ slowly starts to build up in the cell. This excess Na^+ is then unloaded from the cell by the Na^+/Ca^{++} exchanger (Fig. 7.13b). As a consequence, Ca^{++} is now loaded into the cell. This increased intracellular calcium results in a greater force of contraction, improving the

Fig. 7.13 (a, b) Ionotropic effect of digoxin

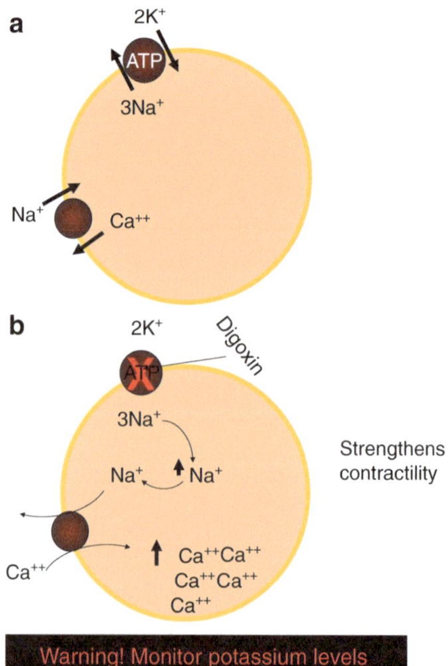

contractile force of the ventricles during each heartbeat. When using this drug however, it is important to maintain adequate K^+ serum levels as the main mechanism that loads K^+ into the cell, the Na/K pump, is impaired.

The second mechanism by which digoxin modulates the heart is via the inhibition of sympathetic nerve discharge. This results in reducing the excitatory effect of the sympathetic nervous system on the SA and AV node and possibly on sites of abnormal automaticity.

Digoxin is cleared by the kidney in a nearly unchanged form, i.e. it experiences little hepatic metabolism; the metabolites produced are active (Lisalo 1977). CYP3A4 has been implicated in its limited metabolism, and its renal clearance is influenced by P-glycoprotein. Therefore, renal dysfunction or drug–drug interactions have significant potential to influence digoxin serum levels. Digoxin has a very narrow therapeutic index (0.5–1.0 μg/L). Therefore, care needs to be taken when this medication is being administered, as it influences serum levels of other drugs and its serum levels are influenced by other medications, including diuretics, calcium-channel blockers, antiarrhythmics and antibiotics.

7.7.2.6 Inhibition of Pacemaker Ion Channels

The action potentials of the SAN and AVN are similar in that they have a slow upward rising baseline before the phase 0 upstroke (Fig. 7.11). This rising baseline is caused by ions moving into the cell by a specific ion channel that is found only in pacemaker cells; the current that these ions produce is known as If or funny current (Fig. 7.11). Inhibition of the ion channel that carries this current is achieved by a drug called ivabradine. Ivabradine has the benefit of reducing the SAN firing rate, i.e. heart rate, without affecting myocardial contractility. This provides a benefit over beta-blockers that are traditionally employed to achieve a reduction in heart rate. Ivabradine is currently prescribed for systolic heart failure and stable chronic angina (Koruth et al. 2017). Ivabradine is metabolised by CYP3A4 and is excreted 4% unchanged in the urine. Adverse effects of ivabradine include bradycardia, new onset AF and phosphenes (experience the perception of light in absence of light) (Petite et al. 2018).

7.7.3 Summary

Antiarrhythmic drugs are currently classified according to their functional effects on ion channels. The majority of which effects ion channels themselves. Classes I, III and IVa and IVb have an effect on sodium, potassium and calcium channels, respectively. Classification II antiarrhythmics are beta-blockers. Class IVb antiarrhythmic medications effect calcium ion channels; they achieve this by opening potassium ion channels. Digoxin, a commonly used antiarrhythmic, does not fall within the typical classification. Adverse effects of antiarrhythmic drugs are primarily Type A. This point is particularly important when considering the use of class II and IV drugs together as they amplify each other's effects on nodal tissue. Also of note is the QT prolongation effect of class III antiarrhythmic medications; this effect limits their clinical use. Amiodarone, one of the most frequently used class III anti-arrhythmics, is further associated with a number of other adverse effects, therefore requiring monitoring with prolonged use.

7.8   HMG-CoA Reductase Inhibitors (Statins)

Simvastatin, atorvastatin, rosuvastatin, pravastatin and fluvastatin

Fats are carried in the blood stream in small particles called lipoproteins that, as their name suggests, contain lipid and protein. There are different kinds of lipoproteins in the blood stream; these range from the very small chylomicrons and different kinds of low-density lipoprotein (LDL) to the larger high-density lipoproteins (HDL). Via the blood stream, LDL delivers cholesterol, a form of lipid, to the cells for structural and energy-related uses. HDL conversely captures cholesterol from the body and brings it back to the liver to be recycled or excreted via the bile. Raised blood levels of low-density lipoprotein (LDL) are important in the formation of atherosclerotic plaques, the cause of cardiovascular diseases such as ischaemic heart disease and stroke.

Cholesterol may be ingested or produced by a complex chain of reactions beginning with the carbohydrate glucose. Therefore, too much cholesterol-containing food or too much sugar (sucrose which contains glucose) can lead to an increase in LDL concentration in the blood stream.

Cholesterol is produced from a metabolite of glucose metabolism (glycolysis) called pyruvate; this substance is enzymatically converted to acetyl-coenzyme A (acetyl-CoA). Acetyl-CoA is the precursor for cholesterol, which is formed following a number of enzymatic reactions (Fig. 7.14). The formation of one of the intermediate substances, mevalonate from 3-hydroxy-3-methylglutaryl-coenzyme A (HMG-CoA), is the rate-limiting step in the formation of cholesterol and is catalysed by the enzyme HMG-CoA reductase (Fig. 7.14).

Following over 20 years of painstaking research, the first commercially available medication to inhibit HMG-CoA reductase, lovastatin, was licenced in 1987 (Endo 2010). This began the reign of one of the most popular groups of medications in pharmaceutical history, statins.

Statins are widely used in prevention of ischaemic heart disease. The overwhelming effect of this medication is ascribed to LDL lowering. However, statins have a number of additional or pleiotropic effects, linked but unrelated to lipid lowering, that reduce the risk of cardiovascular disease. These pleiotropic effects include atherosclerotic plaque stabilisation, vascular smooth muscle proliferation and inhibition of platelet aggregation.

7.8.1   Adverse Reactions of Statins

Despite the adverse effects associated with statins, their use has been widely adopted in clinical practice. The most common adverse effects include muscle pain (myalgia) and joint pain (arthralgia). Under certain circumstances, this group of

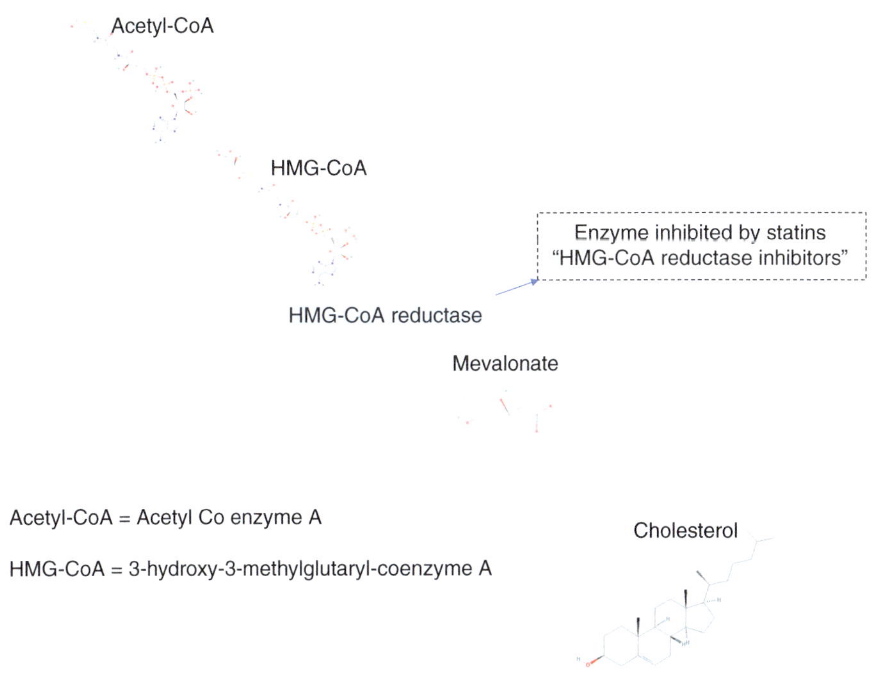

Fig. 7.14 Selected steps in cholesterol formation. Acetyl-CoA Acetyl coenzyme A, HMG-CoA 3-hydroxy-3-methylglutaryl-coenzyme A

medications may cause rhabdomyolysis or muscle breakdown. Although it is not absolutely clear what causes these effects, the muscle abnormalities (myopathy) associated with statins have been linked to changes in the neuromuscular junction and cellular mitochondrial function (Sirtori 2014). Rhabdomyolysis is of concern as pigments liberated into the blood stream following muscle degradation are nephron (kidney) toxic. Although rare today, if rhabdomyolysis occurs, this may lead to acute and persistent kidney dysfunction. A survey of Eudravigilance, the European suspected adverse effect database, from January 2004 to July 2021 found that for atorvastatin, rosuvostatin and simvastatin there were 8965 events link to psychiatric adverse drug reactions. The most common psychiatric adverse effects were; insomnia (37.7–46.9%), depression (28.78–55.23%) and anxiety 9.6–55.64%), with lesser reports of nightmares (5.8%). Hallucinations (2.1%), suicidal ideation and attempts together were reported in smaller numbers (5.4%) (Pop et al. 2022). Statins may precipitate diabetes due to a possible opening of potassium ion channels in the pancreatic beta cells which will inhibit insulin secretion. Other adverse effects that have been associated with statins include liver dysfunction and transient/reversible changes in liver enzyme levels such as transaminase. There have been inconclusive reports of statins being associated with cataracts and erectile dysfunction (Yu et al. 2017; Alves et al. 2018; Kostis and Dobrzynski 2019).

7.8.2 Pharmacokinetics of Statins

The pharmacokinetics of statins includes a range of cytochrome P450 enzymes, commonly including the 3A4 variant (Table 7.19) and together with enzymatic metabolism, drug efflux plays a significant role in pharmacokinetic manipulation of this drug class. Together with different modes of clearance (Table 7.19), these mechanisms regulate statin drug levels in the body. Variations in the efficacy of these pharmacokinetic systems result in individual variation, including differences in lipid-lowering efficacy as well as adverse effects. Owing to single nucleotide mutations or polymorphisms (SNPs) in genes that produce CYP enzymes and drug efflux proteins, there are a wide range of clinical effects observed when using these medications in practice. Drug levels are linked to efficacy as well as the degree of myopathy; currently however, there are no biochemical markers available that can predict which person may experience muscular adverse effects from these medications (Sirtori 2014).

Table 7.19 Pharmacokinetics of some popular statins

Statin	Absorption	PPB	Met	Clearance	$T1/2$
Simvastatin	Plasma concentration peaks 1.3–2.4 h (passes the BBB)	95% bound	3A4 substrate	13% renal 60% faecal	3 h
Atorvastatin	Plasma concentration peaks 1–2 h	98%	3A4,5 70% of drug effect is via active metabolites	Primarily biliary <2% renal	14 h But active metabolites 20–30 h
Rosuvastatin hydrophilic	Plasma concentration peaks 3–5 h	88%	Hydrophilic drug 2 C9 not clinically significant	70–90% faecal	19 h
Pravastatin hydrophilic	Plasma concentration peaks 1–1.5 h	50%	2C9 main, 2D6 and 3A4	Oral primarily faecal IV 47% renal	77 h
Fluvastatin	<1 h (tablet empty stomach) ~6 h (extended release tablet with high-fat meal) ~6 h	98%	2C9 75% 3A4 20% 2C8 5%	Primarily faecal	3 h

BBB blood–brain barrier, *PPB* plasma protein binding, *Met* metabolism, *T1/2* half-life

7.8.3   Summary

Statin drugs are a pivotal strategy to help reduce cardiovascular disease. This is directly related to their efficacy in lowering cholesterol in the blood stream as well as additional pleiotropic effects that help reduce the risk of atherosclerosis and plaque degradation. The main clinical concern with their use is association with muscle damage that results in myalgia and arthralgia, which may result in poor compliance. Drug levels of these medications that may help predict the occurrence of adverse effects are, however, significantly liable to polymorphisms in metabolic and drug efflux pathways. These genetic variations lead to significant person-to-person variability when prescribing statins in clinical practice.

Multiple Choice Questions

1. Which of the following is the most common adverse effect of organic nitrates:
   (a) Constipation
   (b) Headache
   (c) Hypertension
   (d) Anaphylaxis
2. The duration of action of glyceryl trinitrate spray is:
   (a) 4–8 h
   (b) 8 h
   (c) 30 min
   (d) 60 min
3. Which of the following is a disadvantage of organic nitrates:
   (a) A cough
   (b) May cause swelling of the ankles
   (c) Risk of tolerance
   (d) Should not be taken with grapefruit juice
4. Which of the following statements are true:
   (a) Verapamil has a greater effect on vascular smooth muscle and a limited effect on conducting tissues
   (b) Verapamil has a greater effect on conducting tissue and a limited effect on vascular smooth muscle
   (c) Verapamil is an agonist and blocks L-type calcium channels
   (d) Verapamil is an antagonist and opens L-type calcium channels
5. Which of the following is a dihydropyridine:
   (a) Diltiazem
   (b) Amlodipine
   (c) Verapamil
   (d) Atenolol

6. Nitrates are used for the treatment of angina and act to:
   - (a) Increase preload and decrease afterload
   - (b) Decrease preload and increase afterload
   - (c) Decrease venous return and decrease myocardial workload
   - (d) Increase venous return and increase myocardial workload

7. Which of the following statements are true:
   - (a) ACE inhibitors may cause hypokalaemia and diuresis
   - (b) ACE inhibitors are recommended in the treatment of chronic kidney disease and renovascular disease
   - (c) ACE inhibitors block the conversion of renin to angiotensin II
   - (d) ACE inhibitors block the conversion from angiotensin I to angiotensin II

8. A patient is prescribed an ACE inhibitor, which of the following can increase the risk of hypotension:
   - (a) Dehydration
   - (b) Overhydration
   - (c) Decreased renin level
   - (d) Hyperkalaemia

9. Which of the following best describes the action of candesartan cilexetil:
   - (a) Acts as an antagonist on adrenoceptors
   - (b) Acts as an antagonist on angiotensin II receptor
   - (c) Acts as an agonist on adrenoceptors
   - (d) Acts as an agonist on angiotensin II receptor

10. Which of the following is a cardioselective beta-adrenoceptor blocking drug:
    - (a) Propranolol hydrochloride
    - (b) Labetalol
    - (c) Nebivolol
    - (d) Pindolol

11. Which of the following would you question before administering a beta-adrenoceptor blocking drug:
    - (a) Prescribed for angina
    - (b) Prescribed for hypertension
    - (c) Prescribed in cardiogenic shock
    - (d) Prescribed for primary open angle glaucoma

12. Which of the following is an example of a beta-adrenoceptor blocking drug:
    - (a) Verapamil
    - (b) Labetalol
    - (c) Isosorbide dinitrate
    - (d) Enalapril maleate

13. The direct mechanism of action of class IVb antiarrhythmic medications is:
    - (a) Inhibition of calcium ion channels
    - (b) Inhibition of potassium ion channels
    - (c) Opening of potassium ion channels
    - (d) Opening of sodium ion channels

14. When treating a patient with digoxin, which electrolyte commonly requires close monitoring:
    (a) Sodium
    (b) Potassium
    (c) Calcium
    (d) Chloride
15. Which of the commonly used antiarrhythmic may cause irreversible lung damage:
    (a) Amiodarone
    (b) Bisoprolol
    (c) Carvidolol
    (d) Digoxin
16. Which class of antiarrhythmic drugs has a limited effect on potassium ion channels:
    (a) Class 1a
    (b) Class 1b
    (c) Class 1c
    (d) Class III
17. Too much inhibition of potassium ion channels leads to developing the risk of:
    (a) Preexcitation
    (b) AV block
    (c) Long QT
    (d) Atrial fibrillation
18. Which statin does not undergo significant metabolic change:
    (a) Simvastatin
    (b) Atorvastatin
    (c) Fluvastatin
    (d) Rosuvastatin
19. The main adverse effect with the usage of statins is:
    (a) Rhabdomyolysis
    (b) Depression
    (c) Weight loss
    (d) Myalgia
20. Pleiotropic effects of statins:
    (a) Are its main clinical effect
    (b) Are additional clinically relevant effects
    (c) Are additional clinically relevant adverse effects
    (d) Describe its main effects on the atherosclerotic plaque

Answers

1. (b)
2. (c)
3. (c)

4. (b)
5. (b)
6. (c)
7. (d)
8. (a)
9. (b)
10. (c)
11. (c)
12. (b)
13. (c)
14. (b)
15. (a)
16. (c)
17. (c)
18. (d)
19. (d)
20. (b)

References

Akel T, Lafferty J (2018) Efficacy and safety of intravenous vernakalant for the rapid conversion of recent-onset atrial fibrillation: a meta-analysis. Ann Noninvasive Electrocardiol 23(3):e12508

Alves C, Mendes D, Batel Marques F (2018) Statins and risk of cataracts: a systematic review and meta-analysis of observational studies. Cardiovasc Ther 36(6):e12480

Anon (1991) Drugs for arrhythmias. Med Lett Drugs Ther 33(846):55–60

Bailey DG, Dresser GK, Kreeft JH, Munoz C, Freeman DJ, Bend JR (2000) Grapefruit-felodipine interaction: effect of unprocessed fruit and probable active ingredients. Clin Pharmacol Ther 68(1):468–477

Baxter K, Stockley IH (2010) Stockley's drug interactions, 8th edn. Pharmaceutical Press, London, Chicago

Bennett PN, Brown MJ (2008) Clinical pharmacology, 10th edn. Churchill Livingstone, London

British Thoracic Society, National institute of health and care excellence & Scottish Intercollegiate Guideline Network (2024) Asthma: diagnosis, monitoring and chronic asthma management. https://www.nice.org.uk/guidance/NG245/chapter/recommendations. Accessed October 2024

Brown NJ, Ray WA, Snowden M, Grithin MR (1996) Black American s have an increased rate of angiotensin converting enzyme inhibitor associated with angioedema. Clin Pharmacol Ther 60(1):8–13

Brunton L, Chabier B, Knollman B (2011) Goodman and Gilman's the pharmacological basis of therapeutics, 12th edn. McGraw Hill Medical, New York

Dicpinigaitis PV (2006) Angiotensin converting enzyme inhibitor induced cough. Chest 129(1 supp):169S–173S

Electronic Medicines Compendium (eMC) (2025) www.medicines.org.uk. Accessed October 2025

Endo A (2010) A historical perspective on the discovery of statins. Proc Jpn Acad Ser B Phys Biol Sci 86(5):484–493

Harrison DG, Bates JN (1993) The nitrovasodilators: new ideas about old drugs. Circulation 87(5):1461–1467

Hubers SA, Brown NJ (2016) Combined angiotensin receptor antagonism and neprilysin inhibition. Circulation 133(11):1115–1124

Joint Formulary Committee (2024) British National Formulary 87 British. Medical Journal & Royal Pharmaceutical Society, London

Kelson K, deSouza I (2019) Procainamide versus amiodarone for stable ventricular tachycardia. Acad Emerg Med. https://doi.org/10.1111/acem.13767

Khan E, Spiers C, Khan M (2012) The heart and potassium: a banana republic. Acute Card Care 15(1):17–24

Koruth JS, Lala A, Pinney S, Reddy VY, Dukkipati SR (2017) The clinical use of ivabradine. J Am Coll Cardiol 70(14):1777–1784

Kostis JB, Dobrzynski JM (2019) Statins and erectile dysfunction. World J Men's Health 37(1):1–3

Lau W, Newman D, Dorian P (2000) Can antiarrhythmic agents be selected based on mechanism of action? Drugs 60(6):1315–1328

Levick RJ (2000) An introduction to cardiovascular physiology, 3rd edn. Arnold, London

Lisalo E (1977) Clinical pharmacokinetics of digoxin. Clin Pharmacokinet 2(1):1–16

Marieb E, Hoehn K (2008) Anatomy and physiology, 3rd edn. Pearson Benjamin Cummings, San Francisco

Marieb E, Hoehn K (2013) Human anatomy and physiology, 9th edn. Pearson, Boston

McDonald MG, Au NT, Rettie AE (2015) P450-based drug-drug interactions of amiodarone and its metabolites: diversity of inhibitory mechanisms. Drug Metab Dispos 43(11):1661–1669

McGavock H (2005) How drugs work pharmacology for healthcare professional, 2nd edn. Radcliffe, Oxford

Miller MR, Withers R, Bhamra R, Holt DW (1986) Verapamil and breast feeding. Eur J Clin Pharmacol 30(1):125–126

Moini J (2012) Cardiopulmonary pharmacology for respiratory care. Jones and Bartlett Learning LLC, Sudbury

Montague S, Watson R, Herbert R (2005) Physiology for nursing practice, 3rd edn. Elsevier, Edinburgh

National Institute for Health and Care Excellence (2013) Hypertension quality standard (QS28). NICE, London

National Institute of Health and Clinical Excellence (2016) Sacubitril Valsartan for treating symptomatic chronic heart failure with reduced ejection fraction. Technology appraisal guidance TA388

National Institute for Health and Care Excellence (2019) Hypertension in adults: diagnosis and management, (NG136). Accessed October 2024

Norton L, Ottoboni LK, Varady A, Yang-Lu CY, Becker N, Cotter T, Pummer E, Haynes A, Forsey L, Matsuda K, Wang P (2013) Phlebitis in amiodarone administration: incidence, contributing factors, and clinical implications. Am J Crit Care 22(6):498–505

Opie LH, Gersh BJ (2009) Drugs for the heart, 7th edn. Saunders Elsevier, Philadelphia

Page C, Curtis M, Walker M, Hoffman B (2006) Integrated pharmacology, 3rd edn. Elsevier, Philadelphia

Petite SE, Bishop BM, Mauro VF (2018) Role of the funny current inhibitor ivabradine in cardiac pharmacotherapy: a systematic review. Am J Ther 25(2):e247–e266

Pop G, Farcaş A, Butucă A, Morgovan C, Arseniu AM, Pumnea M, Teodoru M, Gligor FG (2022) Post-marketing surveillance of statins-a descriptive analysis of psychiatric adverse reactions in EudraVigilance. Pharmaceuticals (Basel) 15(12):1536

Rang HP, Dale MM, Rutter JM, Flower RJ, Henderson G (2011) Pharmacology, 7th edn. Elsevier Churchill Livingstone, Edinburgh

Schwartz JB, Upton RA, Lin ET, Williams RL, Benet LZ (1988) Effect of cimetidine or ranitidine administration on nifedipine pharmacokinetics and pharmacodynamics. Clin Pharmacol Ther 43(6):673–680

Sirtori CR (2014) The pharmacology of statins. Pharmacol Res 88:3–11

Walker R, Whittlesea C (2011) Clinical pharmacology and therapeutics, 5th edn. Churchill Livingstone, Edinburgh

Yu S, Chu Y, Li G, Ren L, Zhang Q, Wu L (2017) Statin use and the risk of cataracts: a systematic review and meta-analysis. J Am Heart Assoc 6(3):e004180

Yu C, Li J, Zhao C, Guan Y, Wu D, Sun B, Wang X (2023) Effectiveness and safety profiles of vernakalant for cardioversion of acute-onset atrial fibrillation: a systematic review and meta-analysis. Clin Ther 45(3):218–231

Medications Used for the Renal System   8

Roseline Elsie Agyekum

Learning Outcomes
At the end of this chapter, you will be able to:

- Explore the mechanism of drug action, clinical indications, pharmacokinetics and contraindications associated with prescribed; carbonic anhydrase inhibitors, osmotic agents, and loop, thiazide, potassium-sparing diuretics, alkalizing agents, vasopressin receptor antagonists (aquaretic) and Sodium-Glucose Co-Transporters Inhibitors 2 ($SGLT_2i$) and the information patients would require, and the information patients would require.
- Identify the common unwanted effects and important drug-to-drug interactions associated with carbonic anhydrase inhibitors, osmotic agents, and loop, thiazide diuretics, alkalizing agents, vasopressin receptor antagonists (aquaretic) and Sodium-Glucose Co-Transporters 2 inhibitors.
- List the routes of administering of different classes of diuretics
- Review the similarities and differences between carbonic anhydrase inhibitors, osmotic agents, and loop, thiazide and thiazide-like and potassium-sparing diuretics, alkalizing agents, vasopressin receptor antagonists (aquaretic) and Sodium-Glucose Co-Transporters2 inhibitors.
- Outline the nursing considerations and the information patients require when prescribed carbonic anhydrase inhibitors, osmotic agents, and loop, thiazide and potassium-sparing diuretics, alkalizing agents, vasopressin receptor antagonists (aquaretic) and Sodium-Glucose Co-Transporters 2 inhibitors.

R. E. Agyekum (✉)
King's College London, London, UK
e-mail: roseline.1.agyekum@kcl.ac.uk

E. Khan, P. Hood (eds.), *Understanding Pharmacology in Nursing Practice*,
https://doi.org/10.1007/978-3-032-03964-4_8

8.1   Introduction

This chapter focuses on the pharmacology of medications that influence renal function by reviewing the underlying renal physiology that supports the pharmacological action and effect on urine production alongside a focus on the pharmacokinetics, clinical indications, contraindications, unwanted effects, and possible drug–drug interactions.

One of the main functions of the kidney is to maintain homeostasis through the excretion of metabolic waste products such as urea, uric acid and creatinine (Marieb 2020). An important function of the renal system in homeostasis is the regulation of the salt and electrolyte and extracellular volume. Additionally, the kidneys are pivotal in the maintenance of electrolyte and acid–base balance. The types of pharmacological agents that affect renal function through their action on the other body system are diuretics which act on renal tubules blocking renal ionic transport, thereby causing increase in sodium and glucose excretion and subsequently naturesis and glucosuria.

Healthcare practitioners are ideally placed to facilitate and enhance service user's understanding of their prescribed medication, therefore an understanding of the mechanisms of drug action and application of this knowledge into clinical practice is an important aspect of a nurse's safe patient-centred care.

8.2   Renal Physiology and the Production of Urine

The formation of urine begins with a passive ultrafiltration process, in which the movement of water and associated dissolved small molecules is determined by hydrostatic and oncotic pressures. The healthy kidneys receive 20–25% of the cardiac output, approximately about 125–130 ml/min, which is filtered from the glomerular capillaries into Bowman's capsule. The filtrate, although routinely free of proteins and blood cells, also contains glucose, sodium bicarbonate, amino acids, and other organic solutes, plus electrolytes, such as sodium, potassium and chloride. The kidney regulates the ionic composition and volume of urine by the reabsorption or secretion of ions and/or water at five functional zones along the nephron, namely the proximal convoluted tubule, the descending loop of Henle, the thick ascending loop of Henle (TAL), the distal convoluted tubule, and the collecting duct via the action of aldosterone, antidiuretic hormone (ADH) and atria natriuretic peptide (Marieb 2020).

1. Proximal convoluted tubule (PCT): almost all of the glucose, bicarbonate, amino acids, and other metabolites are reabsorbed in PCT. Approximately two thirds of the sodium and 100% of glucose is also reabsorbed in PCT; chloride and water are passively reabsorbed to maintain electrical and osmolar equality.
2. Descending loop of Henle: this segment is permeable only for water, so the osmolarity increases along the descending portion of the loop of Henle. This results in a tubular fluid with a three-fold increase in sodium concentration.

3. Ascending loop of Henle is impermeable to water. Active reabsorption of sodium, potassium and chloride is mediated by a sodium/potassium/chloride co-transporter. The ascending loop is a diluting region of the nephron. Approximately 25–30% of the tubular sodium chloride is reabsorbed into the interstitial fluid maintaining the fluid's high osmolarity.
4. Distal convoluted tubule (DCT): about 10% of the filtered sodium chloride is reabsorbed via sodium/chloride transporter.
5. Collecting tubule and ducts are responsible for sodium/potassium exchanges, Hydrogen secretion, and potassium reabsorption. Stimulation of aldosterone receptors results in sodium reabsorption and potassium secretion. ADH receptors promote the reabsorption of water from the collecting tubules and ducts. Vasopressin increases water absorption by regulating aquaporin-2 which enhances water permeability in the collecting duct.

8.2.1 Measurement of Renal Function

Typical glomerular filtration rate (GFR) is ~ 180 L/day, or 125 ml/min. Of this amount, only 1–2 L/day are excreted as urine daily, implying that 99% of the filtered volume is reabsorbed. The volume filtered by the kidneys is 125–130 ml/minute, i.e. 180 L/24 h whereas urinary elimination is approximately 0.5–1 ml/kg/minute. Diluted (hypoosmotic urine production), occurs when there is reabsorption of solute from tubular fluid without water within the ascending limb of the loop of Henle, distal tubule and collecting duct. Conversely, concentrated (hyperosmotic urine production), is said to occur during reabsorption of water from tubular fluid without solute within the late distal tubule and collecting duct. The dilution and concentration of urine is facilitated mainly by ADH or vasopressin, the medullary interstitial osmotic gradient (counter current multiplication), by the loop of Henle and the different solute and water permeability and transport of the nephron segment (Marieb 2020).

8.3 Diuretics

Diuretics are agents that enhance the secretion and a net loss of sodium and water from the body through their action on the five functional zones along the nephron (Ives 2009; Kaufman 2020). The primary effect leads to decrease the reabsorption of sodium and chloride from the filtrate, increase the excretion of sodium, bicarbonate and water. Clinical indications of diuretics include the management of conditions that are associated with the retention of excessive amounts of fluid such as hypertension, the aim is to decrease pulmonary and peripheral oedema associated with heart failure, renal and liver disorder (Edwin 2006; Braunwald 2014).

Diuretics can be categories into five distinctive classes due to their sites of action (Fig. 8.1): loop diuretics, thiazide diuretics and potassium-sparing diuretics (Bennett 2008; Kaufman 2013; Ashley and Dunleavy (2014)

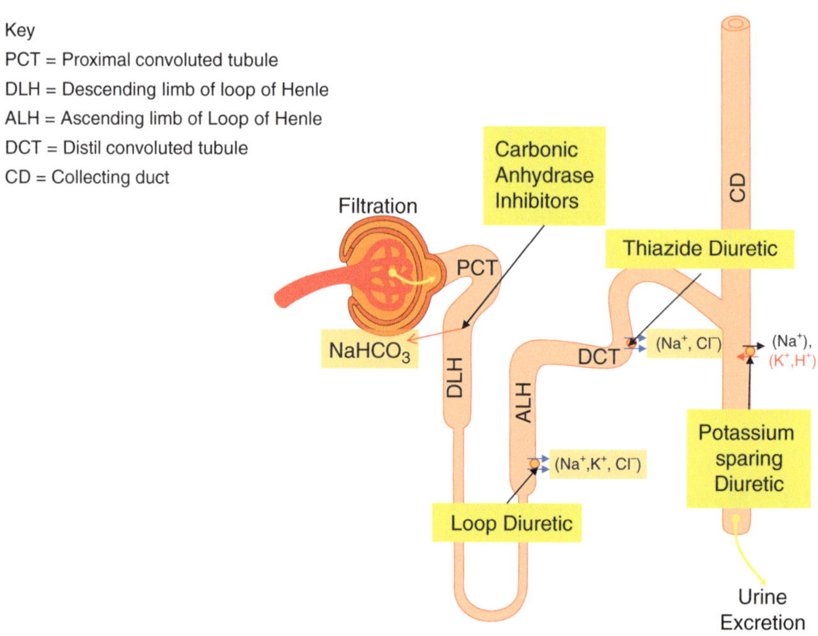

Fig. 8.1 Sites of action of the classes of diuretics

Volume Overload and Oedema

Volume overload which occurs as a result of an increased total body sodium content with a resultant increase in total body water, is defined by a percentage of an individual's body weight; a cut-off of 10% is associated with an increased mortality. A cascade of alterations in the sympathetic nervous system; renin-angiotensin-aldosterone, antidiuretic as well as atrial naturetic peptide, have been reported to initiate volume overload. These disturbances are then translated at the renal perfusion and tubular level, consequently leading to retention of sodium and water. The effect of compromised regulatory mechanisms of sodium and water has been implicated in the occurrence of oedema associated with congestive heart failure (CHF), kidney failure, and liver failure (Palazzuoli et al. 2020).

Capillary hydrostatic pressure and therefore capillary fluid filtration correlates with venous pressure. Diuretics, by reducing blood volume and venous pressure, lower capillary hydrostatic pressure with a subsequent decline in net capillary fluid filtration and subsequent tissue oedema, whether pulmonary and or systemic

8.3.1 Effect of Diuretics on the Cardiovascular System

Diuretics decrease blood volume and venous pressure through their effects on sodium and fluid balance (Gheorghiade 2010; Kaufman 2013). This decreases preload and by the Frank-Starling mechanism, decreases ventricular stroke volume and cardiac output, which leads to a drop in arterial pressure. The decrease in venous pressure decreases capillary hydrostatic pressure which in turns leads to a decline in capillary fluid filtration; subsequently promoting capillary fluid reabsorption and thereby reducing oedema, if present. Loop diuretics are reported to cause vasodilatation, which potentially contribute to the lowering of venous pressure. A decline in systemic vascular resistance has been reported with the long-term use of diuretics which helps to sustain the reduction in arterial pressure.

Diuretics have been used effectively with patients who have hypertension, of which 90–95% has primary or essential hypertension. The use of diuretics as an adjunctive therapy in hypertensive patients is particularly effective when reduced dietary sodium intake is incorporated. The efficacy of these drugs is achieved through their ability to reduce blood volume, cardiac output, and systemic vascular resistance when used as a long-term therapy. Most hypertensive patients are treated with thiazide diuretics (Klabunde 2011). Potassium-sparing, aldosterone-blocking diuretics (e.g. spironolactone), are used in hyperaldosteronism associated secondary hypertension and occasionally used as an adjunct to thiazide treatment for primary hypertension to prevent hypokalaemia.

8.3.2 Heart Failure

Klabunde (2015), Felker et al. (2013) and Ponikowski et al. (2016) argued that physiologically, heart failure results in the activation of the renin-angiotensin-aldosterone system, subsequently leading to increased sodium and water retention by the kidneys. The resultant increased blood volume contributes to the elevated venous pressures associated with heart failure, which can contribute to the development of pulmonary and systemic oedema. Primarily, the use of diuretics in heart failure aims to reduce pulmonary and/or systemic congestion and oedema, and its associated clinical symptoms, such as dyspnoea (Klabunde 2011). Long-term treatment with diuretics may also reduce the afterload on the heart by promoting systemic vasodilatation, which can lead to improved ventricular ejection (Fig. 8.2).

During management of heart failure with diuretics, it is imperative to ensure a gradual offload of circulating volume to prevent the incidence of a depressed cardiac output. For example, if pulmonary capillary wedge pressure is high and

Fig. 8.2 Effects of long-term use of diuretics on afterload

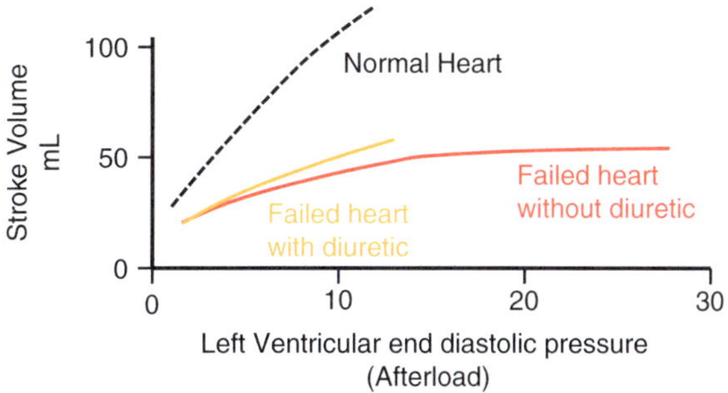

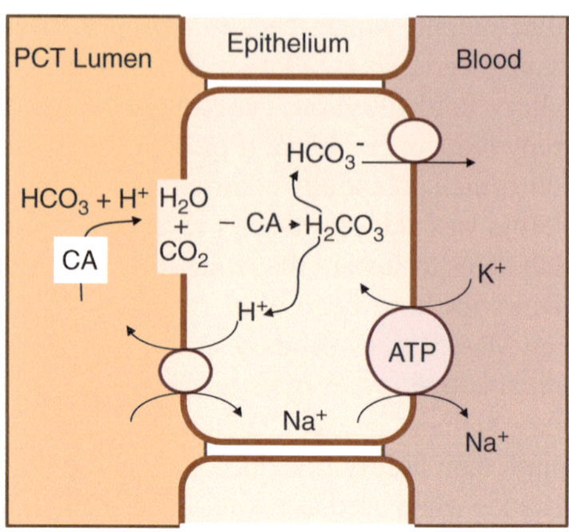

Fig. 8.3 Apical membrane sodium/hydrogen exchanger and bicarbonate reabsorption in the PCT-cell

pulmonary congestion is present, a diuretic can safely reduce that elevated pressure to an acceptable level as depicted in Fig. 8.3. This ensures a decline in pulmonary pressures without negatively altering ventricular stroke volume. Heart failure secondary to systolic dysfunction is associated with a depressed, flattened Frank–Starling curve. However, high circulating volume can lead to decreased stroke volume, the rationale being that the heart will operate on the ascending limb of the Frank–Starling relationship. Conversely, in diastolic dysfunction associated heart failure, diuretics must be used with caution to reduce the probability of impairing ventricular filling (Klabunde 2011; Felker et al. 2013; Ponikowski et al. 2016).

8.4 Classes of Diuretics

The different classes of diuretics differ in their effectiveness due to their site of actions and degree of ability to alter renal handling of sodium and water (Table 8.1).

8.4.1 Carbonic Anhydrase Inhibitors

Examples: Acetazolamide, Dichlorophenamide
Carbonic anhydrase inhibitors are sulphonamide derivatives that impede the activity of the enzyme carbonic anhydrase on the apical membrane of the proximal convoluted tubular (PCT) epithelium, leading to interference of the carbon dioxide to carbonic acid subsequent ionization of hydrogen ions and bicarbonate. Additionally, these agents reduce the production of aqueous humour and often used as an adjunctive treatment in glaucoma (Sugrue 2000; Aung et al. 2014).

For example, the decreased ability to exchange sodium for hydrogen ions in the presence of acetazolamide results in mild diuresis accompanied by potassium

Table 8.1   Classes of diuretics

Carbonic anhydrase inhibitors	Osmotic diuretics	Loop diuretics	Thaizide diuretics	Potassium-sparing diuretics	Combined diuretics
Acetazolamide Dichlorophenamide Dorzolamide Brinzolamide	Mannitol	Furosemide Bumetanide Torasemide	Bendroflumethiazide Metolazone Chlortalidone Indapamide	Spironolactone Eplerenone Amiloride Triamterene	Co-Amilofruse

Source: Bennett 2008; Kaufman 2013; Ashley and Dunleavy 2014

secretion resulting in hypokalaemia. Additionally, bicarbonate is retained in the lumen with marked elevation of urinary pH. The loss of bicarbonate causes a hyperchloraemic metabolic acidosis which carbonic anhydrase, leading to tolerance to the diuretic action of acetazolamide.

8.4.1.1 Pharmacokinetics

Carbonic anhydrase inhibitors (CAI) decrease production of hydrogen and bicarbonate ions in the portion of the proximal convoluted tubule closer to the Bowman's capsule, thereby reducing bicarbonate absorption. Increased distal delivery of bicarbonate exceeds the absorptive threshold of the distal convoluted tubule resulting in bicarbonate, potassium, water and sodium loss is minimal. Tolerance develops as serum bicarbonate level declines; hence the diuretic effect of carbonic anhydrase is transient. Carbonic anhydrase, especially, Acetazolamide, has been reported to reduce frequency of seizures; especially petit mal), possibly by lowering of pH of the brain tissues (Aung et al. 2014; Supuran 2016; Shukralla et al. 2022). Following oral administration CA inhibitors are well absorbed. They are eliminated unchanged by the kidney. It is secreted into the proximal renal tubule via the organic acid transport mechanisms (Table 8.2)

Examples of Carbonic Anhydrase Inhibitors

8.4.1.2 Acetazolamide

Acetazolamide is a derivative of the sulfonamide antibiotic sulfanilamide, which induces diuresis with metabolic acidosis as an adverse effect due to inhibition of carbonic anhydrase. Its clinical use as a diuretic is limited because of its weak effect and the subsequent metabolic acidosis which occurs with chronic use.

Mechanism of Action

The exact mechanism by which acetazolamide suppresses convulsions is unknown. Potent inhibitor of brain carbonic anhydrase, the enzyme irreversibly catalyses the hydration of CO_2 and the dehydration of carbonic acid (Bennett 2008; Ives 2009; Shukralla et al. 2022).

Acetazolamide is a potent carbonic anhydrase inhibitor effective in inducing fluid loss due to its reversible reaction action on the kidney involving hydration of carbon dioxide and dehydration of carbonic acid. (e.g. some types of glaucoma), in

Table 8.2 Clinical indications of carbonic anhydrase

1. Adjunctive treatment of drug-induced oedema or oedema due to congestive heart failure refractory to single therapy
2. Adjunctive treatment of glaucoma (open-angle, secondary glaucoma, pre-operative narrow-angle) to lower intraocular pressure
3. Adjunctive treatment of petit mal epilepsy
4. Prophylaxis management of high-altitude and motion sickness
5. Treatment of cystinuria, and enhance excretion of uric acid and other organic acids
6. Metabolic alkalosis

the treatment of certain convulsive disorders (e.g. epilepsy) and in the promotion of diuresis in instances of abnormal fluid retention (e.g. cardiac oedema).

Acetazolamide is not a mercurial diuretic. Rather, acetazolamide also induces an inhibitory action leading to decrease in the secretion of aqueous humour, with a resultant decline in intraocular pressure in cases of glaucoma.

It has been reported that acetazolamide is effective as an adjuvant treatment of certain dysfunctions of the central nervous system (e.g. epilepsy). It is thought that carbonic anhydrasc Inhibition in this area potentially slows the release of abnormal, paroxysmal neural activity from the central nervous system (Bennett 2008; Ives 2009; Shukralla et al. 2022).

8.4.1.3 Dichlorophenamide

This medication is sulphonamide and carbonic anhydrase, prescribed for the treatment of elevated intraocular pressure associated with glaucoma.

Mechanism of Action

It reduces intraocular pressure by partially suppressing the secretion of aqueous humour (inflow), although the mechanism by which they do this is not fully understood. Evidence suggests that bicarbonate ions are produced in the ciliary body by hydration of carbon dioxide under the influence of carbonic anhydrase and diffuse water is to the posterior chamber by osmosis (Bennett 2008; Ives 2009: Sansone et al. 2016).

Dorzolamide and Brinzolamide are topical carbonic anhydrase inhibitors. They are licensed for use in patients resistant to beta-blockers or those in whom beta-blockers are contra-indicated (Table 8.3).

8.4.2 Osmotic Diuretics Examples: Mannitol, Glycerol

Osmotic agents induce a shift of water between body fluid compartments because of their high permeability properties through biologic membranes compared with water (Bennett 2008; Ives 2009; Sam and Pearce 2023). Their primary site of action is the loop of Henle and through osmotic effects, they also oppose the action of ADH in the collecting tubule. The normal pressure within the kidneys is determined by the concentration of sodium, other electrolytes and urea. In conditions that do not require water conservation, the luminal, cellular and interstitial osmotic pressure remains equal. Osmotic diuretics which are filtered but not reabsorbed, remain in the lumen creating an osmotic gradient that causes reabsorption of water from the cell and the interstitium (Fig. 8.4). Their effectiveness as a diuretic varies from relatively high (urea) to very low (mannitol). They have no direct effect on ion transport but often cause shifts of ions by inducing bulk water flow and changing steady-state water concentration in body compartments.

Table 8.3 Summary of carbonic anhydrase

Examples	Dose	Onset and peak times	Adverse effects	Drug interaction	Contraindications
Acetazolamide Glaucoma Epilepsy Diamox: Sustained-release capsules glaucoma	Oral/IV 0.25–1 g daily in divided doses Oral/IV 0.25–1 g daily in divided doses 250–500 mg daily	Onset: 60–90 min; 2 h Peak times: 1–4 h 3–6 h	Anorexia, Nausea, Vomiting, electrolyte imbalance, haematuria, glycosuria, urinary frequency, renal colic, renal calculi, malaise, nervousness, drowsiness, depression, thrombocytopaenic purpura, hepatic insufficiency, haemolytic anaemia Pruritus, Stevens–Johnson syndrome, transient myopia	Cyclosporine ↑ levels possible nephrotoxicity and neurotoxicity Ephedrine ↑ Ephedrine effect Lithium carbonate/↓ Lithium effect	Hyponatraemia and hypokalaemia, Renal and hepatic dysfunction, hyperchloraemic acidosis, adrenal insufficiency, hypersensitivity to thiazide diuretics, cirrhosis. Chronic use in presence of non-congestive angle-closure glaucoma
Dichlorophenamide	25–50 mg 1–3 times daily	Onset: 30–60 min Peak times: 2–4 h	Hepatic insufficiency Renal failure Adrenocortical insufficiency Acidosis Hyponatraemia hypokalaemia Severe Pulmonary obstruction Hypersensitivity	Anorexia, tachypnoea, lethargy and coma have been rarely reported due to a possible drug interaction with high-dose aspirin	liver or kidney failure, adrenocortical insufficiency, acidity, lung obstruction, low level of minerals in blood and hypersensitivity

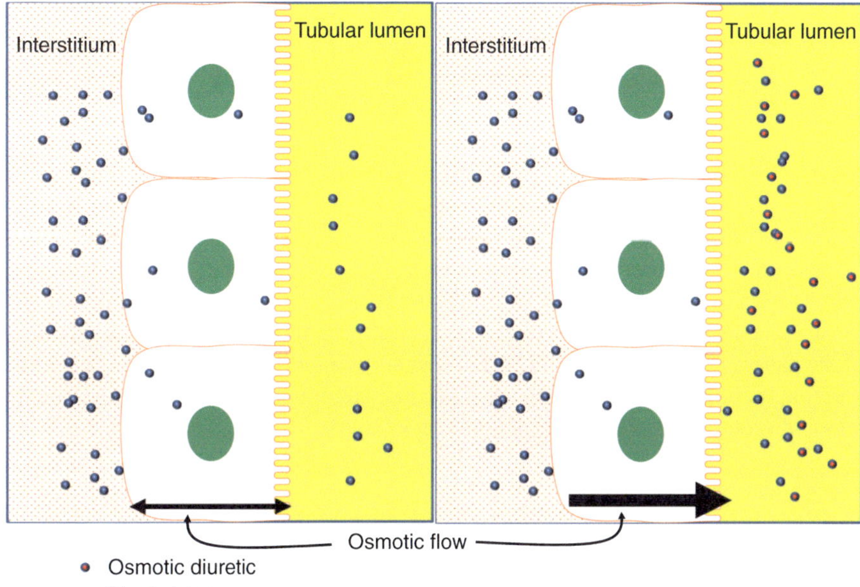

Fig. 8.4 Mechanism of action of osmotic diuretic

Table 8.4 Clinical indications of osmotic diuretics

1. To increase urine volume with limited effect on electrolyte or acid–base balance as an aspect of postoperative care, or after accidents, or haemolysis, e.g. increased pigment load due to transfusion reaction, and to promote excretion of toxic substances
2. Reduction of intracranial and intraocular pressure and cerebral oedema

8.4.2.1 Pharmacokinetics of Osmotic Diuretics

Mannitol and urea are used intravenously. Glycerol is usually given orally and is restricted to the extracellular space. These agents have short half-lives and are all freely filtered at the glomerulus. Glycerol is well absorbed orally, but mannitol is not. The latter is normally administered intravenously. Glycerol is significantly metabolised and eliminated by the liver, while mannitol is excreted by the kidney (Table 8.4).

8.4.2.2 Mannitol

Mannitol is an osmotic agent that is freely filterable nonmetabolized sugar alcohol at the glomerular level, but it is not reabsorbed by the renal tubules (Witherspoon an Ashby 2017). By virtue of its primary site and mechanism of action, mannitol has a high diuretic potential and can markedly increase GFR in all nephron segments including the proximal tubule. Additionally, mannitol acts as a protectant against further renal tubular damage and initiates an osmotic diuresis. It also causes release of renal prostaglandins that lead to renal vasodilation and an increase in tubular urine flow that is believed to protect against renal injury by reducing tubular obstruction (Shawkat et al. 2012; Sam and Pearce 2023). It also acts as a free-radical scavenger and reduces the harmful effects of free radicals during ischaemia–re-perfusion injury.

Consequently, when administered early during acute kidney injury failure (AKI), mannitol tends to facilitate the excretion of cellular debris and prevent tubular cast formation. This action may be responsible for the conversion of oliguric ARF to non-oliguric ARF. Although there is no evidence that the use of mannitol in critically ill patients improves GFR, it does reduce the need for renal replacement therapy. More importantly, converting oliguric AKI to non-oliguric AKI facilitates the management of fluid and electrolyte imbalance, drug therapy, and nutritional needs of the patient (Shawkat et al. 2012). To prevent a compensatory increase in ion reabsorption in the loop of Henle, mannitol is usually administered in combination with a loop diuretic. Mannitol is contraindicated in anuric patients.

Mechanism of Action

Mannitol is filtered at the glomerulus but not reabsorbed from the renal tubule. It exerts osmotic activity within PCT and the descending limb of the loop of Henle and limits passive tubular water reabsorption, causing diuresis. Water loss produced by osmotic diuretic is accompanied by a variable natriuresis (Bennett 2008; Ives 2009; Sam and Pearce 2023).

Pharmacokinetics

Mannitol is not absorbed orally and is given IV as a 20% solution. The drug is distributed in the extra cellular space and extracts water from the intracellular compartment. It is rapidly excreted by the kidney and action starts 30–60 min after administration. Duration of action is 1.5–3 h (Table 8.5).

8.4.2.3 Glycerol

Glycerol is a naturally occurring trivalent alcohol, an essential compound of the human cell membrane, a hyperosmolar agent, and an osmotic diuretic. And was long used in neurosurgery, neurology, and ophthalmology to reduce raised tissue pressure.

Table 8.5 Clinical indications of mannitol

1. Reduction in raised intracranial pressure and preservation of perioperative renal function in patients undergoing major vascular and cardiac surgery and in those with jaundice
2. To promote diuresis and minimise the risk of acute kidney injury in patients after renal transplantation
3. Preservation of renal function in rhabdomyolysis secondary to crush injuries and compartment syndrome
4. Bowel preparation before colorectal surgery and colonoscopy
5. Promotion of urinary excretion of toxic materials

Mechanism of Action

Glycerol (glycerine) helps reduce intraocular pressure by increasing plasma osmotic pressure, thereby drawing water into the blood from extravascular spaces (Bennett 2008; Ives 2009). It also reduces intraocular fluid volume independently of routine flow mechanisms, decreasing intraocular pressure; it may cause tissue dehydration and decreased CSF pressure. Topically applied glycerin produces a hygroscopic (moisture-retaining) effect that reduces oedema and improves visualization in ophthalmoscopy and gonioscopy (an eye test examining for signs of glaucoma). Glycerin reduces fluid in the cornea via its osmotic action and clears corneal haze. It has been reported that a single dose of one gram/kg of glycerol will raise serum osmolality from 295 to 320 mOsm/L in 90 min and reduce CSF pressure for 3–5 h.

As a laxative agent, glycerol suppositories produce laxative action by causing rectal distention, thereby stimulating the urge to defecate; by causing local rectal irritation; and by triggering a hyperosmolar mechanism that draws water into the colon.

Pharmacokinetics

When administered rectally, glycerol is poorly absorbed; after rectal administration the laxative effect occurs in 15–30 min, glycerol is distributed locally and not metabolised. Glycerol is excreted in faeces (Bennett 2008; Ives 2009). The drug is rapidly absorbed from the GI tract following oral administration, with serum levels peaking in 60–90 min. Intraocular pressure decreases in 10–30 min. Action peaks in 30 min–2 h, with effects persisting for 4–8 h. Intracranial pressure (ICP) decreases in 10–60 min; effect persists for 2–3 h. It is distributed throughout the blood but does not enter ocular fluid, however, the drug may enter breast milk. Generally, about 80% metabolised in liver, 10%–20% in kidneys and excreted in faeces and urine (Tables 8.6 and 8.7).

8.4.3 Loop Diuretics

Examples: Frosemide (Lasix®), Bumetanide (Bumex®), Torsemide (Demadex®).

These diuretics block the luminal receptor which is responsible for the reabsorption of sodium, potassium, in conjunction with chloride ions leading to increased sodium, potassium, and chloride and water excretion (Fig. 8.5). Since the thick ascending limb is responsible for about 20% of the sodium chloride reabsorption, loop diuretics are extremely potent diuretics (Kushner et al. 2009; Musini et al. 2014).

They are often described as 'high ceiling' diuretics due to their high diuretic potential; they can cause up to 20% of the filtered load of sodium chloride and water to be excreted in the urine (Peters et al. 2022). They also interfere with the

Table 8.6 Clinical indications and dosages

1. Constipation
2. Reduction of intraocular pressure
3. Reduction of corneal oedema

Table 8.7 Summary of osmotic diuretics

Examples	Dose	Onset and peak times	Adverse effects	Drug interaction	Contraindications
Mannitol	Initial: 0.25–0.5 g/kg IV over 3–5 min 6–8 h continuous infusion of 2–5 mL/min of a 5%–10% solution	30–60 min 30–45 min	Nausea, vomiting, fever, chills, headache, runny nose, swelling, rapid weight gain, chest pain, skin rash, dizziness, blurred vision	Treprostinil ↑ hypotensive effect. Monitor antihypertensive therapy during concomitant use	Established anuria due to severe renal disease, severe pulmonary congestion or frank pulmonary oedema, active intracranial bleeding except during craniotomy severe dehydration progressive renal damage or dysfunction, heart failure
Glycerol constipation Increased intraocular pressure Reduction of corneal oedema	1.5–3 g as a suppository or 5–15 ml as an enema 1–2 g/kg orally 1–1.5 h before surgery 1–2 drops of ophthalmic solution topically before eye examination; 1–2 drops 3–4 h	Rapid 60–90 min	Mild headache, dizziness, eye pain, irritation; cramping pain, thirst, nausea, diarrhoea, rectal hyperaemia and discomfort, mild hyperglycaemia	Diuretics: may cause additive effects	Intestinal obstruction, anuria, severe dehydration, frank or impending acute pulmonary oedema, severe cardiac decompensation, undiagnosed abdominal pain, vomiting

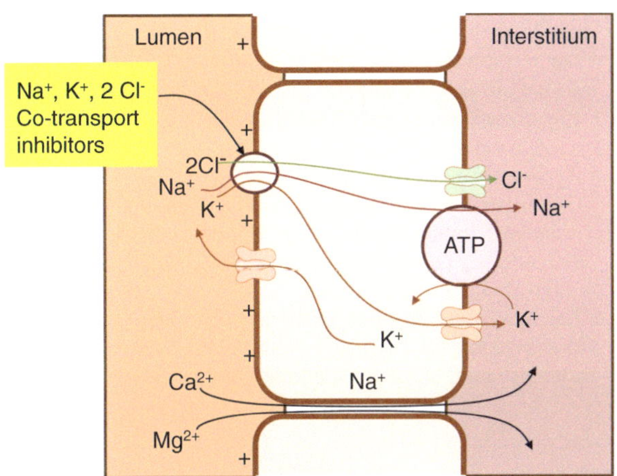

Fig. 8.5 Mechanism of action of loop diuretics

reabsorption of potassium, calcium and magnesium in the Loop of Henle. Two common examples are furosemide and bumetanide, with bumetanide 40 times more potent than furosemide. Both medications are administered orally and are readily absorbed. They are partly eliminated through metabolism and partly eliminated by renal excretion. Drug action is independent of acid–base balance and has a rapid onset of action (within 10–20 min given IV).

Mechanism of Action

The action of loop diuretics is the inhibition of sodium chloride reabsorption in the thick ascending limb of the loop of Henle. Inhibition of the sodium potassium chloride transport system in the luminal membrane subsequently leads to a reduction in sodium chloride reabsorption. Loop diuretics also decreases normal lumen-positive potential secondary to potassium recycling diuretics (Kushner et al. 2009; Musini et al. 2014; Peters et al. 2022).

Due to positive lumen potential which drives calcium magnesium reabsorption, loop diuretics increase magnesium and calcium excretion. Hypomagnesaemia may occur in some patients; however, hypocalcaemia does not usually develop because calcium is reabsorbed in the distal convoluted tubule. In circumstances that result in hypercalcaemia, calcium excretion can be enhanced by administration of loop diuretics with saline infusion (Table 8.8).

8.4.3.1 Furosemide

Furosemide, a loop diuretic, inhibits water reabsorption in the nephron by blocking the sodium-potassium-chloride cotransporter in the thick ascending limb of the loop of Henle. This is achieved through competitive inhibition at the chloride binding site on the cotransporter, thus preventing the transport of sodium from the lumen of the loop of Henle into the interstitium (McMahon and Chawla 2021; Wargo and Banta 2009). Consequently, the lumen becomes more hypertonic while the interstitium becomes less hypertonic, which in turn diminishes the osmotic gradient for water

Table 8.8 Clinical indications of loop diuretics

1. Fluid overload/oedema: congestive heart failure (CHF), acute pulmonary oedema, hepatic ascites, nephrotic syndrome, acute kidney injury and chronic kidney disease
2. Hypertension, especially when accompanied by renal impairment
3. Acute treatment of hypercalcemia
4. Hyperkalaemia: loop diuretics increase potassium excretion, the effect increased by concurrent administration of sodium chloride and water
5. Acute renal failure: may increase rate of urine flow and increase potassium excretion. Loop diuretics may convert oliguric to non-oliguric failure {easier clinical management} renal failure duration—not affected
6. Anion overload: bromide, chloride, iodide are all reabsorbed by the thick ascending loop-systemic toxicity may be reduced by decreasing reabsorption. Concurrent administration of sodium chloride and fluid is required to prevent volume depletion

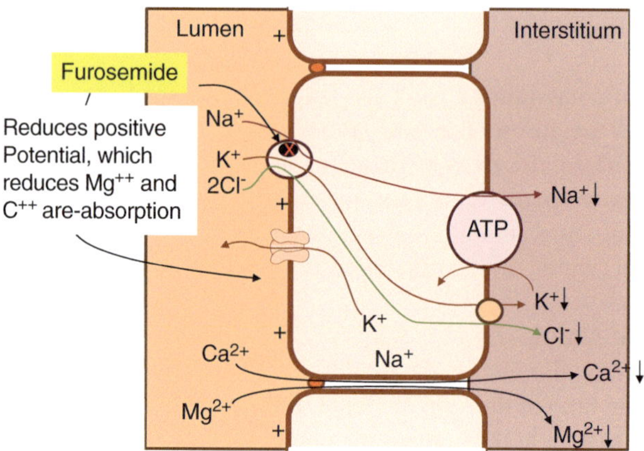

Fig. 8.6 Mechanism of action of furosemide

reabsorption throughout the nephron. As the thick ascending limb is responsible for 25% of sodium reabsorption in the nephron, furosemide is a very potent diuretic.

Mechanism of Action

Furosemide inhibits the sodium-potassium-chloride cotransporter in the thick ascending limb of the loop of Henle (Fig. 8.6). Thus, the ability of the nephron to dilute urine is lost. Additionally, furosemide inhibits the positive potential of the lumen, which then reduces the reabsorption of magnesium and calcium ions (Bennett 2008; Ives 2009; McMahon and Chawla 2021).

Pharmacokinetics

Furosemide is a weak carboxylic acid, existing mainly in the dissociated form in the GIT. It is rapidly but partially absorbed (60–70%) following oral administration and its effect is largely complete within 4 h. The optimal absorption site is the upper duodenum at pH 5.0. Furosemide is bound to plasma albumin with little biotransformation. Elimination is mainly (80–90%); a small fraction of the dose is eliminated via the biliary system. Biliary elimination can be reduced by up to 50% during hepatic impairment. Elimination time of furosemide is increased with residual renal function less than 20% (Bennett 2008; Ives 2009; McMahon and Chawla 2021) (Table 8.9).

8.4.3.2 Bumetanide

Bumetanide is potent, high ceiling loop diuretic with a rapid onset and a short duration of action. The primary site of action is the ascending limb of the Loop of Henle where it exerts inhibiting effects on electrolyte reabsorption causing the diuretic and natriuretic action observed.

Mechanism of Action

Bumetanide inhibits sodium reabsorption in the ascending limb of the loop of Henle, leading to marked reduction of fluid excretion during hydration and vice versa during dehydration Reabsorption of chloride in the ascending limb is also blocked by bumetanide.

Pharmacokinetic

Bumetanide is well absorbed after oral administration with the bioavailability reaching between 80 and 95%. 94–96% of the drug is protein bound. Bumetanide is partially metabolised in the liver with the elimination half-life ranging between 0.75 and 2.6 h. No active metabolites are known (Bennett 2008; Ives 2009; McMahon and Chawla 2021). The drug is mainly excreted by the kidneys (81%), and 2% in faeces. Renal excretion accounts for approximately half the clearance with hepatic excretion responsible for the other half. There is an increase in half-life and a reduced plasma clearance in the presence of renal or hepatic disease. With people who have chronic renal failure the liver is important as an excretory pathway (Table 8.10).

Table 8.9 Clinical indications of furosemide

1. Treatment of CHF, ascites, acute pulmonary oedema, and other oedematous states
2. Hypertension (second line to thiazides)
3. Severe hypercalcaemia (in conjunction with fluid and electrolyte therapy)

Table 8.10 Clinical indications of bumetanide

1. Treatment of oedema associated with congestive heart failure, hepatic and renal disease, including the nephrotic syndrome
2. To the reducing fluid retention refractory to thiazides or with impaired renal function
3. Used as an option if patient is allergic to furosemide

8.4.3.3 Torsemide

Torsemide is the most active of a new series of anilinopyridine sulfonylurea derivatives. Its' actions can be mediated by several mechanisms operating within the thick, medullary segment of the ascending loop of Henle. These include interference with the sodium potassium chloride co-transporter at the luminal surface and the sodium potassium pump and anion exchange.

Mechanism of Action

Torsemide selectively blocks the active sodium and chloride reabsorption in the thick ascending loop of Henle promoting rapid excretion of water, sodium, and chloride. Torsemide has a higher bioavailability, greater potency and a longer duration of action than furosemide (Bennett 2008; Ives 2009; McMahon and Chawla 2021).

Pharmacokinetic

Plasma protein binding of torsemide is 97–99%. The duration of diuresis is independent of the route of administration and lasts for 6–8 h. The volume of distribution of torsemide is 12–15 litres in normal adults or in patients with mild-to-moderate renal failure or congestive heart failure. In patients with cirrhosis, the volume of distribution is approximately doubled. Metabolism and elimination: torsemide is metabolized by the liver. About 73% is excreted through liver metabolism, and 27% is excreted in urine (Tables 8.11 and 8.12).

8.4.4   Thiazides and Thiazide-Like Diuretics

Examples: Bendroflumethazide, Metolazone, Chlortalidone, Indapamide
Thiazide diuretics have been used predominantly as pharmacological agents of choice for the treatment of hypertension. The evolution of thiazide diuretics started during the 1950s, through analysis of the derivatives of sulfonamide-based carbonic anhydrase inhibitor (Bennett 2008; Ernst and Fravel 2022; Ives 2009). The main objective was to identify medications that enhance sodium with chloride excretion rather than sodium bicarbonate. Some of the medications within this class of diuretics are derived from benzothiadiazine. Although indapamide, chlorthalidone and

Table 8.11 Clinical indications of torsemide

1. Acute pulmonary oedema: torsemide increases median fractional sodium excretion significantly along with hourly urine output. This results in significant improvement in both pulmonary rales and orthopnoea
2. Congestive heart failure (CHF): torsemide is well-tolerated in the treatment of sodium and fluid retention resulting from moderate-to-severe CHF. Torsemide reduces pulmonary congestion, peripheral oedema, ascites, jugular venous pressure, and body weight. Consequently, it improves cardiac function and exercise tolerance
3. Chronic renal failure (CRF): torsemide increases fractional excretion of urinary volume, sodium and chloride. It is found to be efficacious even in patients with haemodialysis

Table 8.12 Summary of loop diuretics

Examples	Dose	Onset and peak times (min)	Adverse effects	Drug interaction	Contraindications
Furosemide Oedema Hypertension Congestive Heart Failure Acute pulmonary oedema	Initial: 20–40 mg IV/ IM over 1–2 min Initial: 80 mg daily (divided twice daily) 250–4000 mg daily (IV or PO) 40 mg IV over 1–2 min	Onset: Oral: 30–60 IM: 10–30 IV: 5 Peak: Oral: 60–120 IM: Unknown IV: 30	Blurred vision, dizziness, headache, vertigo, hearing loss, tinnitus, hypotension, anorexia, constipation, diarrhoea, dry mouth, dyspepsia, dehydration, ↑ liver enzymes, nausea, hyponatraemia, metabolic alkalosis, pancreatitis, vomiting, hyperuricaemia, hypercholesterolaemia, hyperglycaemia, electrolyte imbalance	Nitrates-↑ risk of hypotension Other diuretics- ↑ risk of hypokalaemia lithium ↓ excretion may cause toxicity Aminoglycosides orcisplatin- ↑ risk of ototoxicity NSAIDS- ↓ effects Methotrexate- May ↑ risk of toxicity cyclosporine- may ↑ risk of gouty arthritis	Hypersensitivity; Cross-sensitivity with thiazides and sulfonamides may occur; Hepatic coma or anuria; Some liquid products may contain alcohol, avoid in patients with alcohol intolerance
Torsemide	5 mg increased stepwise up to 20 mg daily	Onset: Oral: 30–60 Peak: 60	As above, in addition to ECG changes, mood changes, muscle pain or cramps, numbness or tingling in hands, feet, or lips, ankles, feet, or lower legs	Same as above	Same as above in addition to cardiac arrhythmias, simultaneous therapy with aminoglycosides or cephalosporins
Bumetanide	5 mg daily, increased by 5 mg increments every 12–24 h	Onset: Oral: 30–60 IV: 2–3 Peak: 15–30	Same as above	Same as above	Same as above
Xipamide	Initially 20 mg daily 40 mg daily increase to 80 mg daily if necessary	Onset: rapid Peak: 3–6 h	Same as above	Same as above	Same as above

metolazone possess similar thiazide pharmacologic action on the kidney, they do not have the thiazide chemical structure, they are therefore known as 'thiazide-like diuretics'.

Mechanism of Action

Thiazide and thiazide-like diuretics inhibit the reabsorption of sodium and chloride ions from the distal convoluted tubules by blocking the thiazide binding sites thereby inhibiting water and sodium, potassium, chloride, bicarbonate, and magnesium reabsorption (Fig. 8.7) (Bennett 2008; Ernst and Fravel 2022; Ives 2009). However, the action of thiazide diuretics leads calcium retention. Thiazides may mobilize sodium and water from arterial walls, resulting in decreased luminal diameter and tone. It has been documented that thiazides diuretics may possess direct vascular smooth muscle dilatory properties (Table 8.13).

8.4.4.1 Bendroflumethazide

Bendroflumethazide is a short acting thiazide diuretic which inhibits the renal tubular absorption of salt and water by its action at the beginning of the distal convoluted tubule. Sodium and chloride ions are excreted in equivalent proportions (Bennett 2008; Ernst and Fravel 2022; Ives 2009).

Mechanism of Action

Bendroflumethazide inhibits active chloride reabsorption at the early distal tubule via the sodium-chloride cotransporter, which results in an increase in the excretion of sodium, chloride, and water. Bendroflumethazide also inhibits sodium ion transport across the renal tubular epithelium through binding to the thiazide sensitive sodium-chloride transporter. This results in an increase in potassium excretion via

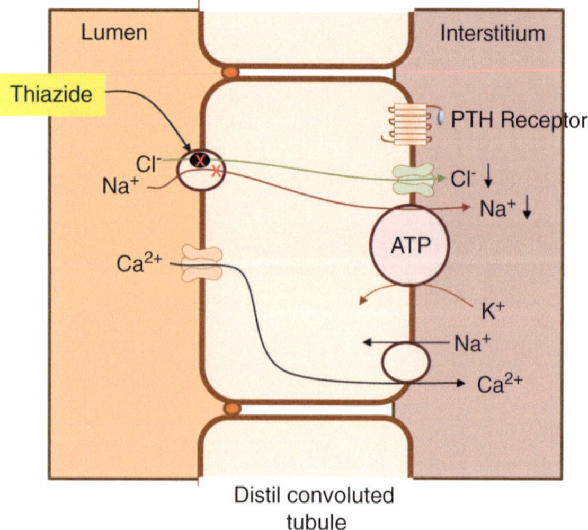

Fig. 8.7 Mechanism of action of thiazide and thiazide-like diuretics

Table 8.13 Clinical indications of thiazide diuretics

1. *Hypertension*: Thiazide diuretics are the most preferred in hypertension because:
   (a) Action of the diuretic (decreased blood volume and cardiac output), is blunted after some time (tolerance) but vasodilatation persistent
   (b) Various studies show that these medications are as effective as the beta blockers or angiotensin converting enzyme inhibitors
2. *Congestive heart failure*
3. *Nephrolithiasis–idiopathic hypercalciuria*: Most of the renal calculi are calcium phosphate. Diuretics lead to increased calcium reabsorption from the nephron, leading to decreased calcium excretion. Consequently renal precipitation of calcium and the formation of renal calculi is reduced
4. *Anion overload*: Bromide and chloride are all reabsorbed by the thick ascending loop. Therefore systemic toxicity may be reduced by decreasing reabsorption

Table 8.14 Clinical indications of bendroflumethazide

1. For the treatment of oedema associated with cardiac, renal, or hepatic origin and iatrogenic oedema

the sodium-potassium exchange mechanism (Bennett 2008; Ernst and Fravel 2022; Ives 2009).

Pharmacokinetics

Bendroflumethazide is absorbed completely from the gastrointestinal tract. The initiation of diuresis commences within 2 h and lasts for 12–18 h or longer. The drug is almost completely (90%) bound to plasma proteins; however, it is extensively metabolised. About 30% of the drug is excreted unchanged in the urine.

Peak plasma levels are reached in 2 h and has a plasma half-life of between 3 and 8.5 h on average (Table 8.14).

8.4.4.2 Metolazone

Metolazone is an intermediate thiazide-like diuretic, its actions result from interference with the renal tubular mechanism of electrolyte reabsorption.

Mechanism of Action

Metolazone inhibits sodium reabsorption in the distal tubules causing increased excretion of sodium and water, as well as, potassium and hydrogen ions (Bennett 2008; Ernst and Fravel 2022; Ives 2009).

Pharmacokinetics

After oral administration, about 65% of a given dose of metolazone is absorbed. However, when the same dose was administered to with cardiac dysfunction, absorption falls to 40%. It must be noted. The absorption rate and extent however, vary depending on preparations. 50%–70% of the drug is bound to erythrocyte and about 33% to protein. Drug crosses the placental barrier and is distributed into breast milk. Its metabolism is reported to be insignificant. Metolazone is predominantly (70%–95%) excreted unchanged in urine (Table 8.15).

Table 8.15 Clinical indications of metolazone

Metolazone is indicated for the treatment of sodium and water retention including:
1. Oedema associated with congestive heart failure; renal diseases, including the nephrotic syndrome and states of diminished renal function
2. Treatment of hypertension, alone or in combination with other different categories of antihypertensive drugs

8.4.4.3 Chlorthalidone

Chlorthalidone is a long-acting oral thiazide-like diuretic with prolonged action (48–72 h) and low toxicity. Its potency at maximum therapeutic dosage is approximately equal to thiazide diuretics. Chlorthalidone may produce diuresis in patients with glomerular filtration rates below 20 mL/min.

Pharmacokinetics

Chlorthalidone is metabolized partially, with 50–70% bound to erythrocytes, and 33% to plasma proteins. The rate and extent of absorption are formulation dependent. Most of the drug is excreted in the unconverted form in the urine. 70–95% is excreted unchanged in urine via glomerular filtration and active tubular secretion. The drug undergoes enterohepatic recycling (Bennett 2008; Ernst and Fravel 2022; Ives 2009; Roush and Sica 2016) (Table 8.16).

8.4.4.4 Indapamide

Indapamide is a long-acting thiazide-like diuretic.

Mechanism of Action

The renal site of action is the proximal part of the distal tubule and the ascending part of Henle's loop (Bennett 2008; Ernst and Fravel 2022; Ives 2009; Roush and Sica 2016). Sodium and chloride ions are excreted in approximately equivalent amounts. The increased delivery of sodium to the distal tubular exchange site results in increased potassium excretion and hypokalaemia. The inhibition of net influx of calcium associated with subsequent inhibition of contractions in vascular smooth muscle has been attributed to the Indapamide primary role in lowering blood pressure. Stimulation of the synthesis of prostaglandin PGE_2 and prostacyclin PGI_2 (vasodilator and platelet antiaggregant) have also been documented as a contributory mechanism for Indapamide's antihypertensive effect (Bennett 2008; Ives 2009; Roush and Sica 2016).

Pharmacokinetics

Indapamide is rapidly and completely absorbed after oral administration. Peak blood levels are obtained after 1–2 h. Indapamide is concentrated in the erythrocytes and is 79% bound to plasma proteins and to erythrocytes (Tables 8.17 and 8.18)

Table 8.16 Clinical indications of chlorthalidone

1. Management of hypertension either as the sole therapeutic agent or to enhance the effect of other antihypertensive drugs in the more severe forms of hypertension
2. Adjunctive therapy in oedema associated with congestive heart failure, hepatic cirrhosis, and corticosteroid and oestrogen therapy
3. Oedema due to various forms of renal dysfunction, such as nephrotic syndrome, acute glomerulonephritis, and chronic renal failure

Table 8.17 Clinical indications of indapamide

1. Management of mild to moderate hypertension: treatment of oedema in congestive heart failure and nephrotic syndrome

8.4.5 Potassium-Sparing Diuretics

Examples: Spironolactone, Eplerenone, Amiloride, Triamterene, Fineronone
Under the influence of aldosterone, potassium is normally secreted in the collecting ducts of the kidney. In circumstances of increased net sodium loss or a decreased circulating volume, the release of aldosterone is activated and sustained. One of the common adverse effects associated with the use of thiazide or loop diuretics is hypokalaemia, which subsequently increases circulating aldosterone level. Two main categories of potassium-sparing diuretics namely adosterone antagonists, also known as indirect acting, are spironolactone and eplerenone and the second category (direct acting); amiloride and triamterene have been documented (Bennett 2008; Ives 2009; Roush and Sica 2016).

Mechanism of Action
The Mineralocorticoid Receptor Antagonists (MRAs) or potassium-sparing diuretics inhibit sodium reabsorption in the collecting duct and hence decreased potassium excretion (Epstein 2021). All are weak diuretics but are effective antihypertensive agents, particularly in low-renin (salt-dependent) hypertension (Fig. 8.8).

8.4.5.1 Spironolactone

Mechanisms of Action
Spironolactone, steroidal MRA, is a specific pharmacologic antagonist of aldosterone; its primary action is to competitively bind the receptors at the aldosterone-dependent sodium-potassium pump in the distal convoluted renal tubule. The effect of spironolactone is increased sodium and water excretion, and retention of potassium. The drug exerts both diuretic and antihypertensive properties by its mechanism. It is used as stand-alone or combined with diuretic agents which with similar mechanism of action (Bennett 2008; Ives 2009; Kolkhof and Bärfacker 2017; Roush and Sica 2016).

Table 8.18 Summary of thiazide and thiazide-like diuretics

Examples	Dose	Onset and peak times (min)	Adverse effects	Drug interaction	Contraindications
Bendroflumethazide Oedema Hypertension	Initial, up to 20 mg orally daily (divided once or twice daily). Maintenance dose: 2.5–5 mg 6 h orally Initial, 5–20 mg orally in one or two divided doses daily. Maintenance dose: 2.5–15 mg 6 h	Onset: Oral: 30–60 IM: 10–30 IV: 5 Peak: Oral: 60–120 IM: unknown IV: 30	Dizziness, hypotension, hyponatraemia, impaired glucose tolerance, gout, impotence, hypokalaemia, hypercalcaemia	Lithium, digoxin, anti-arrhythmics, ciclosporin, corticosteroids, NSAIDs, acetazolamide, antidiabetic agents, alcohol, barbiturates, opioids, antihypertensive	Severe renal and hepatic impairment. Refractory hypokalaemia, hyponatraemia, hypercalcaemia. Symptomatic uraemia, Addison's disease. Lactation
Chlortalidone Hypertension Elderly	25–100 mg/day or 100 mg 3 times/ week 12.5–25 mg/day 12.5–25 mg/day or every other day; there is little advantage to using doses >25 mg/day	Onset: Oral: 30–60 Peak: 60	Hypotension, hyponatraemia, impaired glucose tolerance, gout, hypokalaemia, hypercalcaemia especially in patients prescribed with calcium supplements and vitamin D analogues	Loop diuretics, Lithium, digoxin, NSAIDs, diabetes medications	Same as above in addition to cardiac arrhythmias, simultaneous therapy with aminoglycosides or cephalosporins

Metolazone Oedema: Hypertension	5–20 mg/dose daily 2.5–5 mg/dose daily 0.5 mg/day; if response is not adequate, increase dose to maximum of 1 mg/day	Onset: Oral: 30–60 IV: 2–3 Peak: 15–30	Dizziness, weakness, restlessness, headache, muscle cramps, joint pain or swelling, constipation, diarrhoea	ACE inhibitors, bile acid sequestrants, diazoxide, and lithium excretion. Hypotensive effect may be increased with alcohol	Anuria; hepatic coma or pre-coma, pregnancy, diabetes mellitus, ventricular arrhythmias
Indapamide Oedema Hypertension	2.5–5 mg/day. Note: There is little therapeutic benefit to increasing the dose >5 mg/day 1.25 mg in the morning, may increase to 5 mg/day by increments of 1.25–2.5 mg at 4-week intervals	Onset: 1–3 h Peak: 2 h	Same as Bendroflumethazide	Same as Bendroflumethazide	Hypersensitivity, Anuria, hypotension, diabetes mellitus, fluid or electrolyte imbalance, hyperuricaemia or gout, SLE, liver disease, renal disease

Fig. 8.8 Mechanism of action of potassium-sparing diuretics

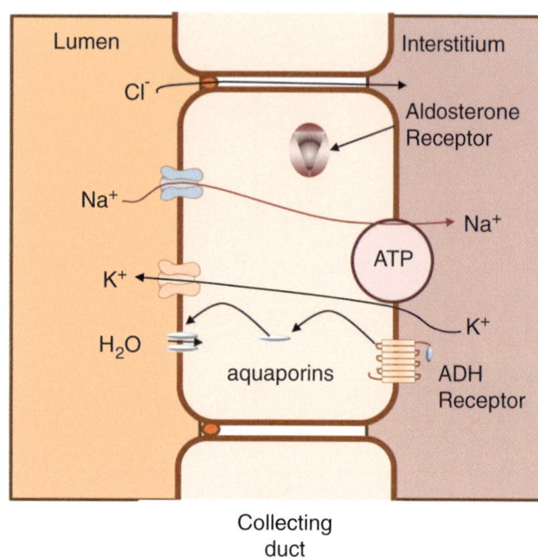

Table 8.19 Clinical indications of spironolactone

1. Oedema and ascites in cirrhosis of the liver; malignant ascites; nephrotic syndrome; congestive heart failure; moderate to severe heart failure resistant hypertension
2. Congestive cardiac failure to treat the sodium and water retention caused by secondary hyperaldosteronism due to diminished intravascular volume
3. Hypertension—as an adjunct to other drugs
4. Hypokalaemia—when other measures are inappropriate

Pharmacokinetics

90% of Spironolactone is bound to plasma proteins. Metabolites of spironolactone are primarily excreted in the urine (47–57%) and secondarily in bile, through faeces (35–41%) (Table 8.19).

8.4.5.2 Eplerenone

Mechanism of Action

Eplerenone selectively inhibits the binding of aldosterone to the mineralocorticoid receptor component of the renin-angiotensin-aldosterone-system (Jansena et al. 2013; Kolkhof and Bärfacker 2017).

Pharmacokinetics

50% of eplerenone is bound to protein. The drug is metabolised primarily in the liver. The bulk (67%) of the drug is excreted in the urine with the rest excreted in the faeces (Table 8.20).

Table 8.20 Clinical indications of eplerenone

1. Adjunct in stable patients with left ventricular ejection fraction $\leq 40\%$ with evidence of heart failure, following myocardial infarction
2. Adjunct in chronic mild heart failure with left ventricular ejection fraction $\leq 30\%$

Table 8.21 Clinical indications of amiloride

1. Oedema; potassium conservation when used as an adjunct to thiazide or loop diuretics for hypertension, congestive heart failure, or hepatic cirrhosis with ascites

8.4.5.3 Amiloride and Triamterene

Mechanism of Action

Amiloride and triamterene interferes with potassium-sodium exchange through active transport in the distal tubule, cortical collecting tubule and collecting duct with a resultant inhibition of the sodium, potassium-pump. This results in the elimination of the driving force for potassium secretion, hence the potential for hypokalaemia is prevented. Their action additionally decreases calcium excretion and increases magnesium loss. However, they exert a moderate diuretic effect (Bennett 2008; Epstein 2021; Ives 2009; Pitt 2021).

Pharmacokinetics

Only 23% of the drug is bound to protein. After oral administration, 15–25% of the drug is absorbed. Amiloride is not metabolized in the liver; no active metabolites are available. 50% of amiloride is excreted in the urine and the remainder, in faeces (Table 8.21).

8.4.5.4 Finerenone

Finerenone is a novel nonsteroidal MRA that is associated with a lower risk of hyperkalaemia than steroidal MRAs (Table 8.22).

Table 8.22 Summary of potassium-sparing diuretics

Examples	Dose	Onset and peak times (min/h)	Adverse effects	Drug interaction	Contraindications
Spironolactone Oedema and ascites in cirrhosis Malignant ascites Nephrotic syndrome Oedema in congestive heart failure and Moderate to severe heart failure Resistant hypertension Primary hyperaldosteronism in patients awaiting surgery	100–400 mg daily, adjusted according to response Initially 100–200 mg daily, increased to 400 mg daily if required; maintenance dose adjusted according to response 100–200 mg daily Initially 100 mg (range 25–200 mg) daily in single or divided doses; maintenance dose adjusted according to response Initially 25 mg once daily, increased according to response to max. 50 mg once daily 25 mg once daily 100–400 mg daily; long-term maintenance if surgery is inappropriate use lowest effective doses	Onset: 2–4 h Peak: 3–4 h	Gastro-intestinal disturbances, hepatotoxicity, malaise, confusion, dizziness, gynaecomastia, benign breast tumour, breast pain, menstrual disturbances, changes in libido, hypertrichosis, electrolyte disturbances, acute renal failure, hyperuricaemia, leucopaenia, agranulocytosis, thrombocytopaenia, leg cramps, alopecia, rash, Stevens–Johnson syndrome	Skeletal muscle relaxants, non-depolarizing (e.g. tubocurarine, lithium, NSAIDS, digoxin	Hyperkalaemia; anuria; Addison's disease

Eplerenone	Initially 25 mg once daily, increased within 4 weeks to 50 mg once daily	Onset: Oral: 30–60 Peak: 1–2 h	As above, in addition to ECG changes, mood changes, muscle pain or cramps, numbness or tingling in hands, feet, or lips, ankles, feet, or lower legs	Same as above	Hyperkalaemia; concomitant use of potassium-sparing diuretics or potassium supplements, avoid in severe hepatic and renal impairment
Triamterene	5–10 mg daily (up to 20 mg)	Onset: 120 Peak: 6–10 h	Headache, nausea or loss of appetite, diarrhoea Vomiting	Same as above	Hyperkalaemia; anuria; Addison's disease Hypersensensitivity
Amiloride With other diuretics in the treatment of congestive heart failure hypertension Cirrhosis with ascites	10 mg daily or 5 mg twice daily, adjusted according to response; max. 20 mg daily Initially 5–10 mg daily Initially 5 mg daily	Onset: initial effect: 2–3 h, max effect: 6–10 h Peak: 3–4 h	Angina, arrhythmias, palpitation, postural hypotension, dizziness, dyspnoea, cough, nasal congestion, confusion, headache, insomnia, weakness, tremor, agitation, dizziness, malaise, paraesthesia, encephalopathy, urinary disturbances sexual dysfunction, hyperkalaemia, arthralgia, visual disturbance, raised intra-ocular pressure, tinnitus, alopecia, pruritus, rash	Quinidine-↑ risk of arrhythmias ACEI & potassium supplements - ↑ risk of hyperkalemia Amoxicillin ↓ effects	Hyperkalaemia Anuria, renal impairment Cr >1.5 Diabetic nephropathy Caution if diabetes mellitus

(continued)

Table 8.22 (continued)

Examples	Dose	Onset and peak times (min/h)	Adverse effects	Drug interaction	Contraindications
Fineronone	Starting dose is 10 mg once daily. The recommended target dose is 20 mg once daily If potassium is 4.8, 10 mg daily If potassium is 4.9–5.0, consider with additional serum potassium monitoring within the first 4 weeks If potassium is >5.0, withhold Finerenone	Onset: immediate Peak: 0.5 and 1.25 h	Confusion, irregular heartbeat Nausea or vomiting, nervousness numbness or tingling in the hands, feet, or lips, stomach pain Trouble breathing, weakness or heaviness of the legs	Boceprevir Ceritinib Clarithromycin Cobicistat Idelalisib Indinavir Itraconazole Ketoconazole	Same as above plus eGFR less than 25

8.4.6   Vasopressin Receptor Antagonists (Aquaretics)

Vasopressin receptor antagonists (VRAs), also known as *aquaretics*, selectively inhibit the action of vasopressin at V2 receptors in the renal collecting ducts. This blockade reduces water reabsorption without affecting sodium or other electrolytes, resulting in *electrolyte-free water excretion* (aquaresis). Clinically, VRAs such as *Tolvaptan* are used to correct *hyponatraemia* in conditions like Syndrome of inappropriate antidiuretic hormone secretion (*SIADH*), *congestive heart failure*, and *cirrhosis*, where inappropriate vasopressin secretion leads to fluid retention.

In addition to fluid regulation, V2 receptor antagonism has shown promise in *autosomal dominant polycystic kidney disease (ADPKD)* by reducing intracellular cAMP levels, thereby slowing cyst growth and preserving renal function.

Examples: Tolvaptan, Conivaptan
Mechanism of Action: Vasopressin receptor antagonists selectively block V2 receptors in the renal collecting ducts, reducing water reabsorption and promoting electrolyte-free water excretion (aquaresis). This mechanism helps correct hyponatremia in conditions such as SIADH, heart failure, and cirrhosis.

Clinical Indications:
- Euvolemic and hypervolemic hyponatremia
- Autosomal dominant polycystic kidney disease (ADPKD)
- Congestive heart failure with fluid retention

Pharmacokinetics: Tolvaptan is orally administered and metabolized by CYP3A4. It has a half-life of 3–12 h and requires careful monitoring of serum sodium levels.

8.4.6.1 Pharmacokinetic Comparison: Tolvaptan Versus Conivaptan

Although Tolvaptan and Conivaptan are both vasopressin receptor antagonists, their pharmacokinetic profiles differ significantly, reflecting their distinct clinical applications

Parameter	Tolvaptan (oral)	Conivaptan (intravenous)
Route of administration	Oral tablet	Intravenous infusion
Absorption	Rapid; bioavailability ~40%	Not applicable (IV administration)
Peak plasma time	~2 h	~1–2 h post-infusion
Half-life	~12 h (dose-dependent)	~5.3–8.1 h
Metabolism	CYP3A4 and P-glycoprotein substrate	CYP3A4 hepatic metabolism
Excretion	Fecal and renal	Primarily hepatic
Steady-state	Achieved after multiple oral doses	Achieved with continuous infusion

Clinical Implication: Tolvaptan is suited for long-term outpatient management, including ADPKD, due to its oral dosing and sustained aquaretic effect. Conivaptan, by contrast, is reserved for acute hospital-based correction of hyponatremia, offering rapid onset via IV infusion.

Examples	Dose	Onset and peak times (min)	Side effects	Drug interaction	Contra-indications
Conivaptan	Loading: 20 mg IV over 30 min Maintenance: 20 mg continuous IV infusion over 24 h for 2–4 days May increase to 40 mg/day if needed	*Onset*: within 1–2 h *Half-life*: ~5.3–8.1 h	Infusion site reactions, fever, headache, hypo-kalaemia Risk of rapid sodium correction: neurological symptoms (e.g., seizures, dysarthria)	Contra-indicated: Strong CYP3A4 inhibitors (e.g., clar-ithromycin, ritonavir) Monitor with diuretics, digoxin, and potassium-altering agents	Anuria Hypovolemic hyponatremia Severe hepatic impairment Concurrent use with strong CYP3A4 inhibitors
Tolvaptan Euvolemic and hypervolemic hyponatremia Congestive heart failure with fluid retention Autosomal dominant polycystic kidney disease (ADPKD)	Initial: 15 mg once daily May increase to 30 mg or 60 mg once daily at ≥24-h intervals 45 mg on waking + 15 mg 8 h later; titrate to 90 mg + 30 mg/day if tolerated	*Onset*: ~2–4 h *Peak*: ~2 h	Thirst, dry mouth, polyuria, hyper-natraemia Rare: hepato-toxicity, osmotic demy-elination (if sodium corrected too rapidly)	Strong CYP3A4 inhibitors (e.g., ketoconazole, clar-ithromycin, ritonavir) *Caution*: ACE inhibitors, ARBs, potassium-sparing diuretics—risk of hyper-kalaemia Avoid use with hypertonic saline	Anuria Inability to respond to thirst Hypovolemic hyponatremia Severe liver disease Pregnancy and breastfeeding (not recom-mended)

Nursing Management of the Patient Receiving Vasopressin Receptor Antagonists

Pre-therapy Assessment
- *Baseline observations*:
  - Blood pressure, heart rate, respiratory rate, weight, and fluid balance
  - Serum electrolytes (Na^+, K^+, Cl^-, Mg^{2+}, Ca^{2+}), renal function (eGFR, creatinine, urea)
- *Medication history*:
  - Review current prescriptions, OTC drugs, herbal supplements
  - Identify potential drug–drug interactions (e.g., NSAIDs, ACE inhibitors, lithium)
- *Clinical indications and contraindications*:
  - Confirm diagnosis (e.g., heart failure, CKD, hypertension)
  - Screen for contraindications (e.g., anuria, hepatic impairment, pregnancy)
- *Patient profile*:
  - Assess hydration status, cognitive ability, and capacity to adhere to therapy
  - Evaluate risk factors for falls, hypotension, or infection

Nursing Interventions and Monitoring During Therapy
- *Vital signs and fluid balance*:
  - Monitor BP, HR, daily weight, and urine output
  - Track signs of volume depletion or overload (e.g., orthostatic hypotension, oedema)
- *Electrolyte monitoring*:
  - Regular blood tests for Na^+, K^+, Mg^{2+}, Ca^{2+}
  - Watch for signs of hypo/hyperkalaemia, hyponatremia, or metabolic acidosis
- *Adverse effect surveillance*:
  - Observe for dizziness, muscle cramps, confusion, polyuria, or rash
  - Monitor serum sodium closely to avoid rapid correction
- *Medication administration*:
  - Administer at appropriate times (e.g., morning dosing to reduce nocturia)
  - Ensure IV infusions (e.g., Conivaptan) are correctly titrated and site monitored
- *Documentation and escalation*:
  - Record all observations and interventions
  - Escalate concerns promptly (e.g., rising creatinine, symptomatic hypotension)

Patient Education
- *Therapeutic purpose and expected outcomes*:
  - Explain how the medication supports fluid balance, blood pressure, or glucose control
  - Reinforce the importance of adherence and regular monitoring
- *Self-monitoring and symptom reporting*:
  - Teach patients to track weight, fluid intake/output, and signs of dehydration

- Encourage reporting of dizziness, palpitations, or unusual fatigue
- *Lifestyle and safety advice*:
  - Promote hydration, balanced diet, and fall prevention strategies
  - Caution against excessive fluid restriction or salt substitutes
- *Empowerment and shared decision-making*:
  - Involve patients in goal setting and medication reviews
  - Provide written resources and visual aids where appropriate

8.4.7 Sodium-Glucose Co-transporter 2 Inhibitors (SGLT2i)

Sodium-glucose co-transporter 2 (SGLT2) inhibitors reduce glucose reabsorption in the proximal renal tubule, promoting glucosuria and mild natriuresis as shown in Fig. 8.9. This mechanism lowers blood glucose levels independently of insulin and contributes to osmotic diuresis, which can reduce volume overload in patients with heart failure and chronic kidney disease (CKD).

Beyond glycaemic control, SGLT2 inhibitors such as dapagliflozin, empagliflozin, and canagliflozin have demonstrated cardiorenal protective effects, including reduced hospitalization for heart failure and slowed progression of CKD. They also lower intraglomerular pressure and reduce albuminuria.

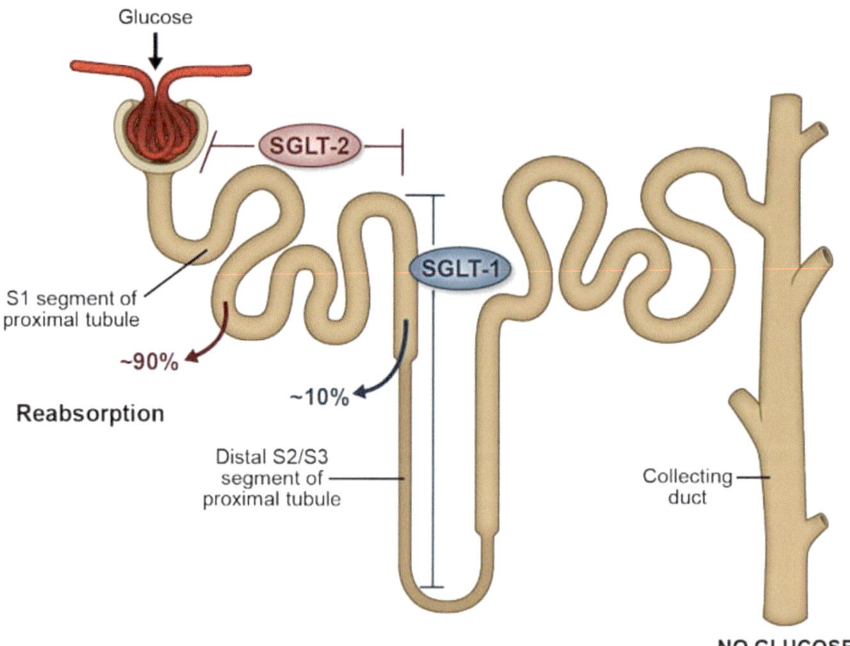

Fig. 8.9 Location and function of Sodium-Glucose Co-transport proteins in the nephron

Examples: Dapagliflozin, Empagliflozin, Canagliflozin
Mechanism of Action: SGLT2 inhibitors block glucose reabsorption in the proximal renal tubule, leading to glucosuria and mild natriuresis. This results in osmotic diuresis and reduced intraglomerular pressure.

Clinical Indications:
- Type 2 diabetes mellitus
- Heart failure with reduced ejection fraction (HFrEF)
- Chronic kidney disease (CKD) with albuminuria

Pharmacokinetics: These agents are orally administered, highly protein-bound, and metabolized via glucuronidation. They have a half-life of 10–13 h. While Dapagliflozin, Empagliflozin, and Canagliflozin all belong to the SGLT2 inhibitor class and share a common mechanism, their pharmacokinetic profiles differ subtly in ways that influence dosing, safety, and renal suitability.

Pharmacokinetic Comparison: Dapagliflozin Versus Empagliflozin Versus Canagliflozin

Parameter	Dapagliflozin	Empagliflozin	Canagliflozin
Route of administration	Oral tablet	Oral tablet	Oral tablet
Bioavailability	~78%	~78%	~65%
Peak plasma time	~2 h	~1.5 h	~1–2 h
Half-life	~12.9 h	~12.4 h	~10.6–13.1 h
Protein binding	~91%	~86%	~99%
Metabolism	UGT1A9, UGT2B4 (glucuronidation)	UGT2B7, UGT1A3, UGT1A8	UGT1A9, UGT2B4; minor CYP3A4
Excretion	~75% renal, ~21% faecal	~54% renal, ~41% faecal	~33% renal, ~42% faecal
Renal suitability	eGFR ≥25 ml/min/1.73 m²	eGFR ≥20 ml/min/1.73 m²	eGFR ≥30 ml/min/1.73 m²

Clinical Implications
- *Dapagliflozin* is preferred in patients with moderate renal impairment due to its renal clearance profile and proven cardiorenal benefits at 10 mg.
- *Empagliflozin* has slightly faster onset and broader approval for heart failure and CKD, even at lower eGFR thresholds.
- *Canagliflozin* has the highest protein binding and a slightly longer half-life, but carries unique risks (e.g., amputation, bone fracture) and requires cautious use in renal impairment

Examples	Dose	Onset and peak times (min)	Side effects	Drug interaction	Contraindications
Dapagliflozin	10 mg once daily	Onset: ~2 h; Peak: ~2 h	Genital infections, dehydration, euglycaemic DKA	Insulin, sulfo-nylureas, diuretics	Type 1 diabetes, eGFR <25, hypersensitivity
Empagliflozin	10–25 mg once daily	Onset: ~1.5 h; Peak: ~1.5 h	UTIs, hypotension, ketoacidosis	Diuretics, insulin	Type 1 diabetes, eGFR <20, hypersensitivity
Canagliflozin	100–300 mg once daily	Onset: ~24 h; Peak: ~1–2 h	Genital infections, hyper-kalaemia, amputation risk	ACE inhibitors	eGFR <30, dialysis, hypersensitivity

Nursing Management of the Patient Receiving Sodium Glucose Co-transporter

Pre-therapy Assessment
- *Baseline observations*:
  - Blood pressure, heart rate, respiratory rate, weight, and fluid balance
  - Serum electrolytes (Na^+, K^+, Cl^-, Mg^{2+}, Ca^{2+}), renal function (eGFR, creatinine, urea)
  - Blood glucose
- *Medication history*:
  - Review current prescriptions, OTC drugs, herbal supplements
  - Identify potential drug–drug interactions (e.g., NSAIDs, ACE inhibitors, lithium)
- *Clinical indications and contraindications*:
  - Confirm diagnosis (e.g., heart failure, CKD, hypertension)
  - Screen for contraindications (e.g., anuria, hepatic impairment, pregnancy)
- *Patient profile*:
  - Assess hydration status, cognitive ability, and capacity to adhere to therapy
  - Evaluate risk factors for falls, hypotension, or infection

Nursing Interventions and Monitoring During Therapy
- *Vital signs and fluid balance*:
  - Monitor BP, HR, daily weight, and urine output
  - Track signs of volume depletion or overload (e.g., orthostatic hypotension, oedema)
- *Electrolyte monitoring*:
  - Regular blood tests for Na^+, K^+, Mg^{2+}, Ca^{2+}
  - Watch for signs of hypo/hyperkalaemia, hyponatremia, or metabolic acidosis
- *Adverse effect surveillance*:
  - Observe for dizziness, muscle cramps, confusion, polyuria, or rash
  - Monitor for genital infections, DKA symptoms, dehydration

- *Medication administration*:
  - Administer at appropriate times (e.g., morning dosing to reduce nocturia)
  - Ensure IV infusions (e.g., Conivaptan) are correctly titrated and site monitored
- *Documentation and escalation*:
  - Record all observations and interventions
  - Escalate concerns promptly (e.g., rising creatinine, symptomatic hypotension)

Patient Education
- *Therapeutic purpose and expected outcomes*:
  - Explain how the medication supports fluid balance, blood pressure, or glucose control
  - Reinforce the importance of adherence and regular monitoring
- *Self-monitoring and symptom reporting*:
  - Teach patients to track weight, fluid intake/output, and signs of dehydration
  - Encourage reporting of dizziness, palpitations, or unusual fatigue
- *Lifestyle and safety advice*:
  - Promote hydration, balanced diet, and fall prevention strategies
  - Advise on hygiene, foot care, and infection signs
- *Empowerment and shared decision-making*:
  - Involve patients in goal-setting and medication reviews
  - Provide written resources and visual aids where appropriate

8.5 Diuretic Resistance

It has been documented that with some people receiving diuretic therapy, failure to decrease the extracellular fluid volume despite liberal use of these agents as stand-alone diuretic therapy, what is termed diuretic resistance, occurs. Recent studies (Felker et al. 2009, 2011; Snigdha et al. 2013; Wilcox et al 2020) suggest a significant association between high-dose diuretics (>160–300 mg daily) and increased mortality. Diuretic resistance may be caused by decreased renal function; and reduced and delayed peak concentrations particularly of loop diuretics in the tubular fluid. A post-diuretic sodium retention and subsequent rebound oedema might occur following the use of short acting diuretics. Additionally, resistance might be observed in the absence of these pharmacokinetic abnormalities. One of the strategies proposed (Kushner et al. 2009; Ponikowski et al. 2016; Trullàs et al. 2023) to overcome diuretic resistance is the use of combination diuretic therapy.

8.6 Combined Diuretics

The combined diuretic therapies in this chapter include Co-Amilofruse.

Table 8.23 Clinical indications

For prompt diuresis especially in conditions where potassium conservation is important: 1. Congestive cardiac failure 2. Fluid retention due to corticosteroid or oestrogen therapy 3. Ascites associated with cirrhosis

8.6.1 Co-amilofruse

This is a combination of Amiloride hydrochloride (Potassium-sparing) and Furosemide (Loop) diuretics, usually in 1:8 ratio, for example Co-Amilofruse 5/40 mg tablets.

8.6.1.1 Mechanism of Action and Pharmacodynamics

See notes under loop and potassium-sparing diuretics (Table 8.23)

8.7 Nursing Management of Patients Receiving Diuretic Therapy

8.7.1 Pre-therapy Assessment

- Assess and record baseline observation necessary for the detection of adverse effects:
  - General: TPR, BP, oedema, weight, skin colour
  - Central nervous system: reflexes, orientation, hearing
  - Cardiovascular: baseline ECG, lying and standing BP, fluid intake
  - Gastrointestinal: liver function test, bowel sounds
  - Genitourinary: output
  - Blood results: electrolytes, liver and renal function, urinalysis, glucose and uric acid
- Review past medical history and documentation that
  - Require cautious use and or contraindicate of individual categories diuretics

8.7.2 Nursing Interventions and Monitoring During Therapy

- Monitor vital signs frequently, monitor infusion rate if medication is administered via the IV route.
- Monitor electrolyte and blood glucose levels and liaise with the medical team appropriately
- Ensure ready access for toileting purposes, especially for elderly patients and those at increased risk of falls
- Provide skin care is required
- Assess patient for adverse effects
- Monitor for possible drug–drug interaction

8.7.3   Patient Education

- For patients who self-administer and or are being discharged from a care setting, provide detailed information about prescribed medication
- Encourage the patient to report any adverse effect of the medication promptly.

Multiple Choice Questions

1. A 35-year-old patient has been admitted to your ward with mild hypertension. Her blood pressure during observations was 145/95 mmHg; there is no other clinically significant complaint. She is otherwise physically fit and adheres to a dietary regimen. She was prescribed antihypertensive drugs on admission, and chlorothiazide was added to her medications. How does this diuretic cause action and effect?
   - (a) Inhibition of sodium and chloride reabsorption in the early distal convoluted tubule
   - (b) Decreases net excretion of chloride, sodium and potassium
   - (c) Increases calcium excretion
   - (d) Inhibits reabsorption of sodium chloride in the thick ascending loop of Henle
   - (e) Interferes with potassium secretion
2. A person presented at A&E with complaints of sharp pain in his flanks and dysuria is admitted to the ward with a diagnosis of idiopathic hypercalcaeuria. What is the common type of medication used for the condition?
   - (a) Loop diuretics
   - (b) Carbonic anhydrase inhibitors
   - (c) Thiazide diuretics
   - (d) Potassium-sparing diuretics
   - (e) Osmotic diuretics
3. A 45-year-old patient with a history of medication-controlled hypertension has been readmitted to the ward with a left painful swollen big toe. A provisional diagnosis of gout has been made. A laboratory analysis of blood requested this morning revealed raised uric acid levels. From the list of his medication below, which of them might be a contributory factor for his current symptoms?
   - (a) Acetazolamide
   - (b) Amiloride
   - (c) Mannitol
   - (d) Hydrochlorothiazide
   - (e) Spironolactone
4. A patient diagnosed with a first episode of congestive heart failure secondary to alcoholic cardiomyopathy has been admitted to the ward. The cardiologist has recommended the inclusion of a diuretic as part of the routine medications, which of the following is the preferred diuretic for this patient?

    (a) Loop diuretics due to their action at the distal convoluted tubule

    (b) Thiazide diuretics due to their effect on the thick ascending limb of the loop of Henle

    (c) Loop diuretics due to its high capacity for sodium chloride reabsorption

    (d) Thiazide diuretics because they increase peripheral vascular resistance

    (e) Thiazide diuretics because they increase cardiac output

5. A patient admitted with myocardial infarction develops respiratory distress. Upon assessment by the medical team, flash pulmonary oedema secondary to myocardial infarction was confirmed. Furosemide was included as part of the pharmacological management. What is the mechanism of action of this diuretic?

    (a) Furosemide inhibits the action of aldosterone

    (b) It inhibits bicarbonate and sodium reabsorption

    (c) Furosemide inhibits active reabsorption of sodium chloride at the distal convoluted tubule

    (d) It alters the diffusion of water relative to sodium and hence reduces sodium reabsorption

    (e) Furosemide inhibits active reabsorption of sodium chloride at the thick ascending loop of Henle

6. Which of the following diuretic cause dizziness and tinnitus?

    (a) Spironolactone

    (b) Mannitol

    (c) Furosemide

    (d) Amiloride

7. Which of the following might not be prescribed for the patient taking potassium supplements?

    (a) Furosemide

    (b) Amiloride

    (c) Mannitol

    (d) Hydrochlorothiazide

8. Which of the below mentioned drug produce its action by competitively inhibiting the sodium-potassium-chloride cotransporter?

    (a) Loop diuretics

    (b) Thiazide diuretics

    (c) Inhibitors of carbonic anhydrase

    (d) Potassium-sparing diuretics

9. Which diuretic drug produces its action by acting on proximal tubules?

    (a) Thiazide diuretics

    (b) Potassium-sparing diuretics

    (c) Loop diuretics

    (d) Inhibitors of carbonic anhydrase

10. Which of the below mentioned diuretic drug produce its action by acting on distal convoluted tubule?

   (a) Carbonic anhydrase inhibitors
   (b) Thiazide diuretics
   (c) Loop diuretics
   (d) Potassium-sparing diuretics
11. What is the primary mechanism of action of vasopressin receptor antagonists (aquaretics)?
   (a) Blockade of V2 receptors in the renal collecting ducts
   (b) Activation of carbonic anhydrase in the nephron
   (c) Inhibition of sodium reabsorption in the proximal tubule
   (d) Stimulation of aldosterone secretion
12. Which of the following is a common adverse effect of SGLT2 inhibitors?
   (a) Hypernatraemia
   (b) Genital infections
   (c) Hepatotoxicity
   (d) Hypokalaemia

Answers

1. (a)
2. (c)
3. (e)
4. (c)
5. (e)
6. (d)
7. (b)
8. (a)
9. (d)
10. (b)
11. (a)
12. (b)

References

Ashley C, Dunleavy A (2014) The renal handbook, 4th edn. Radcliffe, London

Aung T, Laganovska G, Hernandez Paredes TJ, Branch JD, Tsorbatzoglou A, Goldberg I, Franco AM (2014) Twice-daily brinzolamide/brimonidine fixed combination versus brinzolamide or brimonidine in open-angle glaucoma or ocular hypertension. Ophthalmology 121(12):2348–2355

Bennett S (2008) Diuretics: use, actions and prescribing rationale. Nurs Prescrib 6(2):72–77

Braunwald E (2014) Responsiveness to loop diuretics in heart failure. Eur Heart J 35:1235–1237

Brunton LL, La Jolla CA, Ronco C, McCullough PA, Anker SD, Anand I, Aspromonte N, Bagshaw SM, Bellomo R, Berl T, Bobek I, Cruz DN, Daliento L, Davenport A, Haapio MH, House AA, Katz N, Maisel A, Mankad S, Zanco P, Mebazaa A, Palazzuoli A, Ronco F, Shaw A, Sheinfeld G, Soni S, Vescovo G, Zamperetti N, Ponikowski P (2009) Cardio-renal syndromes: report from the consensus conference of the acute dialysis quality initiative. Eur Heart J 31(6):703–711

Edwin K (2006) Diuretics. In: Brunton LL et al (eds) Goodman & Gilman's the pharmacological basis of therapeutics, 11th edn. McGraw-Hill, New York

Epstein M (2021) Aldosterone and mineralocorticoid receptor antagonists: therapeutic advances and challenges. Kidney Int Suppl 11(1):1–8.

Ernst ME, Fravel MA (2022) Thiazide diuretics in hypertension: mechanisms and clinical applications. Curr Hypertens Rep 24(2):123–130.

Felker GM, O'Connor CM, Braunwald E (2009) Loop diuretics in acute decompensated heart failure-necessary? Evil? A necessary. Circ Heart Fail 2(1):56–62

Felker GM, Lee KL, Bull DA, Redfield MM, Stevenson LW, Goldsmith SR (2011) Diuretic strategies in patients with acute decompensated heart failure. N Engl J Med 364:797–805. https://doi.org/10.1056/NEJMoa1005419

Felker GM, Ellison DH, Mullens W, Cox ZL, Testani JM (2013) Diuretic therapy for patients with heart failure: JACC state-of the-art review. J Am Coll Cardiol 61(19):2145–2153.

Gheorghiade M (2010) The role of diuretics in the treatment of heart failure. Am J Cardiol 105(7):S3–S7.

Ives HE (2009) Chapter 15: Diuretic agents. In: Katzung's basic and clinical pharmacology, 11th edn. McGraw-Hill/Lange, New York. ISBN:978-0-07-160405-5

Jansena PM, Frenkelb WJ, van den Bornb BH, de Bruijnec ELE, Deinumd J, Kerstense MN, Arnoldusf JHA, Woittiezg AJ, Wijbengah JAH, Zietsea R, Jan Dansera AH, van den Meiracker AH (2013) Determinants of blood pressure reduction by Eplerenone in uncontrolled hypertension. J Hypertens 31(2):404–413

Kaufman J (2020) Diuretics: mechanisms and clinical use. Clin J Am Soc Nephrol 15(5):737–739.

Kaufman G (2013) Prescribing and medicines management in older people. Nurs Older People 25(7):33–41

Klabunde RE (2011) Cardiovascular physiology concepts. 2nd ed. Philadelphia: Lippincott Williams & Wilkins.

Klabunde RE (2015) Cardiovascular pharmacology concepts. Diuretics. http://www.cvpharmacology.com/diuretic/diuretics. Accessed 20 Feb 2015

Kolkhof P, Bärfacker L (2017) Mineralocorticoid receptor antagonists: 60 years of research and development. J Med Chem 60(17):7101–7115.

Kushner FG, Hand M, Smith SC Jr, King SB III, Anderson JL, Antman EM, Bailey SR, Bates ER, Blankenship JC, Casey DE Jr, Green LA, Jacobs AK, Hochman JS, Krumholz HM, Morrison DA, Ornato JP, Pearle DL, Peterson ED, Sloan MA, Whitlow PL, Williams DO (2009) 2009 focused updates: ACC/AHA guidelines for the management of patients with ST-elevation myocardial infarction (updating the 2004 guideline and 2007 focused update) and ACC/AHA/ SCAI guidelines on percutaneous coronary intervention (updating the 2005 guideline and 2007 focused update): a report of the American College of Cardiology Foundation/American Heart Association task force on practice guidelines. Catheter Cardiovasc Interv 74(7):E25–E68

Marieb EN (2020) Human anatomy & physiology. 11th ed. Pearson Education.

McMahon BA, Chawla LS (2021) Diuretics in acute kidney injury. Clin J Am Soc Nephrol 16(6):943–951.

Musini VM, Nazer M, Bassett K, Wright JM (2014) Blood pressure-lowering efficacy of monotherapy with thiazide diuretics for primary hypertension. Cochrane Database Syst Rev 5:CD003824

Palazzuoli A, Ruocco G, Pellegrini M et al (2020) The role of diuretics in acute heart failure: new insights and open questions. Heart Fail Rev 25(1):123–134.

Peters N, Bhandari S, Kalra PA (2022) Loop diuretics in chronic kidney disease: balancing efficacy and safety. Nephrol Dial Transplant 37(4):678–685.

Pitt B (2021) The use of potassium-sparing diuretics in cardiovascular disease. Eur Heart J 42(3):234–240.

Ponikowski P, Voors AA, Anker SD, Bueno H, Cleland JG, Falk V, González-Juanatey JR, Harjola VP, Jankowska EA, Jessup M, Linde C, Nihoyannopoulos P, Parissis JT, Pieske B, Riley JP, Rosano GM, Ruilope LM, Ruschitzka F, Rutten FH, van der Meer P, ESC Scientific Document Group (2016) ESC guidelines for the diagnosis and treatment of acute and chronic heart failure: the task force for the diagnosis and treatment of acute and chronic heart failure of the European Society of Cardiology (ESC) developed with the special contribution of the Heart Failure Association (HFA) of the ESC. Eur Heart J 37(27):2129–2200

Roush GC, Sica DA (2016) Diuretics for hypertension: a review and update. Am J Hypertens 29(10):1130–1137

Sam R, Pearce D (2023) Osmotic diuretics: mechanisms and clinical applications. Kidney Int 103(2):215–223

Sansone T, Di Marco M, De Angelis C (2016) Carbonic anhydrase inhibitors in glaucoma therapy. Ophthalmol Ther 5(2):123–134.

Shawkat H, Westwood M, Mortimer A (2012) Mannitol: a review of its clinical uses continuing education in anaesthesia, critical care & pain. Br J Anaesth 12(2):82–85

Shukralla A, Ahmed M, Khan S (2022) Carbonic anhydrase inhibitors: pharmacology and clinical applications. J Clin Pharmacol 62(3):345–352.

Snigdha M, Kumar SS, Deepa K, Lalit S, Tanuja S (2013) Review on recent advances in a modern-day treatment: diuretic therapy. Int Res J Pharm 4(6):25–30

Sugrue MF (2000) Pharmacological and ocular hypotensive properties of topical carbonic anhydrase inhibitors. Prog Retin Eye Res 19(1):87–112

Supuran CT (2016) Carbonic anhydrase inhibitors and their therapeutic potential. Nat Rev Drug Discov 15(5):345–356.

Trullàs JC, Comín-Colet J, Enjuanes C et al (2023) Diuretic resistance in heart failure: mechanisms and management. ESC Heart Fail 10(1):123–134.

Wargo KA, Banta WM (2009) A comprehensive review of loop diuretics: should Furosemide be the first choice? Ann Pharmacol 43(11):1836–1847

Haya Abu Ghazaleh and Ehsan Khan

Learning Outcomes

At the end of this chapter, you will be able to

- Distinguish between Type 1 and Type 2 diabetes.
- Differentiate between the mechanisms of action of frequently used medications for managing diabetes.
- Identify and provide a rationale for the most significant adverse effects associated with medications used for diabetes management.

9.1 Introduction

Aetiology and Pathophysiology of Type 1 and Type 2 Diabetes

"Are they so different and why do you need to know?" The World Health Organization (2025) defines diabetes as:

> Diabetes is a chronic disease that occurs either when the pancreas does not produce enough insulin or when the body cannot effectively use the insulin it produces.

The term *diabetes* originates from the word diabainein (Greek = a syphon), first coined by the Greek physician Aretaeus in the first century BC to describe the frequency of urination associated with this condition. It was not until the 1600s that

H. A. Ghazaleh (✉)
Florence Nightingale Faculty of Nursing, Midwifery & Palliative Care, King's College London, London, UK
e-mail: Haya.Abu_Ghazaleh@kcl.ac.uk

E. Khan
Faculty of Nursing Midwifery and Palliative Care, King's College London, London, UK
e-mail: eu.khan@kcl.ac.uk

© The Author(s), under exclusive license to Springer Nature Switzerland AG 2026
E. Khan, P. Hood (eds.), *Understanding Pharmacology in Nursing Practice*,
https://doi.org/10.1007/978-3-032-03964-4_9

mellitus (Greek = like honey) was added to diabetes to describe the sweet-tasting urine of patients suffering from the illness.

9.2   Type 1 Diabetes

Type 1 diabetes is an autoimmune disease characterised by the destruction of insulin-producing pancreatic beta cells. Individuals with Type 1 diabetes are unable to produce insulin or metabolise glucose for energy and must be administered insulin to survive. Insulin has been available to treat Type 1 diabetes since 1920, but despite almost 100 years of insulin replacement therapy, there is still comparatively little known about the cause of this condition. Many causes, such as stress and exposure to cow's milk, have been suggested, but some research points to viral and genetic triggers (Robinson and Kessling 1992; Filippi and von Herrath 2008). The prevalence of Type 1 diabetes is increasing, but at a much slower rate than Type 2 diabetes, and represents approximately 8% of all diabetes diagnoses (National Diabetes Audit 2023). According to the UK National Diabetes Audit 2021–2022 Report 1, there are approximately 280,000 people in the United Kingdom who have Type 1 diabetes (National Diabetes Audit 2023). Traditionally, Type 1 diabetes was believed to occur mainly in children; however, this notion is no longer accurate and Type 1 diabetes can occur in different age groups, albeit with different symptom presentation. In 2022, the International Diabetes Federation (IDF) estimated that globally 64% (5.56 million) of newly diagnosed cases of Type 1 diabetes occurred between 20 and 59 years of age, and approximately 200,000 new cases were reported in less than 20 years (Ogle et al. 2022). Type 1 diabetes is a long-term condition where people can experience a normal life expectancy, albeit this requires medical supervision, commitment and effective self-management.

If a person with Type 1 diabetes is administered insufficient insulin, they are unable to metabolise glucose, their blood glucose will rise, and the cells are forced to get energy from fats. The waste products of fat metabolism are ketones. The build-up of ketones can lead to diabetic ketoacidosis. This can be life-threatening. The onset can be very rapid—hours in the case of an insulin pump malfunctioning and days if doses are not large enough via bolus. It is essential that a person with Type 1 diabetes has adequate insulin replacement.

9.3   Type 2 Diabetes

Type 2 diabetes is a progressive condition marked by insulin insensitivity and loss of beta cell function. Glucose metabolism involves a feedback loop between beta cells and insulin-sensitive tissues. During insulin resistance, beta cells increase insulin output to maintain glucose homeostasis (Kahn et al. 2014). However, a simultaneous decline in insulin secretion as a result of a decrease in beta cell mass and or dysfunction (Weyer et al. 2001), together with loss of insulin response, causes a rise in glucose concentration and promotes the onset of a hyperglycaemic state. Alteration in beta cell gene expression (Frayling et al. 2001) and accumulation of glucose (Fonseca 2009), lipid (Tushuizen et al. 2007) and amyloid deposition (Kahn et al. 1999) in the pancreas are associated with beta cell failure and progression of Type 2 diabetes.

The aetiology of Type 2 diabetes is influenced by environmental, genetic and clinical factors. Individuals with a high basal metabolic index ($\geq$30 kg/m^2, White population; 23.9 kg/m^2, South Asians; 28.1 kg/m^2, Black population; 26.9 kg/m^2, Chinese; and 26.6 kg/m^2, Arabs), hypertension and who are obese are at risk of disease progression (Bellou et al. 2018; Caleyachetty et al. 2021; Ismail et al. 2021). Moreover, age and ethnicity were also reported as determinants in disease onset, such that Afro-Caribbeans, Black Africans and South Asians show earlier diagnosis of diabetes ($\geq$25 years) compared to white British ($\geq$40 years) (Diabetes UK 2025). In contrast, a 1-year longitudinal study demonstrated that younger adults with glycated haemoglobin (HbA1c) levels $\geq$7% had greater odds of disease progression and that each decade of increasing age lessened the risk of diabetes progression by 15% (Pani et al. 2008). These findings suggest that younger patients with Type 2 diabetes, and who are prone to weight gain, require earlier and more rigorous treatment than older individuals with diabetes to better manage their condition.

The central nervous system (CNS) and intestinal flora are also proposed to play a fundamental role in the pathophysiology of Type 2 diabetes. Changes in the composition and activity of gut microbiome alter metabolic processes (Diamant et al. 2011) and are shown to affect insulin sensitivity (Vrieze et al. 2012), suggesting a link to the progression of diabetes. The CNS also regulates endocrine function, such that severance of the vagus nerve to the pancreas in humans diminishes insulin release (Miller 1981).

Diabetes treatment focuses on normalising blood glucose levels for prolonged periods of time and different therapeutic agents are currently available, including oral and injectable drugs. Due to the heterogeneity of the condition, individual responses to antidiabetic drugs will vary. Moreover, a decline in beta cell function and the inevitable gradual increase in HbA1c levels during treatment (~1% every 2 years) often preclude monotherapy due to a reduction in drug efficacy with time (Fonseca 2009). Hence, multidrug therapies are usually prescribed to enhance diabetes management.

9.4 Insulin

Edward Sharpey-Schefer, popularly understood to be the founder of endocrinology, was one of the first physiologists to suggest a glucose-lowering substance to be secreted by the pancreas in the late 1800s. However, it was not until Fredrick Banting's and John MacLeod's (who coined the term insulin) collaborative endeavours in 1922 that the hormone was isolated and extracted in clinically useful concentrations. A year later, Ely Lilly was the first company to mass-produce insulin, making it commercially available. Insulin is a peptide made up of two amino cid (AA) chains; chain A is shorter (21 AA) compared to chain B (30 AA) (Fig. 9.1).

Fig. 9.1 Insulin

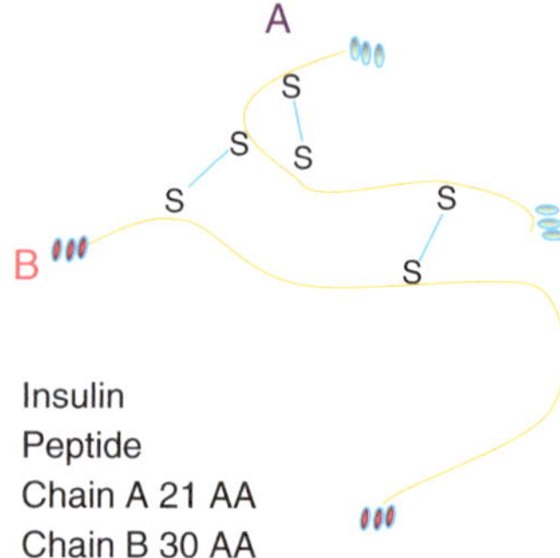

9.4.1 Physiology of Insulin Secretion and Mechanism of Action

Insulin reduces plasma glucose levels primarily by enhancing glucose transport into the cell. Being a water-soluble substance, glucose cannot diffuse across the lipid cell membrane and requires a transport mechanism to carry it across. Glucose is transported by transport proteins known as glucose transporters, which are named GLUT in short. Although there are a large number of different GLUT transporters, GLUT 4, which is mainly found in muscle and fat cells (adipocytes), is the main insulin-dependent glucose transport mechanism and is widely understood to be the key GLUT transporter involved in diabetes mellitus (Mueckler and Thorens 2013).

9.4.1.1 Insulin Secretion

As a number of antidiabetic medications influence insulin secretion, an understanding of the mechanism by which insulin is released will be elucidated.

Once glucose is ingested, it travels via the bloodstream to the beta cells of the Islets of Langerhans in the pancreas. The process of insulin secretion then begins. Insulin secretion can be divided into a number of steps (Fig. 9.2).

1. Glucose is transported into these cells by GLUT 2 or possibly GLUT 1 transporters. Glucose entering the beta cell combines with phosphate (phosphorylation). This is a significant step in insulin secretion, as this step is catalysed by an enzyme known as glucokinase. This enzyme works best at a glucose concentration in the region of 8mM. If the glucose level is below this concentration, then the reaction is limited. Therefore, this step forms the "glucose-sensing" step of insulin secretion, as insulin secretion increases significantly when the glucose level in the bloodstream reaches near this concentration. Phosphorylation of glucose ultimately leads to increasing amounts of adenosine triphosphate (ATP) in the cell.

2. The increased ATP blocks a potassium ion channel, which otherwise allows potassium to leave the cell according to its concentration gradient. Blocking of this potassium ion channel by glucose-derived ATP leads to an accumulation of positive potassium in the cell, leading to the cell becoming internally positive, i.e. depolarising the cell.

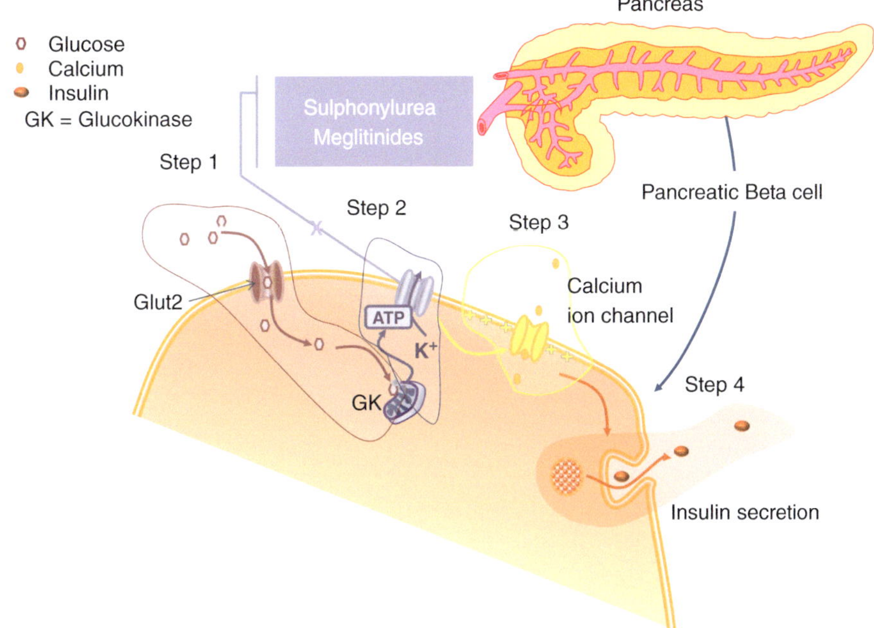

Fig. 9.2 Insulin secretion

3. Depolarisation of the cell leads to opening of a calcium ion channel which allows calcium into the cell.
4. An intracellular calcium increase triggers the liberation of stored insulin from the cell.

Once secreted, insulin binds to receptors on different types of cells, including muscle cells, endothelial cells, fat cells (or adipocytes) and or liver cells (or hepatocytes). Once bound to the receptor, insulin initiates a number of effects in the cell; the primary one of which is the translocation of GLUT 4 from inside the cell to its insertion in the cell membrane (Fig. 9.3). Additional effects of insulin include stimulation of gene expression and protein synthesis as well as inhibition of fat breakdown (lipolysis); as such insulin acts as a growth hormone. Insulin comes in many forms; however, currently all of these are injectable as insulin orally administered is broken down by first pass metabolism in the liver, rendering this route of administration redundant. Therefore, the pharmacodynamics of insulin depend upon the form of insulin used (Table 9.1).

9.4.2   Insulin Safety

The most significant concern regarding the safe administration and use of insulin is hypoglycaemia. New medications are frequently available in clinical practice; it is,

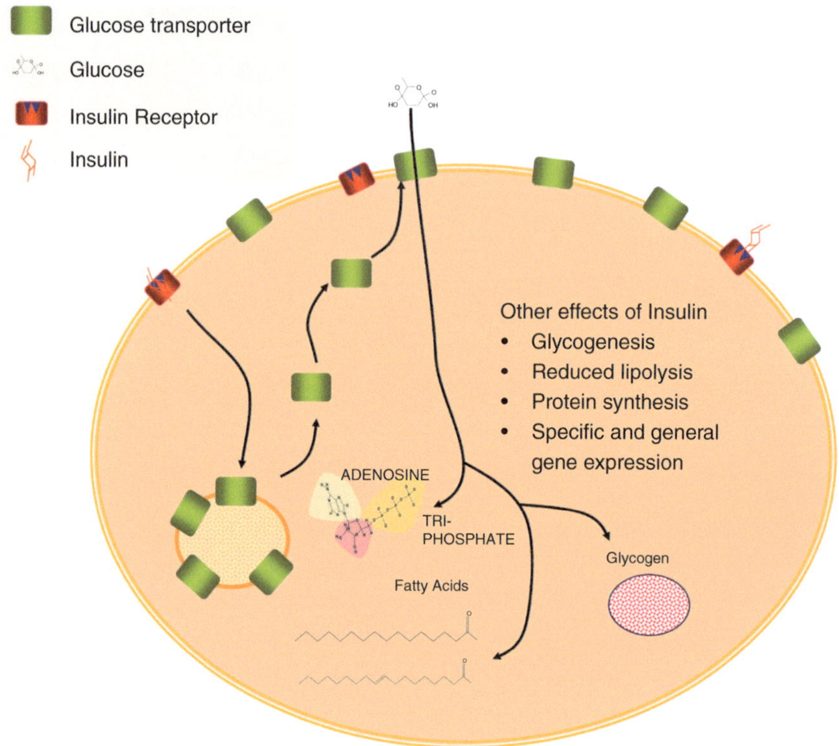

Fig. 9.3 Mechanism of action of insulin

therefore, not within the scope of this text to provide detailed guidelines regarding the use of insulin, as such guidelines are updated internationally, nationally and locally. It is, however, imperative that the person responsible for administering the medication is compliant with relevant policies and guidelines.

Given that insulin is a peptide, it cannot be frozen but must be refrigerated. The practitioner must ensure they do not administer degraded insulin. From the list in Table 9.1, most insulin preparations are clear solutions with the exception of the two intermediate-acting preparations that are generally cloudy (Table 9.1). Change in colour and translucence may be an indicator of degradation depending upon the excipients in the preparation.

It is important to remember that insulin formulations differ in effect depending upon strength, brand, method of manufacture (recombinant DNA vs. animal sourced), and type. Therefore, a person should not be transferred from one insulin to another unless under medical supervision.

By far the most common adverse effect of prescribed insulin is hypoglycaemia. This may present as a wide range of symptoms, depending upon the degree of glucose reduction in the bloodstream, such as cold sweats, cool pale skin, fatigue, nervousness, anxiousness, aggression, tiredness or weakness, confusion, difficulty

Table 9.1 Different preparations of insulin

Generic name	Type	Onset	Peak	Colour	Duration	Delivery system
Fast acting		**−15 min**	**60–90 min**		**3–4 h**	
Lispro	Analogue	5–15 min	2 h	Clear	4–5 h	Vial, cartridge, pen
Aspart	Analogue	15 min	45–90 min	Clear	3–5 h	Vial, cartridge, pen
Glulisine	Analogue	10–20 min	40–60 min	Clear	3–5 h	Vial, cartridge, pen
Short acting		**30–60 min**	**120–180 min**		**3–6 h**	
Soluble	Human	~30 min	90–150 min	Clear	7–8 h	Vial, cartridges
Intermediate		**60–120 min**	**4–10 h**		**10–16 h**	
Isophane	Bovine Porcine Human	60–120 min	8–10 h	Cloudy	20–24	Vial, cartridge
Insulatard	Analogue	~90 min	4–12 h	Cloudy	~24 h	Vial, cartridge, prefilled insulin doser
Long acting		**60–120 min**	**None**		**20–40 h**	
Glargine	Analogue	120–240 min		Clear	~24 h	Vial, cartridge, pen
Detemir	Analogue	60–120 min		Clear	20–24 h	Cartridge, pen, prefilled insulin doser
Degludec	Analogue	60–120 min		Clear	>40 h	Cartridge, pen, prefilled insulin doser

in concentrating, drowsiness, excessive hunger, vision changes, headache, nausea and palpitation (Cryer et al. 2003). Severe hypoglycaemia may present as convulsions, loss of consciousness which may, if not corrected, lead to irreversible brain damage or death (Cryer et al. 2003). With severe hypoglycaemia, initially, glucagon is given, followed by an oral carbohydrate once the person has recovered sufficiently to ingest food.

Although the recipient may be allergic to insulin itself, many excipients such as protamine sulphate and metacresol used in different forms of insulin are allergenic. Owing to these constituents, insulin may generate a range of allergic reactions. Severe allergies are typically limited to 1:10,000, but mild allergies and skin reactions may be more common. Table 9.2 illustrates the frequency of the main adverse effects of the insulin preparations listed in Table 9.1.

Table 9.2 Adverse effects

Insulin type	Severe anaphylaxis	Localised reactions	Lipodystrophy
Lispro	Rare	Common	Uncommon
Aspart	Not known	Common	Common
Glulisine	Uncommon	Common	Rare
Actrapid (soluble insulin)	Very rare	Uncommon	Uncommon
Isophane	Rare	No data	No data
Insulatard	Very rare	Uncommon	Uncommon
Glargine	Rare	Common	Common-uncommon
Detemir	Very rare	Common	Uncommon
Degludec	Common	Not known	Not known

Common >1:100 to <1:10
Uncommon >1:1000 to <1:100
Rare >1:10,000 to <1:1000
Very rare <1:10,000, not known
Data source: Rodbard et al. (2017) and Turk Wensveen et al. (2020)

Other adverse effects of insulin may relate to rapid plasma glucose correction. These include oedema and transient worsening of any neuropathy and retinopathy the patient may have.

Drug interactions with different forms of insulin depend upon the preparation used. Publications such as the British National Formulary provide continually revised lists of these interactions that ensure the practitioner has up-to-date information at hand to best ensure patient safety National Institute of Health Care Excellence (NICE 2025). Other considerations include particular conditions such as pregnancy, breastfeeding, liver and kidney disease.

Although insulin administration is not contraindicated by pregnancy, as insulin does not pass the placental barrier, hormonal changes in pregnancy increase the risk of destabilising glycaemic control, requiring more stringent monitoring and/or adjustment of insulin regimen. This is true for all the insulin preparations listed in Table 9.1. Although, lack of data for long-acting insulin preparations suggests caution with its use. Similarly, breastfeeding does not restrict the use of insulin. However, nutritional requirements of the lactating mother may require adjustments to the insulin regimen. Both renal and hepatic disease may require a reduction in insulin requirements as the liver loses its ability to metabolise insulin, together with reduced capability of gluconeogenesis and a reduced renal clearance of insulin (reversible by dialysis) with impaired kidney function.

Most pharmacokinetic parameters for clinically used insulins are similar to human insulin, as the majority of currently available insulin preparations utilise recombinant techniques to generate human insulin analogues. The pancreas normally generates 50 units of insulin a day. This insulin is degraded effectively by insulin proteases or insulin-degrading enzymes that primarily cleave Chain B of the insulin peptide.

The half-life of insulin is, therefore, not elimination dependent, as the half-life of insulin in plasma is only 3–4 min. The half-life of insulin is, thus, governed by its

Table 9.3 Pharmacokinetics

Insulin	Distribution	Biotransformation	Half-life ($T1/2$)
Lispro	–	–	–
Aspart	Low plasma binding (<10%)	No active metabolites	57 min
Glulisine	Low plasma binding		42 min
Actrapid (soluble insulin)	Low plasma binding	No active metabolites	2–5 h
Isophane	–	–	2 h (IM) 4 h (SC)
Insulatard	Low plasma binding, insulin antibodies may be present	No active metabolites	5–10 h
Glargine	Steady state 2–4 days after initial dose	Two active metabolites (M1 and M2)	$T_{1/2}$ similar to human insulin when administered IV
Detemir	Low plasma binding	No active metabolites	5–7 h

absorption from the site of injection or administration route into the body. The pharmacokinetic profile for the different types of insulin, including their half-lives, are given in Table 9.3.

Apart from the novel administration mechanisms (e.g. transdermal administration, subcutaneous infusion pumps and inhaled insulin), insulin is commonly administered subcutaneously (SC). Intramuscular (IM) and intravenous (IV) routes of administration of insulin are delivered in emergency cases, such as diabetic ketoacidosis (DKA) (see Box 9.1 for information on DKA). As the half-life of most insulin preparations is dependent upon the rate of absorption from the site of administration, variations in injection technique, and needle length choice can also influence drug delivery.

9.4.3 Choice of Needle Size

Muscle is well vascularised, and, therefore, provides rapid absorption and distribution compared to the subcutaneous administration route. Using a skin fold method in insulin administration, predominantly in children, has been advocated to reduce the risk of administering subcutaneous formulated insulin into the muscle (Hofman et al. 2010). With the introduction of insulin pens with shorter needles, the controversy over appropriate needle length continues. Most of the existing evidence suggests that variances in needle length provide similar glycaemic control (Kreugel et al. 2007; Hirsch et al. 2010; Ji and Lou 2014). Findings on insulin needle lengths and insulin pharmacokinetics remain inconsistent due to limitations in assessing insulin leakage in their study designs (Hirsch et al. 2010; Miwa et al. 2012; Ji and Lou 2014; de la Peña et al. 2015). Therefore, further robust studies are needed to clarify whether a correlation between needle length and insulin activity does exist.

9.5 Oral Hypoglycaemic Agents

9.5.1 Biguanides

The only currently available oral biguanide in clinical practice is also the most abundantly prescribed antidiabetic medication available and is namely dimethylbiguanide or more commonly known as metformin. Metformin is extracted from French lilac (*Galega officinalis*). The plant extract (metformin) has been used since medieval times to treat frequent urination associated with glycosuria in diabetes mellitus. With the advent of pharmaceutical insulin in the early twentieth century, research into biguanides was curtailed as insulin was effective in treating both Type 1 and Type 2 diabetes. The full potential of metformin was further masked by analogues of metformin, such as phenformin, that were associated with significant lactic acid generation. Metformin was formally introduced into clinical practice in Europe in 1957 and in the United States in 1995.

9.5.2 Mechanism of Action

Metformin has a number of effects that reduce glucose levels in the bloodstream. However, it does not stimulate the pancreas to secrete more insulin. One of the main effects of metformin is to enhance the secretion of glucagon-like peptide-1 (GLP-1), partly by inhibition of GLP-1 degradation (Mulherin et al. 2011) and/or stimulation of intestinal Muscarinic 3 (M3) and Glucose-Releasing Peptide (GRP) receptors (Mannucci et al. 2001). The GLP-1 peptide is of certain importance to current clinical pharmacology as a number of newer medications used in diabetes influence this hormone (incretins).

Apart from enhancing the secretion of GLP-1, metformin in the liver reduces glucagon action and reduces gluconeogenesis and glycogenolysis. Together, these effects reduce the liberation of glucose from different substrates from within the liver, as well as shifting energy production from fatty acid to glucose utilisation (Tahrani et al. 2016). In the muscle, metformin enhances insulin-mediated uptake of glucose via the GLUT 4 transporter to help reduce circulating glucose. Finally, metformin appears to modulate metabolic processes linked to circadian rhythm in the liver and muscle (Barnea et al. 2012).

9.5.3 Pharmacokinetics

Metformin enters the cell via a transport protein known as organic cation transporter (OCT1) due to its low fat solubility. It is not a candidate for interaction with most drug-metabolising enzymes, including most forms of cytochrome P450 and P-glycoprotein. It has a half-life of 4–9 h and has limited plasma binding. It is secreted largely unchanged via the kidney (Gong et al. 2012).

9.5.4 Cautions and Adverse Effects

The main adverse effect of this drug is gastrointestinal disturbance, which may lead to poor compliance and non-adherence. Although not a candidate for CYP3A4 metabolism, its transport by OCT1 presents potential for drug interaction with other medications, such as fluoxetine and diphenhydramine, that also interact with this protein transporter (Boxberger et al. 2014). The main caution with metformin is its use in severe renal dysfunction (creatinine clearance <30 mL/min) and severe heart failure (in particular, if administered within 48 h of the patient having received iodinated contrast dye), as it increases the risk of lactic acidosis and renal damage.

However, recent analysis of this risk suggests hypoxia as a trigger for lactic acidosis in patients with an estimated GFR <60 mL/17.3 m^2, but not in those who had no episode of hypoxia (Lee et al. 2017), suggesting the need to further research this aspect of metformin use to help define better clinical guidance.

9.5.5 Nursing Considerations

Robust medication history taking is important when patients are taking metformin to help reduce the risk of OCT1-related drug interactions. Given the association between cardiac disease, diabetes, and related renal dysfunction, appropriate monitoring of patients, particularly under hypoxaemia conditions, is important as long-term cardiac and respiratory disease are frequent comorbidities. There is an important role to play regarding patient education. Although not normally associated with hypoglycaemia in monotherapy, a combination of metformin with other antidiabetic medications can potentiate their effect to cause hypoglycemic episodes.

9.6 Sulphonylureas

This class of medications was first identified in the 1940s and has now been categorised into three generations. First-generation medications include tolbutamide, acetohexamide and tolazamide. Second-generation drugs include medications such as glibenclamide, glipizide and gliclazide. Lastly, third-generation drugs include glimepride (Table 9.4).

9.6.1 Mechanism of Action

Sulphonylureas stimulate the pancreas to secrete more insulin in a manner similar to circulating glucose. This is achieved by the drug blocking the ATP-sensitive potassium ion channels (Fig. 9.2, step 2). Inhibition of these ion channels enhances cell depolarisation, leading to an increase in calcium-mediated insulin release. As this medication depends upon functioning beta cells, it has limited use in Type 1 diabetes.

Table 9.4 Sulphonylurea pharmcokinetics

Drug	Absorption	Distribution	Biotransformation	Elimination
Tolbutamide	Rapid following oral admin	95% plasma bound	Liver CYP 2C19, 2C9	$T1/2$ 7 (4–25) h renal 75–85%
Acetohexamide	Rapid following oral admin	90% plasma bound	Hydroxyhexamide. Active metabolite	$T1/2$ 1.3 h $T1/2$ 5–6 h metabolite
Tolazamide	Rapid following oral admin	–	Five major active metabolites, with effects ranging from 0 to 70%	$T1/2$ 7 h Renal 85%, 7% Fecal
Second generation				
Glibenclamide	Onset of action 1 h	99% plasma-bound	CYP3A4, 2 metabolites, are only weakly active unless retain due to renal dysfunction	$T1/2$ 1.4–1.8 h Renal, clearance significantly reduced in patients with creatinine clearance <29 mL/min/1.73 m^2
Glipizide	Rapid GI tract absorption	~99% plasma bound	Liver CYP 2C9	$T1/2$ 2–5 h
Gliclazide	Rapid GI tract absorption, but wide inter/intra individual variability	94% plasma bound	Liver CYP 2C9, 18, 19 also phase 2 glucuronic acid conjugation	$T_{1/2}$ 10–24 h renal (60–70%) Faecal (10–20%)
Third generation				
Glimepiride	100% following	99.5%	Liver	$T1/2$ 5–8 h
	Oral	Plasma	CYP 2C9	Renal (~60%)
	Administration	Bound	Alcohol-dehydrogenase	Faecal (~40%)

9.6.2 Pharmacokinetics

The pharmacokinetics of this class of medications vary significantly. A number of medications have active metabolites (Table 9.4). Importantly, the second-generation glibenclamide is metabolised by CYP3A4, increasing its risk of interaction with other medications. Other enzymes commonly involved in the biotransformation of these medications belong to the 2C CYP subfamily, particularly 2C9, 18, and 19. These medications are primarily cleared by the kidney, with the potential for renal dysfunction to potentiate their hypoglycaemic effect. Half-lives of these medications mainly range between 1.3 and 8 h with the exception of gliclazide, which has an average half-life of 10.4 h (range 10–24 h).

9.6.3   Cautions and Adverse Effects

As these medications directly stimulate pancreatic beta cells to produce insulin, they are at risk of causing hypoglycaemia. The anabolic effect of insulin and reduced glycosuria is associated with weight gain of 1–4 kg, which normally stabilises 6 months after initiation of drug treatment (Tahrani et al. 2016).

9.6.4   Nursing Considerations

The main concern with sulphonylurea medications is hypoglycaemic episodes. When compared to patients taking metformin monotherapy, the adjusted hazard ratio (Duerden 2009) for hypoglycaemia to occur is 2.50 (95% CI, 2.23–2.82) (Van Dalem et al. 2016). This risk further increases with a reduction in kidney function; with eGFR <30 mL/kg/1.73 m^2, the hazard ratio is 4.96 (95% CI, 3.78–6.55). These effects tend to be dose-dependent. However, patients taking glibenclamide exhibit some of the highest risk of hypoglycaemic events (7.48, 95% CI, 4.89–11.44) (Van Dalem et al. 2016). It has been suggested that 1–7% of patients receiving sulphonylureas may experience a severe hypoglycaemic episode requiring third-party intervention (Tahrani et al. 2016).

Taken together, it is clear that patients taking sulphonylurea medications need to be informed about the risks of hypoglycaemia, how to recognise it, and how to manage their diet effectively to reduce the risk of hypoglycaemic attacks. Given the propensity of glibenclamide to cause such episodes, particular attention needs to be taken with managing this medication. CYP3A4 biotransformation may contribute to the observed risk with this medication, so patients with polypharmacy and unstable liver/renal function require extra vigilant monitoring and care. Due to the progressive nature of this disease, improvement of glycaemic homeostasis requires a more patient-centred, structured multidisciplinary approach to ensure appropriate management of this adverse effect (Iqbal and Heller 2016).

9.7   Meglitinides (Glinides)

9.7.1   Mechanism of Action

This class of medications works similarly to sulphonylurea medications; however, they bind to a separate binding site from sulphonylureas. Their mode of action is similar to sulphonylureas by ultimately inhibiting the ATP-sensitive potassium ion channels in pancreatic beta cells, leading to depolarisation and calcium-mediated insulin release (Fig. 9.2). They have a more rapid onset and shorter duration of action compared to sulphonylurea medications.

9.7.2 Pharmacokinetics

Both main medications in this drug class (repaglinide and nateglinide) are CYP3A4 and CYP 2C8/9 substrates. Genetic mutations associated with these two enzymes have been associated with individual variations in how these medications are biotransformed, varying their drug interaction profiles. Interestingly, some of the strongest drug interactions resulting in potentiation of nateglinide have been associated with CYP 2C8 inhibitors such as gemfibrozil (Scheen 2007). Otherwise, the two compounds have similar plasma-binding profiles and similar half-lives (Table 9.5).

9.7.3 Cautions and Adverse Effects

The major caution with glinides is that they stimulate insulin secretion at normal or low blood glucose levels, and hence precipitating hypoglycaemic events (International Hypoglycaemia Study Group 2015). Their use with similar medications that also stimulate insulin secretion at normal or low plasma glucose levels, such as sulphonylureas, and most forms of insulin is contraindicated. However, there is evidence to suggest that combination therapies with glinides (repaglinide) and metformin are as safe as metformin alone in terms of hypoglycaemic events and provide better glycaemic control than metformin monotherapy (Yin et al. 2014). Similarly, in the large Chinese STRATEGY trial, when used as an adjunct to double therapy (metformin + sitagliptin), repaglinide provided an effective, well-tolerated reduction in HbA1c <7% in Type 2 diabetes patients, who were inadequately controlled on previous dual therapies (Xu et al. 2017).

9.7.4 Nursing Considerations

Apart from the risk of hypoglycaemia in some combinations and weight gain associated with improved glucose metabolism, glinides are considered to be safe medications. Owing to their rapid onset of effect and short duration of action, these medications are well suited to patients with erratic meal patterns or to patients at high risk of hypoglycaemia (Tahrani et al. 2016). Their use does, however, warrant self-monitoring of blood glucose (SMBG). It is, therefore, important that the person taking these medications has the physical and cognitive ability to undertake these tests or has arrangements for someone else to undertake them.

Table 9.5 Metiglanides pharmacokinetics

Drug	Distribution	Biotransformation	Elimination
Repaglinide	98% plasma bound	CYP3A4 and 2C8	$T1/2$ 60 min, 90% faecal excretion
Nateglinide	98% plasma bound	CYP3A4 and 2C8 and? 2C9	$T1/2$ 90 min

9.8   SGLT2 Inhibitors

9.8.1   Mechanism of Action

To maintain adequate blood glucose levels, glucose has to be concentrated in the bloodstream. This function is performed by a sodium-dependent glucose co-transport (SGLT) mechanism. In this mechanism, passive movement of sodium coincides with glucose transport into the cell, against its concentration gradient, using the same protein (Fig. 9.4). Similar sodium-dependent cotransport mechanisms are found in many places in the body, where they transport different substances against their concentration gradients by harnessing passive sodium concentration gradients. Such transport is known as secondary active transport. Secondary active SGLTs are found in a number of places in the body, importantly in the intestinal lumen, where they load glucose from the gut, and in the kidney, where glucose is reabsorbed from the filtrate by the proximal tubule. In this location, two different forms of SGLT are found: SGLT2 is found in the first part of the proximal tubule and is responsible for 90% of glucose reabsorption from the nephron filtrate, and SGLT1 is found in the terminal end of the proximal tubule and is responsible for 10% reabsorption of glucose from the filtrate (Fig. 9.4). SGLT2 inhibitors reduce the tubular reuptake of glucose from section 1 of the proximal tubule. These medications are not influenced by insulin, and their effect is dependent upon the presence of filtered glucose in the nephron. As glucose levels in the filtrate drop, the effect of these medications is reduced as there are fewer molecules of glucose being transported back into the bloodstream. Thus, the effect of these drugs becomes self-limiting and, as such, do not cause hypoglycaemia. However, as they have no effect on the underlying cause of hyperglycaemia, i.e. reduced insulin secretion or insulin resistance, this still may have to be addressed by other means. Common SGLT2 inhibitors in clinical use include empagliflozin, canagliflozin, dapagliflozin and ertugliflozin.

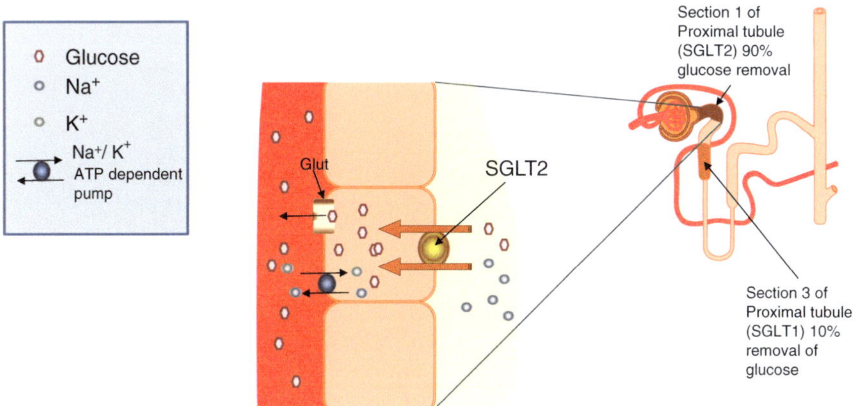

Fig. 9.4 Renal SGLT-dependent glucose reabsorption and associated sodium transport

9.8.2 Pharmacokinetics

SGLT2 inhibitors have half-lives in the range of 10–12 h and are significantly plasma bound (Table 9.6). They are all primarily metabolised by phase II conjugation by 5′-diphospho-glucuronosyltransferases isoforms. Only canagliflozin demonstrates weak inhibition of different CYP isoforms, including CYP3A4.

9.8.3 Cautions and Adverse Effects

The most commonly reported adverse effects of SGLT2 inhibitors are glucosuria-related conditions, including urinary tract infections and female genital mycotic infections (Scheen 2015). Owing to the osmotic diuresis effect from this medication, there is a risk of dehydration and hypovolaemia with its associated symptoms of hypotension, syncope, and tachycardia (Scheen 2015). As the drug depends on normal renal function for its optimal effect, its use is contraindicated in severe renal dysfunction (eGFR less than 30 mL/min/1.73 m^2). The use of SGLT2 inhibitors should not be initiated in a person with eGFR <60 mL/min/1.73 m^2. However, patients already receiving and showing good tolerance to canagliflozin or empagliflozin may wish to continue with these medications at eGFR values as low as 45 mL/min/1.73 m^2 (Tahrani et al. 2016). The Medicines and Healthcare Products Regulatory Agency (MHRA 2016) recommended healthcare professionals educate patients regarding the risk of DKA (Box 9.1). Other adverse effects associated with SGLT2 are the increased risk of terminal proximity, which normally results in large toe amputation in high cardiovascular risk patients.

Table 9.6 SGLT2 inhibitor pharmacokinetics

Drug	Distribution	Biotransformation	Elimination
Canagliflozin	99% plasma-bound	Liver phase II glucuronidation	$T_{1/2}$ 11.8 h, mostly faecal excretion
Dapagliflozin	91% plasma bound	Mainly liver phase II glucuronidation	$T1/2 \sim 12$ h renal 76% Faecal 21%
Empagliflozin	86% plasma bound	Liver phase II glucuronidation	$T_{1/2} \sim 12$ h renal 54.4% Faecal 41.2%
Ertugliflozin	94% plasma bound	Liver phase II glucuronidation	$T_{1/2}$ 11–17 h renal 50% Faecal 41%

Box 9.1 Diabetic Ketoacidosis

- This is a life-threatening condition associated with an abnormally high blood glucose level typically >14 mmol/L. Owing to this, there is a significant osmotic diuresis that leads to severe dehydration and electrolyte derangement, mainly potassium. Owing to a lack of available cellular glucose (as glucose is confined within the bloodstream, in the absence of effective insulin apparatus), cells use alternate methods of energy production, primarily fat, which generates ketones, that induce a drop in blood pH, i.e. cause acidosis.
- Together, these main factors act together to further complicate the person's biochemistry by hypovolaemia reducing tissue perfusion and further compounding ketone-induced systemic acidosis (drop in blood pH). A drop in pH will induce an increase in respiratory rate, leading to a further insensible water loss because of rapid breathing.
- Important signs and symptoms of DKA are:
  - Polyuria (large volume of urine formation associated with excessive thirst (polydipsia) and enuresis (frequency of urine causing urinary incontinence.
  - Dehydration causes hypotension and tachycardia.
  - Abdominal disturbances due to stress and electrolyte imbalance are further complicated by nausea and vomiting.
  - Acetone (sweet) breath because of ketone build-up in the bloodstream.
  - Altered mental state:
  Aggressive
  Incoherent
  Comatose
- Treatment of DKA is linked to rehydration and reestablishing adequate blood glucose control. This, however, is complicated as potassium and glucose are closely linked. Insulin helps remove potassium from the bloodstream. Also, a low serum potassium renders insulin ineffective as potassium is required to aid depolarisation coupled insulin secretion (Fig. 9.2). Therefore, when the potassium level is below 3.5 mmol/L in the bloodstream, it is normal practice to raise the potassium levels before initiating insulin therapy and in most instances administration of both substances will occur in tandem until the serum potassium is in the region of 5 mmol/L.

Euglycaemic DKA

- On occasion DKA can occur in absence of elevated glucose levels. The cause for the ketone rise in the bloodstream as well as the acidosis is unclear, but is suggested to occur in patients who take some form of insulin combined with adequate hydration but inadequate carbohydrate intake (Thawabi and Studyvin 2015).

9.8.4 Nursing Considerations

As with all medications, it is the nurse's responsibility to educate the patient regarding the adverse effects of their medications and provide information regarding when a sign or symptom may need medical attention. SGLT2 inhibitors are relatively safe medications with few drug – drug interactions. Owing to their glycosuria effect, it is important that the patient is educated towards the signs and symptoms of urinary tract infections associated with this medication. Although patients with Type 1 diabetes as well as patients with Type 2 diabetes may be familiar with the risk, signs, and symptoms of DKA, it is important that nurses reiterate these with the patient and their family. As the drug depends upon adequate renal function, the patient needs to be informed regarding recognising and/or monitoring their renal function/output, such as urine output, as well as blood pressure, as these are both intricately linked.

9.9 Incretins (GLP-1 Receptor Agonists)

Together with gliptins, dipeptidyl-peptidase-IV (DPP-IV) antagonists, incretins prolong GLP-1-mediated pre-regulatory action on glucose metabolism.

9.9.1 Mechanism of Action

Glucagon-like peptide 1 has an important role to play in facilitating glucose metabolism. GLP-1 is secreted by L cells of the intestine by a mechanism not dissimilar to insulin secretion (Lim and Brubaker 2006) with the main difference being an apparent lack of ATP-sensitive potassium channel linked cell depolarisation as well as loading of glucose via a different glucose transport mechanism, including GLUT 1 and 5 together with the sodium-dependent glucose transporter (SGLT) (Fig. 9.5). Stimuli for release of GLP-1 include the presence of glucose, protein, and fatty acid in the intestinal lumen, together with an important influence of parasympathetic nerve stimulation via the vagal nerve (Nadkarni et al. 2014). Released GLP-1 has a number of important effects on glucose regulation. One important aspect of this is the so-called gut-brain axis (Burcelin 2010). This mechanism interconnects the brain and gut to help orchestrate normal glucose levels in the bloodstream. This is an anticipatory reflex mediated by GLP-1 on GLP receptors (GLP-R) found on cholinergic neurons, which prepares the body for a glucose load after a meal. These medications also slow down gastric emptying, thus reducing the carbohydrate load in the intestine and reducing glucose absorption into the bloodstream.

The overall effect of GLP-1 is an enhancement of insulin secretion and a reduction in pancreatic glucagon secretion. Additionally, GLP-1 has been shown to increase beta cell proliferation and suppress apoptosis in these cells (Nadkarni et al. 2014), further prolonging beta cell lifespan and possibly function. GLP-1 is broken down or metabolised by the enzyme DPP-IV. Inhibition of DPP-IV leads to a

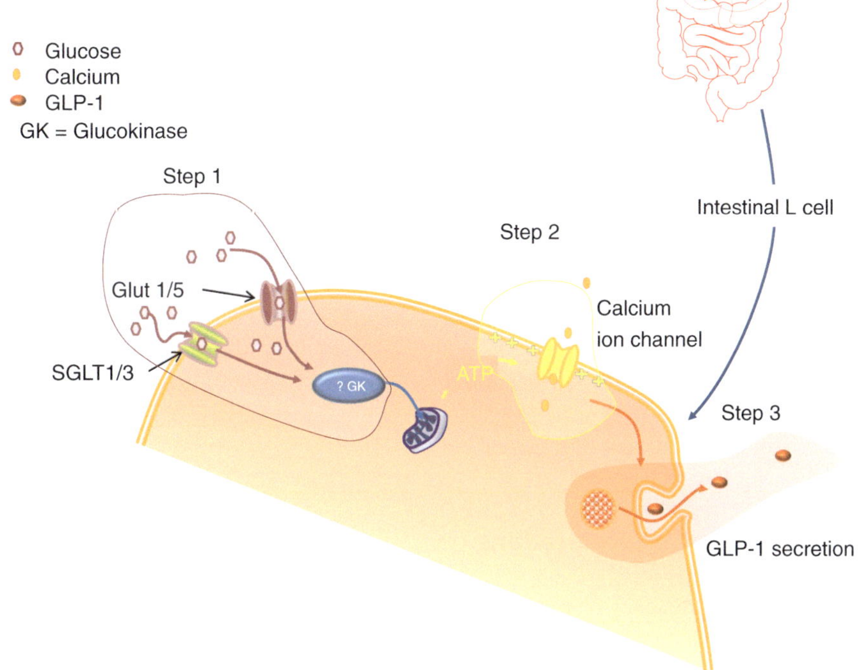

Fig. 9.5 Renal SGLT-dependent glucose reabsorption and associated sodium transport

prolongation of the GLP-1 effect, which forms the basis for the mechanism of action of another class of antidiabetic medications known as the gliptins.

9.9.2   Pharmacokinetics

Being analogues of GLP-1, incretins are peptide structures. As mentioned, GLP-1 is degraded rapidly by the enzyme DPP-IV, giving it a half-life of a couple of minutes. The subtle differences in incretin peptide structure generally protect them from DPP-IV degradation. This provides an enhanced duration of action from 2 to 4 h to an intermediate of 13 h for liraglutide and 90 h for dulaglutide (Table 9.7). Importantly, lixisenatide excretion is reduced by 30% in severe renal dysfunction, eGFR less than 30 mL/min/1.73 m^2 (Gupta 2013), potentially enhancing the medication's effect.

9.9.3   Cautions and Adverse Effects

The main adverse effects associated with incretins include gastrointestinal (GI) disturbances, including nausea, diarrhoea and vomiting. Instances of injection site

Table 9.7 Incretin pharmacokinetics

Drug	Distribution	Biotransformation	Elimination
Exenatide (peptide)	–	General proteolysis	$T1/2$ 2.4 h, renal
Lixisenatide	–	General proteolysis	$T1/2$ 2–3 h, renal
Dulaglutide	–	General proteolysis	$T1/2$ 90 h
Liraglutide	98% plasma protein bound	DPP4/endopeptidase	$T_{1/2}$ 13 h

reactions (nodules, pruritus, and erythema) may vary for different incretins, with exenatide having higher instances compared to liraglutide and dulaglutide (Madsbad 2016). There has been concern that incretin therapy may cause pancreatitis, pancreatic cancer, and thyroid cancer (Elashoff et al. 2011). However, pooled evidence from a narrative review (Forsmark 2016; Karp et al. 2019) and primary data from a retrospective cohort study (Liang et al. 2018) suggest that incretin use was not associated with increased risk of these cancers.

9.9.4 Nursing Considerations

Given the high frequency of gastrointestinal disturbances such as nausea and vomiting when using incretins, it is salient to educate the patient regarding this possible occurrence. As highlighted, lixisenatide clearance may be influenced by severe renal dysfunction, therefore, warranting dose adjustment or drug replacement if renal impairment occurs while the person is taking this drug. Although no clear link has so far been associated with incretins and endocrine tumours, it would be advisable for a person to seek specialist advice, particularly if they have a family history of such tumours and were prescribed incretins.

9.10 Dipeptidyl Peptidase-4 (DPP-IV) Inhibitors

9.10.1 Mechanism of Action

Incretin hormones, GLP-1 and glucose-dependent insulinotropic polypeptides (GIP), have a number of effects on glucose and fat metabolism and influence basic biochemical reactions. Incretins affect regions in the brain that are associated with memory and learning which may improve cognitive function (Gault 2018) (Fig. 9.6). While GLP-1 has more widespread effects than GIP, they both have important effects on the pancreas by which they enhance insulin secretion by improving beta cell function rather than just increasing depolarisation alone as is the case with sulphonylurea medications. Together, these effects enhance glucose metabolism while at the same time improve beta cell health and function. The DPP-IV enzyme rapidly breaks down these hormones, limiting the effect of these hormones to less than 10 min. Inhibition of this proteolytic enzyme results in prolongation of incretin hormones, therefore, enhancing glucose metabolism and long-term improvement of beta cell health and function.

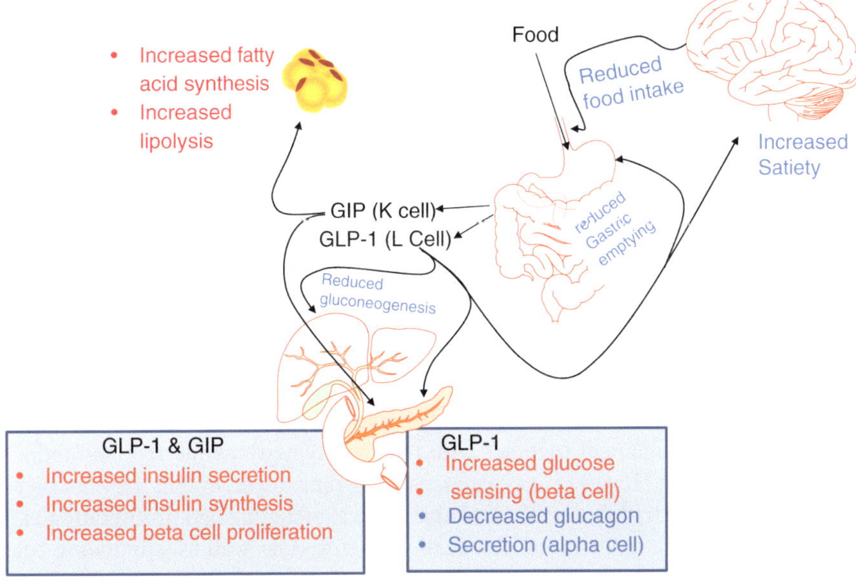

Fig. 9.6   Incretin hormone function

Table 9.8   DPP-1 (gliptin) pharmacokinetics

Drug	Distribution	Biotransformation	Elimination
Vildagliptin	9.3% plasma protein bound	–	T1/2 90 min
Sitagliptin	38% plasma protein bound	CYP3A4/2C8	8–14 h Renal 80%
Linagliptin	75–90% plasma protein bound	Mostly excreted unchanged	80% hepato/faecal 5% renal T1/2 12 h
Saxagliptin	<10% plasma protein bound	CYP3A4/5	T1/2 2.5 h T1/2 3.1 h (active metabolite)

9.10.2 Pharmacokinetics

The pharmacokinetic effects of these drugs vary (Table 9.8). Plasma binding varies from less than 10% to up to 90%. Similarly, half-life varies from 1.5 h to 12 h. Some drugs are known to be bio-transformed by traditional phase I CYP, including CYP3A4, for sitagliptin, which produces an active metabolite with half the potency of the parent drug. As such, these medications do not strongly interact with other medications commonly used in patients with diabetes.

9.10.3 Adverse Effects and Cautions

Despite the range of effects of DPP-IV on a number of substrates associated with inflammation and immunological responses, as well as a number of growth-related hormones, this group of drugs is well tolerated. Saxagliptin has been reported to slightly increase the risk of upper respiratory tract infection, urinary tract infection, and headache compared to placebo. The effect of this drug group on cardiovascular outcomes has been variable, with the majority of retrospective cohort studies demonstrating no significant risk compared to placebo (Tahrani et al. 2016).

9.10.4 Nursing Considerations

Pharmacological manipulation of the incretin hormone pathway provides effective blood glucose management together with reduced hypoglycaemic risk and reduction in body weight. However, it is also now becoming apparent that these medications are associated with beta cell protective effects, including cell proliferation and differentiation, and a reduction in cell death (apoptosis), as well as stimulating beta cell function. As such, they have the capability to limit disease progression and maintain beta cell health. There is now a growing opinion that initiation of these drugs at an early stage helps preserve beta cell function. Introducing them at a later stage in the disease process, once beta cell degradation has occurred, results in chronic irreversible damage to the glycaemic control system (Cernea and Raz 2011; Kaneto et al. 2016).

9.11 Summary

Diabetes has, over many generations, significantly increased globally. Whereas the pharmacological treatments of insulin and metformin remain widespread, a reduction in sulphonylurea usage is apparent. The introduction of GLP-1, SGLT2 and incretin pathway manipulation over the last decade provides a portfolio of safe adjunct therapies that increasingly reduces the risk of hypoglycaemic events. The protective benefits of these exciting new medications may provide a promising tool to help delay the progression of the disease and reduce the long-term effects of diabetes and its associated complications.

Multiple Choice Questions

1. The onset of action of fast-acting insulin is normally:
   - (a) Up to 10 min
   - (b) Up to 15 min
   - (c) Up to 20 min
   - (d) Up to 30 min

2. Most insulin is clear and translucent except for some:
   - (a) Fast-acting preparations
   - (b) Short-acting preparations
   - (c) Intermediate-acting preparations
   - (d) Long-acting preparations
3. Metformin's main mechanism of action involves:
   - (a) Stimulation of insulin secretion
   - (b) Insulin receptor upregulation
   - (c) Enhancing secretion of glucagon-like peptide-1 (GLP1) secretion
   - (d) Inhibiting secretion of glucagon-like peptide-1 (GLP1) secretion
4. Use of metformin is cautioned in which condition:
   - (a) Liver dysfunction
   - (b) Kidney dysfunction
   - (c) GI tract dysfunction
   - (d) Cardiac dysfunction
5. Sulphonylurea medications' main mechanism of action involves:
   - (a) Stimulation of insulin secretion
   - (b) Insulin receptor upregulation
   - (c) Enhancing secretion of glucagon-like peptide-1 (GLP1) secretion
   - (d) Inhibiting secretion of glucagon-like peptide-1 (GLP1) secretion
6. A common adverse effect of sulphonylurea medications such as glibenclamide is:
   - (a) Tachycardia
   - (b) Hypoglycaemia
   - (c) Polyuria
   - (d) Myalgia
7. Glinides such as repaglinide are safe to use in combination with which other medication:
   - (a) Most forms of insulin
   - (b) Tolbutamide
   - (c) Metformin
   - (d) Glibenclamide
8. Together with metformin, which oral antiglycaemic drug may not cause hypoglycaemia?
   - (a) Sulphonylureas
   - (b) Glinides
   - (c) SGLT inhibitors
   - (d) Insulin
9. Together with metformin, which antiglycaemic drug is commonly associated with gastro-intestinal disturbances as an adverse effect?
   - (a) Sulphonylureas
   - (b) SGLT inhibitors
   - (c) Incretins
   - (d) Insulin

10. Glucose secretion from pancreatic beta cells is caused by:
    (a) Beta cell depolarisation following ATP formation
    (b) Beta cell repolarisation following ATP formation
    (c) Beta cell depolarisation following ATP depletion
    (d) Beta cell repolarisation following ATP depletion

Answers

1. (c)
2. (c)
3. (c)
4. (b)
5. (a)
6. (b)
7. (c)
8. (c)
9. (c)
10. (a)

References

Barnea M, Haviv L, Gutman R, Chapnik N, Madar Z, Froy O (2012) Metformin affects the circadian clock and metabolic rhythms in a tissue-specific manner. Biochim Biophys Acta 1822(11):1796–1806

Bellou V, Belbasis L, Tzoulaki I, Evangelou E (2018) Risk factors for type 2 diabetes mellitus: an exposure-wide umbrella review of meta-analyses. PloS One 13(3):e0194127

Boxberger KH, Hagenbuch B, Lampe JN (2014) Common drugs inhibit human organic cation transporter 1 (OCT1)-mediated neurotransmitter uptake. Drug Metab Dispos 42(6):990–995

Burcelin R (2010) The gut-brain axis: a major glucoregulatory player. Diabetes Metab 36(Suppl 3):S54–S58

Caleyachetty R, Barber TM, Mohammed NI, Cappuccio FP, Hardy R, Mathur R, Banerjee A, Gill P (2021) Ethnicity-specific BMI cutoffs for obesity based on type 2 diabetes risk in England: a population-based cohort study. Lancet Diabetes Endocrinol 9(7):419–426

Cernea S, Raz I (2011) Therapy in the early stage: incretins. Diabetes Care 34(Suppl 2):S264–S271

Cryer PE, Davis SN, Shamoon H (2003) Hypoglycemia in diabetes. Diabetes Care 26(6):1902–1912

de la Peña A, Yeo KP, Linnebjerg H, Catton E, Reddy S, Brown-Augsburger P, Morrow L, Ignaut DA (2015) Subcutaneous injection depth does not affect the pharmacokinetics or glucodynamics of insulin lispro in normal weight or healthy obese subjects. J Diabetes Sci Technol 9(4):824–830

Diabetes UK (2025) Diabetes risk factors. https://www.diabetes.org.uk/Preventing-Type-2-diabetes/Diabetes-risk-factors/ Accessed 27 Feb 2025

Diamant M, Blaak EE, De Vos WM (2011) Do nutrient–gut–microbiota interactions play a role in human obesity, insulin resistance and type 2 diabetes? Obes Rev 12(4):272–281

Duerden M (2009) What are hazard ratios? http://www.bandolier.org.uk/painres/download/whatis/What_are_haz_ratios.pdf. Accessed 5 May 2019

Elashoff M, Matveyenko AV, Gier B, Elashoff R, Butler PC (2011) Pancreatitis, pancreatic, and thyroid cancer with glucagon-like peptide-1–based therapies. Gastroenterology 141(1):150–156

Filippi CM, von Herrath MG (2008) Viral trigger for type 1 diabetes: pros and cons. Diabetes 57(11):2863–2871

Fonseca VA (2009) Defining and characterizing the progression of type 2 diabetes. Diabetes Care 32(Suppl 2):S151–S156

Forsmark CE (2016) Incretins, diabetes, pancreatitis and pancreatic cancer: what the GI specialist needs to know. Pancreatology 16(1):10–13

Frayling TM, Evans JC, Bulman MP, Pearson E, Allen L, Owen K, Bingham C, Hannemann M, Shepherd M, Ellard S, Hattersley AT (2001) Beta-cell genes and diabetes: molecular and clinical characterization of mutations in transcription factors. Diabetes 50(Suppl 1):S94

Gault VA (2018) RD Lawrence lecture incretins: the intelligent hormones in diabetes. Diabet Med 35(1):33–40

Gong L, Goswami S, Giacomini KM, Altman RB, Klein TE (2012) Metformin pathways: pharmacokinetics and pharmacodynamics. Pharmacogenet Genomics 22(11):820

Gupta V (2013) Glucagon-like peptide-1 analogues: an overview. Indian J Endocrinol Metab 17(3):413–421

Hirsch LJ, Gibney MA, Albanese J, Qu S, Kassler-Taub K, Klaff LJ, Bailey TS (2010) Comparative glycemic control, safety and patient ratings for a new 4 mm× 32G insulin pen needle in adults with diabetes. Curr Med Res Opin 26(6):1531–1541

Hofman PL, Derraik JGB, Pinto TE, Tregurtha S, Faherty A, Peart JM, Drury PL, Robinson E, Tehranchi R, Donsmark M, Cutfield WS (2010) Defining the ideal injection techniques when using 5-mm needles in children and adults. Diabetes Care 33(9):1940–1944

International Hypoglycaemia Study group (2015) Minimizing hypoglycemia in diabetes. Diabetes Care 38(8):1583–1591

Ismail L, Materwala H, Al Kaabi J (2021) Association of risk factors with type 2 diabetes: A systematic review. Comput Struct Biotechnol J 19:1759–1785

Iqbal A, Heller S (2016) Managing hypoglycaemia. Best Pract Res Clin Endocrinol Metab 30(3):413–430

Ji J, Lou Q (2014) Insulin pen injection technique survey in patients with type 2 diabetes in mainland China in 2010. Curr Med Res Opin 30(6):1087–1093

Kahn SE, Andrikopoulos S, Verchere CB (1999) Islet amyloid: a long-recognized but underappreciated pathological feature of type 2 diabetes. Diabetes 48(2):241–253

Kahn SE, Cooper ME, Del Prato S (2014) Pathophysiology and treatment of type 2 diabetes: perspectives on the past, present, and future. Lancet 383(9922):1068–1083

Kaneto H, Obata A, Shimoda M, Kimura T, Hirukawa H, Okauchi S, Matsuoka TA, Kaku K (2016) Promising diabetes therapy based on the molecular mechanism for glucose toxicity: usefulness of SGLT2 inhibitors as well as incretin-related drugs. Curr Med Chem 23(27):3044–3051

Karp I, Sivaswamy A, Booth C (2019) Does the use of incretin-based medications increase the risk of cancer in patients with type-2 diabetes mellitus? Pharmacoepidemiol Drug Saf 28(4):489–499

Kreugel G, Beijer HJM, Kerstens MN, Ter Maaten JC, Sluiter WJ, Boot BS (2007) Influence of needle size for subcutaneous insulin administration on metabolic control and patient acceptance. Eur Diabetes Nurs 4(2):51–55

Lee EY, Hwang S, Lee YH, Lee SH, Lee YM, Kang HP, Han E, Lee W, Lee BW, Kang ES, Cha BS (2017) Association between metformin use and risk of lactic acidosis or elevated lactate concentration in type 2 diabetes. Yonsei Med J 58(2):312–318

Liang C, Bertoia ML, Ding Y, Clifford CR, Qiao Q, Gagne JJ, Dore DD (2018) Exenatide use and incidence of pancreatic and thyroid cancer: a retrospective cohort study. Diabetes Obes Metab 21(4):1037–1042

Lim GE, Brubaker PL (2006) Glucagon-like peptide 1 secretion by the L-cell. Diabetes 55(Suppl 2):S70–S77

Madsbad S (2016) Review of head-to-head comparisons of glucagon-like peptide-1 receptor agonists. Diabetes Obes Metab 18(4):317–332

Mannucci E, Ognibene A, Cremasco F, Bardini G, Mencucci A, Pierazzuoli E, Ciani S, Messeri G, Rotella CM (2001) Effect of metformin on glucagon-like peptide 1 (GLP-1) and leptin levels in obese nondiabetic subjects. Diabetes Care 24(3):489–494

Medicines and Healthcare Products Regulatory Agency (2016). https://www.gov.uk/drug-safety-update/sglt2-inhibitors-updated-advice-on-the-risk-of-diabetic-ketoacidosis. Accessed 21 May 19

Miller RE (1981) Pancreatic neuroendocrinology: peripheral neural mechanisms in the regulation of the islets of Langerhans. Endocr Rev 2(4):471–494

Miwa T, Itoh R, Kobayashi T, Tanabe T, Shikuma J, Takahashi T, Odawara M (2012) Comparison of the effects of a new 32-gauge× 4-mm pen needle and a 32-gauge× 6-mm pen needle on glycemic control, safety, and patient ratings in Japanese adults with diabetes. Diabetes Technol Ther 14(12):1084–1090

Mueckler M, Thorens B (2013) The SLC2 (GLUT) family of membrane transporters. Mol Asp Med 34(2–3):121–138

Mulherin AJ, Oh AH, Kim H, Grieco A, Lauffer LM, Brubaker PL (2011) Mechanisms underlying metformin-induced secretion of glucagon-like peptide-1 from the intestinal L cell. Endocrinology 152(12):4610–4619

Nadkarni P, Chepurny OG, Holz GG (2014) Regulation of glucose homeostasis by GLP-1. Prog Mol Biol Transl Sci 121:23–65

National Diabetes Audit (2023) Incidence and prevalence of diabetes, 2017–18 to 2021–22. https://digital.nhs.uk/data-and-information/publications/statistical/national-diabetes-audit/report-1-care-processes-and-treatment-targets-2021-22-full-report/section-1%2D%2D-incidence-and-prevalence-17-18%2D%2D-21-22-copy#prevalence. Accessed 27 Feb 2025

National Institute for Health and Care Excellence (2025) British national formulary. https://bnf.nice.org.uk/. Accessed 27 Feb 2025

Ogle GD, Wang F, Gregory GA, Jayanthi M (2022) IDF Atlas reports: type 1 diabetes numbers in children and adults. https://diabetesatlas.org/idfawp/resource-files/2022/12/IDF-T1D-Index-Report.pdf. Accessed 27 Feb 2025

Pani LN, Nathan DM, Grant RW (2008) Clinical predictors of disease progression and medication initiation in untreated patients with type 2 diabetes and A1C less than 7%. Diabetes Care 31(3):386–390

Robinson S, Kessling A (1992) Diabetes secondary to genetic disorders. Bailliere Clin Endocrinol Metab 6(4):867–898

Rodbard HW, Bode BW, Harris SB, Rose L, Lehmann L, Jarlov H, Thurman J (2017) Dual Action of Liraglutide and insulin degludec (DUAL) IV trial investigators. Safety and efficacy of insulin degludec/liraglutide (IDegLira) added to sulphonylurea alone or to sulphonylurea and metformin in insulin-naïve people with Type 2 diabetes: the DUAL IV trial. Diabet Med 34(2):189–196

Scheen AJ (2007) Drug-drug and food-drug pharmacokinetic interactions with new insulinotropic agents repaglinide and nateglinide. Clin Pharmacokinet 46(2):93–108

Scheen AJ (2015) Pharmacodynamics, efficacy and safety of sodium–glucose co-transporter type 2 (SGLT2) inhibitors for the treatment of type 2 diabetes mellitus. Drugs 75(1):33–59

Tahrani AA, Barnett AH, Bailey CJ (2016) Pharmacology and therapeutic implications of current drugs for type 2 diabetes mellitus. Nat Rev Endocrinol 12(10):566–592

Thawabi M, Studyvin S (2015) Euglycemic diabetic ketoacidosis, a misleading presentation of diabetic ketoacidosis. N Am J Med Sci 7(6):291

Turk Wensveen T, Fučkar Čupić D, Jurišić Eržen D, Polić B, Wensveen FM (2020) Severe lipoatrophy in a patient with type 2 diabetes in response to human insulin analogs glargine and degludec: possible involvement of CD4 T cell–mediated tissue remodeling. Diabetes Care 43(2):494–496

Tushuizen ME, Bunck MC, Pouwels PJ, Bontemps S, Van Waesberghe JHT, Schindhelm RK, Mari A, Heine RJ, Diamant M (2007) Pancreatic fat content and beta-cell function in type 2 diabetic and non-diabetic males. Diabetes 30(11):2916–2921

Van Dalem J, Brouwers MC, Stehouwer CD, Krings A, Leufkens HG, Driessen JH, de Vries F, Burden AM (2016) Risk of hypoglycaemia in users of sulphonylureas compared with metformin in relation to renal function and sulphonylurea metabolite group: population based cohort study. Br Med J 13(354):i3625

Vrieze A, Van Nood E, Holleman F, Salojärvi J, Kootte RS, Bartelsman JF, Dallinga-Thie GM, Ackermans MT, Serlie MJ, Oozeer R, Derrien M (2012) Transfer of intestinal micro-biota from lean donors increases insulin sensitivity in individuals with metabolic syndrome. Gastroenterology 143(4):913–916

Weyer C, Tataranni PA, Bogardus C, Pratley RE (2001) Insulin resistance and insulin secretory dysfunction are independent predictors of worsening of glucose tolerance during each stage of type 2 diabetes development. Diabetes Care 24(1):89–94

World health organisation (WHO) https://www.who.int/news-room/fact-sheets/detail/diabetes, accessed 2025

Xu W, Mu Y, Zhao J, Zhu D, Ji Q, Zhou Z, Yao B, Mao A, Engel SS, Zhao B, Bi Y, Zeng L, Ran X, Lu J, Ji L, Yang W, Jia W, Weng J (2017) Efficacy and safety of metformin and sitagliptin based triple antihyperglycemic therapy (STRATEGY): a multicenter, randomized, controlled, non-inferiority clinical trial. Sci China Life Sci 60(3):225–238

Yin J, Deng H, Qin S, Tang W, Zeng L, Zhou B (2014) Comparison of repaglinide and metformin versus metformin alone for type 2 diabetes: a meta-analysis of randomized controlled trials. Diabetes Res Clin Pract 105(3):e10–e15

Medications Used for the Respiratory System

10

Shelley Peacock

Learning Outcomes
At the end of this chapter, you will be able to:

- Identify the mechanisms of action of medications used to treat common conditions and diseases of the respiratory system
- Identify the adverse effects of the medications discussed
- Appreciate the nursing responsibilities associated with the medication, treatment and care identified and reviewed in this chapter

10.1 Introduction

To understand how diseases and other conditions of the respiratory system can be treated pharmacologically, it is necessary to understand the normal function and structure of the respiratory system and the mechanism of breathing and gas exchange. Air must be able to enter and leave the lungs efficiently, and adequate gaseous exchange must be achieved; any condition that interferes with these processes will cause respiratory disorder and or disease.

Medication that acts on the respiratory system focuses on keeping the airways open and gases moving effectively. This chapter focuses on common upper respiratory tract conditions (allergic rhinitis and sinusitis), lower respiratory tract conditions (asthma and chronic obstructive pulmonary disease [COPD]) and the key medications used to manage these disorders.

S. Peacock (✉)
Florence Nightingale Faculty of Nursing, Midwifery & Palliative Care, King's College London, London, UK
e-mail: shelley.2.peacock@kcl.ac.uk

© The Author(s), under exclusive license to Springer Nature Switzerland AG 2026
E. Khan, P. Hood (eds.), *Understanding Pharmacology in Nursing Practice*,
https://doi.org/10.1007/978-3-032-03964-4_10

Figure 10.1 identifies the key structures and conditions of the upper respiratory tract and Fig. 10.2 the key structures and conditions of the lower respiratory tract.

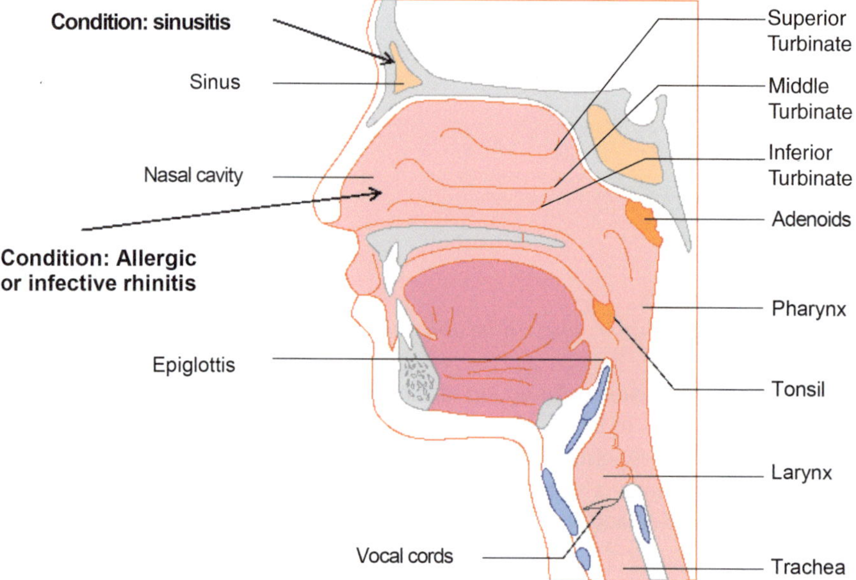

Fig. 10.1 The upper respiratory tract and common conditions. (Copyright © motifolio.com)

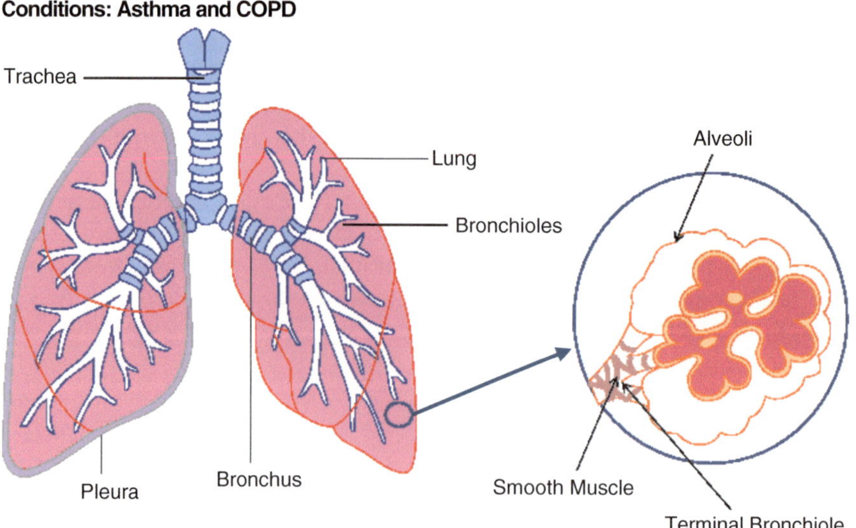

Fig. 10.2 The lower respiratory tract and common conditions. (Copyright © motifolio.com)

10.2   Allergic Rhinitis

10.2.1 Pathophysiology

Allergic rhinitis is an inflammatory condition of the nasal mucosa, the membrane that lines the nasal cavity, and is caused by the immune system reacting to an allergen, a substance that is foreign to the body and can cause an allergic reaction. The immune system will react by attacking allergens in the same way it attacks invading organisms such as viruses and bacteria. Known allergens include house dust mite, mould spores, pollen, wood dust, animal hair or fur (Akhouri and House 2023). A person with allergic rhinitis typically suffers from symptoms such as sneezing, nasal itching and/or clear discharge, postnasal drip and or blockage. Genetic predisposition is also an important factor in rhinitis development (Scadding et al. 2017).

An allergic immune response begins with sensitisation to an allergen. An allergen such as inhaled pollen can cause antigen-presenting cells, such as the Langerhans cells within the nasal mucosa, to express these allergens on their cell surfaces. The allergens are then presented to cells such as T lymphocytes, which are involved in transforming B lymphocytes into plasma cells. Plasma cells produce Immunoglobulin E (IgE), which is specific to that allergen, in this case, pollen. Re-exposure to pollen causes binding of the allergen to IgE, which triggers the degranulation of mast cells, and cell walls rupture, releasing histamine and other mediators such as leukotrienes and prostaglandin activating factor into the surrounding tissue, which, in turn, causes an inflammatory response (Akhouri and House 2023).

10.2.2 Inflammatory Response

Histamine is a chemical produced in the body and stored in cells, such as mast cells and basophils, and is released in response to allergens. Histamine binds to the histamine (H1) receptor, which is present on various cells in the nasal mucosa, causing blood vessels to dilate, become leaky, and the surrounding skin to swell. This is known as inflammation. The inflammatory response allows specialised cells and chemicals that defend the body to access the area. While this is helpful, it also causes nasal discharge (rhinorrhoea), redness (erythema) and swelling (oedema), which often affects the nerves in the surrounding area, making the nasal mucosa feel itchy which causes people to sneeze (Fig. 10.3).

There are two phases to an allergic response. The early phase, which occurs within minutes of reexposure to the allergen and the late phase which begins at the same time as the early phase, but symptoms occur 3–10 h later. The symptoms can remain for up to 24 h before subsiding.

Allergic rhinitis may occur for a few months in those sensitive to seasonal allergens, such as tree or grass pollen. Some people experience allergic rhinitis throughout the year.

Allergic rhinitis is currently classified by its duration and severity.

Duration

- *Intermittent*: Symptoms are present less than 4 days a week or for less than 4 weeks.
- *Persistent*: Symptoms are present at least 4 days a week and for at least 4 weeks.

Severity

- *Mild*: No disturbance of sleep or daily living activities.
- *Moderate to severe*: Sleep and/or daily living activities affected (sleep disturbance, impairment of school, work, leisure, or sport, or otherwise troublesome symptoms National Institute of Health and Care Excellence (NICE 2024a).

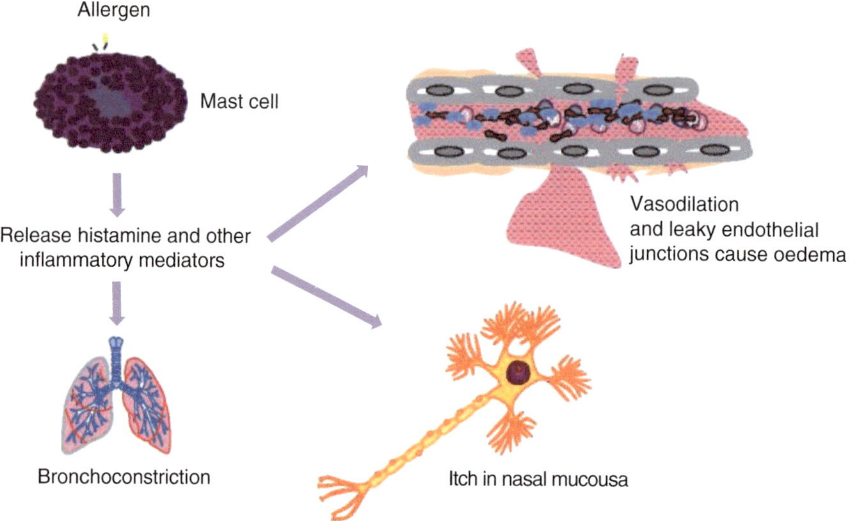

Fig. 10.3 Allergic immune

Seasonal or perennial rhinitis terms are also used, but NICE (2024a) suggests that intermittent or persistent classification provides more clarity.

Allergic rhinitis is not a severe condition, but the symptoms can significantly affect a person's quality of life (Greiner et al. 2012), and there are some complications of allergic rhinitis such as sinusitis. This is possibly due to persistent nasal mucosa swelling, which causes obstruction and prevents sinus drainage and predisposes to potential infection (Scadding et al. 2017). Children's learning and sleep patterns can be adversely affected if the symptoms remain uncontrolled (Lipworth et al. 2017).

10.2.3 Management of Allergic Rhinitis

This is dependent on the duration and severity of the symptoms. Management of allergic rhinitis includes advice on sources of information, nasal irrigation, allergen avoidance measures and pharmacological treatment.

Provide advice on sources of information and support, such as:
- The Allergy UK factsheets
- The NHS patient information leaflets

Nasal Irrigation

This may provide some relief, it is well tolerated, inexpensive, easy to use, and is unlikely to cause adverse effects. The British Society for Allergy & Clinical Immunology (BSACI) guideline (Scadding et al. 2017) notes that there is limited evidence on the effectiveness of nasal saline irrigation but the NICE (2024a) allergic rhinitis guidance suggests this as an option.

Allergen Avoidance

Provide advice on allergen avoidance techniques if there is a specific identified allergen, NICE (2024a)

Pharmacological Treatment

If nasal irrigation and allergen avoidance are not effective, then medication is required.

Mild, intermittent, or both: considering patient preference, age, severity of symptoms and persistence of symptoms
- Intranasal corticosteroids and antihistamines (intranasal or non-sedating oral antihistamines), either alone or in combination. Intranasal corticosteroids are the most effective treatment for allergic rhinitis, but patients may prefer oral medication. The onset of action for intranasal corticosteroids is 6–8 h after the first dose, but the maximal effect may not be seen until after 2 weeks.
- The combination of an intranasal corticosteroid and an oral antihistamine is no more effective than the intranasal corticosteroid alone. However, the combination of an intranasal corticosteroid with an intranasal antihistamine is more effective than an intranasal corticosteroid alone.
- In children, an antihistamine (intranasal or oral non-sedating antihistamine) (NICE 2024a).

Moderate to Severe
- An intranasal corticosteroid or the combination of an intranasal corticosteroid with an intranasal antihistamine.
- Nasal drops may be preferred if there is severe nasal obstruction (NICE 2024a).

If drug treatment provides adequate symptom control, treatment should continue until exposure to the suspected allergen has stopped. If there are recurrent episodes of symptoms controlled by intranasal corticosteroids, advise the person to restart treatment 2 weeks before reexposure to causative allergens.

If there are Additional Eye Symptoms:
- Antihistamine eye drops or chromone eye drops (sodium cromoglycate, nedocromil).

If a person has uncontrolled symptoms following initial self-management strategies and drug treatment:

- Check compliance with self-management strategies, drug treatments and whether the correct nasal administration technique is being used.
- An alternative diagnosis should be considered
- Treatment may need to be enhanced

Severe nasal congestion; an intranasal decongestant such as xylometazoline for up to 5–7 days, depending on the person's age and the preparation used.

In W*atery Rhinorrhoea,* despite a combined use of an intranasal corticosteroid and oral antihistamine, add an intranasal anticholinergic such as ipratropium bromide in adults or young people aged 12 or older.

Persistent nasal itching and sneezing; options are to add an oral antihistamine to be used regularly rather than 'as needed', or a combination preparation containing an intranasal antihistamine and an intranasal corticosteroid.

If the person has ongoing symptoms and a history of asthma, consider adding a leukotriene receptor antagonist such as montelukast to an oral or intranasal antihistamine (NICE 2024a).

For severe, uncontrolled symptoms that are significantly affecting quality of life: Consider a short course of oral corticosteroids to provide rapid symptom relief, such as:

- For adults: prednisolone 0.5 mg/kg in the morning for 5–10 days
- For children: seek advice from a specialist if considering prescribing an oral corticosteroid in this situation.

Consider arranging referral for specialist assessment and management to an allergy or Ear, Nose and Throat (ENT) specialist if:

- There are unilateral symptoms, blood-stained nasal discharge, recurrent epistaxis, or nasal pain—arrange an urgent 2-week wait referral to ENT
- There is predominant nasal obstruction and/or a structural abnormality such as a deviated nasal septum, which makes intranasal drug treatment difficult—arrange referral to ENT
- There are persistent symptoms

- The diagnosis is uncertain—consider referral to an allergy or ENT specialist, depending on clinical judgement.
- The person would like to consider specialist immunotherapy treatment rather than take medication long term (NICE 2024a).

10.3   Acute and Chronic Sinusitis

10.3.1 Pathophysiology

Sinusitis is a common condition that can affect people of any age. It is often caused by irritants such as smoke and air pollution, viral or bacterial infections, allergens and occasional anatomical structural problems. These causative agents lead to inflammation of the lining of the paranasal sinuses. Although not universally accepted, the term rhinosinusitis, rather than sinusitis, is often used since the nasal cavities and parasinuses are lined with a continuous mucous membrane (Fokkens et al. 2020).

There are four pairs of sinuses in the skull that assist in the control of the temperature and humidity of the air reaching the lungs. Each sinus is named after the bone in which they are found: the frontal, ethmoid, maxillary and sphenoidal (Fig. 10.4).

They are connected to the nasal cavity through narrow openings or 'ostia' and drain into the nasal cavity. A mucociliary system helps in moving fluid and micro-organisms out of the sinuses into the nasal cavity.

Allergens can irritate the lining of your sinuses in the same way they irritate the nasal lining. If a person has a blocked or congested nose or copious nasal discharge,

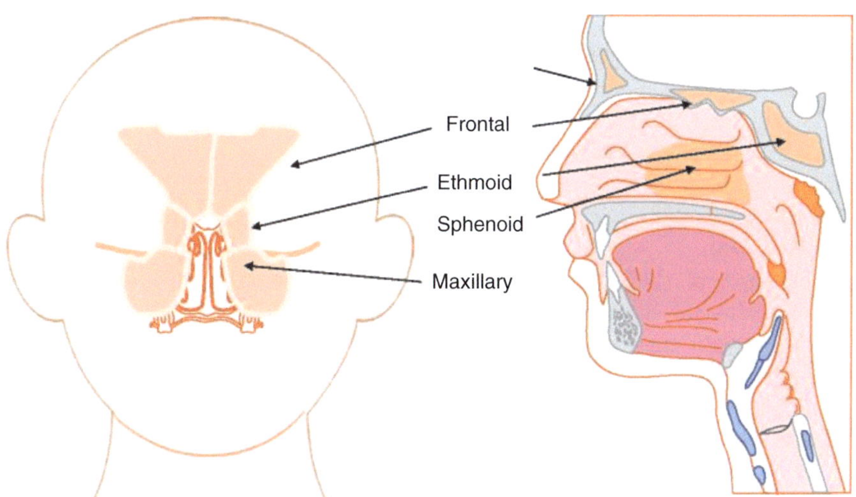

Fig. 10.4 Paranasal sinuses

it can prevent the sinuses from draining properly into the nose. Mucus in the sinuses then becomes blocked, stagnant and can easily become infected.

Fokkens et al. (2020) classifies sinusitis into two main types.

1. ***Acute sinusitis. Defined by symptoms that completely resolve within 12 weeks.***
   Fokkens et al. (2020) classifies acute sinusitis as:

   - Acute viral (or common cold): symptoms last for less than 10 days.
   - Acute post-viral: symptoms worsen after 5 days or persist for more than 10 days (but less than 12 weeks).
   - Acute bacterial: secondary bacterial infection that develops in about 0.5–2% of people with acute viral sinusitis.

2. ***Chronic sinusitis. Defined by symptoms lasting 12 weeks or longer.***
   Fokkens et al. (2020) classifies chronic sinusitis as.
   Primary chronic sinusitis. Which is further classified by endotype dominance as type 2 or non-type 2 inflammation.
   - For localised disease, the two phenotypes are allergic fungal rhinosinusitis and isolated sinusitis.
   - For diffuse disease, the clinical phenotypes are predominantly eosinophilic chronic sinusitis and non-eosinophilic chronic sinusitis.

   Secondary chronic sinusitis is further classified into four categories depending on local pathology, mechanical, inflammatory and immunological factors.
   - For localised disease, the phenotypes include odontogenic, fungal ball and tumour.
   - For diffuse disease, the phenotypes include primary ciliary dyskinesia and cystic fibrosis, granulomatosis with polyangiitis (previously known as Wegener's disease), eosinophilic granulomatosis with polyangiitis (Churg-Strauss disease) and selective immunodeficiency.

Sinusitis is also classified as uncomplicated where there is no evident extension of inflammation outside the paranasal sinuses. Acute exacerbation of a chronic state causing worsening of symptom intensity, often after intervention with corticosteroids or antibiotics and, recurrent acute, where four or more episodes of acute sinusitis per year with distinct symptom-free intervals between each episode (NICE 2024b).

Fokkens et al. (2020) recommends that at least one episode of acute post-viral sinusitis is diagnosed with an endoscopy or CT scan before a diagnosis of recurrent acute sinusitis is considered.

10.3.2 Management of Acute Sinusitis

1. Refer to hospital immediately if a severe systemic infection, signs of sepsis, periorbital oedema or cellulitis, a displaced eyeball, double vision, ophthalmo-

plegia, or newly reduced visual acuity or swelling over the frontal bone, symptoms or signs of meningitis, severe frontal headache, or focal neurological signs.

2. If symptoms last for 10 days or less, advise that acute sinusitis is usually caused by a virus and resolves within 12 weeks, and most people will get better without antibiotics. If the cause is bacterial, this is usually self-limiting and does not routinely need antibiotics.

3. Fever and pain can be managed with paracetamol or ibuprofen. Some people may want to consider a trial of nasal saline or nasal decongestants but NICE (2024b) states there is limited evidence to support their use.

4. If symptoms last for more than 10 days for people over the age of 12, consider prescribing a high-dose nasal corticosteroid for 14 days (e.g. mometa-sone 200 µg twice a day ('off-label use'),[1] being aware that nasal corticosteroids may improve symptoms but are not likely to affect how long they last and could cause systemic effects, particularly in people already taking another corticosteroid and may be difficult for people to use correctly.

5. Consider no antibiotic or a back-up antibiotic prescription as the evidence suggests that antibiotics make little difference to how long symptoms last or the proportion of people with improved symptoms (Falagas et al. 2008; Rosenfeld et al. 2015; Ahovuo-Saloranta et al. 2014)

6. Evidence (Falagas et al. 2008; Rosenfeld et al. 2015; Ahovuo-Saloranta et al. 2014) suggests that withholding antibiotics is unlikely to lead to complications and there are possible adverse reactions of antibiotics, mainly diarrhoea and nausea.

7. Factors that might make a bacterial cause more likely symptoms for more than 10 days, discoloured or purulent nasal discharge, severe localised pain (often unilateral, particularly pain over teeth and jaw), fever greater than 38 °C, and marked deterioration after an initial milder phase.

8. A back-up antibiotic may be preferred when a bacterial cause is more likely.

9. If a reinforcement antibiotic prescription is given, advise the person to take the antibiotic if symptoms do not improve within 7 days or worsen rapidly or significantly, at any time.

10. Seek medical help if symptoms worsen rapidly or significantly despite taking the antibiotic or if the antibiotic has been stopped because it was not tolerated (NICE 2024b).

Consider referral to an ear, nose and throat (ENT) specialist or immunologist for people with acute sinusitis and:

- Doubt about the diagnosis
- Treatment failure after extended courses of antibiotics
- Unusual or resistant bacteria
- Anatomic defect(s) causing obstruction
- Immunocompromise

---

[1] An 'off-label' use of a medication is when it is utilised in a way other than specified in the licence.

- A suspected allergic or immunological cause
- Comorbidities complicating management, such as nasal polyps (NICE 2024b)

10.3.3 Management of Chronic Sinusitis

1. *Hospital admission may be required if sinusitis is associated with a severe systemic infection, or a serious complication including*:
   - Orbital involvement—indicated by periorbital oedema or cellulitis, a displaced eyeball, double vision, ophthalmoplegia or reduced visual acuity
   - Intracranial involvement—indicated by severe frontal headache, swelling over the frontal bone, symptoms or signs of meningitis or focal neurological signs
   - Reduced consciousness (NICE 2024b)
2. *Inform the person that chronic sinusitis may last for 12 weeks or more, and antibiotics are not normally required.* If they have an associated disorder, such as allergic rhinitis or asthma, good control of these is also likely to benefit their sinusitis symptoms.
3. *Advise the person to*:
   - Practise good dental hygiene to reduce the risk of dental infection (which can be associated with chronic sinusitis)
   - Stop smoking and avoid passive smoking, where applicable
   - Avoid allergic triggers if possible, and underwater diving if there are prominent symptoms
4. *Consider nasal irrigation with a saline solution* to relieve congestion and nasal discharge.
5. *Consider a course of intranasal corticosteroids for up to 3 months*, especially if there is suspicion of an allergic cause (such as concomitant allergic rhinitis).
6. *A referral to an ENT specialist or immunologist may be required* if there are unilateral symptoms, persistent symptoms, symptoms that impact on an individual's quality of life, nasal polyps that cause nasal obstruction, treatment is ineffective, the person is immunocompromised, or there is suspected allergic, immunological or anatomic defect (Scadding et al. 2017; NICE 2024b).

10.4 Antihistamines

10.4.1 Pharmacodynamics

Antihistamines are chemically similar to histamine and compete with histamine for the receptor sites known as H1 and H2. An antihistamine blocks the action of histamine. These receptor sites are found in tissue cells, with H1 receptors located throughout the body and H2 receptor sites found in the gastric mucosa. The majority of available antihistamines are H1 antagonists. H1 antagonists are believed to cause action and effect by physically blocking the H1 receptor sites, preventing histamine from reaching its target receptor site. This interrupts the sequence of the allergic reaction and decreases the body's response to such allergens, which helps to reduce troublesome nasal symptoms. Antihistamines tend to be more effective if present in the nasal mucosa when mast cells release histamine. Since mast cells release many other active chemicals, such as leukotrienes and prostaglandin activating factor (Galli and Tsai 2012), antihistamines cannot completely block an allergic reaction; they simply diminish it.

Antihistamine medication can be classified as *systemic* (tablets, solutions, or capsules) or *topical* (nasal spray or drops), depending on how they are administered.

Antihistamine medication peak effectiveness is typically within 1–2 h after being taken and is generally more effective when taken daily rather than intermittently. They are metabolised in the liver and mainly excreted in urine. Azelastine is mainly excreted via faeces eMC (2025) and has different durations of action (Table 10.1).

10.4.2 Adverse Reactions

Oral non-sedating antihistamines:

- Drugs classified as 'non-sedating' antihistamines, including cetirizine, loratadine and azelastine, are described as having a low incidence of drowsiness and sedation.
- An individual taking non-sedating antihistamines should be advised that they may experience feelings of sedation, which may affect their ability to drive or undertake other activities, and that the sedative effects are enhanced if combined with alcohol.
- Dizziness, headache, nausea, fatigue and skin reactions.

Table 10.1 Pharmacokinetics—Antihistamines

Generic drug name	Route	Duration
Cetirizine hydrochloride	Oral (tablets or solution)	12–24 h depending on dose
Fexofenadine	Oral (tablet special-order manufacturers include: oral suspension, oral solution) BNF (2025)	24 h depending on dose
Loratadine	Oral (tablets or solution)	24 h
Azelastine hydrochloride	Intranasal and eye drops	20 h

Electronic Medicines Compendium (eMC) (2025)

Intranasal Antihistamines:

- A bitter taste may be experienced after administration. This is often due to incorrect administration technique (British National Formulary 2025).
- Irritation of the nasal mucosa causes itching, stinging, sneezing or epistaxis.
- Pruritus, rash and urticaria.

10.4.3 Nursing Considerations

- Discuss with the patient which medication they believe is most effective. They may experience a poor response to one drug but an effective response to another.
- Drowsiness may occur and affect the ability to drive or operate machinery; advise the patient accordingly.
- Advise an increase in fluid intake and humidity if possible, to decrease thickened secretions and nasal dryness.
- Some OTC drugs may contain elements of antihistamine drugs; therefore, patients should be cautioned to seek advice before considering whether to self-administer such drugs while taking other prescribed antihistamines.
- Inform the patient about the prescribed dosage, frequency, route, and possible adverse reactions, and who to contact if symptoms persist or adverse effects occur. This approach enhances patient knowledge and understanding about drug therapy and promotes concordance.
- Ensure the intranasal spray/drop technique is correct. Details of the intranasal inhalation technique can be located in Appendix 1

10.5 Corticosteroids

10.5.1 Pharmacodynamics

A topical corticosteroid usually acts effectively to clear all the nasal symptoms (itching, sneezing, watering and congestion).

Topical corticosteroids are highly effective in diseases where there is eosinophil-dominated inflammation (allergic rhinitis, nasal polyposis, allergic fungal sinusitis) and in diseases with neutrophil-dominated inflammation (acute and chronic rhinosinusitis). They are highly effective, and there are few adverse reactions; therefore, these drugs are considered the first-line treatment for allergic and non-allergic, non-infectious rhinitis and acute and chronic rhinosinusitis. Topical corticosteroids are used in addition to antihistamines if symptoms are not fully controlled by either alone.

Corticosteroids are synthetic analogues of natural hormones that are produced by the adrenal cortex and have multiple mechanisms of action, including anti-inflammatory activity, immunosuppressive properties and anti-proliferative actions. They are highly effective in mitigating inflammation, acting primarily by regulating protein synthesis. The unbound steroid molecule enters the cytoplasm of corticosteroid-responsive tissues by passively diffusing across the cell membrane. In the cytoplasm, it binds to a glucocorticoid receptor. This interaction mediates an inhibitory effect on phospholipase A2, the enzyme that produces arachidonic acid, the precursor lipid for inflammatory mediators. Glucocorticoid receptors also mediate an inhibitory effect on cyclooxygenase 2 (COX2), the enzyme that converts arachidonic acids to inflammatory prostaglandins, as well as having an inhibitory effect on COX2 enzyme production in the cell.

The basic pharmacokinetic parameters of a selection of corticosteroids are found in Table 10.2.

Significant improvement in symptoms usually becomes apparent within a few days. Relief or maximum benefit may not occur in some patients until 2 weeks after initiation of therapy.

10.5.2 Contraindications and Cautions

- As corticosteroids block the inflammatory response, their use is contraindicated in the presence of an acute infection and recent nasal surgery. They are used with caution in people who are immunosuppressed, transferred from systemic corticosteroids, and when used in high doses for prolonged periods (as systemic absorption may occur) (BNF 2025).

10.5.3 Adverse Reactions

- Common: altered smell, epistaxis, nasal ulceration, headache, altered taste and throat irritation.
- Rare: glaucoma, nasal septum perforation and blurred vision.
- Systemic corticosteroids and when used in high doses for prolonged periods. Concomitant use of other corticosteroids: take into account the use of other systemic and topical corticosteroids (e.g. creams, ointments and inhalers). The effect of these drugs is probably cumulative, and, therefore, requires close monitoring (BNF 2025).

Table 10.2 Pharmacokinetics—Corticosteroids

Generic drug name	Route	Duration
Fluticasone, 50 µg per dose nasal spray Mometasone, 50 µg per dose pump nasal spray	Intranasal	24 h 24 h

Electronic medicines compendium (eMC) (2025)

10.5.4 Nursing Considerations

- Monitor the height of children receiving high doses of intranasal corticosteroids over extended periods (more than 3 months), and review treatment if any effect on growth restriction is observed.
- Explain and demonstrate how to administer nasal spray and drops to ensure a therapeutic effect (Appendix).

10.6 Common Lower Respiratory Tract Conditions: Asthma and Chronic Obstructive Pulmonary Disease (COPD)

10.6.1 Asthma

10.6.1.1 Pathophysiology

Asthma is a chronic lung disease caused by inflammation (swelling) in the airways, which then causes muscles in the surrounding airways to tighten (Fig. 10.5), leading to wheezing, shortness of breath, chest tightness and coughing.Asthma is a common condition and affects people of all ages, but it most often starts during childhood. In the United Kingdom, 7.2 million people have asthma. This is about 8 in every 100 people (British Lung Foundation 2025).

The cause of asthma remains unclear (British Lung Foundation 2025). In those who have sensitive airways, asthma symptoms can be triggered by breathing in allergens or triggers. Common asthma triggers include animals (pet hair or dander), certain medicines (aspirin and other NSAIDS), changes in weather (most often cold

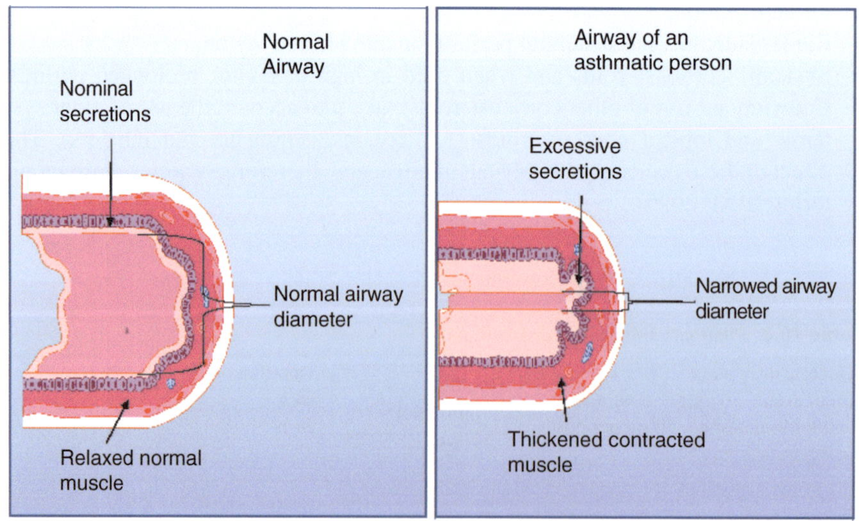

Fig. 10.5 Structure of a normal airway and an airway of a person with asthma

weather), exercise, obesity, low birth weight, exposure to tobacco smoke, air pollution, occupational hazards, low Vit D, female sex hormones oestrogen and proges-
terone, particularly around puberty, menstruation, pregnancy and the menopause
(British Lung Foundation 2025). Many people with asthma have a personal or family history of allergies, such as hay fever (allergic rhinitis) or eczema.

Individuals with asthma have over-sensitive, irritable, or 'hyper-reactive' airways. When the airways are irritated, the airway lining becomes inflamed, and the
bronchial muscles go into spasm.

10.6.1.2 Management of Confirmed Asthma

The aim of asthma management is control of the disease.

Advice

- Explain the condition, treatment and lifestyle changes and medication are meant
  to manage asthma symptoms and prevent an exacerbation.
- Advise the person on avoiding asthma trigger factors.
- Provide advice about sources of information and support, such as Asthma and
  Lung UK, the British Lung Foundation and Beat Asthma
- Ensure an appropriate delivery device is prescribed based on convenience, cost
  and suitability, and demonstrate how to use an inhaler and or a spacer device
  where appropriate.
- Routinely assess adherence in a non-judgemental way whenever medication is
  reviewed.
- The patient should have an action plan to use at home to monitor symptoms and
  recognise an exacerbation. The plan should be reviewed at every asthma-related
  healthcare attendance and at annual review.
- Where appropriate, ensure that the person has their own peak flow meter and
  measures their peak flow regularly as part of their action plan.
- Advise how to recognise early signs of an asthma exacerbation, what action to
  take, including specific instructions about changes to reliever and/or maintenance medications, and when and how to use oral prednisolone, if needed.
- Advise what to do if symptoms do not improve, and how and when to seek urgent
  medical attention.
- Ensure that all routine vaccinations, including all childhood immunisations, and
  the annual influenza vaccination, are up to date.
- Advise about smoking cessation, including parents and carers of children
  with asthma.
- Advise about weight management if the person is overweight or obese.
- Encourage regular physical activity. If the person gets exercise-induced symp-
  toms, advise them to take reliever medication before or during exercise.
- Manage any coexisting comorbid conditions, including emotional stress, anxiety
  or depression (NICE 2025a).

Drug Treatment
Initial treatment for newly diagnosed asthma in people aged 12 years and over:

- A low-dose inhaled corticosteroid (ICS)/long-acting beta-2 agonist (LABA) combination inhaler as an ICS/formoterol combination inhaler to be taken as needed for symptom relief (as-needed 'anti-inflammatory reliever' [AIR] therapy). Consider using AIR therapy before exercise or allergen exposure if needed.
- If the person has regular night-time waking or needs to use AIR therapy three times a week or more, offer low-dose 'maintenance and reliever therapy' (MART) with an ICS/formoterol combination inhaler.
- If low-dose MART is not controlling symptoms, offer moderate-dose MART. If moderate-dose MART is not controlling symptoms despite good adherence to treatment, measure the fractional exhaled nitric oxide (FeNO) level if available and blood eosinophil count. If either of these is raised, refer to a respiratory asthma specialist.
- If neither the FeNO level nor blood eosinophil count is raised, consider a trial of either a leukotriene receptor antagonist (LTRA) or a long-acting muscarinic receptor antagonist (LAMA) used in addition to moderate-dose MART for 8–12 weeks.
- If symptom control is improved but still inadequate, continue the treatment and start a trial of the other medication (LTRA or LAMA).
- If symptoms remain uncontrolled despite treatment with moderate-dose MART and trials of an LTRA and a LAMA, refer to a respiratory asthma specialist (NICE 2025a)

- For children aged 5–11 years and under 5 years of age, seek guidance from NICE (2025a)

10.6.2 Chronic Obstructive Pulmonary Disease (COPD)

Chronic obstructive pulmonary disease (COPD) is an umbrella term for individuals with chronic bronchitis, emphysema or both. Emphysema is a pathological term referring to loss of parenchymal lung texture and chronic bronchitis is a clinical term referring to cough and sputum production for at least 3 months in each of 2 consecutive years Global Initiative for Chronic Obstructive Lung Disease (GOLD) (2024).

Symptoms include persistent cough with mucous and breathlessness primarily due to the narrowing of airways which cause airflow obstruction. Airflow obstruction is usually progressive, not fully reversible, and does not change markedly over several months.

COPD usually affects people over the age of 35, although most people are not diagnosed until they are in their fifth decade. In the United Kingdom, it is estimated that more than 3 million people currently have COPD, and an estimated 2 million people have COPD, which remains undiagnosed (NICE 2025b).

10.6.2.1 Pathophysiology

One of the main risk factors for developing COPD is significant exposure to noxious particles or gases and tobacco smoking (GOLD 2024). The likelihood of developing COPD increases the more people smoke tobacco and the longer they smoke. This is because smoking irritates and inflames the lungs, which results in scarring and over many years causes permanent changes in the lung. The walls of the airways thicken and more mucus is produced. Damage to the delicate walls of the air sacs in the lungs causes emphysema and the lungs lose their normal elasticity (Fig. 10.6). The smaller airways also become scarred and narrowed. These changes cause the symptoms of breathlessness, cough, and phlegm associated with COPD. Some cases of COPD are, however, caused by fumes, dust, air pollution, and genetic disorders, but these are rarer (Halpin et al. 2012).

With emphysema, the walls between many of the air sacs are damaged. As a result, the air sacs lose their shape and become floppy. This damage also can destroy the walls of the air sacs, leading to fewer and larger air sacs instead of many tiny ones (Fig. 10.6). If this happens, the amount of gas exchange in the lungs is reduced.

A primary characteristic of chronic bronchitis is that the lining of the airways is constantly irritated and inflamed. This causes the lining to thicken and thick mucus forming in the airways, making breathing difficult.COPD is treatable but not curable. There are treatments and lifestyle changes that can help people feel better, stay more active and slow the progress of the disease and potential complications.

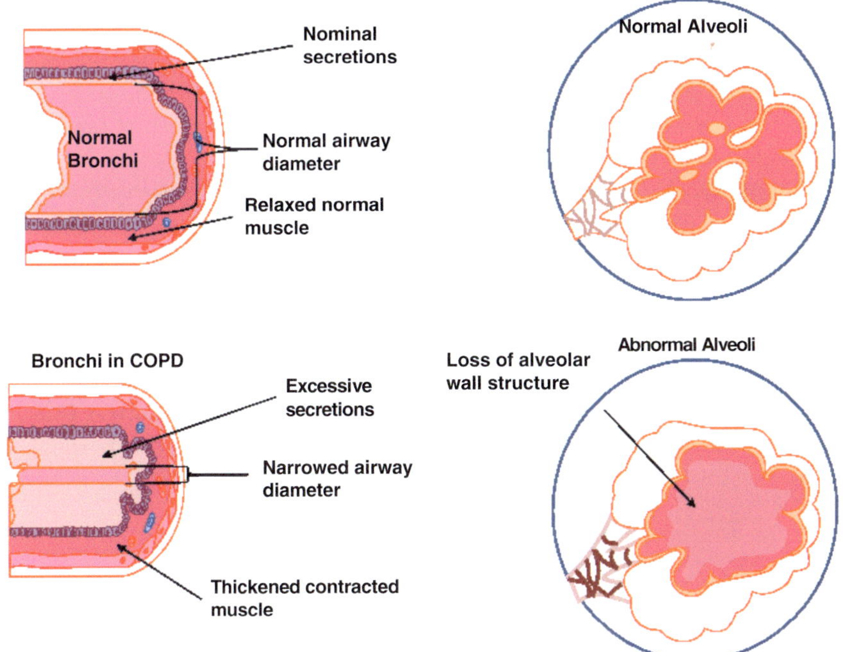

Fig. 10.6 Chronic obstructive pulmonary disease

Complications include depression and anxiety, cor pulmonale (right heart failure secondary to lung disease), frequent respiratory infections, polycythaemia (a high concentration of red blood cells), respiratory failure, pneumothorax due to abnormal lung parenchyma, and muscle wasting and cachexia, due to factors such as breathlessness and anorexia (Park et al. 2020; Sandelowsky et al. 2021; Kahnert et al. 2023).

10.6.2.2 Management of Stable COPD

Advice

- Explain the diagnosis, risk factors for progression, and the importance of a healthy diet and physical activity.
- Provide or advise about support for people with COPD, such as the British Lung Foundation.
- Advise an annual influenza vaccination and pneumococcal vaccination
- Advise about, exercise, weight loss and smoking prevention and cessation, if necessary.
- Routinely assess adherence in a non-judgemental way whenever medication is reviewed.
- Consider pulmonary rehabilitation if indicated.
- Develop a personalised self-management plan in conjunction with the person.
- Consider if treatment for comorbidities requires optimisation and psychological interventions.
- Advise on recognising early signs of exacerbations, how to prevent them and seeking help from healthcare professionals.
- *For people who have frequent exacerbations consider prescribing a supply of 'rescue' medication* (oral corticosteroids and antibiotics to keep at home) and provide written information advising them:
- To start oral corticosteroid therapy if increased breathlessness interferes with activities of daily living
- To start antibiotics if sputum becomes discoloured or increases in volume
- To contact a primary healthcare professional if; they start a treatment, and or are uncertain about whether to start treatment or become more unwell.

Drug treatment

Gold (2024) guidance on drug treatment is dependent on the phenotype. Either 2 or more moderate exacerbations or 1 or more exacerbations leading to hospitalisation or 0 or 1 moderate exacerbation not leading to hospitalisation.

2 or more moderate exacerbations or 1 or more exacerbations leading to hospitalisation. Individuals are classified as group E
Group E

- Long-acting beta-2 agonist (LABA) and Long-acting muscarinic receptor Antagonist (LAMA) combination treatment is first-line therapy in the absence of issues with adverse effects or availability.
- Addition of an inhaled corticosteroid inhaled corticosteroids (ICS) to a LABA and LAMA combination may be considered if the patient's blood eosinophil count is greater than 300 cells/microlitre (triple therapy).
- Use of ICS with LABA alone is not recommended.

0 or 1 moderate exacerbation not leading to hospitalisation. Individuals are classified as group A or B.
Group A: Modified Medical Research Council (MRC) questionnaire 0–1. COPD assessment test (CAT) 0–10.

- Should be offered bronchodilator treatment based on its effect on breathlessness.
- This can be either a short- or a long-acting bronchodilator. If available and affordable a long-acting bronchodilator is the preferred choice except in patients with very occasional breathlessness.
- This should be continued if a benefit is documented.

Group B: Modified MRC questionnaire 2 or more. COPD assessment test (CAT) >10.

- Should be offered treatment with a LABA and LAMA combination
- This has been shown to be superior to LAMA alone on several outcome measures
- If this combination is not acceptable there is no evidence to recommend either LABA or LAMA over the other
- Choice should be guided by patient perception of symptoms.

Further treatment is determined by the patient's symptoms and frequency of exacerbations after treatment and is independent of the patient's GOLD (2024) group at diagnosis. GOLD (2024) recommends different treatment pathways depending on whether the goal is relieving dyspnoea or reducing exacerbations. If treatment is required for both purposes, clinicians should follow the exacerbation pathway (NICE 2025b)

Before any adjustment in treatment, patients should be reviewed for symptoms and exacerbation risk, and their inhaler technique and treatment adherence should be assessed. Other medications that might be considered are oral corticosteroids, theophylline, mucolytic, anti-tussive or antimicrobial drugs (NICE 2025b)

10.7   Bronchodilators

10.7.1 Beta-2 Adrenoceptor Agonists and Muscarinic Receptor Antagonists

To understand the action of beta-2 adrenoceptor agonists and muscarinic antagonists, and their potential adverse reactions, an understanding of the physiology of the autonomic nervous system is required.

The autonomic nervous system consists of the sympathetic and parasympathetic nervous systems. The lungs are innervated by the sympathetic and parasympathetic systems, which entails the activation of adrenergic receptors or adrenoceptors (sympathetic nervous system) and muscarinic receptors (parasympathetic nervous system).

10.7.2 Sympathetic Nervous System

There are two main groups of adrenergic receptors: alpha (α) and beta (β) with several subtypes. The receptors found in the lungs are the β2-adrenergic receptors; they are expressed on the airway smooth muscle and activation causes bronchodilation. The adrenergic receptors are a class of G-protein-coupled receptors that are targets of catecholamines (Fig. 10.7), especially the neurotransmitters norepinephrine (noradrenaline) and epinephrine (adrenaline).

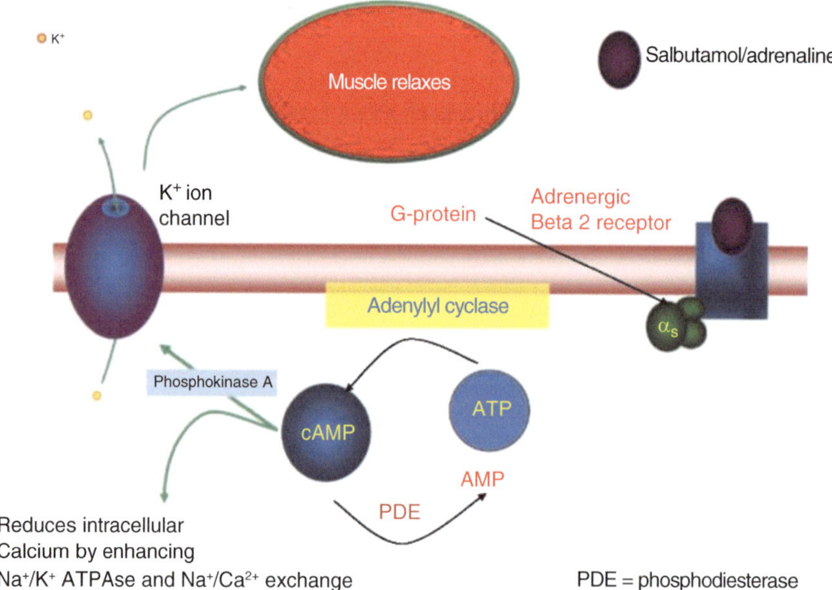

Fig. 10.7 Adrenergic beta 2 receptor activity

10.7.3 Parasympathetic Nervous System

The parasympathetic nerve supply to the lungs comes via the tenth cranial nerve—the vagus nerve. The neurotransmitter is acetylcholine, and the airway smooth muscle receptors are termed muscarinic receptors. There are five different types of muscarinic receptors: M1–M5, and M3 receptors are found on the airway smooth muscle (Fig. 10.8).

Acetylcholine released from the parasympathetic fibres activates the M3 muscarinic receptors located on the airway smooth muscle, causing bronchoconstriction.

β2 Adrenocepter agonists are also known as β2-adrenergic receptor agonists and β2 agonists.

10.7.4 Pharmacodynamics

β2 Agonists are described as sympathomimetic or adrenergic agents as they mimic adrenaline and a normal sympathetic nervous system response.

These drugs cause a response by binding to β2 receptors in airway smooth muscle. β2 Adrenergic receptors are coupled to the stimulatory G protein. The alpha subunit of the G-protein activates adenylyl cyclase, which causes the production of cyclic adenosine monophosphate (cAMP) and subsequent chain of events that leads to decreased intracellular calcium, increased membrane potassium and decreased

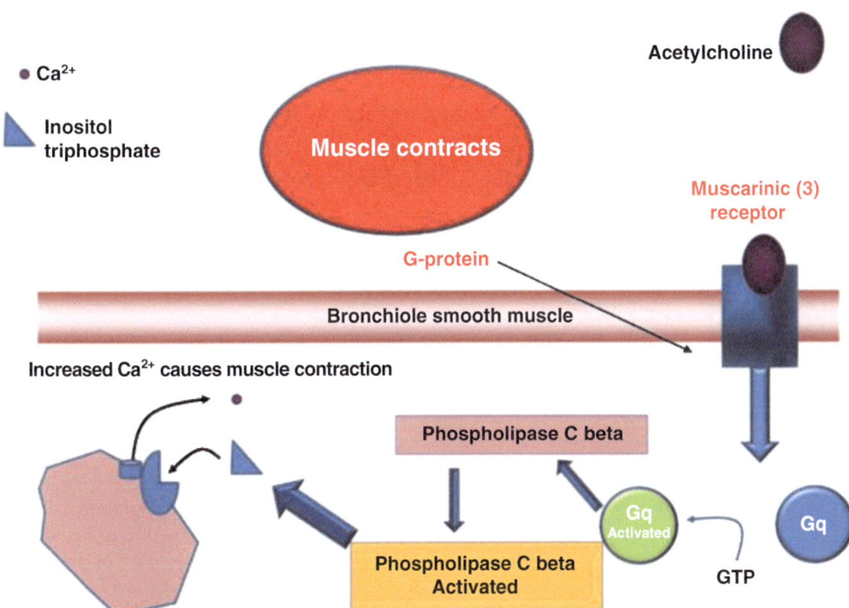

Fig. 10.8 Parasympathetic nervous system mediated bronchoconstriction

myosin light chain kinase activity, which leads to smooth muscle relaxation and bronchodilation (Fig. 10.7).

β2 agonist bronchodilators are designed to bind selectively to β2 receptors in the lungs. However, β2 agonists are not completely selective and can bind to other sympathetic receptors, β1 in other sites such as the heart and skeletal muscle. This occurs particularly when high doses are administered, such as those given orally, intravenously or via a nebuliser.

It is this unwanted binding to receptors that causes adverse reactions. Stimulation of sympathetic receptors in the heart can cause tachycardia or arrhythmia, and stimulation of receptors in skeletal muscle can result in tremor. Other possible adverse reactions include muscle cramp and headache.

There are two classes of β2 adrenoceptor agonists: short-acting drugs that act rapidly and provide immediate relief and longer acting drugs which are often used with a corticosteroid as prophylactic therapy.

10.7.5 Pharmacokinetics

The preferred route of administration is inhalation which is rapidly absorbed into the lung tissue. These drugs can also be administered by subcutaneous, intramuscular, or intravenous injection or orally. The absorbed drug is excreted unchanged in the urine and the remainder transformed into metabolites by the liver and excreted in the urine (Table 10.3).

10.7.6 Adverse Reactions

These are usually dose related and include the following:

- Tachycardia secondary to peripheral vasodilation and cardiac stimulation, sometimes accompanied by palpitations
- Fine tremor, particularly the hands
- Headache, dizziness
- Nervousness, agitation
- Hypokalaemia and potentially hyperglycemia when using formoterol but this is rare

Table 10.3 Route, onset and duration of β2 adrenoceptor agonists

Generic drug name examples	Route	Duration
Short-acting such as salbutamol and terbutaline	Inhaled	3–6 h
Long-acting such as formoterol and salmeterol	Inhaled	12 h or more

Electronic medicines compendium (eMC 2025)

- Acute angle-closure glaucoma has been reported in people taking nebulised short-acting beta-2 agonists
- eMc (2025)

10.7.7 Nursing Considerations

- Observe the individual's inhaler technique; if required, demonstrate and explain correct inhaler device technique. This will assist in achieving the best drug deposition.
- β2 Agonists should be used with caution for people with:
  - *Hyperthyroidism*—β2 agonists may stimulate thyroid activity.
  - *Diabetes mellitus*—there is a rare risk of ketoacidosis, especially after intravenous beta-2 agonist administration. Additional blood glucose measurements are recommended when treatment with a β2 agonist is commenced.
  - *Cardiovascular disease* (including hypertension)—β2 agonists may cause an increased risk of arrhythmias and significant changes to blood pressure and heart rate.
  - *Hypokalaemia*—plasma potassium concentration can be reduced by β2 agonists, particularly high doses, and this can be increased by other potassium-depleting drugs, such as corticosteroids, loop diuretics and theophylline.
- *Digoxin*—monitor potassium levels and be alert to signs of digoxin toxicity, such as loss of appetite, nausea, vomiting, bradycardia, visual disturbance and drowsiness.

10.8 Muscarinic Receptor Antagonists (Anticholinergic Bronchodilators)

10.8.1 Pharmacodynamics

Anticholinergic bronchodilators (or muscarinic receptor antagonists) bind to muscarinic receptors (M3) and block the acetylcholine neurotransmitter that causes the airways to constrict, and so allow the air passages to remain open. There are two classes of muscarinic receptor antagonists: short- and long-acting.

10.8.2 Pharmacokinetics

Ipratropium bromide is short-acting. It takes 30–45 min to reach maximum effect, so these preparations are not suitable for rapid symptom relief. Effects last 6–8 h, and it is generally used regularly three to four times a day (Table 10.4). Ipratropium is not well absorbed, and, therefore, the effects are localised to the airways.

Table 10.4 Pharmacokinetics of muscarinic receptor antagonists

Generic name examples	Route	Duration
Short acting		
Ipratropium bromide 20 µg per dose Ipratropium bromide 250 µg/mL	Metered dose inhaler Liquid for nebuliser	6–8 h 6 h
Long acting		
Tiotropium 18 µg green capsule	Inhaled via inhaler device	24 h

Electronic Medicines Compendium (eMC) (2025)

Tiotropium has a 24-h duration of action and takes about 20 min to cause action and effect; therefore, it is taken only once a day for maintenance (Table 10.4). Tiotropium is excreted unchanged via the kidneys.

10.8.3 Adverse Effects

- Dry mouth, throat irritation and cough
- Abnormal taste in the mouth
- Nasal congestion
- Dryness of nasal mucosa
- Acute angle-closure glaucoma has been reported in people on nebulised ipratropium
- Nausea, vomiting, constipation and diarrhoea.
- Headache and dizziness.
- Urinary disorders such as bladder outflow obstruction and prostatic hyperplasia.

10.8.4 Nursing Considerations

- Observe the individual's inhaler technique, and, if required, demonstrate and explain correct inhaler device technique; this will assist in achieving the best drug deposition and minimise exposure of the eyes.
- Use a mouthpiece rather than a mask with a nebuliser, if possible, to minimise the risk of exposure of the eyes to the drug.
- Advise people on correct administration of dry powder and aerosol inhalers to avoid accidental release of the contents into the eye.
- Advise patients with angle-closure glaucoma who are using muscarinic antagonists to stop and consult an ophthalmologist immediately if they experience eye pain or discomfort, visual halos or coloured images or temporary blurring of vision.

Antimuscarinics should be used with caution in:

- Men with prostatic hyperplasia and bladder-outflow obstruction—worsened urinary retention has been reported in older men.
- People with moderate to severe renal failure (creatinine clearance of 50 mL/min or less)—because of the risk of drug toxicity.
- People with angle-closure glaucoma—nebulised mist of anticholinergic drugs can precipitate or worsen acute closed-angle glaucoma. This may also occur with aerosols or dry powders if these agents accidentally penetrate the eyes.
- People with cardiac rhythm disorders, heart failure or myocardial infarction in the last 6 months should use tiotropium with caution. There is an increased risk of all-cause mortality in this group of people following the use of this product (NICE 2025b).

10.9   Inhaled Corticosteroids

Corticosteroids are a class of chemicals that include the steroid hormones that are produced in the adrenal cortex. Synthetic pharmaceutical drugs such as glucocorticoids with corticosteroid-like effects are used in a variety of conditions, including asthma and COPD.

10.9.1 Pharmacodynamics

Glucocorticoids suppress the inflammatory response in the airways through numerous pathways. Glucocorticoid-specific receptors in the cell cytoplasm bind with steroid ligands to form hormone–receptor complexes that eventually translocate to the cell nucleus. There these complexes bind to specific DNA sequences and alter their expression. The complexes may induce the transcription of mRNA, leading to synthesis of new proteins. These new proteins block the synthesis of prostaglandins, leukotrienes and platelet activating factor (PAF). Glucocorticoids also inhibit the production of other mediators, metabolites such as those produced via COX activation (both COX-1 and COX-2) (Fig. 10.9), cytokines, the interleukins, adhesion molecules, and enzymes such as collagenase leading to profound anti-inflammatory effects.

10.9.2 Pharmacokinetics

As with the majority of inhaled medications, the ability of the drug to enter systemic circulation is limited; the small amounts that enter systemic circulation are not normally a concern regarding excretion. The effects of metabolic enzyme interactions associated with these medications depend upon the medication. Beclomethasone diproprionate is metabolised by tissue esterase enzymes. The newer prodrug,

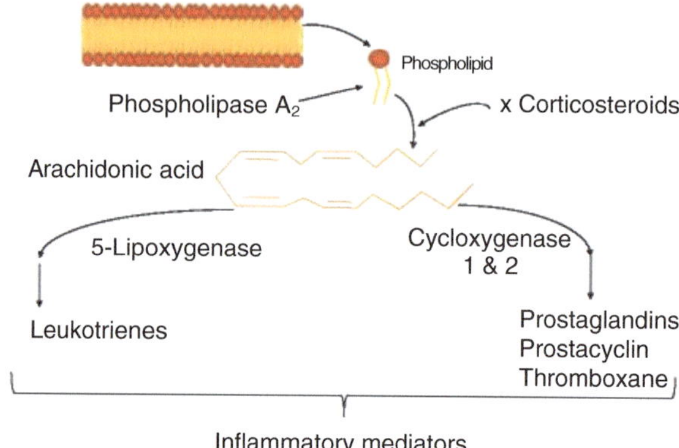

Fig. 10.9 An overview of the action of a corticosteroid

cicle-sonide, is converted by pulmonary epithelium esterases into its active metabolite that provides the main drug action. Although this metabolite is acted on by CYP3A4, owing to its poor bioavailability and localised pulmonary deposition, this drug does not cause systemic CYP3A4 interactions (Derendorf 2007). Budesonide (Pulmicort) and fluticasone propionate (Flixotide), although inhaled, may both enter systemic circulation and owing to metabolism by CYP3A4 have the potential to cause drug–drug interactions.

10.9.3 Adverse Reactions

Local adverse effects include the following:

- Oral candidiasis, sore mouth, dysphonia and hoarseness, especially with high doses.
- Paradoxical bronchospasm—very rarely occurs and is usually mild.
- Mild bronchospasm may be prevented by changing from an aerosol inhaler to a dry powder inhaler.
- There is an increased risk of pneumonia in people with chronic obstructive pulmonary disease treated with inhaled corticosteroids this should be discussed with the person before prescribing.
- Drug–drug interactions and systemic adverse effects are rare but may occur if high doses are prescribed for prolonged periods.

Possible systemic adverse effects include the following:

- Adrenal suppression, reduced bone mineral density, bruising, cataract and glaucoma
- Some initial slowing of growth—may occur in children on high doses of inhaled corticosteroids, but final adult height does not seem to be affected

- Adrenal crisis, coma and death—very rarely in children
- Psychological and behavioral effects
- Local adverse effects include the following:
- Increased susceptibility to infection.
- Reduced bone mineral density.

10.9.4 Nursing Considerations

- Observe the patient's inhaler technique for accuracy. If required, demonstrate and explain inhaler device technique; this will assist in achieving the best drug deposition.
- Consider a large-volume spacer with a pressurized metered-dose inhaler (pMDI) if high doses of inhaled corticosteroid are needed.
- Advise the person to rinse their mouth with water after using the inhaler. Oral candidiasis is dose-related; it is not frequently a major problem and can usually be prevented by gargling, washing and spitting out after taking the inhaler. In some cases, local antifungal treatment may be needed.
- If a hoarse voice and dysphonia are problematic a pMDI and a spacer device maybe prescribed. Steroids being deposited on the vocal cords cause a myopathy of the arytenoid muscles, which causes these symptoms. Since all inhaled steroids must cross the vocal cords to be active, this is the most difficult adverse reaction to overcome; gargling with water after inhaling may help.
- An individual receiving long-term treatment with high doses of inhaled corticosteroids should carry an 'alert' bracelet or information card.
- In children taking inhaled corticosteroids, height should be monitored regularly (BNF 2025)

10.10 Leukotriene Receptor Antagonist (LTRA)

10.10.1 Pharmacodynamics

LTRAs are a class of oral medications that are non-steroidal. They cause action and effect by blocking a chemical reaction that can lead to inflammation in the airways. Although not the preferred first choice therapy, LTRAs can be tried when an inhaled steroid cannot, or will not, be used, or if the dose cannot be increased.

Montelukast is an LTRA. They selectively and competitively block receptors for the leukotrienes C4, D4 and E4 (Fig. 10.9) released during the inflammatory response, block neutrophil and eosinophil migration, neutrophil and monocyte aggregation, increase capillary permeability, smooth muscle contraction and factors that contribute to inflammation and bronchoconstriction.

Table 10.5 Pharma-cokinetics—Leukotriene receptor antagonists

Generic name	Route	Duration
Montelukast	Oral	24 h

Electronic Medicines Compendium (eMC) (2025)

10.10.2 Pharmacokinetics

These drugs are absorbed from the GI tract, metabolised in the liver by P450 enzyme system and excreted in faeces (Table 10.5).

10.10.3 Contraindications and Cautions

- Aspirin can cause toxicity to occur, and the effects of LTRAs can also be reduced by erythromycin, primidone and phenobarbital.
- These drugs should be used cautiously for patients with hepatic or renal impairment as these conditions can affect drug metabolism and excretion. Additionally, both drugs can cross the placenta and enter breast milk.

10.10.4 Adverse Reactions

Headache, vomiting, diarrhoea, abdominal pain, and rarely, Churg-Strauss syndrome may occur, causing vasculitis, eosinophilia and deterioration of pulmonary symptoms.

10.10.5 Nursing Considerations

- Identify conditions that could be cautions or contraindications to using LTRAs.
- Advise patients that LRTA medication is to be taken continuously and not to stop the medication during symptom-free periods; this will ensure therapeutic levels are maintained.
- Advise patients to avoid over-the-counter preparations containing aspirin.
- Patients should inform a health professional if nausea, vomiting, malaise or jaundice occur; these are potential signs of liver dysfunction.

10.11 Summary

This chapter has focused on the pathophysiology of common upper respiratory tract conditions, rhinitis and sinusitis, lower respiratory tract conditions and asthma and chronic obstructive pulmonary disease. The pharmacokinetics and pharmacodynamics of the drugs used to treat and manage these disorders have been explored, as well as the nursing considerations.

Multiple Choice Questions

1. Terbutaline is a type of bronchodilator known as:
   (a) Corticosteroid
   (b) Beta-2 adrenoceptor antagonist
   (c) Beta-blocker
   (d) Beta-2 adrenoceptor agonist
2. High doses of beta-2 adrenoceptor agonist can cause:
   (a) Hypokalaemia
   (b) Anaemia
   (c) Vitamin B12 deficiency
   (d) Scabies
3. Muscarinic receptor antagonists are used as bronchodilators because of their antagonism of muscarinic acetylcholine receptors in the:
   (a) Sympathetic nervous system
   (b) Parasympathetic nervous system
   (c) Cerebral cortex
   (d) Organ of Corti
4. Common adverse reactions of corticosteroids include which of the following:
   (a) Blinking
   (b) Hoarseness
   (c) Dehydration
   (d) Candidiasis
5. Montelukast belongs to which class of drug:
   (a) Muscarinic receptor antagonist
   (b) Calcium channel blocker
   (c) Leukotriene receptor antagonist
   (d) Decongestant
6. How many pairs of sinuses are there in the skull?
   (a) One
   (b) Two
   (c) Three
   (d) Four
7. Which one of the following is a corticosteroid?
   (a) Beclometasone dipropionate
   (b) Amoxicillin
   (c) Salbutamol
   (d) Pseudoephedrine
8. When should intranasal corticosteroids be avoided?
   (a) In acute rhinitis
   (b) In chronic rhinitis
   (c) In those with an untreated nasal infection
   (d) Immediately after surgery

Answers

1. (d)
2. (a)
3. (b)
4. (b) and (d)
5. (c)
6. (d)
7. (a)
8. (c) and (d)

Appendix 1

Nasal spray and technique (ENT UK 2025a)

- Wash your hands, gently blow the nose to try and clear.
- Gently shake the bottle well.
- Keep your head upright. Insert the nozzle tip into one nostril. Keep your other nostril open.
- Try to direct the spray away from the septum (the middle part inside the nose). You may find it easier to use your right hand for spraying your left nostril and vice versa (Fig. 1b).
- Squeeze a fine mist into the nose while breathing in slowly. Do not sniff hard as the spray then travels past the nose into the throat.
- After spraying both nostrils, clean the nozzle and replace the cap

Nasal drop technique (ENT UK 2025b)

- *Wash your hands and* gently blow the nose to try and clear.
- Shake the container well.
- *Lie on your back, with your head just off the bed. Tilt your head backwards so that your chin is pointing upward.*
- *Breathe normally through your mouth while putting the prescribed number of drops into each nostril.*
- *Lie in this position for 2 min after inserting the drops.*
- *Clean the nozzle and replace the cap.*
- Wash your hands after using the drops.

References

Ahovuo-Saloranta A, Rautakorpi U-M, Borisenko OV et al (2014) Antibiotics for acute maxillary sinusitis in adults. Cochrane Database Syst Rev 2:CD000243. https://www.cochranelibrary.com/cdsr/doi/10.1002/14651858.CD000243.pub3/abstract. Accessed 20 Mar 25

Akhouri S, House SA (2023) Allergic rhinitis. In: StatPearls (Internet). National Library of Medicine

British Lung Foundation (2025) What is Asthma? https://www.asthmaandlung.org.uk/conditions/asthma/what-asthma#how-serious-is-asthma Accessed 30 Mar 2025

British National Formulary (2025) British Medical Association and Royal Pharmaceutical Society. https://bnf.nice.org.uk/drugs/fexofenadine-hydrochloride/#indications-and-dose. Accessed 30 Mar 2025

Derendorf H (2007) Pharmacokinetic and pharmacodynamic properties of inhaled ciclesonide. J Clin Pharmacol 47(6):782–789

Electronic Medicines Compendium (eMC) (2025). https://www.medicines.org.uk/emc. Accessed 21 Mar 2025

ENT UK (2025a) How to use nasal sprays. https://www.entuk.org/patients/conditions/79/how_to_use_nasal_sprays. Accessed 30 Mar 2025

ENT UK (2025b) How to use nasal drops. https://www.entuk.org/patients/conditions/77/how_to_use_nasal_drops. Accessed 30 Mar 2025

Falagas ME, Giannopoulou KP, Vardakas KZ, Dimopoulos G, Karageorgopoulos DE (2008) Comparison of antibiotics with placebo for treatment of acute sinusitis: a meta-analysis of randomised controlled trials. Lancet Infect Dis 8(9):543–552

Fokkens WJ, Lund VJ, Hopkins C, Fokkens et al (2020) European position paper on rhinosinusitis and nasal polyps 2020. Rhinology 58(Suppl S29):1–464. https://doi.org/10.4193/Rhin20.600

Galli SJ, Tsai M (2012) IgE and mast cells in allergic disease. Nat Med 18(5):693–704

Global Initiative for Chronic Obstructive Lung Disease (GOLD) (2024) Global strategy for prevention, diagnosis and management of COPD: 2024 report. Global initiative for chronic Obstructive Lung Disease. https://goldcopd.org. Accessed 30 Mar 2025

Greiner AN, Hellings PW, Rotiroti G, Scadding GK (2012) Allergic rhinitis. Lancet 378(9809):2112–2122

Halpin DM, Decramer M, Celli B (2012) Exacerbation frequency and course of COPD. Int J Chron Obstruct Pulmon Dis 7:653–661

Kahnert K, Jörres RA, Behr J, Welte T (2023) The diagnosis and treatment of COPD and its comorbidities. Dtsch Arztebl Int 120(25):434–444

Lipworth B, Newton J, Ram B (2017) An algorithm recommendation for the pharmacological management of allergic rhinitis in the UK: a consensus statement from an expert panel. NPJ Prim Care Respir Med 27(3):1–8

National institute for health and care excellence (2024a) Allergic rhinitis. https://cks.nice.org.uk/topics/allergic-rhinitis/. Accessed 30 Mar 2025

National institute for health and care excellence (2024b) Sinusitis. https://cks.nice.org.uk/topics/sinusitis/. Accessed 30 Mar 2025

National institute for health and care excellence (2025a) Asthma. https://cks.nice.org.uk/topics/asthma/. Accessed 30 Mar 2025

National institute for health and care excellence (2025b) COPD. https://cks.nice.org.uk/topics/chronic-obstructive-pulmonary-disease/. Accessed 30 Mar 2025

Park HY, Kang D, Shin SH et al (2020) Chronic obstructive pulmonary disease and lung cancer incidence in never smokers: a cohort study. Thorax 75(6):506–509

Rosenfeld RM, Piccirillo JF, Chandrasekhar SS, Brook I, Ashok Kumar K, Kramper M, Orlandi RR, Palmer JN, Patel ZM, Peters A, Walsh SA, Corrigan MD (2015) Clinical practice guideline (update): adult sinusitis. Otolaryngol Head Neck Surg 152(2 Suppl):S1–S39

Sandelowsky H, Weinreich UM, Aarli BB et al (2021) COPD – do the right thing. BMC Fam Pract 22(1):224

Scadding GK, Kariyawasam HH, Scadding G, Mirakian R, Buckley RJ, Dixon T, Durham SR, Farooque S, Jones N, Leech S, Nasser SM, Powell R, Roberts G, Rotiroti G, Simpson A, Smith H, Clark AT (2017) BSACI guideline for the diagnosis and management of allergic and non-allergic rhinitis (revised edition 2017; first edition 2007). Clin Exp Allergy 47(7):856–889

Medications Used for the Gastrointestinal System

11

Ehsan Khan

Learning Outcomes

At the end of this chapter, you will be able to:

- Understand the basic function of the gastrointestinal tract in relation to peristalsis, gastric acid secretion and vomiting
- Describe the mechanism of action of commonly used laxatives, stomach acid-reducing medications and anti-emetics
- Identify common and significant adverse reactions of the medications described and relate these to nursing practice

11.1 Introduction

Drugs acting on the gastrointestinal tract (GIT) are commonly prescribed. Nevertheless, drugs acting on the GIT carry cautions and contraindications. This chapter explores three classes of medication (laxatives, acid-reducing medications and anti-emetics). The aim of this chapter is to promote knowledge and the subsequent safe use and administration of GIT medications in practice.

E. Khan (✉)
Faculty of Nursing Midwifery and Palliative Care, King's College London,
London, UK
e-mail: eu.khan@kcl.ac.uk

© The Author(s), under exclusive license to Springer Nature
Switzerland AG 2026
E. Khan, P. Hood (eds.), *Understanding Pharmacology in Nursing Practice*,
https://doi.org/10.1007/978-3-032-03964-4_11

11.2   Laxatives

Laxatives are medications that facilitate defaecation or evacuation of the bowels. This is achieved either by increasing bulk in the intestine and or by increasing gastric motility. Laxatives are taken primarily to treat or prevent constipation.

Constipation can occur for many reasons. Frequently, a number of factors combine together to induce or exacerbate constipation. The use of pharmacological interventions will alleviate constipation, but non-pharmacological interventions can possibly prevent constipation, therefore, negating the need for pharmacotherapy.

11.2.1 Prevalence of Constipation

Constipation has been defined in a number of ways; however, a practical definition provided is 'a reduced frequency or ease of stool passage from what is deemed the normal or expected pattern for that individual' (Gray 2011:1). Prevalence of constipation ranges from 2% to 27% in the general population, with women experiencing nearly a threefold higher incidence compared to men (Schmidt et al. 2015; Vazquez and Bouras 2015; Barberio et al. 2021). Older age is a significant risk factor for constipation (Shi et al. 2015; Schmidt et al. 2015; Vazquez and Bouras 2015). Obesity, although related to constipation in pregnancy (Shi et al. 2015), is not associated with constipation as an independent risk factor in the general population (Eslick and Talley 2016).

11.2.2 Pathology of Constipation

Constipation, particularly in the older person, may arise due to two main mechanisms: poor colonic transport and pelvic floor dysfunction (Vazquez and Bouras 2015). The function of the colon is to dehydrate faeces and store it before defaecation. During defaecation, typically only one aspect of the colon, the descending colon, is emptied, transmitting the stool to the rectum for evacuation. Many factors may contribute to poor colonic transport, including age, dehydration, lack of exercise and poor diet (Taba Taba Vakili et al. 2015). Drug-induced reduction in colonic transit may be associated with medium- to long-term use of opioids and anticholinergic drugs that directly affect gastrointestinal (GI) tract musculature, as well as some calcium channel antagonists and anti-psychotic and anti-depressant medications. Drugs that influence the consistency (hardening) of faeces include antacids, diuretics and supplements such as iron and calcium.

The pelvic floor has a complex arrangement of involuntary and voluntary innervated muscle structures that assist in the expulsion of faeces from the rectum. Pelvic floor dysfunction is a common feature of constipation and may contribute to its prevalence in women (following childbirth) and to constipation occurring in older age, owing to senescence-related cellular degradation that leads to poor muscle and nerve function.

11.2.3 Non-pharmacological Self-Help Strategies

Self-management strategies are typically used as a preventative measure when the risk of short-term constipation may arise, or they may be used as an adjunct to traditional constipation pharmacotherapy. Such self-help strategies include exercise (Costilla and Foxx-Orenstein 2014; Shi et al. 2015) and a high-fibre diet, although this may aggravate chronic constipation (Costilla and Foxx-Orenstein 2014). As dehydration and the consequent electrolyte imbalance are associated with constipation in both the general population and pregnancy (Maughan 2012; Trottier et al. 2012), it is important that individuals susceptible to constipation are encouraged to remain hydrated.

Biofeedback therapy is a relatively new non-pharmacological strategy to alleviate constipation. This therapy has been shown to be as effective as a number of commonly used laxatives and has been suggested to be the therapy of choice for constipation due to dyssynergic defecation (Vazquez and Bouras 2015; Moore and Young 2020).

11.2.4 Pharmacological Interventions Commonly Used for Constipation

Although there are numerous pharmacological treatments available for constipation, this discussion will be limited to those frequently encountered in clinical practice.

Vazquez and Bouras (2015) list the following classification for laxative medications:

- Bulk-forming laxatives
- Osmotic laxative
- Bi-modal laxatives (stimulant laxatives)
- Lubricants
- Guanylate cyclase activators
- Serotonin agents

The first three classes will be examined in detail.

11.2.4.1 Bulk-Forming Laxatives

This group of laxatives includes a number of primarily plant-based substances that do not absorb into the intestinal wall. Owing to the presence of these cellulose-based hydrophilic (affinity for water) gels, these laxatives increase their volume after absorbing water from the gut wall. The increased volume stretches the intestinal wall, which acts as a stimulus to cause muscles behind the faeces to contract and muscles in front to dilate, therefore propelling the faeces forward (Fig. 11.1).

Bulk-forming laxatives include the following:

Fig. 11.1 Bulk forming laxatives

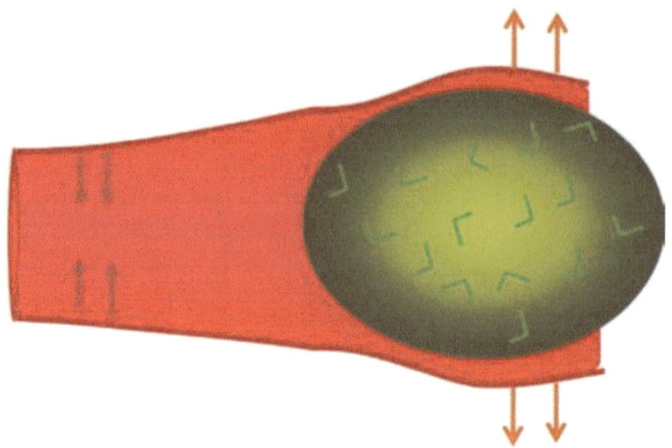

- Bran
- Ispaghula husk
- Methyl cellulose
- Sterculia

It is suggested that bulk-forming laxatives are beneficial for the treatment of pelvic floor dysfunction that sometimes leads to constipation (Khalid et al. 2009). They have few adverse effects but have been reported to cause abdominal discomfort and flatulence. It is important to maintain adequate hydration when using these medications as such laxatives aggravate chronic constipation in a dehydrated person. Therefore, prescribing bulk-forming laxatives when there is reduced colonic transit may be questionable. This limitation may become of consequence when fluid restrictions are required, such as for people with heart failure. As these preparations are not absorbed into the bloodstream, they have limited pharmacokinetic importance. However, there is little understanding of their ability to bind other medications in the gut, therefore potentially reducing absorption of other medications from the intestine.

11.2.4.2 Osmotic Laxatives

This group of laxatives encompasses a range of dissimilar substances that have a similar mechanism of action in relation to their laxative effect. Osmotic laxatives include the following:

- Sulphate salts (saline laxatives)
- Alcohols
- Lactulose
- Polyethylene glycol (Movicol®)

Osmotic laxatives have a similar mechanism of action to bulk-forming laxatives in that they also soften the stool. However, they differ in how they achieve this. Osmotic laxatives depend upon their osmotic pull to attract water from the intestinal wall, causing the intestinal lumen to swell up and expand. All osmotic laxatives are largely insoluble, so they do not traverse the intestinal wall.

Saline-laxatives consist of a small group of insoluble sulphate salts commonly including NaSO4 (Glauber's salts) and MgSO4 (Epsom salts). These salts exert an osmotic pull, drawing water from the intestine, leading to a stretch-induced increase in peristalsis (Fig. 11.2).

Poorly absorbed sugars (alcohol laxatives) include substances such as mannitol and sorbitol, both of which do not permeate the intestinal wall appreciably and, therefore, draw fluid from the intestinal wall into its lumen.

Lactulose is one of the most commonly used laxatives in clinical practice. However, there is limited evidence to demonstrate its efficacy over alternate osmotic laxatives and placebo in children (Gordon et al. 2012), with fewer if any, studies evaluating its efficacy and safety in adults (Ruston et al. 2013; Alsalimy et al. 2018). It is a disaccharide sugar that is not absorbed into the intestinal wall. In addition to its apparent clinical benefit, acids generated by bacterial fermentation of lactulose in the intestine acidify the intestinal contents (Sahota et al. 1982). The consequent reduction in intestinal pH reduces bacterial-derived formation of ammonia from ammonium. The decreased ammonia may reduce the risk of hepatic encephalopathy (Nath et al. 2018).

Polyethylene glycol, macrogol, is commonly used osmotic laxative in clinical practice, for example, Movicol®. Although not as commonly used as lactulose in clinical practice, there is growing evidence to suggest that together with the stimulant Senna there is benefit of using macrogol in chronic constipation (Rao and

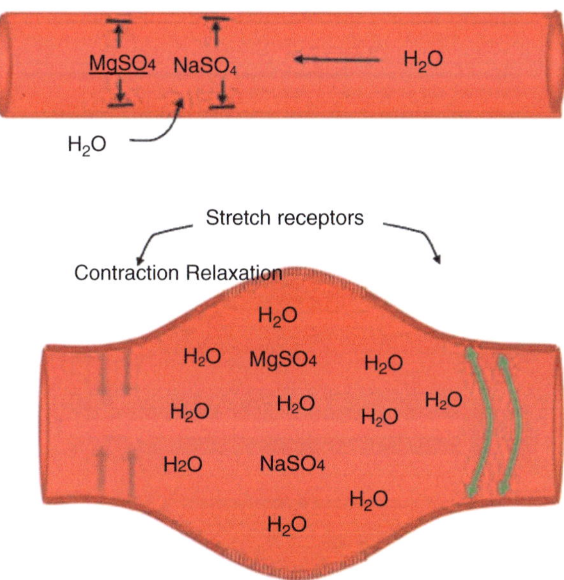

Fig. 11.2 Osmotic laxatives (saline laxatives)

Brenner 2021) as well as being effective in children compared to other commonly used laxatives such as lactulose (Gordon et al. 2012; Southwell 2020).

General Cautions When Using Osmotic Laxatives

Although these medications are relatively safe, sodium-containing Glauber's salts should be given with caution in heart failure owing to the potential of adding to the patient's sodium and, consequently, fluid load. Similarly, Epsom salts should not be taken if the patient has renal dysfunction, as their use may lead to hypermagnesemia.

Sugar-based laxatives such as sorbitol and lactulose are not associated with any risk of plasma glucose elevation in diabetes as the medication is not absorbed by the intestine. There is, however, limited potential for lactulose to cause an acid-related insult to a person's teeth as oral bacteria are capable of fermenting lactulose to release small amounts of acid with regular use of the medication (Moynihan et al. 1998).

11.2.4.3 Bi-modal Laxatives (Stimulant Laxatives)

These laxatives were traditionally known as stimulant laxatives as their main mode of action was by stimulating or irritating intestinal smooth muscle, which led to an increase in peristalsis (Fig. 11.3). However, these laxatives possess other characteristics that contribute towards their effect. The main secondary effect includes an anti-absorptive function. Water passage through the colon's epithelium is promoted by the introduction of small water channels known as aquaporins (Fig. 11.3). In this respect this terminal section of the GI tract functions similarly to the terminal section of the nephron, the collecting duct, where under the influence of anti-diuretic hormone (ADH) aquaporins are inserted into the collecting duct epithelium, thus facilitating the movement of water from the collecting duct lumen back into the

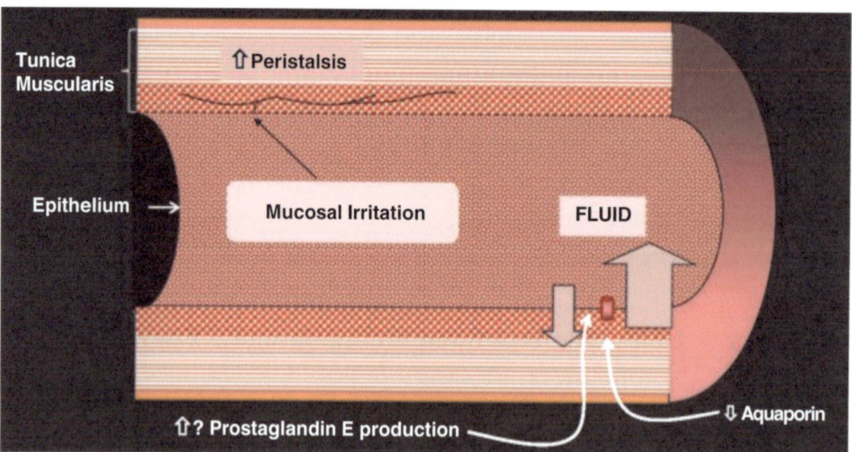

Fig. 11.3 Mechanism of action of stimulants or bi-modal laxatives

blood stream. As a consequence, the fluid volume of urine is reduced and it becomes concentrated, similar to the function of the colon is to reabsorb water from faeces. The anti-absorptive property of these laxatives relates to their ability to limit absorption of fluid from the intestinal lumen by limiting the number of aquaporin's in the intestinal wall, thus keeping the intestinal contents soft (Fig. 11.3). Two commonly used laxatives associated with two different drug classes belong to this bi-modal group of laxatives; these are bisacodyl and senna.

Bisacodyl

Bisacodyl belongs to a family of medications known as the diphenyl methanes. As suggested their main function is to stimulate peristalsis by irritating nerves found between the muscle layers in the colon. Bisacodyl reduces water reabsorption by inhibiting the colon's ability to dehydrate the stool. This is achieved by a bisacodyl-derived increase of prostaglandin E2 (PGE2) that has the effect of reducing aquaporin population in colonic epithelium (Ikarashi et al. 2011). A reduction in colonic aquaporins results in a reduction of water reabsorption from the colon allowing water to remain in a stool, consequently keeping it soft and enhancing its propulsion.

Senna

Senna belongs to a group of drugs known as the anthraquinones. These drugs are one of the most ancient remedies for constipation and were originally extracted from the *Senna alexandrina* plant. Similar to bisacodyl, the senna extract or senna glycosides have a direct effect on gastric motility as well as having an effect on intestinal fluid secretion. The mechanism by which this happens appears to be similar, at least in principle, to that of bisacodyl, as senna also stimulates the release of prostaglandin E following immune cell interaction with colonic epithelium (Geboes et al. 1993). As with bisacodyl, released prostaglandin E should reduce the intestinal aquaporin population, leading to increased water retention in the intestine and a softer stool.

11.2.5 Laxative Dependence: The Myth?

The presence of laxative dependence is based upon the premise that laxatives empty the entire colon, unlike normal defaecation, which only empties the descending colon (Fig. 11.4). Once laxative-induced defaecation occurs, the person would need to wait for a number of days or even a week before the colon has distended enough to initiate defaecation. This period of waiting is uncharacteristic of the person's normal defaecation pattern and if not informed, the individual may take another dose of laxative before the colon is properly filled to instigate defaecation. It was thought that both osmotic and stimulant laxatives lead to a loss of electrolytes, particularly potassium. This is because fluid loss-related dehydration stimulates the kidney to conserve water because of aldosterone secretion; this is achieved at the expense of losing potassium. Water loss further contributes to the loss of potassium via the laxative-related semi-fluid faeces. It was thought that such potassium loss

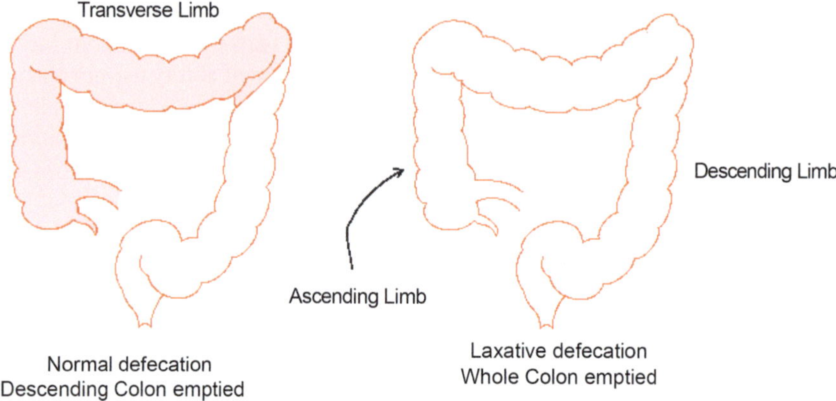

Fig. 11.4 Laxative-derived emptying of the colon. (The empty colon takes 24–48 h to fill; in that time, the patient thinks they are constipated again, as they do not defecate, and subsequently take more laxatives, which leads to expulsion of material from the ascending and transverse colon, leading to a vicious cycle of laxative use)

led to weak peristalsis potentiating further constipation (Fig. 11.5). There is some anecdotal merit to this theory in that Movicol® (PEG + electrolytes, including K^+) is more effective at reducing recurrence of constipation than many other non-electrolyte-containing laxatives, suggesting that replenishment of electrolytes does improve gastric motility and/or defaecation.

Together, these two mechanisms (Figs. 11.4 and 11.5) have popularised the concept of laxative dependence. This adverse effect is still being evaluated (Guijarro et al. 2010). However, scrutiny of data challenges the presence of this phenomenon (Leung et al. 2011; Krammer et al. 2014), suggesting that with patient education and titration of dose, dependence does not develop.

11.2.6 Implications for Clinical Practice

Constipation is common in older age (Barberio et al. 2021). It is important before initiating treatment to ascertain the form of constipation, that is, slow transit or pelvic floor dysfunction, as this will direct the appropriate choice of therapy/medication. This assessment should be followed by a monitoring and evaluation process to help optimise the laxative treatment. Patient education regarding laxative-derived altered bowel habits is appropriate to reduce the risk of laxative abuse. It appears that laxatives such as Movicol® that contain electrolytes are associated with improved outcomes. Although relatively safe, some laxatives, particularly those of the osmotic group, need to be taken with due consideration of co-morbidities such as heart and renal dysfunction.

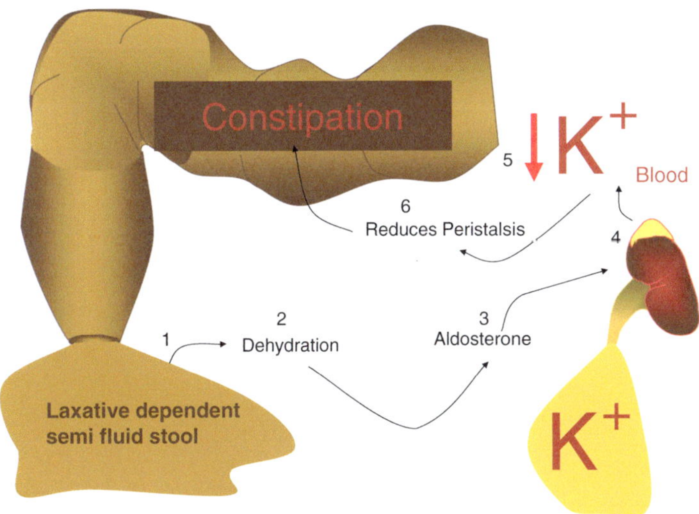

Fig. 11.5 Laxative-derived constipation

11.2.7 Summary

- Constipation may occur because of slow gut transit time and or pelvic floor dysfunction.
- Biofeedback therapy is the recommended therapy for pelvic floor dysfunction and chronic constipation.
- Bulk-forming, osmotic and stimulant laxatives are the main treatment for slow transit constipation in well-hydrated patients. As most laxatives possess a degree of osmotic effect, their use in a dehydrated patient may aggravate the patient's condition further.
- Laxative dependence may be an outcome of poor bowel management requiring focused management of the patient with pharmacotherapy.

11.3   Antacids, Histamine-2 Receptor Antagonists (H2RA) and Proton Pump Inhibitors (PPIs)

The stomach epithelium contains parietal cells that secrete hydrochloric acid (HCl) in response to a number of stimuli, including the hormones, histamine, gastrin and the neurotransmitter acetylcholine (Fig. 11.6). Acid has a number of functions in the stomach. It assists in the metabolism of protein by activating the proteolytic enzyme pepsin, which needs a low pH (1–2) for maximal activity. Acid also acts as an anti-bacterial agent and sterilises the contents of the stomach.

To protect the gut epithelium, the gastric pit (Fig. 11.6) possesses two mucous-secreting cells: the surface and neck mucous-secreting cells that cover the surface of the stomach with a thick tenacious mucous that acts as a barrier between the

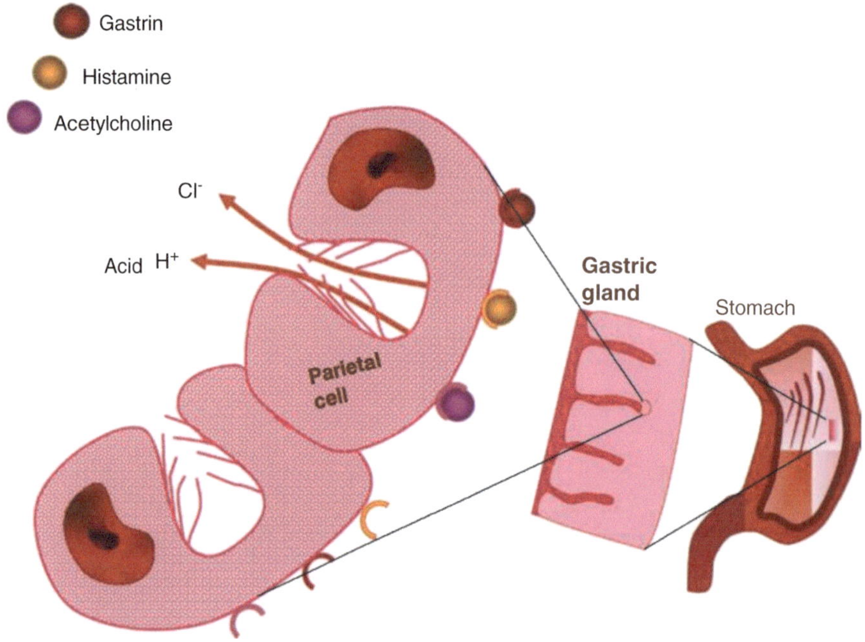

Fig. 11.6 Gastric acid secretion

stomach's HCl and the delicate stomach wall. Mucous secretion and blood flow to the stomach epithelium are regulated by a number of mechanisms, of which the cyclo-oxygenase 1 enzyme (COX1) is of particular importance. This enzyme, in addition to maintaining epithelial blood flow and mucous secretion, limits HCl secretion; the COX1 enzyme is inhibited by non-steroidal anti-inflammatory medications, resulting in an inhibition of the beneficial effects of the COX1 enzyme in the stomach. This leads to a reduction in epithelial blood flow and a reduction in mucus secretion together with a dis-inhibition of HCl secretion. Together, these effects increase the risk of ulceration of the gastric mucosa.

11.3.1 Pathologies That Require a Reduction in Gastric Acid

Under certain conditions, the delicate stomach epithelium can be exposed to gastric HCl. Such situations include peptic ulcers or ulcerations of the stomach epithelium that are caused by a number of factors, the most important of which includes the bacteria *Helicobacter pylori* and the continuous use of non-steroidal anti-inflammatory medications.

Normally acid does not travel to the oesophagus; however, with gastro-oesophageal reflux disease (GORD) acid does enter the oesophagus where it may cause temporary or permanent mucosal damage. Likewise, mild indigestion or dyspepsia may also be associated with abnormal acid secretion in the stomach.

11.3.2 Antacids

Antacids are the simplest pharmacological solution to remedy an increase in gastric acid. Antacids utilise the acid–base equation to neutralise acid in the stomach; this is why they are also known as acid neutralisers.

Most 'over-the-counter' (OTC) indigestion remedies include antacids in their active ingredients. They work on the basic principle that when you mix an acid with a base, a salt is formed. The base tends to be a form of metal base, including aluminium (Alka-Seltzer®), magnesium (Milk of Magnesia), sodium (Enos®, Gaviscon®) or calcium (Gaviscon®). When these combine with gastric HCl, they form the corresponding metal chloride salt, for example, $MgCl_2$, $AlCl_3$ or $CaCl_2$, thus neutralising the gastric acid. Some antacids also have additional ingredients to help contain the acidic gastric contents; this is useful with GORD where gastric contents will be propelled up into the oesophagus. Gaviscon®, for example, has an alginate that covers the surface of the gastric contents; if any content impacts the oesophageal wall, the particles are coated with the alginate base mix so even if the acid is not completely neutralised, the alginate acts as a physical barrier between the gastric contents and the oesophageal wall.

Given antacids' popularity, it is interesting to find there is evidence to suggest that antacids are little better than a placebo in effect (Talley and Vakil 2005; Leiman et al. 2017). However, use of the double-action preparations that contain an alginate together with an antacid seems to be superior to placebo and antacid monotherapies (De Ruigh et al. 2014; Thomas et al. 2014.

11.3.2.1 Antacid–Drug Interactions

Although now infrequently prescribed owing to more effective drugs such H2 receptor antagonists and proton pump inhibitors, the availability of antacids 'over-the-counter' together with the increase in combination therapies has perpetuated the use of these medications. On their own, they are relatively safe; however, when used in combination, they can cause some significant drug–drug interactions that may be of clinical consequence. Owing to the metallic nature of their ingredients, they readily bind other substances, a process known as chelation. These chelated complexes cannot be absorbed and, therefore, the bioavailability of medication is reduced, potentially reducing or removing the effect of the chelated medication. Importantly, some drugs that require stable plasma drug levels for their therapeutic effect, such as antibiotics, are known to be chelated by antacids; this includes antibiotics such as tetracyclines and fluoroquinones (ciprofloxacin) (Del Rosso 2009; Ogawa and Echizen 2011). Similarly, anti-tuberculosis drugs isoniazid, rifampicin and ethambutol, but not pyrazinamide, have been reported to be influenced by antacids either because of chelation or delay in absorption (Arbex et al. 2010). The simplest solution to reduce the risk of chelation if antacids are needed is to separate the administration of these medications by at least 30–60 min (Arbex et al. 2010; Ogawa and Echizen 2011).

11.3.2.2 Clinical Implications of the Use of Antacids

It is important that a detailed medication history, including self-administered 'over-the-counter' medications, is obtained from the patient before prescribing antacids. Special mention should be made of the use of antacids, particularly when patients are to commence antibiotics or other drugs with crucial drug levels such as digoxin. Given the unclear benefit of single-action antacids, repetitive use of them may be futile, necessitating the patient to seek an alternative acid-reducing therapy, or they may require further specialist assessment. It should be ensured that when necessary, an antacid should not be administered at the same time as an oral antibiotic. If unsure of the risk of chelation, refer to the pharmacist, who will be able to verify any interactions. It is important to educate the patient regarding the risk of chelation interactions so that they do not increase the risk of this occurring. In addition to chelation, sodium-containing antacids such as those containing sodium bicarbonate may cause a rise in plasma sodium levels; this may aggravate underlying cardiovascular disease, such as hypertension or heart failure.

Other specific adverse reactions of antacids may include the following:

- Diarrhoea (MgSO4) (Milk of Magnesia)
- Formation of renal stones (long-term use with some silicone-containing antacids)
- Constipation (Al(OH)3) (Alka Seltzer®)
- Metabolic alkalosis (NaHCO3 containing antacids)

11.3.3 Proton Pump Inhibitors

Hydrogen ions (H^+) contain only a positive charge owing to the presence of one proton in their nucleus, as they are devoid of negatively charged electrons; for this reason, ionic hydrogen may also be referred to as a proton. Proton pump inhibitors (PPIs) inhibit the pumping of H^+ (protons) from the parietal cells into the gastric lumen (Fig. 11.7). This effectively reduces the $[H^+]$ concentration, causing the acidity of the gastric contents to diminish, that is, increase the pH in the stomach to a more alkaline value.

Proton pump inhibitors, pantoprazole and omeprazole, are now the drug of choice to treat GORD and its associated oesophagitis. A meta-analysis of two proton pump inhibitors, esomeprazole and omeprazole, found that esomeprazole demonstrated superiority over omeprazole in oesophageal healing at week 8 of treatment (Teng et al. 2015).

11.3.3.1 Drug–Drug Interactions with Proton Pump Inhibitors

Having been widely used for nearly three decades a number of PPI adverse effects have been recorded. These interactions are derived from two aspects of the drugs' pharmacokinetic profile. The first factor associated with PPIs is their ability to effectively raise the pH of the stomach. The second reason to expect interactions with PPIs and with omeprazole, in particular, is that omeprazole has a high affinity for the 2C19 isoform of the phase 1 enzyme cytochrome P450 (CYP) (Wedemeyer

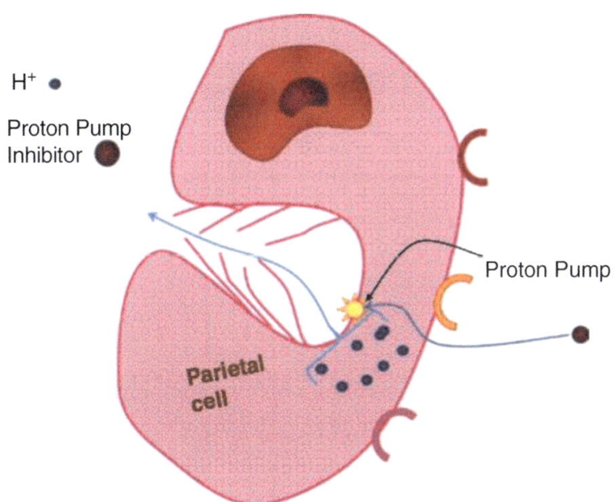

Fig. 11.7 Proton pump Inhibitors

and Blume 2014) and a moderate interaction with CYP3A4 (Chap. 2 for details). CYP3A4-interacting medications also frequently interact with drug efflux pumps such as P-glycoprotein, further potentiating their risk of drug–drug interactions resulting in a change in drug plasma levels.

The use of gastric pH-increasing drugs such as omeprazole with anti-retroviral drugs such as rilpivirine has demonstrated reduced drug absorption, potentially reducing the anti-viral effect of the medication (Crauwels et al. 2013). Although not a drug–drug interaction, one of the benefits of a low pH in the stomach is destroying bacteria; use of PPIs has demonstrated that a rise in pH above 4 in the stomach is associated with an increased survival of GI bacteria, including *Clostridium difficile* (Mezoff and Cohen 2013).

In relation to CYPs, interactions between omeprazole and commonly prescribed medications may occur, including diazepam, phenytoin and clopidogrel (Ogawa and Echizen 2010; Wang et al. 2015). Based upon CYP2C19 interactions, general class interactions with omeprazole and many other PPIs include benzodiazepines and selective serotonin reuptake inhibitors (including fluoxetine) may occur.

This data demands the need for pharmacovigilance in patients who have polypharmacy. Changes to drug regimens and sudden alteration of liver or kidney function may further destabilise an otherwise stable drug regimen.

11.3.4 Histamine-2 Receptor Antagonists

The histamine-2 (H2) receptors on gastric parietal cells stimulate the proton pump to liberate H⁺ into the gastric lumen. H2 receptor antagonists (H2RAs) effectively reduce H⁺ concentration in the stomach, increasing stomach pH, consequently alleviating acidity-related symptoms and disease (Fig. 11.8). H2RAs have typically been replaced by PPIs owing to the overall better outcomes associated with this medication group (Nagahara et al. 2010).

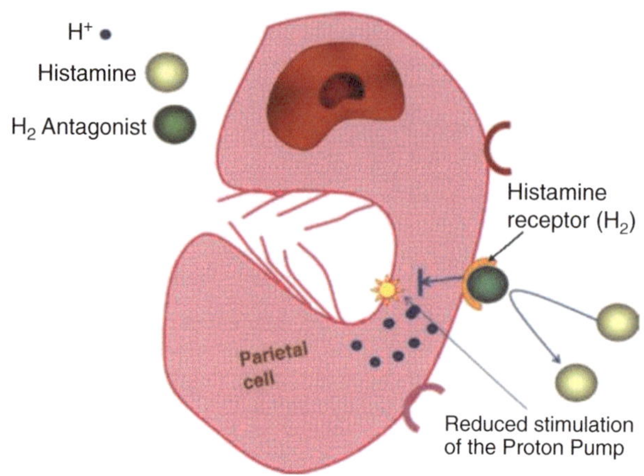

Fig. 11.8 Histamine (H2) receptor antagonists

11.3.4.1 Histamine-2 Receptor Antagonists and QT Prolongation

Another reason for the reduced use of histamine-2 receptor antagonist arises from their perceived ability to prolong the QT interval (LQT) on the electrocardiograph. A drug-induced prolongation of this electrocardiogram measurement is pro-arrhythmic and may lead to Torsade de Pointes (TdP), a potentially fatal form of ventricular tachycardia (Spears and Gollob 2015). The prototype anti-histamine, terfenadine (Seldane®), was discontinued because of this interaction. There are a number of websites that compile up-to-date lists of medications that are known to or may cause TdP, for example, https://www.crediblemeds.org/index.php/login/dlcheck. According to this site, there are currently no listed H2 receptor antagonists that have a published known risk of TdP. However, famotidine has been listed as a medication with a potential risk to cause TdP under certain conditions, such as renal dysfunction, electrolyte imbalance and concomitant administration of other QT pro-longing drug. Similarly, cimetidine has also been added to the conditional risk list. Commonly used ranitidine (Zantac®) has no recent reports of use associated with arrhythmia (database accessed 03–2025), other than in a neonate who had congenital long QT syndrome, a genetic disposition to have a prolonged QT interval (Alliët and Devos 1994).

11.3.5 General Adverse Effects of Proton Pump Inhibitors and Histamine-2 Receptor Antagonists

A number of specific adverse effects and contraindications for proton pump inhibitors and histamine-2 receptor antagonists have been discussed. Owing to many of these effects being related to pharmacokinetic issues, pharmacokinetic parameters for omeprazole and ranitidine are provided (Table 11.1). A list of generic adverse reactions is given in Table 11.2.

Table 11.1 Pharmacokinetic parameters

	Omeprazole	Ranitidine
Metabolism	Hepatic (CYP2C19, 3A4)	Hepatic (CYP1A2; CYP2C19; CYP2D6)
Half life	1–1.2 h	2–3 h
Excretion	Renal 80%	30–70% renal

Table 11.2 Adverse effects

Omeprazole	Ranitidine
Diarrhoea	Diarrhoea
Constipation	Liver impairment
Flatulence	Abnormal heart rhythms
Nausea and vomiting	Blood disorders
Hypersensitivity reaction	Hallucinations in the very old and very ill
Blood disorders	

11.3.6 Clinical Implications for Practice

Proton pump inhibitors are commonly prescribed medications and are available 'over-the-counter'. They are also frequently prescribed for persistent indigestion and as an adjunct to NSAID usage, together with more specific use in gastro-oesophageal reflux disease (GORD) and its associated pathologies. This use requires that healthcare professionals be cognisant of their mechanism of action and potential risk to generate adverse effects and the potential to modulate the effect of co-administered medications. Unlike antacids, PPI or H2RA administration may not be usefully segregated from other medications. Consequences of a pH increase in relation to concomitant drug absorption need to be factored into prescribing. Metabolism enzyme-related drug–drug interactions need to be considered on altering the prescription of medications and the pharmacist needs to be consulted regarding the potential for interactions. Importantly, patient education is significant with these drugs, in relation to monitoring for adverse effects. As both omeprazole and ranitidine are available as 'over–the-counter' purchases, it is important to verify whether patients are taking these medications, as the presence of these drugs may alter further prescribing. Similarly, occasional use of these medications, prescribed or otherwise, may also influence drug concentrations of other medications, particularly with polypharmacy.

11.4   Anti-emetics

There are a large number of anti-emetics available that employ a plethora of mechanisms resulting in a variety of associated adverse effects. The main effects of these drugs, regardless of their use, are to maintain an anterograde peristaltic movement (prokinetic) and to limit the retrograde movement of GI tract contents. The effects the drugs have may be central (CNS) or local. To help categorise the drug's action, their effects and adverse effects, Table 11.3 provides an overview of commonly used anti-emetics in clinical practice.

11.4.1 Physiology of Nausea and Vomiting

Although associated with pathological circumstances, nausea and vomiting are primarily a physiological response that protects the body from harm. Nausea and vomiting are generated by a multitude of conditions and disturbances in the body. These stimuli congregate in two areas in the brain stem: the chemoreceptor trigger zone (area postrema) and the emetic centre, which encompasses the nucleus tractus solitarius.

11.4.1.1 Chemoreceptor Trigger Zone

The chemoreceptor trigger zone (CTZ), as the name suggests, responds to chemicals. The CTZ is a bilateral set of nerve nuclei located just below the terminal point of the fourth ventricle (Fig. 11.9). Unlike most areas in the brain, blood vessels that supply this structure are devoid of blood-brain barrier (BBB) properties. Subsequently, substances that would otherwise not be able to enter the brain, such as dopamine, have access to nerves in the CTZ. This feature enables the CTZ to continuously monitor the bloodstream for noxious substances. Substances that may influence the CTZ may be blood-borne toxins that have been ingested or accumulated in the bloodstream owing to impaired excretion as seen in uraemia.

Table 11.3 Antiemetic

Drug	Target	Structures	Effective in N&V caused by
Ondansetron	5-HT3	Emetic Centre, CTZ, peripheral (intestinal and spinal)	Some emetogenic cytotoxic drugs Post radiation and post-operative
Metoclopramide	D2 antagonist 5-HT3, 5-HT4	CTZ Crosses the BBB	GI disturbances, chemical toxins radiation Migraines Pregnancy Post-operative
Domperidone	D2 Antagonist 5-HT3	CTZ Does not cross the BBB	Similar to metoclopramide
Cyclizine	H1, M1	Emetic Centre CTZ, vestibular apparatus	Motion sickness Opioid nausea Post operative
Diphenhydramine	H1, M1		Motion sickness
Hyoscine	M1		Motion sickness Post operative

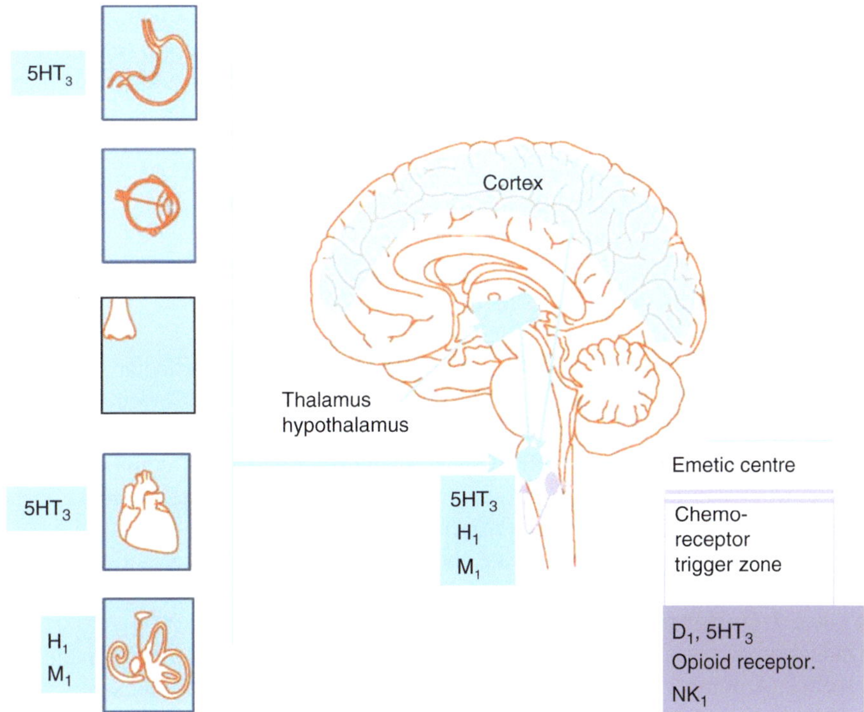

Fig. 11.9 Inputs for the emetic centre

Pregnancy causes nausea and vomiting by the release of cytokines and prostaglandins in areas linked to emesis (Zhong et al. 2021); hypoxia and diabetic ketoacidosis also influence the CTZ. Opioids and chemotherapies act on the CTZ.

11.4.1.2 The Emetic Centre

The emetic centre is a group of nerves that receives input from a number of areas (Fig. 11.9), of which the CTZ exerts considerable influence. The other main areas that directly influence the emetic centre include the GI tract via both vagal and sympathetic nerve inputs. Other important organs that stimulate the emetic centre include the heart, liver and bile duct. Significant sensory inputs are received by the emetic centre, including both olfactory and visual stimuli; together with these sensory stimuli, the vestibular apparatus stimulates the emetic centre, forming the basis for motion sickness.

Emetic centre stimulation by the cerebral cortex is associated with the generation of nausea from fear and anxiety. Finally, the thalamus and hypothalamus, the neurohumoral homeostatic centres of the brain, also stimulate the emetic centre. Outputs from the emetic centre are complicated and are largely conveyed by the reticular formation. This is a network of nerves that arises from the brain stem and has widespread connections to many parts of the brain, including significant pathways to the cortex, particularly to the motor and premotor areas.

A number of receptors are associated with the aforementioned structures and organs, the majority of which include serotonin (5-HT), cholinergic (muscarinic) and histamine (H1) receptors. The subtle exception to these is the additional receptors found in the CTZ which include the D2 dopamine receptor subtype, neurokinin (NK1) receptors that bind the pain neuro-peptide, substance P and a range of opioid receptors. Owing to their prevalence in either the emetic centre or CTZ, these receptors are potential drug targets for anti-emetic medications.

11.4.2 Anti-emetic Medications

Use of an anti-emetic is determined by its effectiveness for a particular pathology and the adverse effect profile of the drug. The benefit of anti-emetics varies significantly from condition to condition, given the significant but, in most instances, infrequent reports of adverse effects. In this context, a number of commonly used anti-emetics will be examined in relation to their main targets and adverse effects profile to help understand the preference for an anti-emetic over another in a particular situation to ensure appropriate choice and monitoring of medication.

11.4.2.1 Ondansetron

Ondansetron is a selective 5-HT3 receptor antagonist and is used widely in clinical practice. A number of studies have demonstrated its effectiveness and safety with children, particularly with adjuncts such as dexamethasone or neurokinin 1 (NK1) receptor antagonists (Kang et al. 2015; Shen et al. 2015). Studies focused upon pregnant women have found that ondansetron is effective and safe after the first trimester (Niebyl and Briggs 2014). Use of ondansetron in pregnancy is not associated with significant birth defects, including heart defects (Huybrechts et al. 2018; Kaplan et al. 2019). Generally, Ondansetron is an effective anti-emetic and safe, although a meta-analysis demonstrated it can reduce the effects of analgesics, such as tramadol (Christofaki and Papaioannou 2015; Onifer et al. 2015; Stevens et al. 2015). In general, ondansetron has a high first-pass metabolism resulting in bioavailability of approximately 60%. Administration of antacids does not affect its absorption and peak drug concentration is reached between 0.5 and 2 h. Ondansetron is moderately plasma bound (70–76%) and has a half-life of 3.8 ± 1 h (Roila and Del Favero 1995). Like many other drugs, the pharmacokinetics of this medication is also influenced by genetic variation, typically of the highly polymorphic CYP 2D6 that causes individual variations in drug response and clearance (Farhat et al. 2015; Moore et al. 2025).

11.4.2.2 Metoclopramide

Metoclopramide is a mixed-effect anti-emetic having both strong dopaminergic and serotonergic effects. Serotonergic effects are mediated via two receptor interactions: 5-HT3 (antagonist) and 5-HT4 (agonist). 5-HT4 receptors in the GI tract enhance peristalsis; therefore, the agonistic effect of metoclopramide on this receptor elicits the prokinetic effect of the drug. Unlike other anti-emetics that have D2 receptor antagonistic interactions, metoclopramide can cross the blood-brain barrier, owing to which this drug is associated with considerable dopamine-related adverse effects, most important of which are extrapyramidal effects that generate Parkinsonian-like tremors in patients. This medication can be used in the second and third trimester of pregnancy (Niebyl and Briggs 2014) and has been shown to be effective in reducing nausea and vomiting post lower segment caesarean section birth in women who underwent regional anaesthesia (neuraxial anaesthesia) (Mishriky and Habib 2012). Owing to its effects on the CTZ, it is also an effective remedy for toxin- and uraemia-related nausea as well as vomiting related to GI disturbances such as gastroenteritis and GORD.

11.4.2.3 Domperidone

Similar to metoclopramide, domperidone is primarily a D2 receptor antagonist, which also has 5-HT receptor activity, leading to a prokinetic effect. Unlike metoclopramide, domperidone does not cross the BBB; therefore, its central nervous system effects, other than those on the BBB-devoid CTZ, are minimal. Domperidone has been associated with a risk of QT prolongation; therefore, it is suggested that this drug should not be administered to those with a known QT prolongation or at risk of generating a QT prolongation (Doggrell and Hancox 2014). Although the risk may be limited in healthy adults (Buffery and Strother 2015), those at risk may include people with cardiac disease, including those with a history of myocardial infarction or those with heart failure. In addition, if the patient has an electrolyte imbalance and or is receiving medications that prolong the QT interval, administering domperidone may exacerbate QT prolongation (Makari et al. 2014; Ehrenpreis et al. 2017). In this respect, assessment for the potential of pharmacokinetic drug interactions is important; drugs that are CYP3A4 metabolised may potentiate the QT-prolonging potential of domperidone. When being prescribed domperidone, assessment of the QT interval at appropriate times may also be considered in patients at risk of QT prolongation.

11.4.2.4 Cyclizine

Cyclizine is an anti-histamine anti-emetic with some anti-cholinergic function; it has an effect on the emetic centre as well as the CTZ. Cyclizine is one of a limited number of anti-emetics that has a significant effect on elements of the vestibular apparatus; as such, this anti-emetic has the potential to alleviate motion sickness, which is one of its main indications for use. Cyclizine is used widely in clinical practice, including palliative care (Vella-Brincat et al. 2012). In relation to its safety profile, there have been reports of it being associated with abuse and suicide (Bailey and Davies 2008; Arnestad et al. 2014; Hatting and Hansen 2017). Effects of cyclizine on cardiac function have also been explored in respect to its potential to cause QT-related arrhythmias and its general effect on cardiac function in states of heart disease. Risk of QT-related arrhythmias has been found for cyclizine (Poluzzi et al. 2015, 2017). There is also evidence (albeit limited) to suggest cyclizine may adversely affect blood pressure, leading May and Kumar (2006) to suggest that this anti-histamine should not be prescribed for people with ischemic heart disease.

Cyclizine prescription is contraindicated in patients who are hypersensitive to the drug and its excipients, in severe liver failure and porphyria. Caution should be exercised when prescribing and administering this drug in patients with urinary retention, glaucoma and pyloroduodenal obstruction, people who have epilepsy or are prone to seizures, and those who have a pheochromocytoma (BNF 2022).

The phase 1 CYP2D6 enzyme is thought to be involved in the metabolism of cyclizine (Vella-Brincat et al. 2012). This is clinically significant because there is genetic variation in how ethnic populations express this enzyme, with poor metabolism being the highest in Caucasians (8%) (Roberts et al. 2002). This information is useful in clinical practice when dealing with polypharmacy. Patients taking other medications such as the anti-depressant venlafaxine demonstrate an age-dependent (>65) drug serum elevation if they are poor CYP2D6 metabolisers (Waade et al. 2014). This pharmacokinetic profile increases the risk of drug–drug interactions in a polypharmacy regimen.

11.4.2.5 Diphenhydramine

Similar to cyclizine, diphenhydramine (Benadryl®) is an H1 antagonist with some central anti-cholinergic effect. This anti-histamine also has a similar pharmacodynamic effect with similar benefits in motion sickness. Owing to its ability to cross the BBB, this medication has a number of central effects related to both its anti-histamine as well as anti-cholinergic actions. Drowsiness is a significant histamine-related effect which enables the medication to be used as a hypnotic, whereas the anti-cholinergic effect of this medication is harnessed in counteracting the anti-Parkinson effects of anti-psychotic medications.

Diphenhydramine has been associated with a risk of causing QT-related cardiac arrhythmias (Poluzzi et al. 2015; Shi et al. 2015). There is also growing evidence of abuse of this 'over-the-counter' medication (Erbe and Bschor 2013). This medication has been linked with other forensic events, such as suicide and drug overdose in combination with other drugs. Botch-Jones et al. (2014), suggesting this medication needs to be monitored and assessed in a drug history. As yet, the evidence is limited, but given its potential for abuse and its associated adverse effect profile, the future of this medication in clinical practice is unclear.

11.4.2.6 Hyoscine

Hyoscine (scopolamine) has limited use as an anti-emetic. In the community, per se, it is licensed primarily as a remedy for travel sickness.

Being a primarily anti-cholinergic preparation, its main adverse effect is a dry mouth. Hyoscine may also cause disturbances with vision, including blurred vision and difficulty in accommodating, as parasympathetic nerve tone causes pupil constriction. Other significant adverse effects of this drug are associated with a reduction of the inhibitory parasympathetic effect on the heart, resulting in tachycardia. This medication has a traditional pharmacokinetic profile with hepatic metabolism and renal clearance and a half-life of 4 h.

11.4.3 Summary and Implications for Clinical Practice

A number of anti-emetics are available; their efficacy in particular forms of nausea is dependent upon their location of function. In general, drugs effective on the CTZ including the two D2 receptor antagonists (domperidone and metoclopramide), are effective on blood-borne toxins, whereas 5-HT receptor antagonists, such as ondansetron are effective in emetogenic events associated with chemotherapy. Anti-emetics containing antihistamines are effective in motion sickness and opioid-related nausea and vomiting. Anti-cholinergic anti-emetics are effective in motion sickness, with diphenhydramine being more suited to long journeys and hyoscine for shorter ones, unless used as a transdermal patch.

Adverse effect profiles limit the use of some anti-emetics long term. Of note are the anti-Parkinson-like effects of metoclopramide and the QT prolongation potential of histamine antagonists and domperidone. Data presented suggests that QT-related adverse effects of medications are related to age and polypharmacy (Khan 2010). Also, the female gender is suggested to be an independent risk factor for QT prolongation (Li et al. 2013). Females are also more prone to drug-adverse reactions (Gochfeld 2017). Together, this suggests female patients must be carefully assessed before prescribing medication that may prolong the QT interval.

11.5 Summary

This chapter has examined a number of drug classes that affect gastrointestinal function. The varied pharmacodynamic mechanisms of laxatives and their osmotic effects are emphasised. It is important to remember that when taking these medications the patient must be well hydrated.

Antacids and other medications that increase gastric pH, such as histamine receptor antagonists and proton pump inhibitors, are an effective measure to reduce stomach acid. Different forms are associated with different adverse effects, many of which are associated with the risk of drug–drug interactions. Therefore, when taking a patient history, note should be taken if they are currently receiving such medications. Antacids and laxatives should not be taken at the same time as other medicines. If co-administration is required, a pharmacist should be consulted to ensure there is no potential for these drugs to alter the absorption of any other medication.

Anti-emetics act on pathways in the emetic centre, the chemoreceptor trigger zone and associated brain structures. Specific anti-emetics act on particular nerve pathways, leading to specific effects for individual medications. Drowsiness is a significant adverse effect that determines the choice of the prescribed anti-emetic. Other salient factors that need to be considered when prescribing an anti-emetic include the potential effects in the first trimester of pregnancy and the possible effect on cardiac function.

Multiple Choice Questions

1. Laxatives may lead to a number of biochemical abnormalities. Select one abnormality that may be aggravated by a bulk forming laxative:
   (a) Dehydration
   (b) Hyperkalaemia
   (c) Oedema
   (d) Hypoglycaemia
2. Most laxatives depend upon this principle for their action:
   (a) Mucosal irritation
   (b) Receptor antagonism
   (c) Osmosis
   (d) Sympathetic agonism
3. Some laxatives share this effect with some antacids:
   (a) Dehydration
   (b) Chelation
   (c) Acidosis
   (d) Muscle fatigue
4. Proper laxative dose titration and patient hydration can reduce the risk of:
   (a) Constipation
   (b) Urinary retention
   (c) Laxative dependence
   (d) Laxative tolerance
5. Which form of substance added to antacids neutralises stomach acid?
   (a) Salt
   (b) Base
   (c) Lipophilic solution
   (d) Milk
6. Antacids are commonly known to bind with which form of medication and reduce its absorption from the intestine?
   (a) Calcium channel blockers
   (b) Beta-blockers
   (c) Broncho-dilators
   (d) Antibiotics
7. Proton pump inhibitors block the transport of which ion into the gastric lumen?
   (a) K^+
   (b) Na^+
   (c) Cl^-
   (d) H^+
8. Medications such as omeprazole should be monitored for drug–drug interactions because they are:
   (a) Strongly plasma-bound
   (b) Nephrotoxic
   (c) Metabolised by CYP3A4
   (d) Hydrophilic

9. Some anti-histamine anti-emetics may increase the risk of which adverse effect?
    (a) Headache
    (b) Urinary retention
    (c) QT prolongation
    (d) Insomnia
10. The action of cyclizine on these structures enables it to alleviate motion sickness:
    (a) Eye and nose
    (b) Basal ganglia
    (c) Visual cortices
    (d) Vestibular organs
11. In which trimester of pregnancy are most anti-emetics contraindicated?
    (a) First
    (b) Second
    (c) Third
    (d) None
12. Domperidone and metoclopramide both work on which receptor for their main anti-emetic function?
    (a) Cholinergic
    (b) Serotonin
    (c) Dopamine
    (d) NK1z

Answers

1. (a)
2. (c)
3. (b)
4. (c)
5. (b)
6. (d)
7. (d)
8. (c)
9. (c)
10. (d)
11. (a)
12. (c)

References

Alliët P, Devos E (1994) Ranitidine-induced bradycardia in a neonate—secondary to congenital long QT interval syndrome? Eur J Pediatr 153(10):781

Alsalimy N, Madi L, Awaisu A (2018) Efficacy and safety of laxatives for chronic constipation in long-term care settings: a systematic review. J Clin Pharm Ther 43(5):595–605

Arbex MA, Varella Mde C, Siqueira HR, Mello FA (2010) Antituberculosis drugs: drug interactions, adverse effects, and use in special situations. Part 1: first-line drugs. J Bras Pneumol 36(5):626–640

Arnestad M, Eldor KB, Stray-Pedersen A, Bachs L, Karinen R (2014) Suicide due to cyclizine overdose. J Anal Toxicol 38(2):110–112

Bailey F, Davies A (2008) The misuse/abuse of antihistamine antiemetic medication (cyclizine) by cancer patients. Palliat Med 22(7):869–871

Barberio B, Judge C, Savarino EV, Ford AC (2021) Global prevalence of functional constipation according to the Rome criteria: a systematic review and meta-analysis. Lancet Gastroenterol Hepatol 6(8):638–648

Botch-Jones SR, Johnson R, Kleinschmidt K, Bashaw S, Ordonez J (2014) Diphenhydramine's role in death investigations: an examination of diphenhydramine prevalence in 2 US geographical areas. Am J Forensic Med Pathol 35(3):181–185

British National Formulary (BNF) (2022) https://bnf.nice.org.uk. Accessed 2022.

Buffery PJ, Strother RM (2015) Domperidone safety: a mini-review of the science of QT prolongation and clinical implications of recent global regulatory recommendations. N Z Med J 128(1416):66–74

Christofaki M, Papaioannou A (2015) Ondansetron: a review of pharmacokinetics and clinical experience in postoperative nausea and vomiting. Expert Opin Drug Metab Toxicol 10(3):437–444

Costilla VC, Foxx-Orenstein AE (2014) Constipation: understanding mechanisms and management. Clin Geriatr Med 30(1):107–115

Crauwels H, Van Heeswijk RPG, Stevens M, Buelens A, Vanveggel S, Boven K, Hoetelmans R (2013) Clinical perspective on drug-drug interactions with the non-nucleoside reverse transcriptase inhibitor rilpivirine. AIDS Rev 15(2):87–101

De Ruigh A, Roman S, Chen J, Pandolfino JE, Kahrilas PJ (2014) Gaviscon double action liquid (antacid & alginate) is more effective than antacid in controlling post-prandial oesophageal acid exposure in GERD patients: a double-blind crossover study. Aliment Pharmacol Ther 40(5):531–537

Del Rosso JQ (2009) Oral antibiotic drug interactions of clinical significance to dermatologists. Dermatol Clin 27(1):91–94

Doggrell SA, Hancox JC (2014) Cardiac safety concerns for domperidone, an antiemetic and prokinetic, and galactogogue medicine. Expert Opin Drug Saf 13(1):131–138

Ehrenpreis ED, Roginsky G, Alexoff A, Smith DG (2017) Domperidone is commonly prescribed with QT-interacting drugs: review of a community-based practice and a postmarketing adverse drug event reporting database. J Clin Gastroenterol 51(1):56–62

Erbe S, Bschor T (2013) Diphenhydramine addiction and detoxification. A systematic review and case report. Psychiatr Prax 40(5):248–251

Eslick GD, Talley NJ (2016) Prevalence and relationship between gastrointestinal symptoms among individuals of different body mass index: a population-based study. Obes Res Clin Pract 10(2):143–150

Farhat K, Iqbal J, Waheed A, Mansoor Q, Ismail M, Pasha AK (2015) Association of anti-emetic efficacy of ondansetron with G2677T polymorphism in a drug transporter gene ABCB1 in Pakistani population. J Coll Physicians Surg Pak 25(7):486–490

Geboes K, Spiessens C, Nijs G, De Witte P (1993) Anthranoids and the mucosal immune system of the colon. Pharmacology 47(Suppl 1):49–57

Gochfeld M (2017) Sex differences in human and animal toxicology: toxicokinetics. Toxicol Pathol 45(1):172–189

Gordon M, Naidoo K, Akobeng AK, Thomas AG (2012) Osmotic and stimulant laxatives for the management of childhood constipation. Cochrane Database Syst Rev 11(7):CD009118

Gray JR (2011) What is chronic constipation? Definition and diagnosis. Can J Gastroenterol 25(Suppl B):7B–10B

Guijarro P, Viqueira A, Alonso-Babarro A, Fernandez G (2010) Health-related quality of life in opioid induced constipation patients in Spain. Value in health. In: ISPOR 13th Annual European Congress, Prague, Czech Republic, 13(7), p A373

Hatting NP, Hansen PM (2017) Intentional suicide with cyclizine. Ugeskr Laeger 179(14):V01170022

Huybrechts KF, Hernández-Díaz S, Straub L, Gray KJ, Zhu Y, Patorno E, Desai RJ, Mogun H, Bateman BT (2018) Association of maternal first-trimester ondansetron use with cardiac malformations and oral clefts in offspring. JAMA J Am Med Assoc 320(23):2429–2437

Ikarashi N, Baba K, Ushiki T et al (2011) The laxative effect of bisacodyl is attributable to decreased aquaporin-3 expression in the colon induced by increased PGE2 secretion from macrophages. Am J Physiol Gastrointest Liver Physiol 01:G887–G895

Kang HJ, Loftus S, Taylor A, DiCristina C, Green S, Zwaan CM (2015) Aprepitant for the prevention of chemotherapy-induced nausea and vomiting in children: a randomised, double-blind, phase 3 trial. Lancet Oncol 16(4):385–394

Kaplan YC, Richardson JL, Keskin-Arslan E, Erol-Coskun H, Kennedy D (2019) Use of ondansetron during pregnancy and the risk of major congenital malformations: a systematic review and meta-analysis. Reprod Toxicol 5(86):1–13

Khalid U, Thomas K, Lalji A, Andreyev J (2009) The use and efficacy of sterculia for patients with defaecatory disorders. In: Annual meeting of the British Society of Gastroenterology, Glasgow, United Kingdom. Conference publication, pp A86–A87

Khan EU (2010) Medicine management: pharmacokinetic update for community nurses. Br J Community Nurs 15(9):436–444

Krammer H, Thomann AK, Rustemeyer T, Ehehalt R (2014) Constipation and myth of laxative abuse. Verdauungskrankheiten 32(3):138–146

Leiman DA, Riff BP, Morgan S, Metz DC, Falk GW, French B, Umscheid CA, Lewis JD (2017) Alginate therapy is effective treatment for GERD symptoms: a systematic review and meta-analysis. Dis Esophagus 30(5):1–9

Leung L, Riutta T, Kotecha J, Rosser W (2011) Chronic constipation: an evidence-based review. J Am Board Fam Med 24(4):436–451

Li G, Cheng G, Wu J, Zhou X, Liu P, Sun C (2013) Drug-induced long QT syndrome in women. Adv Ther 30(9):793–802

Makari J, Cameron K, Battistella M (2014) Domperidone-associated sudden cardiac death in the general population and implications for use in patients undergoing hemodialysis: a literature review. Can J Hosp Pharm 67(6):441–446

Maughan RJ (2012) Hydration, morbidity, and mortality in vulnerable populations. Nutr Rev 70(Suppl 2):S152–S155

May G, Kumar R (2006) Best evidence topic report. Use of intravenous cyclizine in cardiac chest pain. Emerg Med J 23(1):61–62

Mezoff EA, Cohen MB (2013) Acid suppression and the risk of Clostridium difficile infection. J Pediatr 163(3):627–630

Mishriky BM, Habib AS (2012) Metoclopramide for nausea and vomiting prophylaxis during and after caesarean delivery: a systematic review and meta-analysis. Br J Anaesth 108(3):374–383

Moore D, Young CJ (2020) Systematic review and meta-analysis of biofeedback therapy for dyssynergic defaecation in adults. Tech Coloproctol 24(9):909–918

Moore C, Williams E, Dyas R, Halman A, Stenta T, Khatri D, Elliott DA, Lange PW, Caudle KE, Conyers R (2025) CYP2D6 genotype and associated 5-HT3 receptor antagonist outcomes: a systematic review and meta-analysis. Clin Transl Sci 18(2):e70108

Moynihan PJ, Ferrier S, Blomley S, Wright WG, Russell RRB (1998) Acid production from lactulose by dental plaque bacteria. Lett Appl Microbiol 27(3):173–177

Nagahara A, Asaoka D, Hojo M, Oguro M, Shimada Y, Ishikawa D, Osada T, Kawabe M, Yoshizawa T, Otaka M, Watanabe S (2010) Observational comparative trial of the efficacy of proton pump inhibitors versus histamine-2 receptor antagonists for uninvestigated dyspepsia. J Gastroenterol Hepatol 25:S122–S128

Nath A, Haktanirlar G, Varga Á, Molnár MA, Albert K, Galambos I, Koris A, Vatai G (2018) Biological activities of lactose-derived prebiotics and symbiotic with probiotics on gastrointestinal system. Medicina (Kaunas) 54(2):E18

Niebyl JR, Briggs GG (2014) The pharmacologic management of nausea and vomiting of pregnancy. J Fam Pract 63(2 Suppl):S31–S37

Ogawa R, Echizen H (2010) Drug-drug interaction profiles of proton pump inhibitors. Clin Pharmacokinet 49(8):509–533

Ogawa R, Echizen H (2011) Clinically significant drug interactions with antacids: an update. Drugs 71(14):1839–1864

Onifer DJ, Butler FK, Gross KR, Otten EJ, Patton R, Russell RJ, Stockinger Z, Burrell E (2015) Replacement of promethazine with ondansetron for treatment of opioid- and trauma-related nausea and vomiting in tactical combat casualty care. J Spec Oper Med 15(2):17–24

Poluzzi E, Raschi E, Godman B, Koci A, Moretti U, Kalaba M, Wettermark B, Sturkenboom M, De Ponti F (2015) Pro-arrhythmic potential of oral antihistamines (H1): combining adverse event reports with drug utilization data across Europe. PLoS One 10(3):e0119551

Poluzzi E, Diemberger I, De Ridder M, Koci A, Clo M, Oteri A, Pecchioli S, Bezemer I, Schink T, Pilgaard Ulrichsen S, Boriani G, Sturkenboom MCJ, De Ponti F, Trifirò G (2017) Use of antihistamines and risk of ventricular tachyarrhythmia: a nested case-control study in five European countries from the ARITMO project. Eur J Clin Pharmacol 73(11):1499–1510

Rao SSC, Brenner DM (2021) Efficacy and safety of over-the-counter therapies for chronic constipation: an updated systematic review. Am J Gastroenterol 116(6):1156–1181

Roberts RL, Begg EJ, Joyce PR, Kennedy MA (2002) How the pharmacogenetics of cytochrome P450 enzymes may affect prescribing. N Z Med J 115(1150):137–140

Roila F, Del Favero A (1995) Ondansetron clinical pharmacokinetics. Clin Pharmacokinet 29(2):95–109

Ruston T, Hunter K, Cummings G, Lazarescu A (2013) Efficacy and side-effect profiles of lactulose, docusate sodium, and sennosides compared to PEG in opioid-induced constipation: a systematic review. Can Oncol Nurs J 23(4):236–246

Sahota SS, Bramley PM, Menzies IS (1982) The fermentation of lactulose by colonic bacteria. J Gen Microbiol 128(2):319–325

Schmidt FM, Santos VL, Domansky Rde C, Barros E, Bandeira MA, Tenório MA, Jorge JM (2015) Prevalence of self-reported constipation in adults from the general population. Rev Esc Enferm USP 49(3):440–449

Shen YD, Chen CY, Wu CH, Cherng YG, Tam KW (2015) Dexamethasone, ondansetron, and their combination and postoperative nausea and vomiting in children undergoing strabismus surgery: a meta-analysis of randomized controlled trials. Pediatr Anesth 24(5):490–498

Shi W, Xu X, Zhang Y, Guo S, Wang J, Wang J (2015) Epidemiology and risk factors of functional constipation in pregnant women. PLoS One 10(7):e0133521

Southwell BR (2020) Treatment of childhood constipation: a synthesis of systematic reviews and meta-analyses. Expert Rev Gastroenterol Hepatol 14(3):163–174

Spears DA, Gollob MH (2015) Genetics of inherited primary arrhythmia disorders. Appl Clin Genet 18(8):215–233

Stevens AJ, Woodman RJ, Owen H (2015) The effect of ondansetron on the efficacy of postoperative tramadol: a systematic review and meta-analysis of a drug interaction. Anaesthesia 70(2):209–218

Taba Taba Vakili S, Nezami BG, Shetty A, Chetty VK, Srinivasan S (2015) Association of high dietary saturated fat intake and uncontrolled diabetes with constipation: evidence from the National Health and Nutrition Examination Survey. Neurogastroenterol Motil 27(10):1389–1397

Talley NJ, Vakil N (2005) Guidelines for the management of dyspepsia. Am J Gastroenterol 100(10):2324–2337

Teng M, Khoo AL, Zhao YJ, Lin L, Lim BP, Wu TS, Dan YY (2015) Meta-analysis of the effectiveness of esomeprazole in gastroesophageal reflux disease and Helicobacter pylori infection. J Clin Pharm Ther 40(4):368–375

Thomas E, Wade A, Crawford G, Jenner B, Levinson N, Wilkinson J (2014) Randomised clinical trial: relief of upper gastrointestinal symptoms by an acid pocket-targeting alginate-antacid (Gaviscon Double Action)—a double-blind, placebo-controlled, pilot study in gastro- oesophageal reflux disease. Aliment Pharmacol Ther 39(6):595–602

Trottier M, Erebara A, Bozzo P (2012) Treating constipation during pregnancy. Can Fam Physician 58(8):836–838

Vazquez RM, Bouras EP (2015) Epidemiology and management of chronic constipation in elderly patients. Clin Interv Aging 2(10):919–930

Vella-Brincat JW, Begg E, Jensen BP, Chin PK, Roberts RL, Fairhall M, Macleod SA, Reid K (2012) The pharmacokinetics and pharmacogenetics of the antiemetic cyclizine in palliative care patients. J Pain Symptom Manag 43(3):540–548

Waade RB, Hermann M, Moe HL, Molden E (2014) Impact of age on serum concentrations of venlafaxine and escitalopram in different CYP2D6 and CYP2C19 genotype subgroups. Eur J Clin Pharmacol 70(8):933–940

Wang ZY, Chen M, Zhu LL, Yu LS, Zeng S, Xiang MX, Zhou Q (2015) Pharmacokinetic drug interactions with clopidogrel: updated review and risk management in combination therapy. J Ther Clin Risk Manag 11:449–467

Wedemeyer RS, Blume H (2014) Pharmacokinetic drug interaction profiles of proton pump inhibitors: an update. Drug Saf 4:201–211

Zhong W, Shahbaz O, Teskey G, Beever A, Kachour N, Venketaraman V, Darmani NA (2021) Mechanisms of nausea and vomiting: current knowledge and recent advances in intracellular emetic signaling systems. Int J Mol Sci 22(11):5797

Medications Used for the Central Nervous System

12

Ehsan Khan and Amira Shaikh

Learning Outcomes

At the end of this chapter, you will be able to:

- Understand the mechanisms of CNS drug action
- Describe the medications used for treating
    - Epilepsy
    - Parkinson's disease
    - Dementia
- Recognise the clinical implications of medication used to treat central nervous system conditions

12.1 Introduction

This chapter explores the therapeutic medications used to treat disorders that arise from the central nervous system (CNS). Drugs designed for the CNS frequently cause a significant drug burden. There are a number of ways to define the central nervous system; for simplicity, it is sufficient to say that the CNS consists of the brain and spinal cord. Pharmacologically, this is a useful definition as it groups the two neuronal structures with the mechanisms that protect them. These protective structures include the membranes covering the brain and spinal cord, as well as the meninges, and the protection provided by CNS capillaries the so called

E. Khan (✉)
Faculty of Nursing Midwifery and Palliative Care, King's College London, London, UK
e-mail: eu.khan@kcl.ac.uk

A. Shaikh
Florence Nightingale Faculty of Nursing, Midwifery & Palliative Care, King's College London, London, UK

© The Author(s), under exclusive license to Springer Nature Switzerland AG 2026
E. Khan, P. Hood (eds.), *Understanding Pharmacology in Nursing Practice*,
https://doi.org/10.1007/978-3-032-03964-4_12

blood–brain barrier, which protects delicate CNS cells from blood-borne toxins. Pharmacologically these protective structures limit drug entry into the CNS, these mechanisms have, therefore, to be breached to achieve a steady state level of therapeutic medication in the CNS.

12.1.1 Action Potential and Its Relevance to CNS Drug Action

CNS medication effects (pharmacodynamics) are based upon two main mechanisms, action potentials and synapses; together these two processes govern nerve firing and communication in the brain and the periphery. Therefore, to understand how CNS drugs act, these two processes will be reviewed.

Nerves, like muscle, are excitable tissues and function because of ion movement in and out of the cell. This ion movement is triggered by very small amounts of voltage in the millivolt range. Nerve cells have a resting and active, i.e. conducting state. The resting phase is known as the polarised state which occurs when the inside of the cell membrane is significantly negatively charged compared to the outside. Conversely, the active or depolarised state is associated with a comparatively positive charge on the inside of the cell membrane (Fig. 12.1). A depolarised cell favours the opening of calcium (Ca^{2+}) ion channels. Calcium entry into the cell then helps propagate the depolarised state of the cell down the length of the nerve or axon (Fig. 12.1).

A nerve fires when it depolarises and stops firing when it is polarised or negatively charged inside the cell. The changes in charge (polarity) inside the cell are mediated by passive ion movement. Owing to differences in ion concentration inside and out of the cell, different ions move passively either into or out of the cell.

Ions that move into the cell according to their concentration gradient include sodium (Na^+) and calcium (Ca^{2+}). Whereas potassium (K^+) is the main ion that moves out of the cell passively (Fig. 12.2), chloride ions (Cl^-) are negatively charged and also have an inward concentration gradient (Fig. 12.2). These ion movements occur due to the opening of ion channels at particular times.

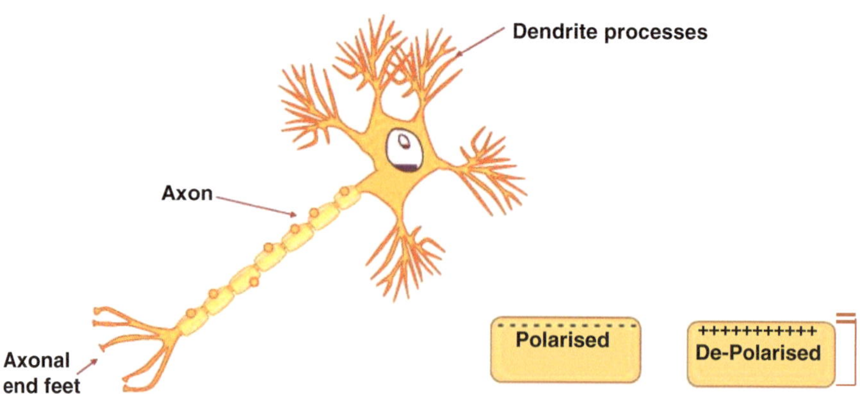

Fig. 12.1 Nerve anatomy and polarity

Fig. 12.2 Passive movement of a selection of ions via ion channels

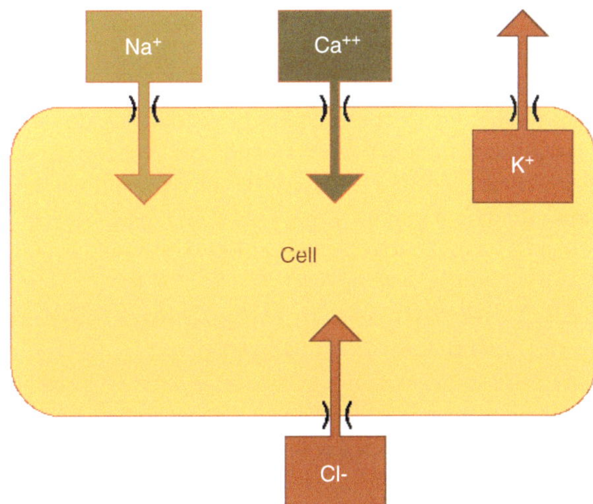

Depolarisation of the cell is sodium-dependent, i.e. passive Na$^+$ entry into the cell via sodium ion channels causes the inside of the cell to become positive or depolarised. Sodium ion channels are opened in response to an electrical stimulus or discharge. Once the cell membrane is depolarised, this triggers Ca^{2+} ion channel opening that further depolarises the nerve membrane and causes it to conduct this depolarisation wave down the length of the axon to the axonal end feet (Fig. 12.1).

Once depolarised, an exit of the positively charged potassium from the cell begins, according to its outward concentration gradient (Fig. 12.2). Movement of this positive charge out of the cell brings it back to a polarised resting state, i.e. potassium re-polarises the cell.

To pharmacologically modulate nerve firing, you can either deter cell depolarisation by reducing Na$^+$ or Ca^{2+} ion entry into the cell by blocking ion channels that conduct these ions, or conversely, the cell can be rendered negatively charged by keeping potassium ion channels open. This enables more positively charged ions to leave the cell (hyperpolarisation of the cell); thus making it difficult to depolarise. Chloride ion channel opening has the same hyperpolarising effect as it causes an inward movement of negatively charged Cl$^-$ ions (Fig. 12.2), rendering the inside of the cell negative.

12.1.2 The Synapse

Once the depolarisation wave arrives at the axonal end feet (Fig. 12.1), these endings communicate the depolarisation wave with other nerves and cells. They achieve this by liberating stored chemicals known as neurotransmitters from their endings. These neurotransmitters communicate with an opposing nerve ending to form a synapse.

The synapse consists of the nerve carrying the depolarising wave (pre-synaptic nerve) to the communication junction, the synapse, where the depolarising nerve promotes the movement of communicating molecules, the neurotransmitter stored in vesicles to move to the nerve membrane and liberate the neurotransmitter into the space between the two nerve endings—the synaptic cleft—the neurotransmitter traverses the synaptic cleft to bind to the nerve receiving the neurotransmitter (post synaptic nerve) via specific binding proteins known as receptors (Fig. 12.3). Binding of neurotransmitters then modulate post synaptic nerve function to either generate a depolarisation of the postsynaptic nerve or reduce the nerve's ability to depolarise thus stopping it conducting (Fig. 12.3).

12.1.3 Neurotransmitter Regulation: A Potent Pharmacological Target

The neurotransmitter is released from its receptor after a specific time, where it may undergo metabolism, as is the case with acetylcholine, which is broken down into its acetyl and choline components by the enzyme cholinesterase, choline is then reloaded into the acetylcholine-releasing presynaptic nerve for incorporation back into acetylcholine molecules. Other neurotransmitters such as catecholamines, i.e. dopamine, serotonin and adrenaline are taken back (undergo re-uptake) directly into the releasing presynaptic nerve by re-uptake transporter proteins (Fig. 12.4). Both these mechanisms clear the synaptic cleft of the neurotransmitter and therefore reduce postsynaptic nerve stimulation. These mechanisms are typically pharmacologically inhibited in a number of CNS disorders to prolong the neurotransmitter effect on their receptors. For example, in Alzheimer's disease, inhibition of acetylcholine breakdown by drugs that inhibit the cholinesterase enzyme prolongs the

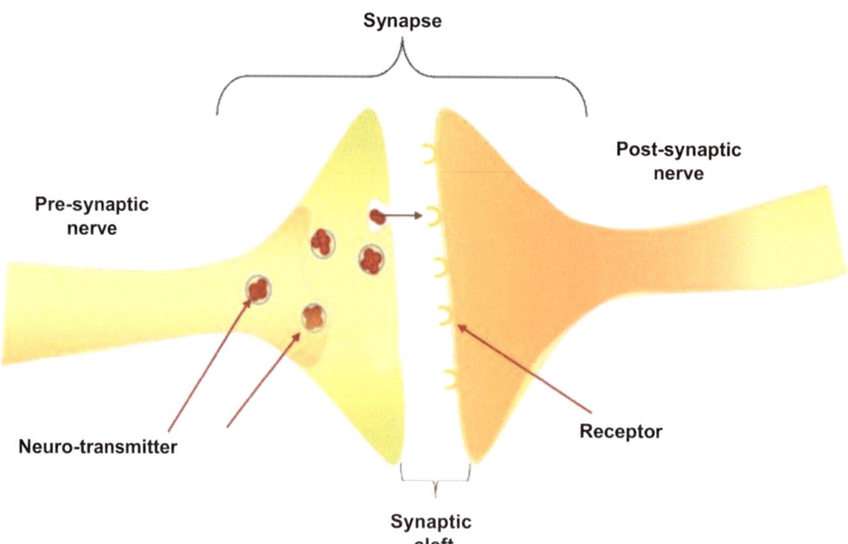

Fig. 12.3 The synapse

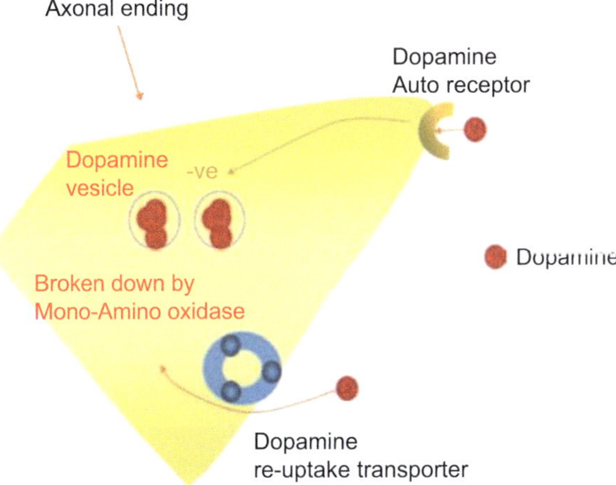

Fig. 12.4 Neuro-axonal ending transmitter regulation mechanisms

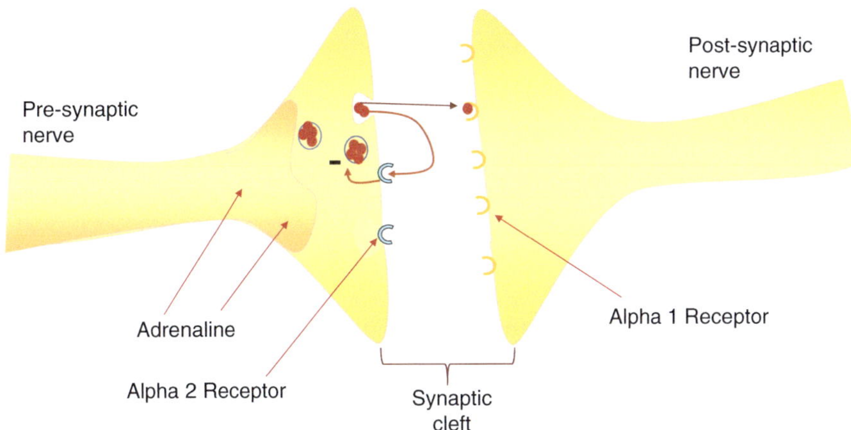

Fig. 12.5 Neurotransmitter autoregulation

effect of acetylcholine, the main neurotransmitter involved in memory formation. Similarly, a number of antidepressants act by inhibiting the reuptake of CNS stimulatory neurotransmitters such as serotonin and adrenaline.

Synapses also have a negative feedback pathway that auto-regulates presynaptic neurotransmitter release (Figs. 12.4 and 12.5). This mechanism normally depends upon a presynaptic receptor that binds the neurotransmitter released, resulting in a reduction of neurotransmitter release from the presynaptic nerve. This mechanism can be exemplified using adrenaline. Postsynaptic adrenergic receptors tend to be of the alpha 1 type, whereas presynaptic adrenergic receptors are of the alpha 2 type.

Adrenaline release from the presynaptic nerve causes postsynaptic nerve stimulation via the alpha 1 receptor. At the same time, binding of adrenaline to the presynaptic nerve alpha 2 receptor attenuates further adrenaline release (Fig. 12.5), therefore modulating the amount of adrenaline released. The more the presynaptic nerve is stimulated, the more adrenaline release is modulated to help regulate nerve function.

12.2 Drug Therapy for Epilepsy

Epilepsy is associated with abnormal and excessive neuronal discharge in the CNS. There are many forms of epilepsy, and the choice of which drug to prescribe depends upon a number of parameters, such as the type of epilepsy, the type of medications already prescribed, and other considerations such as pregnancy. An epileptic seizure is a consequence of different pathological mechanisms, and while the exact causes vary, there is substantial understanding of the mechanisms underlying epilepsy (e.g. genetic predispositions, structural brain abnormalities). These mechanisms, however may not be apparent at the time of initial treatment, so prescription of a drug may not be aligned with a particular mechanism. Therefore, to be effective, most medications prescribed for epilepsy aim to reduce CNS activity. They achieve this by either generally inhibiting the excitatory nerves or by enhancing or potentiating the inhibitory nerve pathways in the brain.

12.2.1 CNS Excitatory Nerve Modulation for Treatment of Epilepsy

There are a number of excitatory nerves in the brain, these include adrenergic (noradrenaline releasing nerves), serotonergic (serotonin releasing nerves) and glutamatergic (L-glutamine releasing nerves). The propagation of any neuronal action potential is Na^+ dependent, whereas the release of neurotransmitter at the axonal endplate is Ca^{2+} dependent. Traditional anti-epileptic medications such as phenytoin and carbamazepine act by inhibiting voltage-gated Na^+ (Fig. 12.6a, b), thus reducing Na^+ and reducing axonal nerve conduction. This effect attenuates abnormally firing nerves that occur in epilepsy. Other mechanisms associated with the modulation of excitatory nerves include inhibition of postsynaptic positive ion (Na^+, Ca^{2+}) entry into the nerve. Small positive ions enter postsynaptic nerves in response to excitatory neurotransmitters such as l-glutamate (Fig. 12.6a), anti-epileptic drugs such as ethosuximide inhibit these ion channels, resulting in inhibition of receptor-mediated post-synaptic nerve stimulation.

More recent medications such as Levetiracetam, licenced in the United States in 1999 and in the United Kingdom (UK) in 2000, acts by stabilising the neurotransmitter vesicle and stopping liberation of neurotransmitter into the synaptic cleft (Fig. 12.6a). Retigabine was a novel first-in-class anti-epileptic medication that opens the neuronal variant of a commonly drug-targeted potassium ion channel. Opening of potassium ion channels leads to a passive movement of K^+ out of the cell according to its concentration gradient (Figs. 12.2 and 12.6a). This renders the nerve endings overtly negative or hyperpolarised, making them harder to depolarise

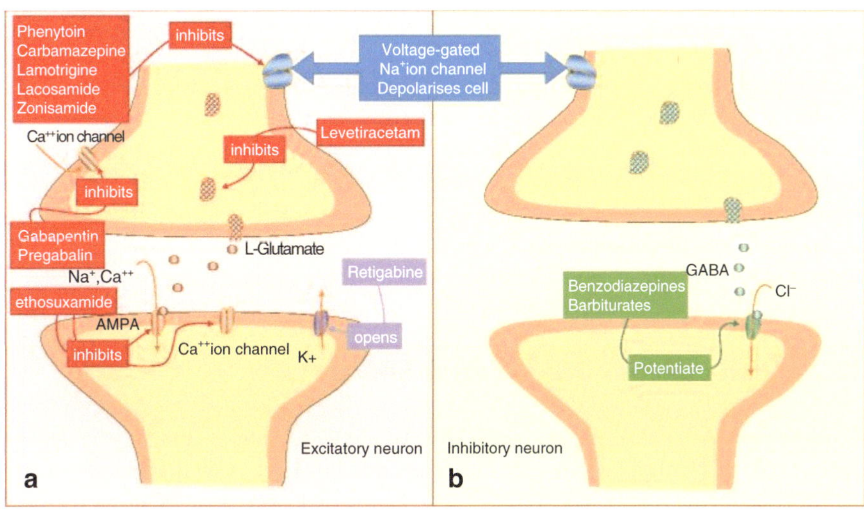

Fig. 12.6 Mechanism of action of anti-epileptic medications. (**a**) Medications effective on excitatory synapses and (**b**) medications effective on inhibitory synapses

and propagate depolarisations. However, this medication has now been withdrawn (EMA 2018) following reports of it causing blue skin discolorations and eye abnormalities by its producer, Glaxo Smith Kline (GSK), and is only mentioned as a first-in-class medication, the mechanism of which may be adopted by future anti-epileptic medications.

Sodium valproate is a first-line commonly prescribed, relatively safe anti-epileptic drug, although primarily a voltage-gated sodium channel blocker. Valproate also affects gamma-aminobutyric acid (GABA) releasing nerves, where it appears to potentiate the effect of GABA by enhancing levels in the brain.

12.2.2 CNS Inhibitory Nerve Modulation for Treatment of Epilepsy

Gamma-aminobutyric acid is the main inhibitory neurotransmitter in the brain. Many medications used in epilepsy potentiate the effect of GABA in the brain. GABA binds directly GABA-A receptors found on chloride ion (Cl$^-$) channels, These channels conduct Cl$^-$ into the cell passively, once open. An increased intraneuronal Cl$^-$ concentration makes the nerve membrane internally more negative, i.e. it polarises the neuron, making it more difficult for the nerve to depolarise (Fig. 12.6b). First-generation anti-epileptics included a combination of ion channel antagonists and GABA agonists, e.g. phenytoin, Na$^+$ channel blocker, ethosuximide, Ca^{2+} channel blocker and phenobarbital GABA agonist. The development and use of many GABA agonist drugs have made available second-generation GABA agonists with diazepam, clonazepam and clobazam and the multi-effect valproate, introduced before the 1980s. The majority of newer anti-epileptics drugs have multiple effects, with only vigabatrin singularly affecting the GABA channel and drugs such as topiramate and the more recently introduced (2002) stiripentol, having a combined GABA and cationic (positive ion) ion channel effect.

The knowledge of drug mechanisms provides an understanding of a drug's adverse effects, a key healthcare consideration in maintaining a safe medication regimen and signposting issues such as drug resistance. Therefore, understanding the mechanisms of anti-epileptic drugs helps predict potential adverse effects and addresses key healthcare considerations such as drug resistance.

12.2.3 Anti-epileptic Drug Adverse Effects

Adverse effects of anti-epileptic drugs (AEDs) are wide-ranging and may be dependent or independent of drug levels. For drugs that have a narrow therapeutic index, monitoring drug serum levels to ensure that the medication is at a safe concentration is imperative. Many factors influence drug serum levels such as polypharmacy and changes to liver and kidney function (Chap. 2).

Three commonly prescribed anti-epileptic drugs have a relatively narrow therapeutic index (Table 12.1) and therefore need monitoring periodically, but more frequently when the patient is undergoing drug regimen changes or when they have experienced degradation of hepatic and or renal function.

Adverse effects of anti-epileptic medication may be associated with somnolence and cognitive impairment. Other adverse effects include behavioural changes and precipitation of psychotic and depressive events, although in relation to mental health-related effects it is not always clear which illnesses precipitated which, as epilepsy and mental health disease are frequent co-morbidities. Another effect of many anti-epileptic drugs is sensitivity reactions. These may range from a benign rash to Stevens-Johnson Syndrome (a rare but potentially fatal reaction affecting the body's mucous membranes) (Levi et al. 2009; Harr and French 2010).

A range of additional, adverse effects associated with anti-epileptic drugs involves blood cells. Aplastic anaemia was a common effect of the older generations of anti-epileptic (particularly felbamate) medication. Aplastic anaemia reduces production of all three blood cell types: erythrocytes, white blood cells, platelets or thrombocytes. With other anti-epileptic drugs, this adverse effect may present as leukopenia (white blood cell deficiency), anaemia (reduced red blood cell counts) or thrombocytopenia (reduced platelet count). Depending upon which form of abnormal blood cell disorder (dyscrasia) prevails, symptoms present accordingly (Table 12.2).

Table 12.1 Therapeutic drug levels for some commonly used anti-epileptics

Drug	Level (µg/mL)
Phenytoin	10–20
Carbamazepine	4–12
Valproate	50–120

Table 12.2 Blood dyscrasia and presenting symptoms

Blood dyscrasia	Symptoms
Anaemia (red blood cell)	Shortness of breath, tachycardia, pale complexion and mucous membranes, tiredness and lethargy
Leukopenia (white blood cell)	Risk of infection (particularly in the mouth and lung) tiredness, behavioural irritability and the desire for warm fluids
Thrombocytopenia	Increased bruising, bleeding from mucous membranes (mouth, nose and rectum). Prolonged bleeding from wounds. Petechiae (rash of pinpoint red-purplish spots)

12.2.4 The Role of the Healthcare Professional in Maintaining Drug and Patient Safety in Epilepsy

All CNS drugs present a significant pharmacological load to the body, taxing liver metabolism and requiring the patient receiving CNS medication to have a robust, stable hepatic and renal function to ensure drug biotransformation and subsequent clearance. Together, these processes, if fully functional, maintain steady drug serum levels. A number of epilepsy medications with narrow therapeutic margins have already been identified (Table 12.1). It is imperative, therefore, when caring for people receiving these particular medications, as well as with anti-epileptic drugs in general, that the healthcare professional closely monitors the patient for any adverse effects. Many of the symptoms of the common adverse effects have been given (Table 12.2). Such effects may happen at any drug concentration; patients with co-morbidities and those receiving polypharmacy are more at risk. Other patients whom this may affect include women and older people. Women have different metabolic enzyme activity from men and therefore may have different responses to medication and expression of adverse effects when receiving polypharmacy (Soldin and Mattison 2009). Also, a number of commonly used AEDs, particularly valproate and to a lesser extent topiramate, are associated with teratogenic effects; therefore, these medications should not normally be given to women of childbearing age.

Older women also require close monitoring for epilepsy. This is because with advanced age, epilepsy-generated falls may become more problematic, as there is an increased risk of bone fractures. Such events have, of course, consequences as regards morbidity and mortality. Fall-related fractures as well as age-related pharmacokinetic impairment are not limited to women but may, to a lesser extent, occur in men. Advanced age may be associated with the development of resistance to AEDs and may occur in up to 40% of people taking such drugs.

12.2.5 Drug Resistance in Epilepsy

The international league against epilepsy (ILAE) defines drug-resistant epilepsy as a 'failure of adequate trials of two tolerated and appropriately chosen and used AED schedules (whether as monotherapies or in combination) to achieve sustained seizure freedom' (Kwan et al. 2010, p. 1073). Some patients experience a number of stable and effective anti-epileptic drug courses but become prone to seizures again. The causes behind drug resistance are unclear and appear to be multifactorial and derived from the interplay of a number of poorly separated factors. These include disease severity and epidemiological factors together with drug and disease-associated alterations in physiological function (Fig. 12.7). These factors may then be influenced (or caused by) genetic variants (Potschka 2013). This rather unclear hypothesis suggests that whereas epilepsy itself may have genetic determinants associated with it, the evolution of drug resistance may present a separate set of genetic variants that lead to its development.

Currently, there is a lack of knowledge regarding drug resistance; overcoming it is challenging. Additional medication may sometimes retrieve a failing drug regimen, but disease drug resistance is frequently intractable.

12.2.6 Summary

Anti-epileptic drugs are chosen for affected individuals in all age groups. Their mechanism of action typically involves modulating depolarisation through ion channel regulation and altering synaptic nerve-to-nerve communication by manipulation of neurotransmitter activity and metabolism. Anti-epileptic drugs need to be typically taken long term and are associated with significant pharmacokinetic loads that increase the risk of drug–drug and pharmacokinetic-based interactions that may precipitate or aggravate drug adverse effects. Women are particularly susceptible to these issues.

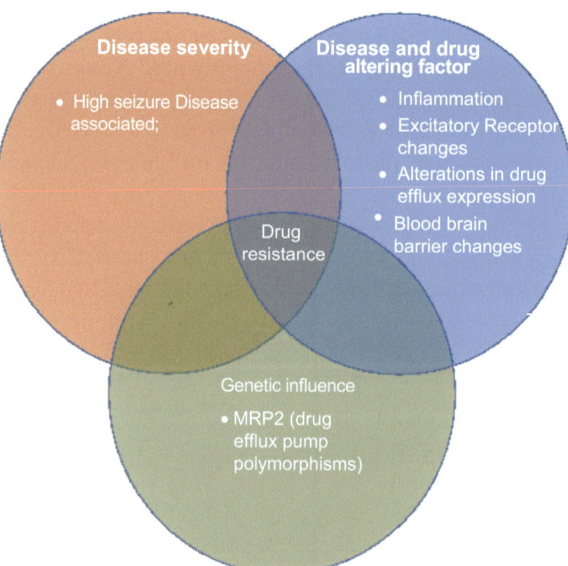

Fig. 12.7 Factors influencing anti-epileptic drug resistance

Epilepsy elicits a dynamic body response that results in drug resistance. Mechanisms of which are probably multifactorial and may include dynamic changes to blood–brain barrier drug efflux potential, disease-related inflammatory changes and genetic determinants linked to the disease and drug pharmacokinetics.

12.3 Anti-Parkinson Medication

12.3.1 Pathology Related to Pharmacology

Parkinson's disease is caused by degeneration of dopamine secreting (dopaminergic) nerves found in a part of the basal ganglia called the substantia nigra. The basal ganglia are a group of nerves found in the base of the cerebrum and divided like most of the brain is divided into two symmetrical hemispheres. The basal ganglia have a number of functions, including motivation, as well as initiating and fine-tuning of movement. The basal ganglia possess a number of nerve circuits that process inputs received from the cerebral motor cortex and output them to muscles via the lateral cortico-spinal tract in the spinal cord. The nerve circuits consist of three types of nerve, glutaminergic (excitatory), GABA releasing nerves (inhibitory) and dopaminergic (excitatory and inhibitory depending upon the receptor-stimulated), with a fourth group of nerves releasing acetylcholine (cholinergic). These nerves are of importance in the basal ganglia and Parkinson's disease, although they constitute a very small amount to the whole number of nerve fibres present in these structures. The interplay between these nerve types leads to an inhibition of muscle movement that is primarily mediated via the cholinergic nerves via muscarinic receptors and a dis-inhibition in particular areas of the basal ganglia that lead to an overall excitatory effect of motor outputs that is mediated by the dopaminergic D1 receptors (Fig. 12.8). It is the degradation of the nerves that leads to difficulty in initiating movement. This is due to a lack of dopamine, which is exacerbated by an inhibition of cholinergic nerves.

Parkinson's disease is a progressive degradation of dopaminergic nerves that leads to a reduction in dopamine availability at the synapse.

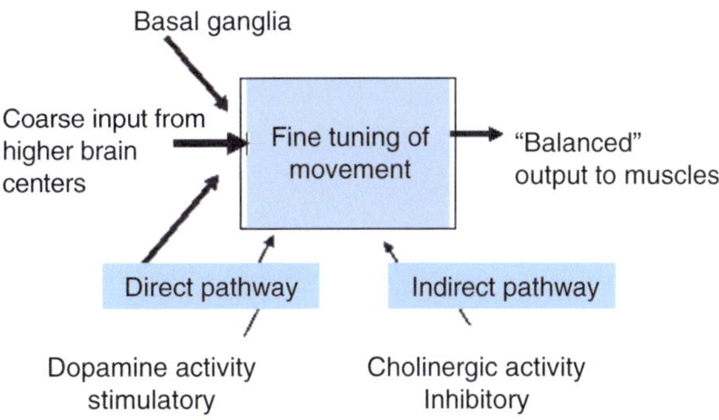

Fig. 12.8 Schematic of basal ganglia disbalance in Parkinson's disease

Therapeutic strategies for the disease have primarily been to enhance the presence of dopamine in the brain. Dopamine, however, does not cross the blood–brain barrier, so it cannot be administered peripherally to enhance brain uptake of this neurotransmitter. Furthermore, large serum concentrations of dopamine peripherally cause significant nausea and vomiting. Dopamine is produced in dopaminergic nerves by the enzymatic action of DOPA-decarboxylase on levodopa (L-Dopa). L-Dopa is transported from the bloodstream into the brain by the large neutral amino acid transport protein (Fig. 12.9).

Given that the disease is caused by a lack of dopamine at nerve terminals strategies to improve Parkinson's disease are primarily associated with the production and maintenance of dopamine at the basal ganglial synapses. A secondary strategy is directed towards reducing the overt cholinergic inhibition that overwhelms the basal ganglia in Parkinson's disease and (or) the elevated motor effects caused by an increased dopamine availability. The primary strategies designed to improve dopamine activity in the brain include the following:

1. Improving brain dopamine concentration by increasing L-Dopa concentration in the blood.
2. Use of dopaminergic agonists.
3. Inhibition of dopamine re-uptake into the dopamine-releasing nerve.
4. Inhibition of the enzyme systems (monoamine oxidase B, MAO-B and catechol-*O*-methyltransferase inhibitor COMT) that break down dopamine in the synaptic cleft and surrounding cell types.

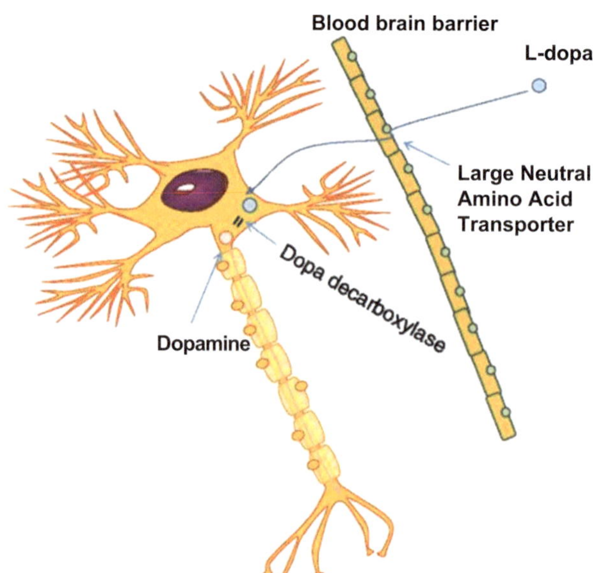

Fig. 12.9 L-Dopa transport and conversion to dopamine in the brain

12.3.2 Improving Brain Dopamine Concentration by Increasing L-DOPA Concentration in the Blood

L-DOPA administration is the primary first-line treatment for Parkinson's disease (NIH 2014; NICE 2017). L-DOPA is always given in combination with carbidopa. The reason for this is that when administered peripherally, L-DOPA gets converted readily into dopamine in the peripheral circulation, leading to many detrimental adverse effects, including cardiovascular and GI tract problems. Also, peripheral conversion of L-DOPA to dopamine reduces the availability of L-DOPA for upload into the brain, reducing its clinical efficacy.

Carbidopa is a dopa decarboxylase inhibitor, preventing the conversion of L-DOPA to dopamine. This effect is limited to the peripheral circulation as carbidopa, unlike L-DOPA, cannot pass through the blood–brain barrier and enter the brain. The dual benefit of using this combination of drugs (L-Dopa and carbidopa) is that peripheral production of dopamine is limited, reducing the deleterious effects of an increased peripheral dopamine serum concentration and secondly, a lack of L-DOPA conversion peripherally improves its availability to be uploaded into the brain.

12.3.3 Use of Dopaminergic Agonists

Dopamine agonists act by binding to and activating dopamine receptors in the basal ganglia (Fig. 12.10). There are a number of dopamine agonists that are licensed for use in Parkinson's disease, these include apomorphine (administered subcutaneously, owing to extensive first pass metabolism via the oral route), bromocriptine, pergolide and rotigotine (Fig. 12.10). According to the National Institute of Health and care Excellence (NICE 2017), dopamine agonists may be used as first line drugs for all stages of Parkinson's disease.

12.3.4 Inhibition of Dopamine Re-uptake into the Dopamine-Releasing Nerve

There are limited medications that modulate the dopamine transporter in the presynaptic neuron. Amantadine is thought to have a dual effect, by which it enhances presynaptic dopamine release together with a possible inhibition of the dopamine transporter (Fig. 12.10). Amantadine also inhibits the cholinergic inhibitory pathway (Agúndez et al. 2013) (Fig. 12.8) in the basal ganglia that may help to alleviate the imbalance of the basal ganglia outputs to improve movement initiation.

12.3.5 Inhibition of Enzymes that Metabolise Dopamine

There are two general enzyme systems that help metabolise dopamine, catechol-O-methyl transferase (COMT) and monoamine oxidase B (MAO B). These enzymes can be found in the presynaptic nerve as well as other cells such as astrocytes and

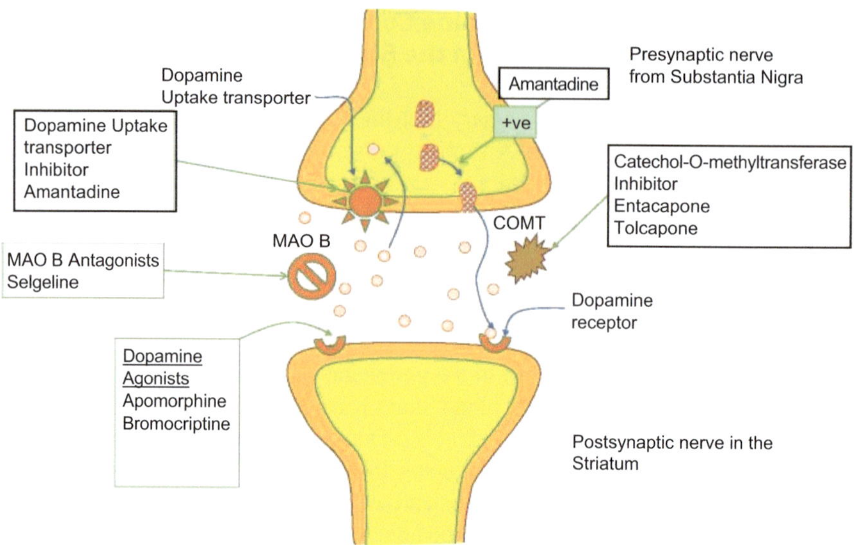

Fig. 12.10 Mechanism of action of medications used for treatment of Parkinson's disease

glial cells that surround the synapse (Fig. 12.10). Together, these enzymes help break down dopamine and reduce its concentration in the synaptic cleft. These enzymes however, are not specific for dopamine alone, as they are also involved in the metabolism of other catecholamines such as nor-adrenaline, serotonin and adrenaline. Selegiline is a commonly used MAO B inhibitor (Fig. 12.10). This medication irreversibly inhibits the MAO B enzyme and, owing to its nearly complete first-pass metabolism, has poor oral availability but good bioavailability when administered via a transdermal patch.

Entacapone and tolcapone are commonly used COMT inhibitors. These drugs inhibit their respective enzymes resulting in an increased availability of dopamine at the synapse. Entacapone acts peripherally, whereas tolcapone is centrally active. Entacapone is available clinically in combination with carbidopa and levodopa in a medicine called Stalevo®.

12.3.6　Adverse Effects of Medications Used to Improve Dopamine Activity in Parkinson's Disease

Adverse effects of medications used in Parkinson's disease are varied owing to the different kinds of drugs being used and the variety of neuro-regulatory targets these drugs modulate. Generally, these adverse effects may be categorised into three to four main groups, including motor complications, impulsive and compulsive behaviours, nausea and hallucinations (Connolly and Lang 2014). A detailed list of adverse effects associated with anti-Parkinson's drugs is provided (Table 12.3).

Table 12.3 Anti-Parkinson's drugs side effects

Drug	Adverse effects
Levodopa/carbidopa	Nausea, orthostatic hypotension, dyskinesia and hallucinations
Bromocriptine	Nausea, orthostatic hypotension, precipitation of Raynaud's phenomenon, elicits psychotic symptoms, owing to potent D2 (neuroleptic receptor) agonism
Apomorphine	Confusion, dizziness, nausea, sedation, vomiting, worsening of psychiatric condition
Rotigotine Pergolide	Nausea, orthostatic hypotension, hallucinations, oedema and increased somnolence
Entacapone	Dark-coloured urine and exacerbation of levodopa adverse effects
Tolcapone	Hepatotoxicity (tolcapone)
Amantadine	Hallucinations, confusion, blurred vision, oedema, livedo reticularis, nausea, dry mouth and constipation
Trihexyphenidyl Benzatropine	Dry mouth, nose and throat, urinary retention, constipation, drowsiness, blurred vision, confusion states, cognitive disturbances

12.3.7 Inhibition of Cholinergic Nerve Activity in the Treatment of Parkinson's Disease

There are two common anti-cholinergic medications used in Parkinson's disease, these include trihexyphenidyl and benzatropine (benztropine). Similar to amantadine, benzatropine has a number of disparate effects that are useful in Parkinson's disease. It is primarily a muscarinic 1 (M1) antagonist that inhibits the basal ganglionic cholinergic inhibitory activity. This aids in addressing the imbalance between the reduced dopamine tone in the Parkinsonian basal ganglia with the unchecked movement inhibitory cholinergic tone; this is the same mechanism of action of trihexyphenidyl. In addition, benzatropine may also inhibit dopamine uptake from the synapse, resulting in an extension of the dopamine effect.

Many of the adverse effects observed with these two anticholinergic medications are associated with the main effects of the parasympathetic nervous system, i.e. digestion (Table 12.3).

The use of anticholinergic drugs is typically associated with a number of gastrointestinal, pulmonary and cardiovascular contraindications Agúndez et al. (2013) include the following:

- Glaucoma, tachycardia, myocardial ischemia, unstable cardiovascular state in acute haemorrhage, partial obstruction of the GI and biliary tracts, prostatic hypertrophy, renal disease, myasthenia gravis, hepatic disease, paralytic ileum, pyloroduodenal stenosis, pyloric obstruction, intestinal atony, ulcerative colitis, obstructive uropathy, with older persons suffering from atherosclerosis or mental impairment.

12.3.8 The Clinical Implications of the Pharmacological Treatment of Parkinson's Disease

Parkinson's disease is a long-term and complicated condition. The complexity of the pharmacotherapeutic management of Parkinson's disease is centred on its progressive nature. Typically, Parkinson's disease becomes particularly difficult to manage in the later years of life, with the adverse effects of the medication limiting its use or further compounding a complicated situation. Symptom deterioration tends to progress with age in Parkinson's disease. This requires changes from mono to multiple therapies. At the same time, the metabolic and clearance capacity of the body is reducing, resulting, in some instances, in a doubling of medication half-lives. Given the propensity of the pharmacokinetic burden with these medications, it is important to be aware of the main pharmacokinetic parameters associated with these drugs (Table 12.4). Factors such as liver function and renal function should be monitored, the frequency of which will be determined by age, gender and presence of polypharmacy and other co-morbidities (Chap. 2).

Individuals with Parkinson's disease frequently display an expressionless and confused demeanour. This can be misinterpreted as psychotic behaviour if the person becomes confused and violent, leading to them becoming labelled as unstable and displaying challenging behaviour. In such instances, many clinicians resort to prescribing antipsychotic drugs in an attempt to keep the patient safe. It is the health professional's responsibility to assess the patient's situation to ascertain reasons behind 'challenging behaviour' and not revert to pharmacological control of behaviour as a first option unless there is a risk to safety.

Table 12.4 Pharmacokinetic parameters of selected drugs used in Parkinson's disease

Drug	Metabolism	Half life	Excretion
Levodopa (L-Dopa)	COMT, DDC	0.8–1.5 h	
Bromocriptine	? CYP3A4	2–8 h	85% Bile (faeces)
Apomorphine	? Phase I and Phase II	~40 min	–
Rotigotine	Liver? Phase II	5–7 h	71% Urine
Pergolide	CYP3A4	27 h	–
Entacapone	Phase II conjugation	0.4–0.7 h	90% Faecal
Tolcapone	Phase II conjugation	2–3 h	60% Urine, 40% Faeces
Amantadine	Phase II N-acetylation	10–31 h	Urine
Trihexyphenidyl	–	3.7–10 h	–
Benzatropine	Phase I CYP2C19, CYP2D6	12–24 h	Urine

12.3.9 Summary

Anti-Parkinson's drugs are primarily associated with increasing dopamine availability in areas associated with the substantia nigra and striatum of the basal ganglia and secondarily with subduing un-hindered cholinergic activity in the basal ganglia. Drug delivery of medications is complicated by the blood–brain barrier and the effects of first-pass metabolism. Adverse effects of medications used in Parkinson's disease further limit drug use. Adverse effects of dopamine-enhancing drugs can be divided into a number of main categories, including nausea and vomiting, hallucinations, psychotic symptoms and problems of blood pressure control. Anticholinergic medications are associated with anticholinergic effects typically associated with digestion, but have a significant number of contraindications. The management of Parkinson's disease is complicated by age, co-morbidities and polypharmacy and effective care requires knowledge of the Parkinson's disease process as well as an understanding of drug pharmacodynamics and kinetics.

12.4   Drugs Used for Dementia

There are three forms of dementia, the most common of which is Alzheimer's dementia, which accounts for approximately two-thirds of the population with dementia. The other two forms are dementia associated with Parkinson's disease and Lewy body dementia (Broadstock et al. 2014). The aetiologies and causes of these three dementias are different; however, they all have a common feature of grey matter loss associated with cholinergic nerve degradations.

12.4.1 Drug-Related Pathology of Dementia

Cholinergic nerves have an important role in dementia. The activity of a small group of cholinergic nerves in the basal ganglia affects disease symptoms, functionally, however, acetylcholine is primarily associated with memory formation in the CNS. There are two relatively large projections of cholinergic nerves radiating from the basal nucleus of Meynert and the pedunculopontine laterodorsal tegmental complex (Fig. 12.11). It is thought that the basal nucleus of Meynert, in particular, is associated with memory formation. Cholinergic neuron imaging in patients comparing Alzheimer's dementia and dementia with Lewy bodies (Whitwell et al. 2007) found that whereas dementia with Lewy bodies was associated with a relatively limited cholinergic nerve loss (Fig. 12.11), cholinergic nerve loss in Alzheimer's dementia was more extensive, encompassing both cholinergic nuclei (substantia innominata) and areas of the temporoparietal cortex.

These findings, together with evidence from drug studies, suggest that Alzheimer's dementia is associated with impaired or loss of cholinergic nerve function. Drug treatment of Alzheimer's dementia utilises only two mechanisms of action; by far the most common is inhibition of acetylcholine breakdown in the synapse.

Acetylcholine is released by depolarisation of the presynaptic nerve and binds to postsynaptic cholinergic receptors (Fig. 12.12). Once released, acetylcholine is broken down by acetylcholinesterase enzymes to liberate an acetyl group and choline (Fig. 12.12). The liberated choline is then taken up by the presynaptic nerve via a choline transporter (Fig. 12.12).

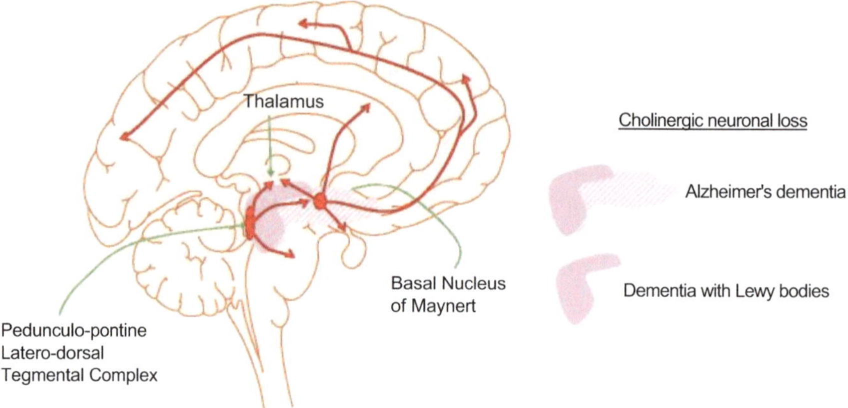

Fig. 12.11 Main cholinergic nuclei and projections in the brain

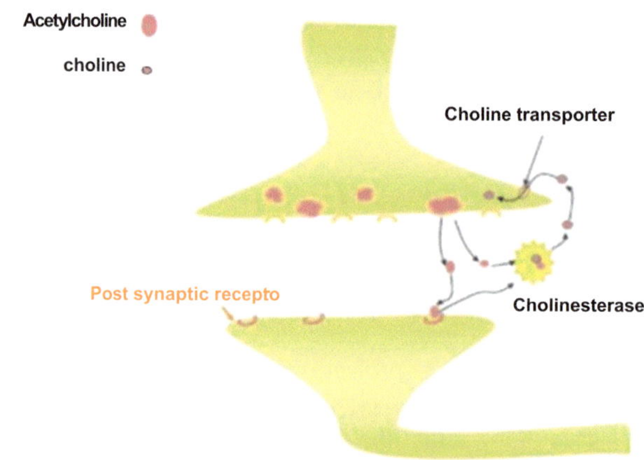

Fig. 12.12 Synaptic acetylcholine release and re-uptake

12.4.2 Anticholinesterases and NMDA Receptor Antagonists

Currently, three cholinesterase inhibitors or anticholinesterases are available, these include: rivastigmine, galantamine and donepezil. Whereas galantamine and donepezil are acetylcholinesterase inhibitors, rivastigmine is a butyl and acetylcholinesterase. The benefit of anticholinesterase medications is well established for Alzheimer's disease. A Cochrane review (Rolinski et al. 2012) found that use of anticholinesterase medications in Parkinson's disease dementia as well as Lewy body dementia improved a number of disease symptoms, including cognitive function, behavioural disturbances and activities of daily living. The same review identified that tremor as an adverse reaction was common with rivastigmine but not with donepezil (Rolinski et al. 2012). Currently, the aforementioned anticholinesterases are licenced for mild-to-moderate Alzheimer's dementia.

Memantine is the only licenced medication for moderate to severe Alzheimer's dementia. Memantine is primarily a glutamate NMDA receptor antagonist; however, it also has serotonin receptor antagonistic activity and dopamine (D2) receptor agonistic effects. A review of clinical trials, however, suggests that donepezil is as good as memantine in moderate-to-severe Alzheimer's dementia (Molino et al. 2013), a similar finding was reported by Yang et al. (2013), who found that memantine was not associated with any significant benefits for Alzheimer's disease in relation to a patient's mental state and daily living activities compared to donepezil. It has therefore been suggested that the choice of drug should be based on drug contraindications, not disease severity (Molino et al. 2013).

12.4.3 Anticholinesterase Pharmacokinetics and Adverse Effects

Adverse effects of anticholinesterase medications include mainly gastrointestinal disturbances such as constipation, nausea, and vomiting, whereas donepezil is also associated with bradycardia.

Both galantamine and donepezil are metabolised by two clinically important phase I enzymes. Galantamine is metabolised by both CYP2D6 and 3A4, whereas donepezil is primarily metabolised by CYP3A4 (Table 12.5) (Noetzli and Eap 2013). Owing to CYP3A4's frequent involvement in drug metabolism, drugs metabolised by this enzyme are at increased risk of interactions. Similarly, CYP2D6 is important in metabolising many medications used in mental health (Seripa et al. 2011). Approximately 7% of Caucasians and 1–2% of other ethnic groups have poor CYP2D6 activity, which increases the risk of drug interactions in this population when using these drugs (Johnson et al. 2006; Stephan et al. 2006).

12.4.4 Memantine Pharmacokinetics and Adverse Effects

Memantine is excreted by the kidney unchanged and has a very long half-life, ranging between 60 and 100 h. Memantine is associated with an increased risk for somnolence, weight gain, confusion, hypertension, nervous system disorders and falling (Molino et al. 2013).

12.4.5 Clinical Implications of Drugs Used in Dementia

Regardless of the type of dementia, currently there is limited treatment, although a number of new drug targets are under trial, including monoclonal antibodies, against

Table 12.5 Anti-cholinesterase drugs pharmacokinetic profile

Drug	Metabolism	Half-life (h)	Excretion
Rivastigmine	Pseudo-cholinesterase in the liver	1.5	Renal
Galantamine	CYP2D6/3A4	7	95% Renal (32% unchanged)
Donepezil	? CYP2D6	70	Renal

beta amyloid and Tau protein, the two causative protein agents associated with Alzheimer's disease; these have not as yet received a licence (Broadstock et al. 2014). Therefore, whereas a reduction in disease progression is currently possible with medications available, regression of illness is currently not possible. Similar to what has been discussed in Parkinson's disease, dementia is a progressive illness. The co-existence of dementia and other forms of mental illness, which require medication, is therefore common and leads to a further drug burden that not only affects drug pharmacokinetics but also increases the risk of drug-drug interactions from a pharmacodynamic perspective. A practitioner should be alert to these issues, particularly when a patient's liver function deteriorates or when they experience a drug regimen change.

Dementia is associated with degradation of cholinergic nerve firing in the brain. This progressive illness currently has no cure, with few if any, currently available disease-modifying medications. The main therapeutic target in dementia is the enzyme that breaks down acetylcholine in the synapse. There are three commonly used inhibitors of this enzyme available, together with a glutamine receptor antagonist, memantine. Given the metabolic profile of these anticholinesterase medications, they have potential to cause drug-drug interactions along with other prescribed drugs a person may be taking juxtaposed with a variable drug response owing to ethnic variation in drug metabolism.

Many new potentially disease-modifying medications are currently being trailed yet until successful approval is achieved, the healthcare professional must manage patients' anti-dementia medication with care and sensitivity in order to optimise drug treatment and quality of life.

12.4.6 Summary

Medications targeted on the central nervous system affect the neuronal action potential together with structures and processes involved in nerve–to–nerve communication at the synapse. With ant-epileptics mainly affecting neuronal ion channels and synapse receptors, whereas medications aimed at alleviating symptoms of dementia are typically cholinesterase inhibitors. Anti-Parkinson medications include a number of dopamine receptor agonists and acetylcholine receptor antagonists. Successful long-term treatment of CNS disease is hampered by a poor understanding of the disease process and the restrictive and adaptive nature of mechanisms that protect the brain.

Multiple Choice Questions

1. Which ion channel was traditionally a target for anti-epileptic medications?
   (a) Calcium
   (b) Sodium
   (c) Potassium
   (d) Magnesium

2. Repolarisation is associated with movement of which ion out of the nerve cell?
   (a) Calcium
   (b) Sodium
   (c) Potassium
   (d) Magnesium
3. Which neurotransmitter exerts the main inhibitory influence in the brain?
   (a) Dopamine
   (b) Acetylcholine
   (c) Serotonin
   (d) Gamma aminobutyric acid
4. What do phenytoin, carbamazepine and sodium valproate have in common?
   (a) They are all GABA agonists.
   (b) They are all used in the treatment of anxiety.
   (c) They all have a narrow therapeutic margin.
   (d) They are all administered intravenously.
5. In Parkinson's disease, dopamine and acetylcholine medications may be prescribed because:
   (a) They both act as inhibitory pathways in the basal ganglia.
   (b) They both act as excitatory pathways in the basal ganglia.
   (c) Dopamine pathways are excitatory and acetylcholine pathways are inhibitory in the basal ganglia.
   (d) Dopamine pathways are inhibitory and acetylcholine pathways are excitatory in the basal ganglia.
6. Mechanistically, treatment of which mental health illness may complicate treatment of Parkinson's disease the most?
   (a) Depression
   (b) Anxiety
   (c) Schizophrenia
   (d) Dementia
7. Why is the co-administration of carbidopa beneficial when administering levodopa for treating Parkinson's disease?
   (a) Because it inhibits conversion of levodopa to dopamine
   (b) Because it enhances the conversion of levodopa to dopamine
   (c) Because it only inhibits the conversion of levodopa to dopamine outside the CNS
   (d) Because it only inhibits the conversion of levodopa to dopamine inside the CNS
8. The function of a cholinesterase enzyme is to:
   (a) Break down esters found in nerve membranes
   (b) Break down acetylcholine
   (c) Increase action of acetylcholine at the synapse
   (d) Aid in acetylcholine binding to its post synaptic receptor
9. Medications that affect cholinergic nerve function will most frequently affect which other system:
   (a) Respiratory
   (b) Digestive

   (c) Olfactory
   (d) Reproductive

Answers

1. (b)
2. (c)
3. (d)
4. (c)
5. (c)
6. (c)
7. (c)
8. (b)
9. (b)

References

Agúndez JA, García-Martín E, Alonso-Navarro H, Jiménez-Jiménez FJ (2013) Anti-Parkinson's disease drugs and pharmacogenetic considerations. Expert Opin Drug Metab Toxicol 9(7):859–874

Broadstock M, Ballard C, Corbett A (2014) Latest treatment options for Alzheimer's disease, Parkinson's disease dementia and dementia with Lewy bodies. Expert Opin Pharmacother 15(13):1797–1810

Connolly BS, Lang AE (2014) Pharmacological treatment of Parkinson disease a review. JAMA J Am Med Assoc 311(16):1670–1683

European Medicines Agency (EMA) (2018). https://www.ema.europa.eu/en/documents/public-statement/public-statement-trobalt-withdrawal-marketing-authorisation-european-union_en.pdf. Accessed 5 May 2019

Harr T, French LE (2010) Toxic epidermal necrolysis and Stevens-Johnson syndrome. Orphanet J Rare Dis 16(5):39–50

Johnson M, Markham-Abedi C, Susce MT, Murray-Carmichael E, McCollum S, de Leon J (2006) A poor metabolizer for cytochromes P450 2D6 and 2C19: a case report on antidepressant treatment. CNS Spectr 11(10):757–760

Kwan P, Arzimanoglou A, Berg AT, Brodie MJ, Hauser WA, Mathern G, Moshé SL, Perucca E, Wiebe S, French J (2010) Definition of drug resistant epilepsy. Consensus proposal by the ad hoc Task Force of the ILAE Commission on Therapeutic Strategies. Epilepsia 51(6):1069–1077

Levi N, Bastuji-Garin S, Mockenhaupt M, Roujeau JC, Flahault A, Kelly JP, Martin E, Kaufman DW, Maison P (2009) Medications as risk factors of Stevens-Johnson syndrome and toxic epidermal necrolysis in children: a pooled analysis. Pediatrics 123(2):e297–e304

Molino I, Colucci L, Fasanaro AM, Traini E, Amenta F (2013) Efficacy of memantine, donepezil, or their association in moderate-severe Alzheimer's disease: a review of clinical trials. Sci World J 29:925702

National Institute of Health (2014) Parkinson's disease: diagnosis and treatment. MedlinePlus 8(4):8–10. https://medlineplus.gov/magazine/issues/winter14/articles/winter14pg8-10.html. Accessed 5 May 2019

National Institute of Health and Care Excellence (NICE) (2017) NG 71. https://www.nice.org.uk/guidance/ng71/chapter/Recommendations#pharmacological-management-of-motor-symptoms. Accessed 5 May 2019

Noetzli M, Eap CB (2013) Pharmacodynamic, pharmacokinetic and pharmacogenetic aspects of drugs used in the treatment of Alzheimer's disease. Clin Pharmacokinet 52(4):225–241

Potschka H (2013) Animal and human data: where are our concepts for drug-resistant epilepsy going? Epilepsia 54(Suppl. S2):29–32

Rolinski M, Fox C, Maidment I, McShane R (2012) Cholinesterase inhibitors for dementia with Lewy bodies, Parkinson's disease dementia and cognitive impairment in Parkinson's disease. Cochrane Database Syst Rev 2012(3):CD006504

Seripa D, Bizzarro A, Pilotto A, D'Onofrio G, Vecchione G, Gallo AP, Cascavilla L, Paris F, Grandone E, Mecocci P, Santini SA, Masullo C, Pilotto A (2011) Role of cytochrome P4502D6 functional polymorphisms in the efficacy of donepezil in patients with Alzheimer's disease. Pharmacogenet Genomics 21(4):225–230

Soldin OP, Mattison DR (2009) Sex differences in pharmacokinetics and pharmacodynamics. Clin Pharmacokinet 48(3):143–157

Stephan PL, Jaquenoud Sirot E, Mueller B, Eap CB, Baumann P (2006) Adverse drug reactions following nonresponse in a depressed patient with CYP2D6 deficiency and low CYP3A4/5 activity. Pharmacopsychiatry 39(4):150–152

Whitwell JL, Weigand SD, Shiung MM, Boeve BF, Ferman TJ, Smith GE, Knopman DS, Petersen RC, Benarroch EE, Josephs KA, Jack CR Jr (2007) Focal atrophy in dementia with Lewy bodies on MRI: a distinct pattern from Alzheimer's disease. Brain 130(3):708–719

Yang Z, Zhou X, Zhang Q (2013) Effectiveness and safety of memantine treatment for Alzheimer's disease. J Alzheimer's Dis 36(3):445–458

Medications Used for Mental Health Illness

Ehsan Khan

Learning Outcomes

At the end of this chapter, you will be able to:

- Develop an understanding of the nerve pathways associated with mental health illness.
- Identify individual drug groups for treating a range of mental health conditions.
- Recognise the adverse reactions associated with medications used for treating mental health conditions.
- Appreciate the need for focused individual care when administering, monitoring and documenting prescribed mental health medication.

13.1 Introduction: Biology of Schizophrenia

Schizophrenia presents a varied and complex array of psychotic symptoms. These have been divided into positive and negative symptoms (Birnbaum et al. 2017):

Positive symptoms

Hallucinations	
Delusions	
Positive formal thought disorder	Incoherent speech and use of particular words
	Distractible speech
Bizarre behaviour	

E. Khan (✉)
Faculty of Nursing Midwifery and Palliative Care, King's College London, London, UK
e-mail: eu.khan@kcl.ac.uk

E. Khan, P. Hood (eds.), *Understanding Pharmacology in Nursing Practice*,
https://doi.org/10.1007/978-3-032-03964-4_13

Negative symptoms

Affective flattening or blunting	Lack or reduced emotional expression
Avolition	Loss of motivation
Alogia	Reduced speech or verbal fluency
Anhedonia	Diminished capacity to experience pleasant emotions
Asociality	Reduced social interaction

13.2 Introduction: Brain Structures and the Circuitry in Schizophrenia

Drugs that are prescribed to treat psychotic episodes (antipsychotic medication) in schizophrenia modulate a number of pathways, the most important of which are the dopamine, serotonin and glutamine pathways. Schizophrenia primarily involves disruptions in dopaminergic pathways within specific brain regions. Dopamine has four nerve pathways in the brain, and although they are not all directly involved in schizophrenia, antipsychotic medications alter all four dopaminergic pathways, leading to both therapeutic effects and significant adverse outcomes (Fig. 13.1). For this reason, a brief overview of the four pathways is provided as follows:

- Nigrostriatal tract; involved in processing movement (Chap. 12 for further detail).
- Tuberoinfundibular tract; an important dopaminergic tract that links the hypothalamus with the pituitary gland. The release of dopamine into the pituitary tonically inhibits prolactin release.

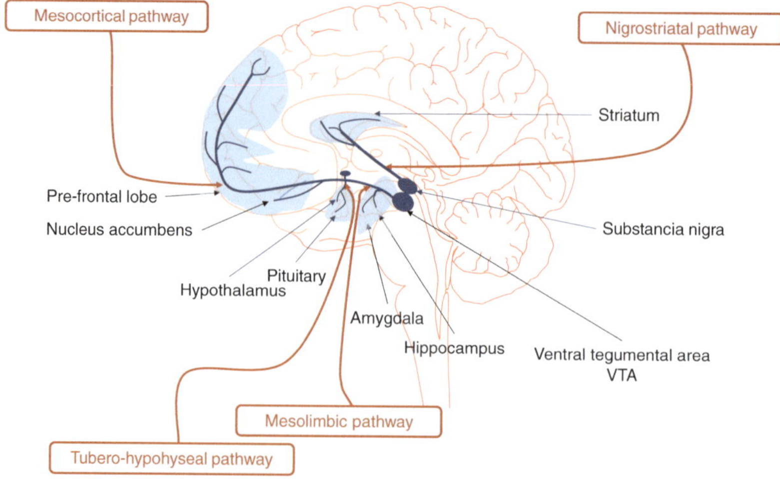

Fig. 13.1 Dopaminergic pathways in the brain

- Mesolimbic tract involved with regulating emotions includes the amygdala, hippocampus and nucleus accumbens. This tract may be associated with the positive symptoms of schizophrenia.
- Mesocortical tract, this pathway is involved with regulating thought and cognition. Hypo-function of this tract may manifest as negative symptoms of schizophrenia (Lammel et al. 2014).

Although these tracts or pathways have been shown as relatively separate entities (Fig. 13.1), they are interconnected and are regulated by a number of nerve pathways, in particular the mesocortical and mesolimbic tracts are interlinked to such an extent that they are typically portrayed together and called the mesocorticolimbic system. This interconnected system, termed the mesocorticolimbic tract, serves as the brain's primary reward circuitry, relying on dopamine as its chief neurotransmitter (Fig. 13.2).

13.2.1 The Mesocorticolimbic Tract

The mesocorticolimbic tract is of prime importance in mental health illness, as it is within these tracts that behaviour, cognition and motivation are processed. Dopamine sends out a number of axons from the ventral tegmental area (VTA) to the hippocampus, amygdala, nucleus accumbens and prefrontal cortex (PFC).

- Hippocampus
    - Memory formation
    - Spatial orientation and processing
    - Behavioural inhibition

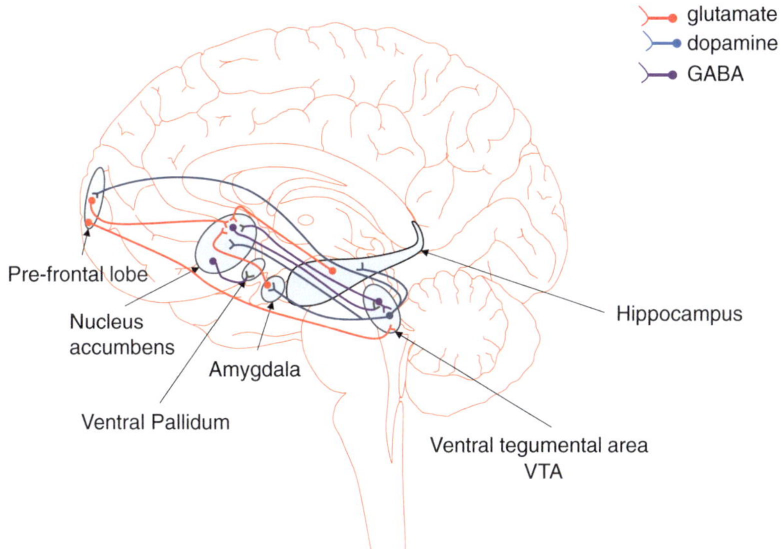

Fig. 13.2 Mesocorticolimbic system

- Amygdala
  - Memory (long term)
  - Emotional decision-making (e.g. fear and anger)
  - Gender bias
  - Social interaction
- Nucleus accumbens
  - Motivation
  - Reward
  - Reinforcement
- Pre-frontal cortex

  - Complex cognitive behaviour
  - Analysis and differentiation of concepts
  - Processes conflicting information and enables extrapolations and future prediction
  - Helps inhibit socially unacceptable urges

13.2.2 Serotonin Pathways in the Brain

Serotonin pathways, though not traditionally involved with schizophrenia symptoms, have gained attention as a target for newer antipsychotic treatments. Serotonin was initially recognised as a vascular constrictor substance that was thought to originate from the blood serum thus its name serotonin; however, serotonin is found in many parts of the body. Serotonin, produced by enterochromaffin cells in the intestinal epithelium, also plays a role in regulating digestive reflexes such as secretion and peristalsis.

In the brain, serotonergic nerves innervate many parts of the brain primarily from four nuclei, the Raphe Nuclei, which are located along the brain stem between the Pons Medulla and Cerebellum (Fig. 13.3). From these nuclei, branches enter the basal ganglia, thalamus, hypothalamus, prefrontal cortex and much of the cortex. The cerebellum is also strongly innervated with serotonin from the Raphe nuclei. Given its profuse and important distribution, serotonin modulates many functions in the brain. With the thalamus and the nearby suprachaismatic nucleus, serotonin is involved in circadian rhythm control and sleep. The hypothalamic involvement links serotonin to endocrine function, which, together with the Raphe Nuclei in general, also involves serotonergic nerves in the autonomic control, thus serotonin has an important role to play in homeostasis. Basal ganglia and cerebellar inputs involve serotonin in motor function and prefrontal cortex and limbic system involvement link serotonin to mood. Finally, the Raphe Nuclei are linked to the reticular formation which has an important sensory and nociceptive role (Fig. 13.3).

Serotonin or 5-hydroxy tryptamine (5-HT), {chemical name}, is produced from the essential amino acid l-tryptophan by the action of the enzyme 5-hydroxytrytophan decarboxylase (Fig. 13.4), unlike most nerves, serotonergic nerves release 5-HT from swellings known as varicosities along the length of the nerve (Fig. 13.4) rather

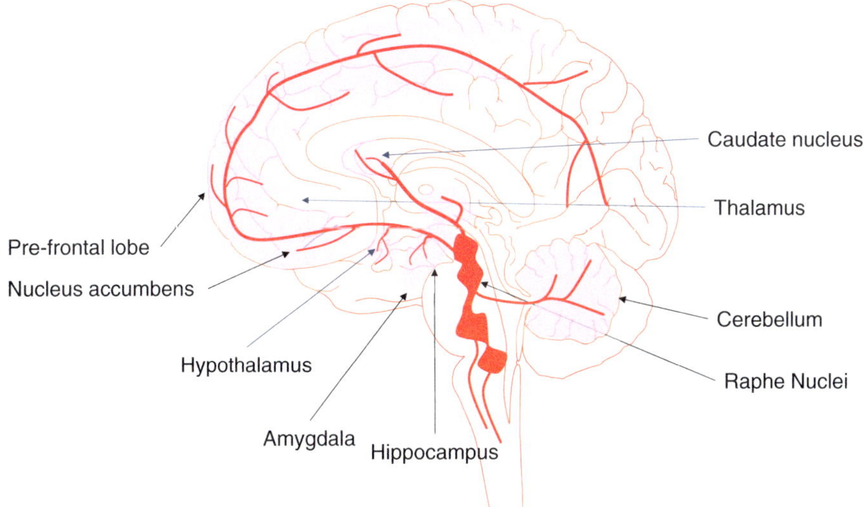

Fig. 13.3 Serotonin pathways in the brain

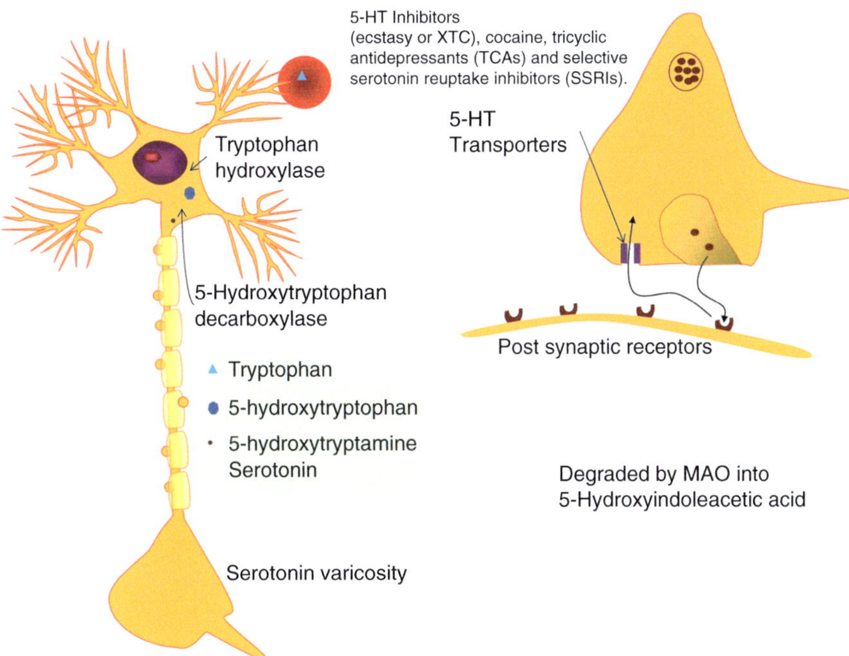

Fig. 13.4 Serotonin production and release

than via axonal end feet, 5-HT then diffuses to receptors on dendrites and synapses to elicit its effects.

13.2.2.1 Serotonin (5-HT) Receptors

Serotonin receptors are among the most diverse receptor types in the nervous system. Examination of the plethora of effects of these receptors and their location is beyond the scope of this chapter nevertheless, there are currently seven 5-HT known receptor subtypes (5-HT$_{1-7}$), of these subtypes the 5-HT$_1$ receptor have a further five subtypes (A, B, D, E and F) and 5-HT$_2$ receptors have a further three subtypes (5-HT$_{2A}$, 5-HT$_{2B}$ and 5-HT$_{2C}$). Together with other functions, the majority of these receptors are involved in mental health disorders, including anxiety, depression and what are referred to as the 'positive and negative' symptoms of schizophrenia (Lindenmayer et al. 2013).

13.2.3 Glutamate and Schizophrenia

Currently, antipsychotic medications utilise dopamine and 5-HT receptors as their primary targets. There is now a small but growing body of knowledge that suggests glutamatergic nerve modulation may enhance treatment of schizophrenia (Lin and Lane 2019). In an extensive review of atypical antipsychotic medications, Horacek et al. (2006) suggest a role for glutamate-related synapse dysfunction in schizophrenia and relate this change to changes in nerve growth factors such as brain-derived neurotrophic factor (BDNF). The notion that atypical antipsychotic medications (Second-generation antipsychotic medications) may have an indirect effect on glutamate in the pre-frontal cortex (PFC) is supported by Di Pietro and Seamans (2007), who suggest that although dopamine receptor blockade may still play an important role in antipsychotic medication drug action, indirect glutamate and GABA modulation via 5-HT may be a substantial drug mechanism. These theories fit with mesocorticolimbic nerve circuitry, particularly between the VTA and PFC nucleus accumbens (Figs. 13.2 and 13.3), where there are strong interactions between dopamine, glutamate, GABA and serotonin. Much more needs to be understood about schizophrenia before these mechanisms can be further elucidated. The use of new imaging techniques that allow real-time in vivo measurements of neurotransmitter activity will contribute to such advances. Indeed, in a review of proton magnetic resonance imaging of glutamate in people with schizophrenia, Poels et al. (2014) found an elevated glutamatergic signal in areas of the PFC and striatum in schizophrenia patients that were medication-free or naïve, which supports a role for glutamatergic neuron dysfunction with this condition.

13.3 Drugs Used for Treating Schizophrenia

Antipsychotic medication has been used since the 1950s with the introduction of chlorpromazine (Shen 1999). Many terms have been used to classify these medications including neuroleptics and dopamine antagonists. Both of these terms relate to what was thought to be the main effect of the medication, i.e. inhibition of dopamine receptors or more specifically the neuroleptic receptor that was later identified as the D_2 receptor. Currently, there are two and some suggest three generations of antipsychotic medications. Generation differences are based upon the presence of extrapyramidal side-effects (EPS) of the drugs rather than underlying drug mechanism as most first-generation (typical antipsychotic medications), and second-generation drugs (atypical antipsychotic medications), have multiple drug effects involving dopamine, serotonin (5-HT), muscarinic, alpha-adrenergic and histamine modulation.

13.3.1 First-Generation Antipsychotic Medications

First-generation antipsychotic medications such as haloperidol, thioridazine and trifluoperazine primarily act by inhibition of dopaminergic receptors. Extrapyramidal effects are drug-induced effects ascribed to nigrostriatal inhibition as a result of direct or indirect D_2 receptor antagonism (Meunch and Hamer 2010). A number of syndromes are observed, the most problematic being Tardive Dyskinesia (Box 13.1).

Box 13.1 Tardive Dyskinesia
Tardive [appearing late] dyskinesia [abnormal movement], is a symptom associated with long-term use of antipsychotic medications. This symptom may be difficult to treat and is sometimes incurable. Although typically associated with facial movements, limb movements are also common. The features of these movements are that such patients are hyperkinetic, i.e. they have an inability to stop moving, in comparison to dyskinesia, which is an inability to start moving, as is seen with Parkinson's disease.

Facial dyskinesia may manifest as excessive blinking, lip sucking and puckering and grimacing (Chang and Fung 2014). Limb dyskinesia may be evident as purposeless repetitive movement of the arms or legs, the severity of which may make walking difficult in some cases.

Interestingly, the prototype antipsychotic medication, chlorpromazine, is associated with fewer extrapyramidal adverse effects than one of the most commonly used first-generation antipsychotic medications still prescribed, haloperidol. This is suggested to be owing to its weaker dopamine receptor binding (Meunch and Hamer 2010).

13.3.2 Second-Generation Antipsychotic Medication Drugs, the Atypical

Because of the increased risk of prolactin secretion associated with dopamine antagonism and the reported extrapyramidal effects of first-generation medications, second-generation (atypical) antipsychotic medications were readily adopted in the

1990s (Shen 1999). The drug effects of atypical antipsychotic medications include a wide range of activities, ranging from single receptor antagonism or partial agonism to dual receptor effects to multi-acting receptor-targeted antipsychotic medications (MARTA) (Horacek et al. 2006) (Table 13.1). Atypical antipsychotic medications are now the most commonly prescribed.

However, atypical antipsychotic medications are not without their problems, owing to the wide-ranging expression of 5-HT receptors in the brain (Fig. 13.3) and the multiple receptor types targeted by atypical antipsychotic drugs (Table 13.1). Atypical antipsychotic medications have a number of effects that influence compliance with drug regimens. These include weight gain, precipitation of diabetes mellitus and anticholinergic effects (Table 13.2).

A secondary analysis of a first and second-generation antipsychotic medication randomised control trial has found that there was little difference between the extrapyramidal adverse effects (EPS) of first- and second-generation antipsychotic medications (Peluso et al. 2012), nevertheless, despite having similar EPS, patients receiving second-generation antipsychotic medications were 30-fold less likely to receive an anticholinergic adjunct to help relieve these adverse effects. Although further studies need to be undertaken to clarify these findings, these data may lead to a potential revision of antipsychotic medication prescribing as cheaper first-generation antipsychotic medications may have more clinical benefits than the

Table 13.1 Atypical antipsychotic receptor activity

Drug	Action
Amisulpride	D_{2-3} antagonist
Paliperidone (MARTA)	D_2, $5HT_{2A}$, $alpha_1$ and $Muscarinic_{1\&3}$ antagonist
Aripiprazole	D_2 (Partial agonist), $5HT_{2A}$ antagonist
Asenapine	D_2, $5HT_{2A\&2C}$ antagonist
Clozapine (MARTA)	$5HT_{2A\&2C}$, $alpha_1$, and $Muscarinic_{1\&3}$ antagonist
Olanzapine (MARTA)	D_{2-3}, $5HT_{2A\&2C}$, $Muscarinic_{1\&3}$, H_1 antagonist
Risperidone	D_2, $5HT_{2A}$, antagonist

Table 13.2 Atypical anti-psychotic medication metabolic adverse effects

Serotonin $5\text{-}HT_{2C}$ antagonism	Weight gain Diabetes mellitus (Citrome and Jaffe 2003)
Serotonin $5\text{-}HT_{1A}$	Weight gain
Histamine H1 antagonism	Weight gain, diabetes, sedation
Dopamine D2 antagonism	Extrapyramidal side effects (EPS), weight gain, and increased prolactin secretion
Muscarinic M1 antagonism	Anticholinergic (dry mouth, blurred vision, constipation)
Muscarinic M3 antagonism	Diabetes

Adapted from Nasrallah (2008)

metabolically disruptive second-generation antipsychotic medications given their similar EPS profile.

Given the current prevalence of second-generation antipsychotic medications in clinical practice, it is important that healthcare professionals ensure appropriate partnerships in clinical decision-making are fostered as the metabolic disturbances caused by these medications may otherwise deter adequate medication is taken and for some people, the body image change (for example, weight gain) and anxiety some adverse effects may produce further trigger or sustain a patient's psychotic disorder.

13.3.3 QT Interval Prolongation and Antipsychotic Medication

Another clinically important adverse effect associated with both first- and second-generation antipsychotic medications is drug-induced prolongation of the QT interval. The QT interval is an electrocardiograph measurement that starts at the beginning of the ventricular depolarisation complex, the QRS and ends at the end of ventricular depolarisation or the end of the T wave (Fig. 13.5). An abnormally prolonged QT interval causes an increased risk of developing a specific form of ventricular tachycardia known as torsade de pointes (Fig. 13.6a).

QT interval prolongation has traditionally been a genetic disorder which is associated with upwards of 15 different gene variants that typically encode different cardiac ion channels, particularly genes that encode for potassium ion channels. More recently, drugs that modulate the same ion channels have caused the so-called drug-induced Long QT syndrome to overtake the genetic variant in clinical practice. Genetic Long QT syndrome is a congenital disease and therefore presents early in life, it is a main contributor to cot deaths and is a significant cause of death in otherwise young and healthy adolescents. Genetic Long QT syndrome can be triggered by a number of stimuli, including competitive exertion, sudden sounds and sleeping. People with an underlying genetic predisposition of Long QT syndrome are at a higher risk of developing drug-induced long QT syndrome. A number of

Fig. 13.5 QT interval prolongation

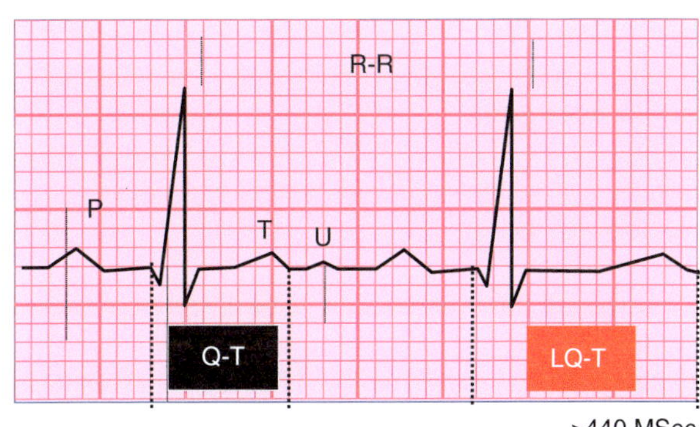

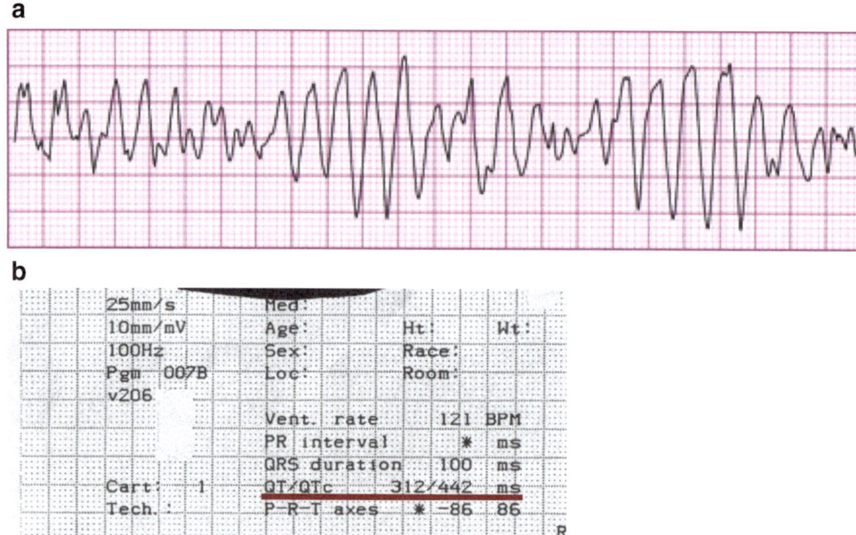

Fig. 13.6 Torsade de pointes and its clinical assessment. (a) Torsade de pointes and (b) QTc identification

medications used in general and mental health care can induce long QT. Commonly used medications that have been reported to induce long QT are given below:

- Clozapine Clozaril® Anti-psychotic
- Quetiapine Seroquel® Anti-psychotic
- Risperidone Risperdal® Anti-psychotic
- Venlafaxine Effexor® Antidepressant

Therefore, when a person is about to commence an antipsychotic medication drug regimen, it is best practice to assess the QT interval beforehand and once again when the medication has reached a steady state serum concentration. The simplest way to do this is to record a 12-Lead electrocardiograph (ECG) and read the heart rate corrected QT interval (QTc) calculated on the ECG (Fig. 13.6b). A normal QTc should be below 0.43 s (430 ms). A QTc approach 0.5 s (500 ms) is of significant clinical concern and the patient needs to be referred to specialist care to review the medication regimen.

There are a number of risk factors associated with drug-induced QT prolongation, most of which are linked directly or indirectly to drug pharmacokinetics. These risk factors include:

- women > men (as women have a different metabolic enzyme concentration than men)
- polypharmacy (more likely to burden metabolic enzymes)
- class 3 antiarrhythmics (potassium channel blockers that prolong QT intervals)

- metabolic disease (impaired drug metabolism and clearance)
- age, either extreme (impaired drug pharmacokinetics, presence of co-morbidities and risk of polypharmacy, increased risk of undiagnosed genetic long QT syndrome in children/adolescents)
- QTc >500 ms (increased risk of prolonged QT to induce torsade de pointes)
- slow HR (QT interval is at its longest at slow heart rates)
- hypokalaemia

An understanding of pharmacokinetic parameters is useful when caring for people taking antipsychotic medications together with other drugs used for mental health illnesses. With the multiple mechanisms of second-generation antipsychotic medications, there is a greater risk of drug–drug interactions occurring, such as when administering an anticholinergic with an atypical antipsychotic medication that also has anticholinergic effects. Issues regarding QT prolongation are also of clinical importance, particularly if the person has heart disease and a number of the identified risk factors. Owing to the blood-brain barrier and lipophilic nature of many of the medications used in psychiatry, these drugs tend to have long half-lives and many of which have narrow therapeutic indices. Many commonly used antipsychotic medications are metabolised by common metabolic enzymes, including CYP3A4 and CYP2D6 (Table 13.3). Such drugs may contribute to the risk of drug-drug interactions in a polypharmaceutical regimen or when there is impairment of liver or renal function. Drugs metabolised by CYP2D6 are of clinical interest because of a polymorphism (genetic variant) that, when present, leads to poor ability of this enzyme to metabolise drugs. This polymorphism is present in 7% of people with white ethnicity and 1–2% other races (Stephan et al. 2006).

Table 13.3 Second-generation antipsychotic pharmacokinetics

Drug	Half life (h)	Primary metabolic pathway
Asenapine (SL)	24	CYP1A2, UGT
Aripiprazole	75	CYP3A4, CYP2D6
Paliperidone (ext. release)	24	UGT & CYP3A4, CYP2D6 (minor/partial)
Olanzapine	33	CYP1A2, UGT & CYP2D6 (minor/partial)
Risperidone	22	CYP3A4, CYP2D6 (minor/partial)
Clozapine	9–17	CYP3A4, CYP1A2, CYP2C19 (minor/partial), CYP2D6 (minor/partial)

13.3.4 Summary

Antipsychotic medication drugs are classified according to their dopamine-mediated side effects. Drugs which are associated with significant extrapyramidal adverse effects and/or prolactin secretion have traditionally been grouped into the first generation. Medications that have other primary modes of action, such as serotonin inhibition or anti-cholinergic effects, are classified as second-generation or atypical antipsychotic medications. Currently prescribed antipsychotic medications utilise a number of different mechanisms of action including dopaminergic, serotonergic, cholinergic and histaminergic pathways, with the evolving potential to modulate the excitatory catecholamine glutamate pathway as an antipsychotic medication drug target.

Atypical antipsychotic medications gained popularity because of a purported lack of EPS, as these drugs used primary modes of action other than dopamine antagonism. However, it has been recently reported that atypical antipsychotic medications have similar extrapyramidal adverse effects to first-generation antipsychotic medications. Given the additional metabolic adverse effect profile of atypical antipsychotic medications, the choice of drug may require a review. In addition to the challenging adverse effect profiles of antipsychotic medications, their propensity to elicit drug–drug interactions requires significant clinical vigilance particularly in older patients with co-morbidities and polypharmaceutical drug burdens. The potential for drug-induced Long QT syndrome is also elevated in such a client group, although because of the traditional genetic nature of some Long QT, this syndrome can occur in adolescents. Therefore, the use of antipsychotic medications for any age may further aggravate or promote the development of a prolonged QT interval, putting the patient at increased risk of developing the potentially fatal torsade de pointes arrhythmia (Berling et al. 2018).

13.4 Antidepressants

13.4.1 The Biology of Depression

The aetiology of clinical depression is complex; many factors may contribute towards its generation, including early age experiences, current life stressors, and environmental and genetic factors (McCrae and Khan 2014). As is the case with other areas of psychiatric medicine much of what we know of the illness is extrapolated from the pharmacodynamic effects of drugs. The effects link disease process to particular nerve pathways based upon the presence or absence of effect of particular drug-target modulation. Depression and its treatment in Europe has for the last five to six decades been explained in terms of the so-called monoamine hypothesis; this suggests depression is a consequence of monoamine neurotransmitter deficiency.

For many years, the brain was thought to have a static internal environment; it is now understood that brain histology changes and adapts in response to environmental changes and injury (Calderón-Garcidueñas et al. 2015). The dynamic nature of neuronal function and connectivity is known as plasticity. Duman (2014) has suggested that stress degrades synaptic structure because of a reduction in brain-derived neurotrophic factor (BDNF), leading to poor synaptic communication. Clinically, such changes may manifest as depression. In support of this theory, Duman (2014) demonstrates that in drug-resistant depressed patients, administration of ketamine, a glutamate system (N-methyl-D-aspartate) NMDA receptor antagonist, provides a rapid and sustained reversal of depression. Studies have shown that ketamine induces BDNF in the brain, and it is postulated that ketamine-induced BDNF rejuvenates the stress-degraded synapse to its original pre-stress state (Wohleb et al. 2017). Further research needs to be undertaken to clarify this mechanism. However, this concept reiterates the issue of plasticity in CNS pharmaco-therapy. Many medications used for treatment of psychiatric illness have a significant mismatch between the time a drug serum level peaks and optimises and the onset of beneficial effect of the drug. If neural plasticity is accepted as a phenomenon, this would explain to some extent the delay, as the drug needs time to rectify the structural anomaly before a functional improved can be observed.

13.4.2 Antidepressants

Currently, the two main mechanisms that contribute towards a clinically useful antidepressant effect are receptor auto-regulation inhibition and catecholamine reuptake inhibition. Both of these mechanisms endeavour to prolong the effect of excitatory monoamines in the brain, thus reversing subdued brain activity that manifests as depression.

13.4.2.1 Receptor Auto-Regulation Inhibition

Most central or peripheral nerves have negative feedback pathways built into their synapses to help automatically regulate presynaptic neurotransmitter release. The basic principle of these mechanisms is that an increase in presynaptic neurotransmitter release will lead to an increase in presynaptic receptor binding, the result of which is a reduction in presynaptic neurotransmitter release.

Adrenergic auto-regulation is a commonly modulated mechanism in clinical depression. Adrenergic pathways in the brain have a significant role in promoting and sustaining alertness and awareness in the brain, the so-called fight-or-flight response. This response is mediated by strong adrenergic stimulation in the area of central autonomic control, the medulla oblongata, via neuronal nuclei known as the locus coeruleus. Adrenergic branches enter most areas of the cortex to elicit its effects of alertness and panic. On depolarisation, the presynaptic nerve releases noradrenaline that binds to a postsynaptic alpha 1 receptor, which then stimulates the postsynaptic nerve. Nor-adrenaline present in the synaptic cleft may, however, also bind to presynaptic alpha 2 receptors. This interaction leads to a reduction in noradrenaline release from the presynaptic adrenergic nerve (Fig. 13.7). Receptor interactions slightly favour alpha 1 stimulation, possibly helped by a slightly higher affinity of nor-adrenaline for the alpha 1 than the alpha 2 receptor.

13.4.2.2 Monoamine Reuptake Inhibition

Catecholamines are metabolised after binding to their postsynaptic receptor either by enzymatic degradation mediated by astrocyte and glial monoamine oxidase enzymes or by being taken back up into the presynaptic nerve via transport proteins

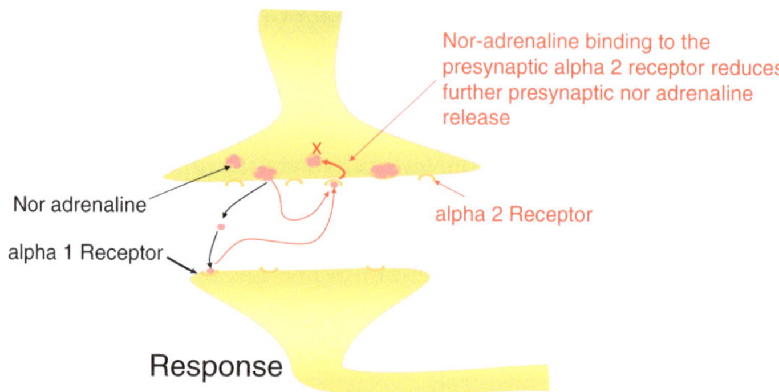

Fig. 13.7 Receptor auto-regulation

(Fig. 13.4). The net effect of this activity is to clear the synaptic cleft of neurotransmitter, thus reducing synaptic communication. A number of drugs, such as Prozac and Reboxetine, can inhibit the effect of these transport proteins leading to an increased availability of these neurotransmitters in the synaptic cleft, where they can then bind again to postsynaptic receptors, thus prolonging the response.

13.4.3 Tricyclic Antidepressants

Tricyclic antidepressants have been used clinically since the 1950s (Hillhouse and Porter 2015) and take their name from the three carbon rings that make up the drug molecule. The prototype tricyclic antidepressant (TCA) was imipramine, which is still in clinical use today. TCAs' mode of action is primarily inhibition of catecholamine transport proteins involved in neurotransmitter re-uptake from the synapse. However, these drugs were never really specific for a single kind of transport protein. TCAs also had an affinity for a number of different receptors and, in some cases, had a stronger affinity for some receptors than for transport proteins (Table 13.4). Owing to this variability and multiple affinities for different targets, TCAs are plagued with a poor and unpredictable adverse effect profile and for this reason have now been superseded by the more selective re-uptake inhibitors.

13.4.3.1 Selective Re-uptake Inhibitors

Selective monoamine transporter (re-uptake) inhibitors have now become the mainstay drugs used in depression. Selective serotonin re-uptake inhibitors (SSRIs) such as fluoxetine, sertraline and citalopram (Table 13.5) are well established and recommended for treatment of most forms of depression, including short-term and chronic mild depression as well as severe to moderate depression. Although this class of drug is normally associated with inhibition of serotonin re-uptake, some newer antidepressants include other modes or action including Mirtazapine (alpha 2 receptor antagonist), and reboxetine (a selective nor-adrenaline re-uptake inhibitor) (Table 13.5).

Table 13.4 TCA receptor binding affinity for receptors and transport proteins

Drug				
Amitriptyline	H_1 >	SERT >	5-HT2C >	M Ach
Clomipramine	SERT ≫	$Alpha_1$ ≫	H_1 >	$5\text{-}HT_{2A}$
Imipramine	SERT ≫	H_1 ≫	NET ≫	$Alpha_1$
Nortriptyline	NET >	H_1 =	$5\text{-}HT_{2C}$ >	SERT

H histamine, *SERT* serotonin transporter, *5-HT* serotonin receptor antagonist, *Mach* muscarinic receptor antagonist, *NET* nor-adrenaline transporter, *Alpha* alpha receptor antagonist
> = Affinity within a tenfold range of the next target, ≫ = affinity more than tenfold of the next target

Table 13.5 Selective re-uptake inhibitors

Drug	Mode of action
Mirtazapine	Alpha 2 inhibitor, ? 5-HT antagonist
Reboxitine	Selective Nor-adrenaline transporter inhibitor
Venlafaxine	Serotonin Nor-adrenaline transporter inhibitor
Fluoxetine	Selective Serotonin transporter inhibitor
Citalopram	Selective Serotonin transporter inhibitor
Fluvoxamine	Selective Serotonin transporter inhibitor
Paroxetine	Selective Serotonin transporter inhibitor
Sertraline	Selective Serotonin transporter inhibitor

13.4.4 Pharmacokinetic Properties of Antidepressants

The majority of antidepressants, regardless of mode of action, are metabolised by two primary metabolic enzymes, CYP2D6 and CYP3A4 (Table 13.6). As has been discussed earlier in this and other chapters, drugs metabolised by CYP3A4 are common and when put into a polypharmaceutical drug mix, they increase the risk of drug-drug interactions. The risk of these drug-drug interactions is further increased owing to the fact that many of these drugs are not just metabolised by these enzymes, but the drugs themselves act as inhibitors of these enzymes. For example, most SSRIs identified are weak to moderate enzyme inhibitors of CYP3A4. Inhibition of the enzyme will lead to an increase in drug half-life (only parent drug half-lives given in Table 13.6) and cause a potentiation of the medication and in some instances cause it to become toxic.

13.4.5 Antidepressant Adverse Effects

Adverse effects of antidepressants depend upon their mode of action. As discussed TCAs have a number of adverse effects that have limited their clinical use. Importantly, nearly all TCAs also act as sodium channel blockers (Class 1a antiarrhythmic, Chap. 7), although this effect may contribute to its neuro-genic pain relief capability, administration of most antiarrhythmic medications to a person with a normal heart rhythm will promote the formation of arrhythmias.

Table 13.6 Pharmacokinetic parameters for a selection of anti depressants

Drug	Half life (h)	Excretion	Metabolism
Amitryptyline	9–27	18% urine	CYP3A4, 2C19, 2D6
Clomipramine	30	Urine 60%, faeces 18%	CYP2D6
Imipramine	30	Urine	CYP1A2, 2C19, 2D6
Nortriptyline	28–31	Urine/faeces	CYP2D6
Citalopram	35–36	15% Urine	CYP3A4, 2C19
Fluoxetine	96–114 (repeated dose)	15% Urine	CYP2D6
Fluvoxamine	18	85% Urine	CYP2D6, 1A2, 3A4, 2C9
Paroxetine	17	64% Urine, 36% faeces	CYP2D6
Sertraline	23–26	40–45% Faeces, urine 12–14% (unchanged)	CYP2B6, 2D6
Venlafaxine	5	87% Urine	CYP2D6
Mirtazapine	20–40	75% Urine, 15% faeces	CYP1A2, 2D6, 3A4
Reboxetine	12–13	78% Urine, 10% unchanged	CYP3A4

13.4.5.1 Suicidal Tendencies

There have been many reports of suicidal thoughts and behaviour associated with antidepressants. Both the US drug monitoring agency, the Food and Drug Administration (FDA) and its UK counterpart the Medicines and Healthcare Products Regulatory Agency (MHRA) have issued a warning regarding the use of antidepressants in 18–25-year-olds in the initial stages of treatment (generally in the first 1–2 months), this statement was last updated for the HMRA in 2008. However, there has been some controversy over these statements, with some commentators critiquing the demographic links made between the data analysed by the FDA (Stone 2014). A large survey involving 8218 respondents found no association between the use of antidepressants and suicidal ideation when other symptoms of depression and anxiety were taken into account (Rissanen et al. 2014). However, this survey was open to all recipients of antidepressants and the age was not limited to adolescents as delineated by the FDA and MHRA statements. A meta-analysis of RCTs examining risk for suicidal ideation and behaviour in adolescents found a small increased risk (odds ratio 1.62) compared to an increasing protective effect in older ages (odds ratio 0.87 for 25–64 and odds ratio 0.37 for 65+) (Brent 2016). Similarly, a survey undertaken in Sweden spanning 14 years found that in young women (15–24-year-olds) there was an increase in completed suicides in those taking antidepressants from 23% in 1999–2003 to 39% in the years 2009–2013 (Larsson 2017). Therefore, a better understanding of the potential of antidepressants to cause suicidal ideas and behaviour is needed, and clearly patients receiving treatment need clinical monitoring and vigilance to ensure their safety, particularly in the 15–25 age group.

13.4.5.2 Sexual Dysfunction

Sexual dysfunction is common in depression and is aggravated by a number of antidepressants. Adverse effects of antidepressants include loss of libido, erectile dysfunction and anhedonic orgasms (pleasureless orgasms). Antidepressants that modulate serotonin uptake (SSRIs and SNRIs) are associated with the most sexual dysfunction-related adverse effects (Bergh and Giraldi 2014; Clayton et al. 2014; Montejo et al. 2019). Whereas antidepressants such as Bupropion (dopamine re-uptake inhibitor) and Buspirone (5-HT_{1A+} antagonist) were associated with the fewest sexual dysfunctional adverse effects.

13.4.5.3 Cardiovascular Adverse Effects

Cardiovascular adverse effects are not a common characteristic of antidepressants; however, when present, they can be very concerning and potentially fatal. In a longitudinal study involving 169,278 patients receiving antidepressants, a German study analysed 198 patients who had experienced cardiovascular adverse effects associated with treatment (Spindelegger et al. 2014). These revealed monoamine oxidase inhibitors (MAOIs), such as moclobemide and selegiline, were most frequently associated with severe hypotension. This effect can, of course, also increase the risk.

13.4.5.4 Antidepressant Discontinuation Syndrome

Antidepressant discontinuation syndrome (ADS), also referred to as 'Antidepressant Withdrawal Syndrome' (ADS), may present in a number of ways, including flu like symptoms, problems with sleeping, gastrointestinal disturbances, problems with coordination and gait, as well as mood disturbances. These symptoms tend to occur after having taken the medication for at least a month and are most commonly seen after the sudden stopping of medication or too rapid a down titration of the drug, suggesting a requisite development of some form of habituation process such as receptor up or down-regulation (Chap. 2). Although the mechanisms behind this phenomenon are not clear, serotonergic dysfunction appears to be central to this syndrome (Harvey and Slabbert 2014).

13.4.5.5 Other Adverse Effects

Given the plethora of modes of action a number of other general adverse effects may be observed with antidepressants, these include problems with:

- Movement and co-ordination: tremors and twitching and jerking limbs
- Sleeping: Sedation and insomnia
- Digestion large anticholinergic effects: dry mouth, GI tract disturbances, blurred vision
- Weight gain, potentially due to return of appetite

- Rash, urticaria and other hypersensitivity reactions

13.4.6 Clinical Implications of the Use of Antidepressants

The use of antidepressants in clinical practice is a relatively new introduction over the last 40 years, one of the reasons for this is that depression was never really recognized as a clinical problem, only after extensive marketing in the 1960s was depression established as a common mental disorder. The appearance of SSRIs in the late 1980s saw the first mass marketing campaign associated with antidepressants (fluoxetine). A recent meta-analysis of the effects of antidepressants on disease severity demonstrated that there was a correlation between disease severity and antidepressant benefit (Fournier et al. 2010). This analysis showed that whereas antidepressants were effective in severe depression, they had minimal to non-existent effect beyond placebo in patients with mild to moderate symptoms of depression. Thus administration and management of antidepressants must be carefully judged and balanced against the benefit-to-harm that such medications may cause. Medications such as MAOIs may be more effective than TCAs. However, MAOIs are associated with severe toxic reactions when eating certain foods containing tyramine. Processed and fermented foods tend to have high concentration of tyramine, including alcoholic beverages and fermented cheese such as stilton and some fruit and vegetables such as red kidney beans, bananas, coconuts and pineapples. Given the pharmacokinetic profile of antidepressants in general, the addition of any of these medications to a drug regimen requires careful monitoring of the patient for overt effects of the antidepressant or adverse effects of medications being co-administered. This is because of antidepressants' propensity to be metabolised by CYP3A4 and CYP2D6 and at the same time act as inhibitors of these same enzymes. This interaction will potentially elevate unchanged drug levels of other medications that the person may be taking.

13.4.7 Summary

Use of selective re-uptake inhibitors has superseded older and more toxic antidepressants such as tricyclic antidepressants and monoamine oxidase inhibitors. The mechanism of action of these medications seems to be based upon neuronal plasticity, which will result in the benefits of the medication being delayed, with the adverse effects of the medication preceding the therapeutic outcome. This phenomenon is significant as a person may choose not to persevere with the prescribed drug regimen if well-being is not initially apparent.

The limited therapeutic outcome of these medications in milder forms of depression may lead to a review of their clinical use, particularly given the potential risk of suicide in adolescents when initiating these medications.

13.5 Drugs Used for Treating Anxiety

Generalised anxiety disorder is commonly encountered in primary practice and is defined as excessive worry and difficulty in managing feelings of anxiety for at least 6 months, together with three or more of the following symptoms (Andrews et al. 2010):

- Restlessness
- Easily fatigued

- Irritability
- Difficulty concentrating
- Muscle tension
- Sleep disturbance

Other forms of anxiety are recognised including panic disorder and different kinds of phobias, together with lower grades of anxiety associated with clinical procedures. All these conditions have anxiety as a common element. Treatment of anxiety may involve the prescription of adrenaline and serotonin re-uptake inhibitors already discussed, particularly when being used long term. This section will focus on the commonly used benzodiazepines. For many years, benzodiazepines, were the most popular anxiolytic drug group used in practice. However, now due to concerns about tolerance and dependence associated with benzodiazepines they should only be prescribed in the short term.

Benzodiazepines are gamma-amino butyric acid (GABA) agonists. GABAergic nerves are the main inhibitory nerves in the brain, accounting for at least 50% of all inhibitory synapses. GABAergic pathways are found in most parts of the brain. GABA binds to a chloride ion channel that enables intracellular passive transport of chloride (Fig. 13.8). Opening of the chloride ion channel by GABA leads to the cell membrane becoming hyperpolarised as negatively charged chloride ions flood into the cell (Figs. 13.8 and 13.9). A hyperpolarised (overtly negatively charged) internal nerve membrane is hard to depolarise, therefore rendering the nerve inactive.

Examples of commonly used benzodiazepines include diazepam, lorazepam, nitrazepam, lorazepam, temazepam and midazolam. These medications cause varying levels of anxiolytic or sedative effect.

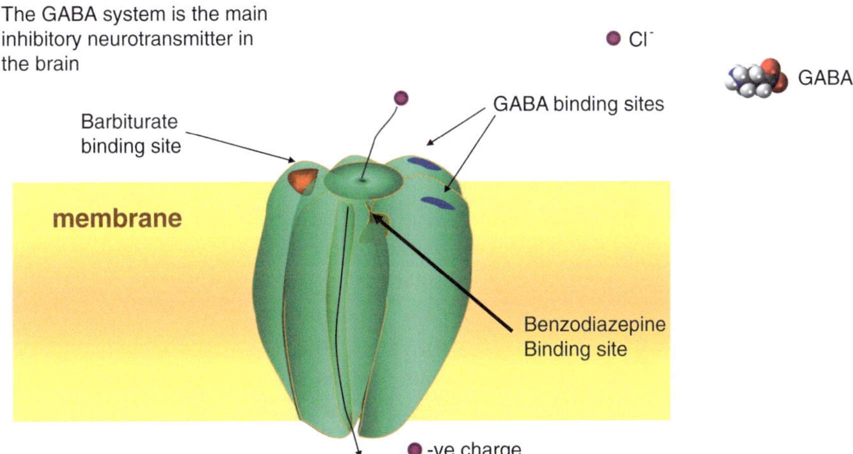

Fig. 13.8 GABA opens a chloride ion channel

Fig. 13.9 GABA activity

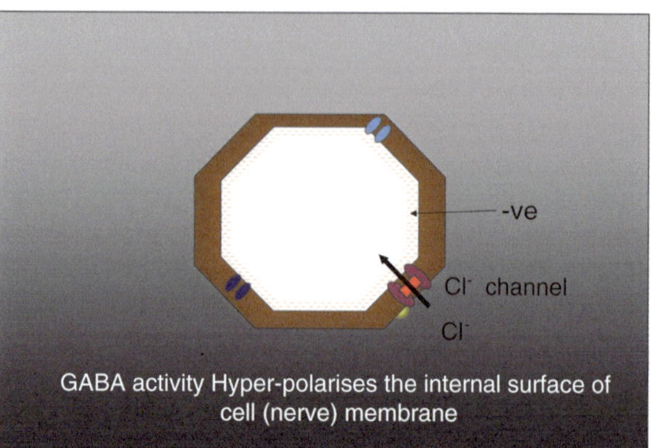

13.5.1 Adverse Effects of Benzodiazepines

Common adverse effects of this group of medications are associated with its subduing effect on the cortex and may include:

- Problems of alertness: drowsiness, dizziness and some general lack of alertness that may influence use of heavy machinery and driving and some leisure activities
- Lack of co-ordination: together with problems of alertness problems with coordination also lead to difficulties in driving and falls, with the older person particularly susceptible
- Cardiovascular effects: normally caused by use of benzodiazepine in hospital-based sedation intravenous regimen, such as intra-procedural midazolam use. These medications can cause a drop in vascular resistance that leads to hypotension and arrhythmias
- Respiratory depression: benzodiazepine may cause a drop in minute volume that is normally compensated by the patients respiratory rate
- Cognitive impairment and anterograde amnesia

13.5.2 Paradoxical Effects

A paradoxical effect of a medication exhibits as the opposite of the desired drug effect, for example, tachycardia caused by a medication that reduces heart rate, or pain being caused by an analgesia medication. These effects are disinhibition reactions associated with benzodiazepine use. These reactions generally manifest as excessive restlessness and talkativeness, as well as acts of aggression (Tae et al. 2014). Reactions are primarily based on acts of aggressive social disinhibition as well as aggression towards one's self and suicide (Saïas and Gallarda 2008). These reactions have a low frequency in the general population (approximately 1%) but are more frequent in people with borderline personality disorders or so-called recreational users of benzodiazepines (Saïas and Gallarda 2008; Jones et al. 2011).

13.5.3 Benzodiazepine Tolerance and Dependence

In addition to its anxiolytic effects, benzodiazepines may be used in other situations such as seizures, alcohol withdrawal and as a muscle relaxant. Tolerance (reduced pharmacological effect of an initially effective drug dose) to benzodiazepines may occur to a number of its therapeutic effects after a period of 4 weeks to 6 months of continual usage. There is however, some controversy over the build-up of tolerance to the anxiolytic effect of the drug (Willems et al. 2013). The mechanism of tolerance and dependence which also feeds into symptoms of withdrawal is founded on the same principle. As suggested, GABA activity is the main inhibitory system in the CNS and is important in conscious and autonomic brain function (Fig. 13.8). Benzodiazepines potentiate this effect. However, in the interest of CNS homeostasis the brain resists the potentiation of the GABA pathway. As the brain cannot limit the concentration of benzodiazepine eventually entering it, the brain may responds by down-regulating GABA receptors, thus reducing the drug-receptor binding, and reducing the drug effect. Together with this particularly in long-term use, there is an up-regulation of excitatory nerve function in the brain; this may involve all excitatory nerves including adrenergic dopaminergic and importantly glutamatergic pathways. Thus clinically the person may be receiving increasing concentrations of benzodiazepine to maintain their anxiolytic effect, the central nervous system is up-regulating its excitatory function in retaliation. Sudden or abrupt cessation or withdrawal from benzodiazepines produces a CNS excitatory overdrive as the inhibitory GABA mechanism has been down-regulated rendering endogenous concentrations of GABA release ineffective, but at the same time adrenergic (adrenergic storm) and glutamatergic pathways have been potentiated and now act unhindered (Fig. 13.9).

13.5.4 Benzodiazepine Overdose and Withdrawal

When used in in combination with other CNS depressants and with alcohol in particular, the potential for benzodiazepine overdose greatly increases combination with other CNS depressants and with alcohol in particular the potential for overdose greatly increases. Women are at more risk of overdose as they normally possess half the concentration of alcohol dehydrogenase, the enzyme that metabolises alcohol, compared to men. People with Asian ethnicity are particularly susceptible to the effects of benzodiazepine and overdose again due to polymorphistic variances and their poor ability to metabolise the drug group (Ajir et al. 1997). Flumazenil is used as an antidote for benzodiazepine use, however, owing to contraindications associated with poor vital signs, history of arrhythmia or seizures, its use is limited.

Benzodiazepine withdrawal is problematic. Symptoms of withdrawal are wide ranging and include signs of central and peripheral excitation and agitation leading to muscles tremors and irritability to CNS excitation resulting in insomnia, agitation and more severe cognitive impairments such as psychosis and suicidal thoughts and behaviour. Frequency and severity of withdrawal symptoms have been linked to the rate of withdrawal. Benzodiazepines should not be withdrawn abruptly. There is no clear consensus on how long it should take to withdraw benzodiazepines as the duration depends upon many factors include dosage, age of patient underlying pathology and environmental issues. Withdrawal can take anywhere from 4–5 weeks to 2–3 years. During withdrawal, it is important to keep the person from using CNS depressants. As already mentioned alcohol can lead to benzodiazepine potentiation. The broad spectrum fluoroquinolones group antibiotics (ciprofloxacin) should also be avoided as they displace benzodiazepines from its ion channel binding site, further reducing the GABA effect in the brain and aggravating withdrawal symptoms.

13.5.5 Benzodiazepine Pharmacokinetics

Benzodiazepines are lipophilic medications and are metabolised by CYP3A4 (Table 13.7). Given the recommended short-term use of this medication, the effects of enzyme-related drug–drug interactions are unclear. However, a number of benzodiazepines are hepatotoxic in their own right and this property is believed to be associated with nitrobenzodiazepines such as flunitrazepam, nimetazepam, and nitrazepam (Mizuno et al. 2009).

Table 13.7 Benzodiazepine pharmacokinetics

Drug	Half life (h)	Metabolism	Clearance	Dependence
Diazepam	20–100	CYP3A4	Urine	Moderate
Midazolam	1.8–6.4	CYP3A4	Urine	–
Temazepam	8–20	Liver	Urine	High
Nitrazepam	16–38	CYP3A4 + Phase II	Urine	–
Lorazepam	9–16	Phase II	Urine	Moderate to high

13.5.6 Clinical Implications of Use of These Medications

Anxiolytic therapies may be divided into short- and long-term therapies. Although benzodiazepines have been used for many years for both short and long durations, concerns regarding tolerance and dependence have now caused most medication regulating agencies including those in Canada, the USA and the UK to only recommend them for short-term use. Conversely SSRIs and SNRIs are recommended for long-term use in anxiety. However, as discussed in antidepressants, these drugs are also associated with considerable adverse effects, particularly in young patients. They also produce withdrawal (discontinuation syndrome) that requires significant clinical management and vigilant monitoring.

Owing to concerns regarding tolerance and dependence benzodiazepines have been somewhat superseded by other medications as long-term anxiolytics. They are however, still commonly used medications for short-term use both in primary, secondary and tertiary care. Drug safety varies according to the potency of the drugs. In primary care, short-term usage of orally administered drugs such as diazepam (Valium) is safe unless prescribed with other CNS depressants or taken with alcohol.

Medications such as temazepam and midazolam, particularly when administered intravenously, are associated with risk of respiratory and cardiovascular depression requiring close continuous monitoring of the patient.

13.5.7 Summary

Medications used for the treatment of mental ill health act on a number of areas in the brain, including the mesocortico limbic reward and motivation centres, together with more general nerve pathways responsible for stimulation and alertness as well as pathways involved in inhibition of brain activity. There is considerable overlap between uses of particular medication classes in different mental health conditions; this signifies the complex nature of mental health disease. Effects of antipsychotic medications have traditionally been based on interactions with dopaminergic nerves, with the more recent addition of serotonergic and glutama-tergic nerve interactions. Common antidepressants affect a person's mood by inhibiting the removal of excitatory monoamine neurotransmitters from the synapse. Short-term use anxiolytics are dominated by the GABA agonist benzodiaz-epine drug class, with long-term therapies being associated with monoamine re-uptake inhibitors. Many medications used for mental health illness may be associated with tolerance, habituation or addiction. Adverse effects of drug classes include extrapyramidal motor and metabolic disturbances with antipsychotic medications, antidepressants have the additional danger of being associated with an increased risk of suicidal behaviours in the adolescent and younger adult age groups. Whereas anxiolytic medications are associated with significant withdrawal syndromes. In combination with CNS depressants such as alcohol and opioids, benzodiazepine anxiolytic medications are associated with a considerable fatality risk.

Multiple Choice Questions

1. Inhibition of dopaminergic nerves by antipsychotic medication medications commonly results in which symptom:
   - (a) Chest pain
   - (b) Parkinsonian symptoms
   - (c) Itching
   - (d) Hyperglycaemia
2. Electrocardiograms (ECGS) are now required for the majority of patients being treated with antipsychotic medications. This is undertaken to identify a variant of which abnormal heart rhythm:
   - (a) Atrial tachycardia
   - (b) Ventricular tachycardia
   - (c) AV Block
   - (d) Atrial fibrillation

3. Dopaminergic-mediated prolactin secretion leading to lactation used to be an adverse effect commonly associated with typical antipsychotic medications:
   (a) True
   (b) False
4. Serotonin re-uptake inhibitors may cause which problematic adverse effect:
   (a) Bradycardia
   (b) Weight gain
   (c) Chest pain
   (d) Bronchospasm
5. Drugs that interact with cytochrome P450 3A4 (CYP3A4), commonly increase the risk of drug interactions. Identify the CYP that is of importance in antidepressant drug metabolism:
   (a) CYP2E1
   (b) CYP2B6
   (c) CYP2D6
   (d) CYP1A2
6. Benzodiazepines act on which form of nerve receptor:
   (a) Glutamatergic
   (b) Cholinergic
   (c) Adrenergic
   (d) GABAergic
7. Use of benzodiazepines is associated with which problem:
   (a) Insomnia
   (b) Diarrhoea
   (c) Withdrawal symptoms
   (d) Tardive dyskinesia
8. Which ethnicity population has difficulty metabolising benzodiazepines, resulting in the risk of elevated drug levels:
   (a) Asian
   (b) Black
   (c) Polynesian
   (d) White

Answers

1. (b)
2. (b)
3. (a)
4. (b)
5. (c)
6. (d)
7. (c)
8. (a)

References

Ajir K, Smith M, Lin KM, Fleishaker JC, Chambers JH, Anderson D, Nuccio I, Zheng Y, Poland RE (1997) The pharmacokinetics and pharmacodynamics of adinazolam: multi-ethnic comparisons. Psychopharmacology 129:265–270

Andrews G, Hobbs MJ, Borkovec TD, Beesdo K, Craske MG, Heimberg RG, Rapee RM, Ruscio AM, Stanley MA (2010) Generalized worry disorder: a review of DSM-IV generalized anxiety disorder and options for DSM-V. Depress Anxiety 27(2):134–147

Bergh SJ, Giraldi A (2014) Sexual dysfunction associated with antidepressant agents. Ugeskr Laeger 176(22):pii: V11130687

Berling I, Gupta R, Bjorksten C, Prior F, Whyte IM, Berry S (2018) A review of ECG and QT interval measurement use in a public psychiatric inpatient setting. Australas Psychiatry 26(1):50–55

Birnbaum ML, Wan CR, Broussard B, Compton MT (2017) Associations between duration of untreated psychosis and domains of positive and negative symptoms. Early Interv Psychiatry 1(5):375–382

Brent DA (2016) Antidepressants and suicidality. Psychiatr Clin N Am 39(3):503–512

Calderón-Garcidueñas L, Calderón-Garcidueñas A, Torres-Jardón R, Avila-Ramírez J, Kulesza RJ, Angiulli AD (2015) Air pollution and your brain: what do you need to know right now. Prim Health Care Res Dev 16(4):329–345

Chang FC, Fung VS (2014) Clinical significance of pharmacogenomic studies in tardive dyskinesia associated with patients with psychiatric disorders. J Pharmgenomics Pers Med 13(7):317–328

Citrome LL, Jaffe AB (2003) Relationship of atypical antipsychotic medications with development of diabetes mellitus. Ann Pharmacother 37(12):1849–1857

Clayton AH, El Haddad S, Iluonakhamhe JP, Ponce Martinez C, Schuck AE (2014) Sexual dysfunction associated with major depressive disorder and antidepressant treatment. Expert Opin Drug Saf 13(10):1361–1374

Di Pietro NC, Seamans JK (2007) Dopamine and serotonin interactions in the prefrontal cortex: insights on antipsychotic medication drugs and their mechanism of action. Pharmacopsychiatry 40(Suppl 1):S27–S33

Duman RS (2014) Neurobiology of stress, depression, and rapid acting antidepressants: remodeling synaptic connections. Depress Anxiety 31(4):291–296

Fournier JC, DeRubeis RJ, Hollon SD, Dimidjian S, Amsterdam JD, Shelton RC, Fawcett J (2010) Antidepressant drug effects and depression severity: a patient-level meta-analysis. JAMA J Am Med Assoc 303(1):47–53

Harvey BH, Slabbert FN (2014) New insights on the antidepressant discontinuation syndrome. Hum Psychopharmacol 29(6):503–516

Hillhouse TM, Porter JH (2015) A brief history of the development of antidepressant drugs: from monoamines to glutamate. Exp Clin Psychopharmacol 23(1):1–21

HMRA (2008) https://www.hma.eu/fileadmin/dateien/Human_Medicines/CMD_h_/Product_Information/PhVWP_Recommendations/Antidepressants/PAR_suicidal_thoughts.pdf (accessed 2026)

Horacek J, Bubenikova-Valesova V, Kopecek M, Palenicek T, Dockery C, Mohr P, Höschl C (2006) Mechanism of action of atypical antipsychotic medication drugs and the neurobiology of schizophrenia. CNS Drugs 20(5):389–409

Jones KA, Nielsen S, Bruno R, Frei M, Lubman DI (2011) Benzodiazepines—their role in aggression and why GPs should prescribe with caution. Aust Fam Physician 40(11):862–865

Lammel S, Lim BK, Malenka RC (2014) Reward and aversion in a heterogeneous midbrain dopamine system. Neuropharmacology 76(Pt B):351–359

Larsson J (2017) Antidepressants and suicide among young women in Sweden 1999-2013. Int J Risk Saf Med 29(1–2):101–106

Lin CH, Lane HY (2019) Early identification and intervention of schizophrenia: insight from hypotheses of glutamate dysfunction and oxidative stress. Front Psych 10:93

Lindenmayer JP, Nasrallah H, Pucci M, James S, Citrome L (2013) A systematic review of psychostimulant treatment of negative symptoms of schizophrenia: challenges and therapeutic opportunities. Schizophr Res 147(2–3):241–252

McCrae N, Khan E (2014) Shooting the messenger: the neurobiology of depression. Br J Neurosci Nurs 10(4):185–190

Meunch J, Hamer AN (2010) Adverse effects of antipsychotic medications. Am Fam Physician 81(5):617–622

Mizuno K, Katoh M, Okumura H, Nakagawa N, Negishi T, Hashizume T, Nakajima M, Yokoi T (2009) Metabolic activation of benzodiazepines by CYP3A4. Drug Metab Dispos 37(2):345–351

Montejo AL, Calama J, Rico-Villademoros F, Montejo L, González-García N, Pérez J, SALSEX Working Study Group (2019) A real-world study on antidepressant-associated sexual dysfunction in 2144 outpatients: the SALSEX I study. Arch Sex Behav 48(3):923–933

Nasrallah HA (2008) Atypical antipsychotic medication-induced metabolic side effects: insights from receptor-binding profiles. Mol Psychiatry 13(1):27–35

Peluso MJ, Lewis SW, Barnes TRE, Jones PB (2012) Extrapyramidal motor side-effects of first- and second-generation antipsychotic medication drugs. Br J Psychiatry 200:387–392

Poels EM, Kegeles LS, Kantrowitz JT, Javitt DC, Lieberman JA, Abi-Dargham A, Girgis RR (2014) Glutamatergic abnormalities in schizophrenia: a review of proton MRS findings. Schizophr Res 152(2–3):325–332

Rissanen I, Jääskeläinen E, Isohanni M, Koponen H, Joukamaa M, Alaräisänen A, Miettunen J (2014) Use of antidepressant medication and suicidal ideation-the Northern Finland Birth Cohort 1966. Hum Psychopharmacol 29(6):559–567

Saïas T, Gallarda T (2008) Paradoxical aggressive reactions to benzodiazepine use: a review. L'Encéphale 34(4):330–336

Shen WW (1999) A history of antipsychotic drug development. Compr Psychiatry 40(6):407–414

Spindelegger C, Papageorgiou K, Grohmann R, Engel RR, Greil W, Konstantinidis A, Agelink MW, Bleich S, Ruether E, Toto S, Kasper S (2014) Cardiovascular adverse reactions during antidepressant treatment: a drug surveillance report of German-speaking countries between 1993 and 2010. Int J Neuropsychopharmacol 18(4):pyu080

Stephan PL, Jaquenoud Sirot E, Mueller B, Eap CB, Baumann P (2006) Adverse drug reactions following nonresponse in a depressed patient with CYP2D6 deficiency and low CYP 3A4/5 activity. Pharmacopsychiatry 39(4):150–152

Stone MB (2014) The FDA warning on antidepressants and suicidality—why the controversy? N Engl J Med 371(18):1668–1671

Tae CH, Kang KJ, Min BH, Ahn JH, Kim S, Lee JH, Rhee PL, Kim JJ (2014) Paradoxical reaction to midazolam in patients undergoing endoscopy under sedation: incidence, risk factors and the effect of flumazenil. Dig Liver Dis 46(8):710–715

Willems IA, Gorgels WJ, Oude Voshaar RC, Mulder J, Lucassen PL (2013) Tolerance to benzodiazepines among long-term users in primary care. Fam Pract 30(4):404–410

Wohleb ES, Gerhard D, Thomas A, Duman RS (2017) Molecular and cellular mechanisms of rapid-acting antidepressants ketamine and scopolamine. Curr Neuropharmacol 15(1):11–20

Medications Used for Cancer

14

Mary Anne Lagmay Tanay

Learning Outcomes
At the end of this chapter, you will be able to:

- Understand how systemic anticancer therapies impact cancer cells.
- Identify types of cytotoxic chemotherapy and routes of administration.
- Describe the principles of cytotoxic chemotherapy administration.
- Identify the most common adverse reactions of cytotoxic chemotherapy.
- Understand the key differences between cytotoxic chemotherapy and some novel cancer therapies.
- Describe measures to ensure patient and staff safety in administration of systemic anticancer therapies.

14.1 Introduction

Cancer is a group of diseases characterised by uncontrolled multiplication and spread of abnormal cells in the body (Yandle 2014). It is one of the most common causes of death in developed nations. Cancer Research UK (2015) reports that between 2017 and 2019, more than 385,000 people were newly diagnosed with cancer in the United Kingdom. There are three main treatment modalities for cancer—surgery, irradiation and systemic anticancer therapies (SACT). SACT has an integral role in the treatment of cancer and despite rapid advances in other treatment strategies, it remains a mainstay treatment modality for many solid tumours and haematological malignancies.

M. A. L. Tanay (✉)
Berkshire Cancer Centre, Royal Berkshire NHS Foundation Trust, Reading, UK
e-mail: mary.tanay@nhs.net

E. Khan, P. Hood (eds.), *Understanding Pharmacology in Nursing Practice*,
https://doi.org/10.1007/978-3-032-03964-4_14

14.2 Pathology of Cancer

The term cancer refers to a malignant neoplasm (new growth). The growth of cancer is called *carcinogenesis* or *tumorigenesis*. The transformation of one normal cell into a cancer cell is caused by one or more mutations in the cell's DNA, which can be acquired or inherited. Examples of carcinogenic (cancer-causing) factors include smoking, radiation and viruses such as human papillomavirus, which cause acquired cell mutation. Epigenetic factors such as hormones and carcinogens do not produce cancer but increase the likelihood that the genetic mutations will eventually result in cancer. An example of an inherited mutation is breast cancer. Women who inherit a single defective copy of either of the tumour suppressor genes BRCA1 and BRCA2 have a significantly increased risk of developing breast cancer (Madariaga et al. 2019). Carcinogenesis is a complex process and usually involves more than one genetic factor and other epigenetic factors.

There are two main categories of genetic changes that may lead to malignancy. These are as follows:

1. *The activation of proto-oncogenes to oncogenes*

   Cell division, apoptosis and differentiation are normally controlled by *proto-oncogenes*. *Oncogenes* are DNA sequences that code the key proteins involved in carcinogenesis. About 100 dominant oncogenes have been identified. When proto-oncogenes are converted to oncogenes, malignant cell change is induced by viral and carcinogenic action.

2. *The inactivation of tumour suppressor genes*

   Normal cells contain *tumour suppressor genes* that have the ability to suppress malignant change. Evidence shows that the loss of function and mutation of these tumour suppression genes are involved in many different cancers. Examples of tumour suppressor genes are *p53* and *rb*. Mutations of these genes are identified in Li-Fraumeni syndrome and retinoblastoma, respectively.

Hanahan and Weinberg (2011) identified six hallmarks of cancer. These are biological capabilities cells acquire as they develop into cancer cells. These include the following:

1. Sustaining proliferative signalling
2. Evading growth suppressors
3. Resisting cell death
4. Enabling replicative immortality
5. Inducing angiogenesis (formation of new blood vessels)
6. Activating invasion and metastasis

14.3   What Is Systemic Anticancer Therapy (SACT)

SACT is an umbrella term for all drug treatments used to treat cancer, including cytotoxic chemotherapy and targeted anticancer treatments. SACT is most often used in combination with other cancer treatment modalities. It is very seldom that SACT is used on its own because for many cancers, SACT alone will not treat the disease. SACTs may be used as adjuvant treatment, meaning 'in addition to'. For example, SACT is often used as an adjuvant treatment following surgery, which is a primary treatment. In this example, SACT is administered after surgical removal of tumour to destroy any remaining cancer cells in the body. As it is delivered systemically, SACT drugs are able to reach most tissues and attack microscopic or inoperable metastatic cancer cells. Radiotherapy is often used as adjuvant treatment to help destroy specific identified areas of cancer growth but unlike chemotherapy, it is used to target specific areas of cancer growth. In some cases, all three treatment modalities can be used to achieve better outcomes.

SACT can also be used as a *neo-adjuvant treatment*. This means that it is used as a supplementary treatment *before* the primary treatment. This is often done in order to shrink the tumour prior to surgery to make it more feasible to surgically remove the entire tumour. SACT can also be given prior to radiotherapy. *Concomitant SACT* is the term used while a patient is receiving another treatment modality such as radiotherapy. SACT may also be used as the primary treatment, mainly for haematological malignancies such as acute leukaemia. As malignant white cells naturally travel throughout the body, the only available option is a systemic treatment such as SACT. *Palliative SACT* is used when the goal of treatment is to alleviate cancer symptoms, such as pain, when no more treatment options are available.

14.3.1 Routes of Administration

SACTs may be administered through various routes such as intravenous, oral, subcutaneous, intramuscular, topical, intrathecal, intra-vesical, intra-ventricular, intra-peritoneal, intra-arterial, intra-ocular and intra-pleural. Administration routes may be influenced by several factors, which include the type of cancer, drug bioavailability, the condition of the patient and any comorbidities they may have, age, health status and patient choice.

14.3.2 Principles of SACT Administration

Patients requiring SACTs are prescribed treatment according to a SACT protocol (or treatment plan), which provides guidance on how the treatment should be given. It also includes supportive treatment that is given before or after SACT administration, which can include pre-hydration, antiemetics and antihistamines. As new drugs are developed and treatments evolve, the use of SACT as a treatment modality for cancer is an area that is constantly changing. Hundreds of different cytotoxic chemotherapy, immunotherapies and targeted anticancer drugs are now available; however, the specific drugs used for the treatment of patients with cancer will depend on both disease and individual patient-related factors. These will include the following:

- Type of cancer
- Grade/stage of cancer
- Goal of treatment (primary, palliative, neo-adjuvant)
- Tumour location and spread
- Tumour characteristics and genomics
- Previous treatments with SACT
- Potential drug side effects and adverse events
- Patient age and performance status
- Comorbidities
- Social circumstances and available support
- Combination with other treatment modalities such as radiotherapy or surgery

In order to maximise its potential, SACT needs to be given repeatedly over an extended period of time (Morgan 2003). The interval between treatments is known as *cycles*. Most SACT cycles are timed to facilitate normal healthy cells to recover from the toxic effects of the drugs. It is also important, however, to prevent long episodes between cycles to elapse as this may lead to the cancer cells repopulating and tumour growth. Recovery times will vary depending on the specific SACTs that are given. However, many cytotoxic chemotherapy cycles are timed to be administered every 21–28 days, as this allows for bone marrow cells to recover to prevent life-threatening complications. Some newer SACTs such as CDK4/6 inhibitors used in metastatic breast cancer are not given in fixed doses but continue until disease progression. Delaying, reducing or discontinuing SACT may be necessary to manage SACT-related adverse reactions. SACT-related adverse reactions may be classified in various ways. These are presented in Table 14.1.

Table 14.1 Classification of SACT-associated adverse reactions

Category	Types
Onset	Immediate
	Late
Length of manifestation	Acute
	Chronic
Severity	Mild to severe
	Life threatening
Dose-related	Cumulative effect
	Unrelated to frequency or number of doses
Reversibility	Reversible/temporary
	Irreversible/permanent

14.4 Cytotoxic Chemotherapy Mechanism of Action

Cytotoxic chemotherapy is the use of drugs that are toxic to human cells, to kill or disable cells, either leading to cell death (apoptosis) or preventing cell replication. The term '*chemotherapy*' is used when referring to cytotoxic chemotherapy in clinical practice, frequently called 'cytotoxics' and 'chemo'.

Different healthy cells in the body have varying rates of division and proliferation. Some cells have little or no capacity to divide and proliferate, such as the neurons, while other cells, such as those in the gastrointestinal mucosa and bone marrow, are rapidly dividing. Normal cell proliferation is balanced by cell death (apoptosis). Apoptosis is a process in which obsolete or damaged cells undergo an organised progression to programmed cell death.

Cancer is a proliferative disease in which cell growth is increased, abnormal and uncontrolled. The main purpose of using chemotherapeutic agents to treat cancer is to prevent cancer cells from multiplying, invading other tissues and metastasising (spreading to another part of the body away from the primary tumour), causing morbidity and mortality. Most cytotoxic chemotherapies discussed in this chapter focus on affecting cancer cell proliferation. Therefore, to understand how chemotherapy operates, it is essential to understand the basic processes of cellular proliferation.

The cell cycle starts and ends with mitosis, a period of nuclear cell division when the cell splits into two identical daughter cells. Mitosis comprises subphases: Prophase, Metaphase, Anaphase and Telophase. The cell prepares the main components of the cell during these phases. Chromatin, chromosomes, centromeres and spindle fibres enable the cell to divide into two daughter cells. After telophase, there is a process of cytokinesis when the cell's cytoplasmic composition is equally reallocated into two equally sized daughter cells. One of these two daughter cells usually matures and takes on a specific function of the tissues or organ that it is intended to become. The other usually remains as a stem cell until it receives a stimulus to reproduce and make a new cell to replace another that has died.

When the cell is not dividing, it is in interphase, a period when the cell is resting from dividing. However, there are various metabolic processes that are taking place; thus, it is not in absolute 'rest'.

It is very common that a cell will leave the cell cycle and will never re-enter the cell cycle. This is called the G zero phase (G0). When cells are in this phase, these are carrying out the function of that particular cell (e.g. liver cells, skin cells, muscle cells) The cell will carry out its function until it dies, which then prompts a signal to the 'other remaining cell' which is in G1 phase to progress to the cell cycle and divide into another two identical daughter cells (Table 14.2). The cell cycle and G0 are illustrated in Fig. 14.1.

Table 14.2 Four stages of cell progression

G1 phase (Gap 1)—characterised by rapid growth and metabolic activity as the cell prepares to double its DNA
S phase (DNA synthesis)—further growth and the amount of DNA is doubled
G2 phase (Gap 2)—the cell makes final preparation for division
M phase (mitosis)—the cell divides into two daughter cells

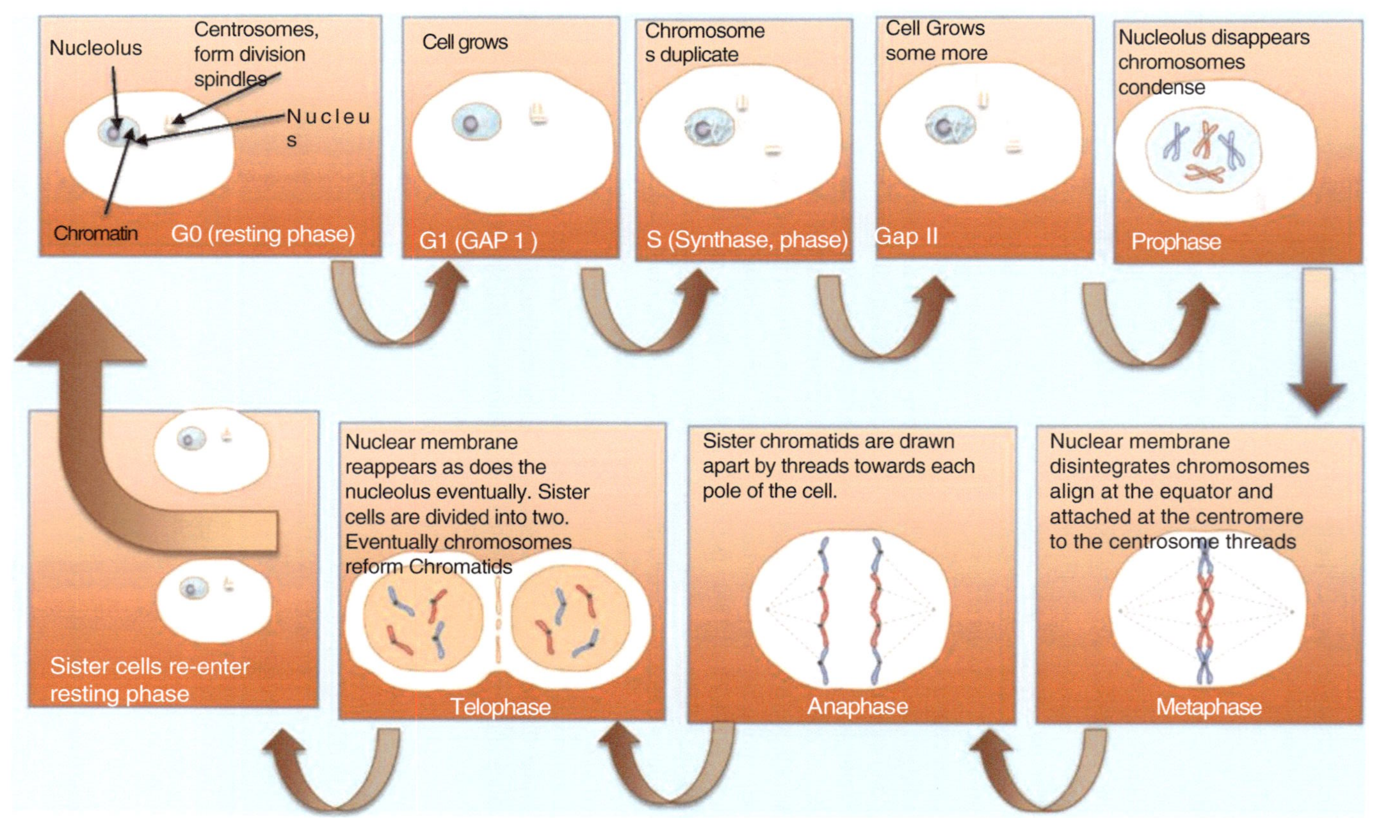

Fig. 14.1 The cell cycle

14.5 Phase and Cell Cycle Specificity

Cell cycle phase specific chemotherapy drugs exert an effect on cells that are actively in the cell cycle and affect specific phases of the cell cycle. This prevents the cell from completing its cycle or leads to its death. These drugs are most effective against rapidly cycling cells and small tumours with a high growth fraction. Because only those cells in the sensitive phase (when chemotherapy drugs are most effective) are killed, there is a limit to the number of cells that can be killed with a single drug exposure. A higher dose of the drug does not kill more cells. Therefore, to kill more cells, prolonged or repeated doses of the drug should be administered to allow more cells to enter the sensitive phase of the cycle. A greater number of cancer cells could be killed by a phase-specific drug if the number of cells in the sensitive phase could be increased. On the other hand, cell cycle-specific (or phase nonspecific) chemotherapy drugs do not rely on the cell to be in a specific phase to be effective, but are actively effective throughout the cycle. Some drugs may have greater activity in one phase than in the other. Cell cycle-nonspecific chemotherapy is effective whether the cells are resting or dividing.

14.6 Types and Classification of Cytotoxic Chemotherapy Drugs

Cytotoxic drugs may be classified into five main categories. These are as follows:

1. Alkylating Agents—Alkylating agents directly damage DNA by interfering with transcription and replication. Their main effect is seen during replication (S phase) when some zones of the DNA are unpaired and more susceptible to alkylation. As a result, G2 phase is blocked, which eventually causes apoptosis (cell death). Examples of alkylating agents are cyclophosphamide, cisplatin, melphalan and chlorambucil.
2. Antimetabolites—interfere with DNA and RNA growth by substituting for the normal building blocks of RNA and DNA. These damage cells during the S phase. Methotrexate, capecitabine, cytarabine and gemcitabine are some examples of antimetabolites.
3. Antitumour Antibiotics—bind with DNA by interfering with enzymes involved in DNA replication, thereby inhibiting DNA and RNA synthesis. These drugs work in all phases of the cell cycle. Bleomycin, mitomycin, daunorubicin, doxorubicin and epirubicin are examples of antitumour antibiotics.
4. Mitotic Inhibitors—these drugs stop mitosis through the inhibition of enzymes from making proteins needed for cell production. These drugs work during M phase of the cell cycle but can damage cells in all cycles. Some of the most commonly used mitotic inhibitors are taxanes (e.g. docetaxel and paclitaxel) and vinca alkaloids (e.g. vincristine, vinblastine and vinorelbine).
5. Topoisomerase Inhibitors—interfere with enzymes called topoisomerases, which are essential in the separation of DNA strands during replication. Examples include irinotecan and etoposide.

Other anticancer drug regimes include hormones. These include steroids such as glucocorticoids, oestrogens and androgens. Drugs that suppress or antagonise hormone secretion are also under this category. Examples include tamoxifen, aromatase inhibitors such as Letrozole (Femara®), Anastrozole (Arimidex®) and luteinising hormone blockers such as Goserelin (Zoladex®) and Leuprorelin (Prosta®). Other SACTs are designed to affect specific tumour-related cell-signalling pathways to stop cancer cell growth.

SACTs may be given as a single agent or in combination with other SACTs. Combination cytotoxic chemotherapy is often more effective than single agents, as combined they can target cells at different stages of the cell cycle or target both cycling and resting cells, as well as different targeted mechanisms of cancer growth. The goal of combination therapy is twofold: (1) to achieve maximal tumour cell kill without excessive toxicity and (2) to reduce the likelihood of resistance and improve response rates. There are several principles that guide clinicians when prescribing combination chemotherapies to achieve their goals but at the same time ensuring patient safety (Skeel et al. 2016). These are summarised below:

Whenever possible,

- Each SACT drug in the combination should be active against the specific type of cancer when used on its own
- The mechanisms of action of the different agents should work together to complement each other. For example, a cell cycle phase-specific chemotherapy may be combined with a cell cycle nonphase-specific agent to produce maximum cell kill
- Chemotherapy agents that produce adverse reactions in different organ systems should be combined so that maximum doses of each can be administered without excessive toxicity
- Drugs that have different adverse reactions occurring at different times should be combined

14.7 Adverse Reactions of Cytotoxic Chemotherapy

Cytotoxic chemotherapeutic agents are unable to target malignant cells exclusively. Rapidly dividing normal cells are also affected when patients receive chemotherapy. As a result, temporary damage occurs to frequently dividing normal cells such as bone marrow, gastrointestinal mucosa, gonads and hair follicles (Barton-Burke and Wilkes 2018). Normal cells have more efficient repair mechanisms than cancer cells therefore damage to normal cells is usually temporary, although in some cases, adverse events may be permanent. This is why it is important to give time for the normal cells to recover by allowing breaks in between chemotherapy cycles.

Prior to administration of the next dose of chemotherapy, it is important to determine if the patient has experienced any adverse reactions with the previous cycle. Depending on the severity of any adverse reactions, chemotherapy may be delayed or dose-reduced. Certain chemotherapeutic agents have an affinity for certain organs in the body. When given over time, these may cause toxicity on that specific organ. An example of this is Doxorubicin, which may cause myofibril damage in the heart, leading to an increased risk of cardiomyopathy.

According to Skeel et al. (2016), there are several factors that may contribute to the severity and nature of adverse reactions with cytotoxic chemotherapy:

(a) A specific chemotherapeutic agent—for example, Cisplatin is more likely to cause nausea and vomiting than Fluorouracil
(b) Dose—higher doses usually result in severe adverse reactions
(c) The administration schedule (infusion rate and frequency of dose)—cycles administered more closely to each other provide less time for normal healthy cells to recover
(d) The route of administration—for example, drugs administered directly into the patient's bladder increase the risk of bladder irritation
(e) Patient's genetic factors— an individual with DPD gene mutation causing decrease in DPYD enzyme secretion will have worse toxicities with Capecitabine.
(f) Preexisting illnesses—older people with existing comorbidities may have severe adverse reactions

Cytotoxic chemotherapy affects normal cells in various systems of the body. An illustration of possible adverse reactions is presented in Fig. 14.2. However, it must be noted that different cytotoxic chemotherapies cause different adverse reactions. It is important to know specific adverse reactions caused by specific cytotoxic dugs prior to administration. Some common adverse reactions are discussed below.

14.7.1 Anaphylaxis

An immediate toxicity that may happen during chemotherapy administration is anaphylaxis. 'Anaphylaxis is a severe, life-threatening, generalised or systemic hypersensitivity reaction. This is characterised by rapidly developing life-threatening airway and/or breathing and/or circulation problems usually associated with skin and mucosal changes' (UK Resuscitation Council 2021, p. 7). The United Kingdom Resuscitation Council (2021) has guidelines for the management of anaphylaxis, which also apply to chemotherapy-related anaphylaxis.

14.7.2 Bone Marrow Suppression

The bone marrow is constantly active as it responds to the body's needs for white blood cells (WBC) to fight infection, red blood cells (RBC) to carry oxygen around the body, and platelets to prevent bleeding (Longenbaker 2017). These different cells are produced from stem cells, which originate from the bone marrow. The stem cells, which divide very frequently, are affected when chemotherapy interferes with

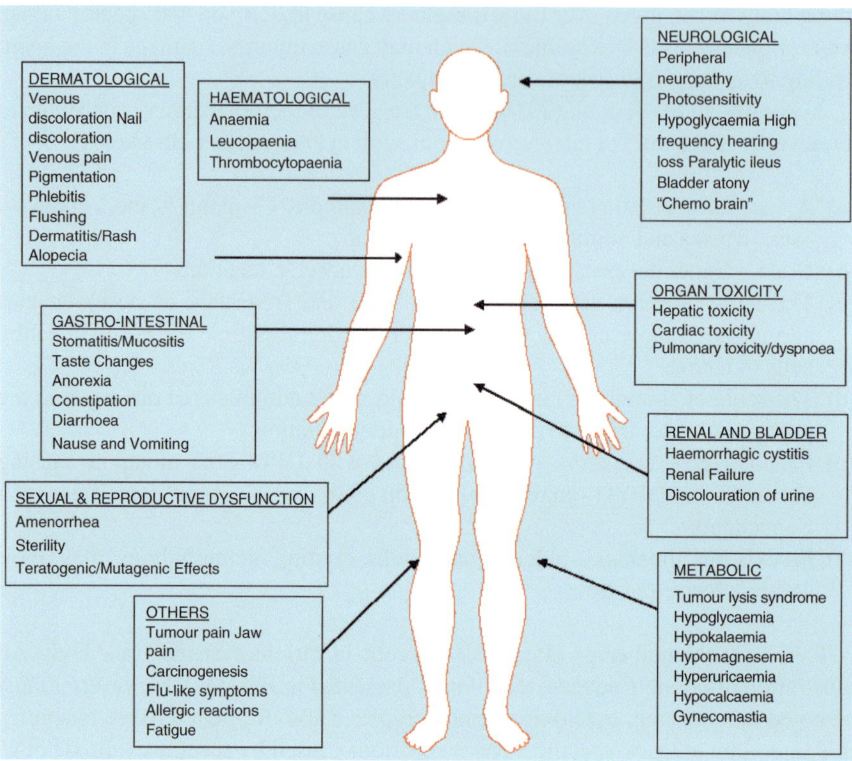

Fig. 14.2 Possible cytotoxic chemotherapy-induced adverse reactions

cell division. The lowest point reached in blood cell count after administration of chemotherapy is called *nadir*, which happens approximately 7–14 days after chemotherapy treatment, depending on the specific drug. The patient may experience leukopaenia, anaemia and thrombocytopaenia (Fig. 14.3).

The term leukopaenia indicates inadequate levels of leukocytes (WBC) in the blood. Fifty to seventy percent of the circulating WBCs are neutrophils. Neutrophils are the first of the WBCs to arrive at a site of injury, and attack and digest bacteria (Longenbaker 2017). They play a very important role in fighting infection. Neutropaenia is characterised by a low neutrophil count. When a patient is neutropaenic, the body's immunity or ability to fight infection is weakened, making the patient more susceptible to infection. If any patient receiving chemotherapy experiences fever or low temperature and/or presents with any obvious signs of infection, rapid assessment and treatment are essential as the patient could deteriorate very quickly when their neutrophil counts are very low. This condition is called neutropaenic sepsis and is considered a medical emergency (National Cancer Action Team 2011). As a preventive measure, patients are reminded to have a thermometer at home and are advised to call the 24-h emergency number when they feel unwell. Infection control measures such as proper handwashing should be taught to patients and their carers.

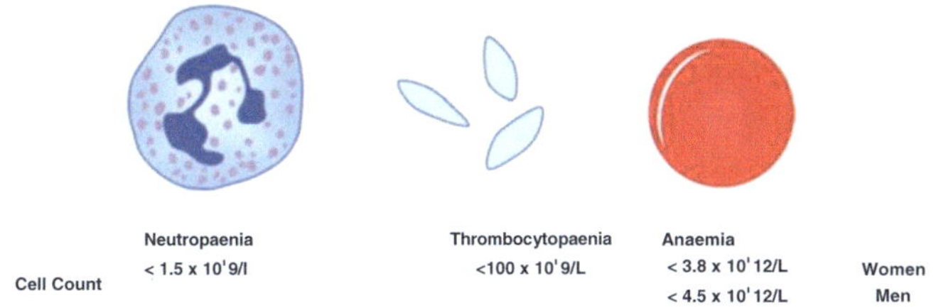

Fig. 14.3 Effects of cancer-related bone marrow suppression on blood cell production

Anaemia is the deficiency in either quality (low haematocrit level) or quantity (low haemoglobin level) of red blood cells and patient may demonstrate symptoms such as pallor, shortness of breath, dizziness and lethargy. Due to the relatively long life cycle of the RBC, which is around 120 days, anaemia caused by cytotoxic chemotherapy can take weeks or months to appear. Anaemia leads to patients feeling tired, lethargic and breathless. Thrombocytopaenia is characterised by a platelet count of less than 100 (adult normal value 150–400 × 10^9/L) and increases patient risk of bleeding or haemorrhage. After chemotherapy, patients are advised to report signs of bleeding such as epistaxis (nosebleed), haematemesis (blood in vomitus), melaena (blood in stool), petechiae (intradermal bleeding), ecchymoses (bruising), gum bleeding, haematuria (blood in urine), purpura and vaginal bleeding or a menstrual period that is heavier than normal.

14.7.3 Nausea and Vomiting

Nausea refers to a vague, uncomfortable sensation and a conscious need to vomit, while vomiting refers to the actual forceful expulsion of gastric contents through the mouth. In cancer patients, other factors such as pain, infection, radiotherapy and cancer itself may cause nausea and vomiting. Vomiting may be classified according to its onset, namely, acute, delayed or anticipatory.

Determining the emetogenicity (potential of drug to cause vomiting) when using chemotherapy agents is an important consideration when planning pharmacological management of nausea and vomiting. Chemotherapies are classified according to their degree of emetogenicity (Herrstedt et al. 2024). Some examples of chemotherapies and their emetogenicity potential are presented in Table 14.3.

However, combining chemotherapies may result in greater emetogenicity of the combined drugs. It is important to assess patients appropriately to ensure pharmacological and supportive therapies are adequately provided. Antiemetics are discussed in more detail in Chap. 11.

14.7.4 Oral Mucositis

Mucositis may occur anywhere along the gastrointestinal tract, which results from the toxic effects of chemotherapy on rapidly dividing cells of the mucosal lining.

Table 14.3 Emetogenic potential of chemotherapy drugs

Degree of emetogenicity (incidence)	Examples of chemotherapy drugs
High (>90%)	Cisplatin, carmustine, dacarbazine
Moderate (30–90%)	Oxaliplatin, carboplatin, doxorubicin, daunorubicin
Low (10–30%)	Paclitaxel, docetaxel, etoposide, pemetrexed
Minimal (<10%)	Bleomycin, vinblastine, vincristine, bevacizumab

Oral mucositis refers to mucosal inflammation and ulceration that occurs in the mouth, which in most cases can be very painful, resulting in a decrease in nutritional and fluid intake (Elad et al. 2020). Patients experience difficulty in swallowing and difficulty with oral communication. Signs and symptoms of oral mucositis include burning sensation in the mouth, sensitivity to hot or cold and spicy or salty food, erythema, cracked lips, difficulty wearing dentures, difficulty swallowing, bleeding, xerostomia (dry mouth) and ulceration.

It is important to keep in mind that bone marrow suppression increases a patient's susceptibility to infection and bleeding. As such, mucositis may become more severe as a result. Equally, mucosal damage is a port of entry for bacteria; therefore, good oral hygiene is paramount after chemotherapy. Patients may be prescribed antibacterial mouthwashes and analgesia for pain.

14.7.5 Alopecia

Hair follicles are rapidly proliferating cells. Loss of hair as a result of chemotherapy can range from hair thinning to partial or total loss of scalp hair. The degree of hair loss depends on (1) drug dose, (2) length of drug exposure and (3) schedule of administration. Two mechanisms may contribute to alopecia with the administration of chemotherapy. Firstly, alopecia may be due to the destruction of rapidly dividing epithelial cells of the hair follicle. Secondly, damage to stem cells at the base of the hair shaft leads to atrophy of the hair follicle, which results in a thinner and weaker hair shaft that can break off. Alopecia usually begins 1–2 weeks after the first cycle of chemotherapy. Loss is temporary and regrowth begins shortly after the end of treatment, approximately about 2–3 months.

Hair regrowth might be softer in texture, curlier, or different in colour. Alopecia may result in altered body image and poor self-esteem. It may affect perceived sexual attractiveness and engagement in social activities, and for many people, a visible reminder of their illness. In some chemotherapies, patients may be offered scalp cooling to prevent the drug from reaching the area by constricting the blood vessels. However, these may become sanctuary sites for cancer cells and therefore are contraindicated for some cases, such as haematological malignancies. Patients may be offered wigs and headwear prior to the start of chemotherapy. Women may also be offered make-up classes to highlight facial features, which may help boost self-esteem during treatment.

14.7.6 Fertility Issues

Cytotoxic chemotherapy may cause some fertility concerns for both male and female patients. With men, fertility may be affected in different ways, such as slowing down or stopping of sperm production. Sperm production may be temporary or permanent, which will affect the patient's ability to reproduce, and this is dependent on the drug(s) dose (higher doses of chemotherapy are more likely to affect fertility), and the combination of drugs. Chemotherapy can also affect the sperm's ability to fertilise a female ovum. Male patients may be offered sperm banking. Some chemotherapy drugs may also cause temporary problems with having and or maintaining an erection. These effects usually disappear gradually once the treatment is finished. It has to be highlighted to patients that chemotherapy drugs do not normally have any permanent effect on sexual performance or enjoyment of sex.

For women, chemotherapy affects the ability of the ovaries to produce oocytes. It may result in fewer or none being produced. Patients may experience early menopause in which menstrual periods become irregular and then stop completely (amenorrhea). Infertility could be permanent or temporary (and may take up to 2 years before the ovaries are fully functional). Although ovum freezing is an option, the process could be lengthy and may not be possible, especially when there is a need to start treatment immediately.

All patients who are about to receive chemotherapy must be encouraged to use contraception during and throughout treatment, as chemotherapy drugs are teratogenic and could harm a developing foetus. Depending on the type of cancer, medical clinicians provide advice about when to best conceive or father a child after chemotherapy. Use of condom during sex will protect their partner from SACT exposure through vaginal secretions or semen.

14.7.7 Diarrhoea

Diarrhoea is the passage of frequent and watery stools resulting from the destruction of actively dividing epithelial cells of the gastrointestinal tract (GI tract) causing water retention into the intestinal lumen, resulting in increased stool volume and weight. This is a more common adverse reaction of anti-metabolites and is a dose-limiting factor (criteria for drug reduction) for chemotherapy drugs such as 5FU and Irinotecan. Supportive management includes administration of anti-diarrhoeals such as Loperamide, adequate hydration and electrolyte monitoring.

14.7.8 Constipation

Constipation is a chronic gastrointestinal disorder consisting of hard stools (fewer than three times per week), or the inability to expel stool, whether soft or hard. Chemotherapy drugs such as Vinca Alkaloids, Etoposide and Cisplatin may cause constipation. For individuals who have cancer, constipation may be caused or aggravated by other factors such as immobility, antiemetics, opioid analgesics and dehydration.

14.7.9 Peripheral Neuropathy

Chemotherapy-induced peripheral neuropathy (CIPN) is characterised by symptoms such as pain, burning, tingling ("pins and needles" feeling) or electric/shock-like pain, burning, loss of feeling and cold sensitivity (Park et al. 2013). It is caused by damage to the peripheral nerves that carry sensations to the brain and control arm and leg movements. It is commonly caused by taxanes such as Docetaxel and Paclitaxel and platinum compounds such as Carboplatin and Oxaliplatin. CIPN can greatly affect the quality of life of patients as they may have difficulties performing simple everyday tasks such as cooking, walking, dressing and picking/holding things (Tanay et al. 2017). Symptoms may linger for a long time after the end of treatment. Unfortunately, CIPN is dose-related; therefore, while it is ideal to administer the full recommended dose of chemotherapy, in some cases it may be necessary to reduce, delay, or discontinue chemotherapy. It is essential to assess presenting symptoms, risk factors such as diabetes and evidence-based management. Management strategies include pharmacologic agents such as steroids, numbing patches or creams, anti-depressants, anti-convulsants and opioids for when the pain is severe. Other management strategies include electrical nerve stimulation, occupational therapy, physical therapy and relaxation exercises.

14.8 Novel Cancer Treatments

Increased knowledge about the complex processes involved when human tumours develop paved the way to targeted cancer treatments (Hanahan and Weinberg 2011). For example, growth signals called vascular endothelial growth factor (VEGF) that are responsible for inducing angiogenesis are inhibited by treatments such as bevacizumab. As the mechanism of action of bevacizumab is targeted at inhibiting VEGF, normal cells are not directly affected. This does not mean that targeted drugs do not have any side effects. They do, but in general, these are fewer in quantity and less severe. For example, the most common side effects of bevacizumab are hypertension and proteinuria (Wilkes 2011). Another group of treatment is immunotherapies. Immunotherapies work by strengthening the immune system and helping the immune system to recognise the cancer cell. Examples of immunotherapies are Nivolumab and Ipilimumab.

14.8.1 Comparison of Cytotoxic Chemotherapy and Immunotherapy

The primary difference between immunotherapy and cytotoxic chemotherapy lies in their targeting mechanisms and modes of action in destroying cancer cells.

Cytotoxic chemotherapy specifically targets rapidly dividing cells, including cancer cells, by disrupting the process of cell division. Unfortunately, this approach can also damage healthy cells that divide quickly, such as those in hair follicles and the gastrointestinal tract. Certain cancers can evade treatment by activating immune checkpoint pathways. In contrast, immunotherapy aims to enhance the body's natural defences by training the immune system to identify cancer cells as threats. This enables a targeted and prolonged response against cancer.

Immune checkpoint inhibitor (ICI) therapy is an innovative form of immuno-therapy that targets immune checkpoints, which serve as crucial regulators of the immune system. These therapies work by preventing the immune system from being deactivated when cancer cells are present, effectively blocking checkpoint proteins and enabling the body to continue fighting the cancer. ICIs specifically target molecules such as CTLA-4, PD-1 and PD-L1. CTLA-4 is a protein receptor that acts as an immune checkpoint, responsible for downregulating immune responses. By blocking CTLA-4, T cells are better able to identify and attack cancer cells. PD-1, or programmed cell death protein 1, is a transmembrane protein that interacts with PD-L1. When the PD-L1 protein on a cancer cell binds to the PD-1 protein on an immune cell, it signals that the cancer cell is healthy and should not be attacked. Certain checkpoint inhibitors are designed to block either PD-1 or PD-L1, thereby exposing the cancer cells to immune attack.

Immunotherapy is typically associated with fewer acute adverse effects compared to cytotoxic chemotherapy; however, it can still present significant risks, and adverse effects may be life-threatening. These side effects can arise at any point, including months after the end of treatment, may affect various parts of the body, and can rapidly worsen, sometimes within days. The range of adverse effects from immunotherapy differs markedly from those associated with cytotoxic chemotherapy due to its distinct mechanism of action. As immunotherapy stimulates the immune system, it can lead to an overactive immune response, resulting in immune cells attacking healthy tissues and triggering a variety of adverse effects. Immune checkpoint inhibitor (ICI)-related adverse effects can result in gastrointestinal, dermatologic, cardiac, hepatic, endocrine and pulmonary toxicities due to inflammation in various organs, such as myocarditis, pneumonitis in the lungs, colitis in the colon and hepatitis in the liver.

Patients may experience multiple toxicities simultaneously, complicating the identification and treatment of side effects. A comprehensive assessment of the patient, from head to toe (Fig. 14.4), is essential, with a focus on potential inflammatory conditions *(-itis)*. While fatigue is the most common adverse effects, it can also be indicative of cancer and other underlying issues. In instances of severe fatigue, it is important to consider causes such as adrenal insufficiency, hypophysitis, hypothyroidism, diabetes, myasthenia gravis and myocarditis.

Immunotherapy may lead to significant but manageable adverse effects, especially if identified early in the course of treatment. Many of these adverse effects are likely to occur while the patient is at home. Prompt and thorough nursing assessments are crucial in identifying the presence of adverse effects, determining the necessary investigations and deciding on appropriate interventions. Based on the

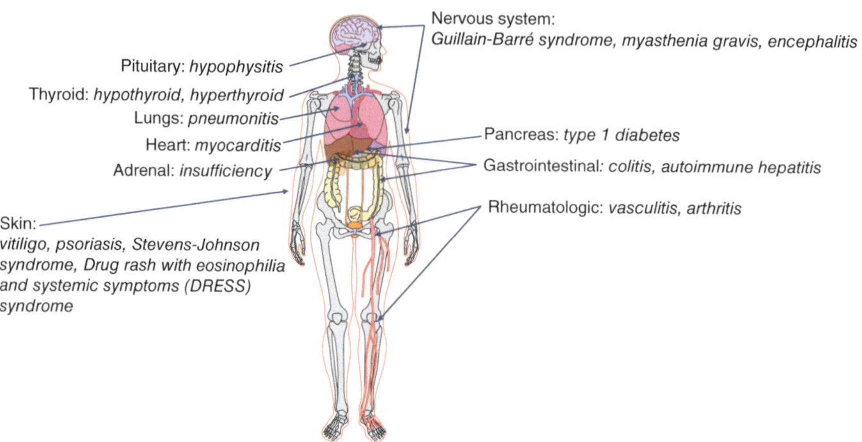

Fig. 14.4 Examples of immunotherapy side effects from head-to-toe

severity of the side effects and the patient's response to treatment, immunotherapy can continue as needed. Effective communication skills are essential for nurses to gather important information from patients regarding their symptoms and overall well-being. Management guidelines should be followed for management. The European Society of Medical Oncology has developed guidelines for the management of toxicities from immunotherapy from diagnosis, treatment and follow-up (Haanen et al. 2022).

14.9 Safety in SACT Administration

SACT may also affect normal cells; thus, safety in chemotherapy practice must be observed. Staff who prepare and handle chemotherapy must wear appropriate personal protective equipment (PPE) according to their hospital or unit policies. Staff must also be aware of their local guidelines when there is chemotherapy spillage. SACT units usually keep spillage kits which contain materials such as plastic aprons or gowns, plastic overshoes, disposable armlets, disposable gloves, particulate respirator (mask), goggles, disposable clinical waste bags, paper towels or absorbent pads, procedure document and an incident form. When chemotherapy is spilled on the skin, this must be washed with soap and running water. Eye splashes may also occur, which must be rinsed with running water. Staff should be advised to go to the occupational health department or the emergency department for further assessment.

14.9.1 Extravasation

Extravasation is the inadvertent administration of *vesicant* medication or solution into the surrounding tissues (Dougherty 2008). Vesicants are cytotoxic or noncytotoxic solutions that cause the formation of blisters with subsequent slough-ing of tissues due to tissue necrosis (Dougherty 2008). Symptoms include burning, stinging, pain and swelling at the cannula site. Examples of cyctotoxic chemother-apy vesicants are vinca alkaloids such as Vincristine, Vinorelbine and Vinblastine, Paclitaxel, Dactinomycin, Daunorubicin, Doxorubicin, Epirubicin, Idarubicin, Mithramycin and Mitomycin C. Extravasation can lead to extensive injury and dis-ability. It should be managed immediately to minimise the severity of injury.

Management depends on the vesicant that extravasated. Local policies and guidelines must be followed, as these may vary in terms of supportive management and which antidotes to use. In some cases, patients may need to undergo debride-ment surgery and plastic reconstructive surgery when extravasation is severe. Preventive measures include good cannulation skills, patient education and identi-fying patients who are at risk such as older people who have fragile and thin veins and patients with existing peripheral nerve morbidities, who may not be able to report pain or abnormal sensations on the cannula site.

Nurses play a central role in the prevention and management of adverse reactions of SACT (Bloomfield and Tanay 2012; Chan et al. 2014). Some adverse events are dose-limiting; therefore, poor management results in delay or even discontinuation of treatment. Many adverse events could also affect the patient's quality of life. Patients must be provided with a 24-h emergency contact number prior to discharge after receiving chemotherapy so they can call the hospital when adverse effects hap-pen at home. Appropriate assessment of adverse effects and patient education are paramount to ensure early detection and prompt management.

Chemotherapy waste must be discarded in a puncture-proof container with a purple lid. Containers must be correctly sealed and labelled cytotoxic, then stored to await removal. After receiving chemotherapy, patient waste such as urine, faeces and vomit may still contain high concentrations of the unchanged chemotherapy drug or active metabolites (Brighton and Wood 2005). Staff must wear appropriate PPE when handling human waste after chemotherapy.

14.10 Summary

Systemic anticancer therapy (SACT) is one of the main treatments for cancer. Although cytotoxic chemotherapy works against cancer cells, it cannot avoid healthy cells and so results in adverse events. Newer treatments are more targeted at stopping molecular processes and pathways that promote tumour growth but are also not without adverse effects. Nurses' knowledge about SACTs and potential adverse events is important to ensure proper assessment, prevention and manage-ment of symptoms and to effectively support patients holistically during and after receiving their treatments. The Multinational Association of Supportive Care in Cancer (2025) provides helpful resources and guidelines for nurses and healthcare professionals about providing supportive care for individuals who develop adverse effects of SACTs. Healthcare teams must follow local and national guidelines and protocols to ensure safety in SACT administration.

Multiple Choice Questions

1. Cell cycle phase-specific chemotherapy are drugs that:
   (a) Exert an effect on cells when they are resting only
   (b) Exert an effect on cells when they are actively in the cell cycle and affect specific phase of the cell cycle
   (c) Exert an effect on cells whether they are cycling or in G0 phase
   (d) Exert an effect on cells during mitosis only
2. Normal cell proliferation is balanced by apoptosis. What is apoptosis?
   (a) Obsolete or damaged cells undergo programmed cell death
   (b) Ability of cancer cells to form new blood vessels
   (c) Ability of malignant cells to evade growth suppressors
   (d) The migration of cells to a different organ
3. The following are examples of chemotherapies except:
   (a) Alkylating agents
   (b) Antitumour antibiotics
   (c) Antiemetics
   (d) Antimetabolites
4. Chemotherapy is given repeatedly over a period of time with intervals called cycles. What is the rationale for this?
   (a) To facilitate the normal cells to recover
   (b) To stop cancer cells from dividing
   (c) To allow cancer cells to rest
   (d) To allow normal cells to self-destruct
5. How does cancer immunotherapy work?
   (a) Disrupts cell division which leads to apoptosis
   (b) Blocks signals that cause formation of new blood vessels
   (c) Enables the immune system to induce programmed cell death
   (d) Enhances the body's natural defences by training the immune system to identify cancer cells as threats.
6. Why do adverse reactions happen when receiving cytotoxic chemotherapy?
   (a) Adverse reactions are caused by cancer cells and not due to anything else
   (b) The body got used to the cancer cells and protects the cancer cells from the chemotherapy
   (c) Cytotoxic chemotherapy cannot distinguish between cancer cells and normal cells, and affects both
   (d) Adverse reactions are basically caused by the interaction of the patient's routine drugs and chemotherapy
7. Several factors which may contribute to the severity and nature of adverse reactions following cytotoxic chemotherapy include all except one:
   (a) Dose
   (b) Route of administration
   (c) Environmental temperature
   (d) Type of drug

8. The emetogenic potential of chemotherapy refers to what?
    (a) Potential of drug to cause vomiting
    (b) Potential of drug to cause constipation
    (c) Potential of drug to cause peripheral neuropathy
    (d) Potential of drug to cause neutropaenic sepsis
9. To ensure safety in the administration of chemotherapy what must the nurse do?
    (a) Discard all chemotherapy waste in a hospital plastic bag
    (b) Wear appropriate personal protective equipment
    (c) When chemotherapy is spilled, wait until the hospital cleaner arrives to clean the spill
    (d) Dispose of chemotherapy waste like any other clinical waste
10. What other cancer treatment modalities may be used alongside chemotherapy?
    (a) Surgery
    (b) Radiotherapy
    (c) Hormonal therapy
    (d) All of the above

Answers

1. (b)
2. (a)
3. (c)
4. (a)
5. (d)
6. (c)
7. (c)
8. (a)
9. (b)
10. (d)

References

Barton-Burke M, Wilkes S (2018) Oncology nursing drug handbook. Jones and Bartlett Publishers, Burlington
Bloomfield J, Tanay M (2012) Chemotherapy in the community: the importance of patient assessment. Br J Community Nurs 17(6):278–283
Brighton D, Wood M (2005) The Royal Marsden Hospital handbook of cancer chemotherapy. Elsevier—Churchill Livingstone, Edinburgh
Cancer Research UK (2015) Cancer statistics for the United Kingdom. Available online on: https://www.cancerresearchuk.org/health-professional/cancer-statistics-for-the-uk. Accessed 26 Mar 2025
Chan A, Lees J, Keefe D (2014) The changing paradigm for supportive care in cancer patients. Support Care Cancer 22:1441–1445

Dougherty L (2008) IV therapy: recognising the difference between infiltration and extravasation. Br J Nurs 17(14):896–901

Elad S, Cheng KKF, Lalla RV, Yarom N, Hong C, Logan RM, Bowen J, Gibson R, Saunders DP, Zadik Y, Ariyawardana A, Correa ME, Ranna V, Bossi P, Mucositis Guidelines Leadership Group of the Multinational Association of Supportive Care in Cancer and International Society of Oral Oncology (MASCC/ISOO) (2020) MASCC/ISOO clinical practice guidelines for the management of mucositis secondary to cancer therapy. Cancer 126(19):4423–4431. https://doi.org/10.1002/cncr.33100

Haanen J, Obeid M, Spain L, Carbonnel F, Wang Y, Robert C, Lyon AR, Wick W, Kostine M, Peters S, Jordan K, Larkin J, ESMO Guidelines Committee. Electronic address: clinicalguidelines@esmo.org (2022) Management of toxicities from immunotherapy: ESMO Clinical Practice Guideline for diagnosis, treatment and follow-up. Ann Oncol 33(12):1217–1238. https://doi.org/10.1016/j.annonc.2022.10.001

Hanahan D, Weinberg RA (2011) Hallmarks of cancer: the next generation. Cell 144:650–674. https://doi.org/10.1016/j.cell.2011.02.013

Herrstedt J, Clark-Snow R, Ruhlmann CH, Molassiotis A, Olver I, Rapoport BL, Aapro M, Dennis K, Hesketh PJ, Navari RM, Schwartzberg L, Affronti ML, Garcia-Del-Barrio MA, Chan A, Celio L, Chow R, Fleury M, Gralla RJ, Giusti R, Jahn F (2024) 2023 MASCC and ESMO guideline update for the prevention of chemotherapy- and radiotherapy-induced nausea and vomiting… participants of the MASCC/ESMO Consensus Conference 2022. Electronic address: clinicalguidelines@esmo.org. ESMO Open 9(2):102195

Longenbaker SN (2017) Mader's understanding human anatomy and physiology, 9th edn. McGraw-Hill Education, New York

Madariaga A, Lheureux S, Oza AM (2019) Tailoring ovarian cancer treatment: implications of BRCA1/2 mutations. Cancers (Basel) 11(3):E416

Morgan G (2003) Chemotherapy and the cell cycle. Cancer Nurs Pract 2(1):27–30

Multinational Association of Supportive Care in Cancer (2019) http://www.mascc.org/. Accessed 26 Mar 2025

National Cancer Action Team (2011) Manual for cancer services: acute oncology—including metastatic spinal cord compression measure. Version 1.0. Department of Health and Social Science. Available online on: https://assets.publishing.service.gov.uk/government/uploads/system/uploads/attachment_data/file/216121/dh_125889.pdf. Accessed 26 Mar 2019

Park S, Goldstein D, Krishnan A, Lin CSY, Friedlander M, Cassidy J, Kolzenburg M, Kiernan M (2013) Chemotherapy-induced peripheral neurotoxicity: a critical analysis. Cancer J Clin 63(6):419–437

Skeel R, Khleif S, Rixe O (2016) Handbook of cancer chemotherapy, 9th edn. Lippincott Williams & Wilkins, Philadelphia

Tanay M, Armes J, Ream E (2017) The experience of chemotherapy-induced peripheral neuropathy in adult cancer patients: a qualitative thematic synthesis. Eur J Cancer Care 26. https://doi.org/10.1111/ecc.12443

United Kingdom Resuscitation Council (2021) Emergency treatment of anaphylactic reactions: guidelines for healthcare providers—annotated with links to NICE guideline. Emergency treatment of anaphylactic reactions: Guidelines for healthcare providers | Resuscitation Council UK Accessed 26 Mar 2025

Wilkes G (2011) Targeted cancer therapy: a handbook for nurses. Jones and Bartlett Publishers, Burlington

Yandle A (2014) Cancer biology. In: Jacobs C, Webb C, Robinson L (eds) Genetics for healthcare professionals in cancer care: from principles to practice. Oxford University Press, Oxford

Ehsan Khan

Learning Outcomes

At the end of this chapter, you will be able to:

- Provide a fundamental understanding of the stages of coagulation.
- Give an account of platelet activation and its consequences.
- Differentiate between anticoagulant and antiplatelet medication.
- Explain important clinical pharmacokinetic and pharmacodynamic considerations of common anticoagulants prescribed in clinical practice.
- Explain important clinical pharmacokinetic and pharmacodynamic considerations of common antiplatelet medications used in practice.

15.1 Introduction

With advances in cardiovascular medicine and an increasingly ageing population there is an ongoing need to sustain people taking different forms of prescribed medication that reduce blood coagulation. This chapter will detail the mechanism of blood coagulation and then present the main groups of medication that are prescribed to attenuate this process.

To understand the different medications that are prescribed to reduce blood coagulation, it is important to understand haemostasis. Haemostasis or thrombus formation is a process that utilises blood components to generate a gel-like clot to help stop or limit blood loss from the cardiovascular circulation.

In essence haemostasis can be divided into cellular components, in particular platelets, erythrocytes leucocytes, and plasma proteins.

E. Khan (✉)
Faculty of Nursing Midwifery and Palliative Care, King's College London, London, UK
e-mail: eu.khan@kcl.ac.uk

© The Author(s), under exclusive license to Springer Nature
Switzerland AG 2026
E. Khan, P. Hood (eds.), *Understanding Pharmacology in Nursing Practice*,
https://doi.org/10.1007/978-3-032-03964-4_15

Based on these components, medications that reduce thrombosis can generally be divided into two main categories: anticoagulant and antiplatelet medications. Although the commonly used term to describe these medications are 'blood thinners', neither of these groups of medications thin or dilute the blood. For this reason, such medications will be collectively termed antithrombotic, as this term improves the description of their action.

15.2 The Clotting Cascade

There are 20 blood proteins that interact to create and modulate the mesh-like gel that forms a blood clot.

These proteins are mainly produced by the liver and circulate within the body as an inactive enzyme termed a zymogen. Once stimulated, they set up a cascade reaction that activates each enzyme in sequence, one activated enzyme activating the next.

The proteins are numbered using roman numerals; the first 13 (I–XIII) have classically been recognised as coagulation cascade proteins. Factors XIV and XV belong to the Kallikrein–Kininogen system, a system that links coagulation to inflammatory and immune responses (Bryant and Shariat-Madar 2009). Factor XVI is termed the von Willebrand factor, and the final four factors have anticoagulant properties that help modulate thrombus formation (Palta et al. 2014).

Before examining the interaction between coagulation proteins and how medication may influence this process, it is important to understand the concepts of what this physiological system is trying to achieve. This has a bearing on the effects and adverse effects of medications used to manipulate this process.

To be an effective mechanism, blood clotting needs to be a very balanced response to the risk of blood loss via a puncture of the blood vessel; too little a response and there is a risk of excessive bleeding, too much of a response and there is a risk of a blocked blood vessel leading to the possibility of ischaemia and infarction. To help minimise these risks, activation of coagulation proteins, at least physiologically, is initiated by exposure of blood to subendothelial tissues. This is known as the physiological or, traditionally, the extrinsic pathway. This pathway is the haemostatic mechanism arising from blood loss when ruptures of blood vessels occur, primarily small arteries and capillaries. Clinically, however, blood coagulation may also be initiated by other stimuli, for example, when blood encounters particular substances, such as the glass of a blood sample vial. In this circumstance, another set of coagulation proteins is activated, and this pathway is known as the intrinsic or contact pathway. This pathway also has a significant role to play in initiating coagulation in disease processes that result in an increased risk of blood clotting, such as deep vein thrombosis and atherosclerosis.

It was initially believed that the two pathways were separate; however, the current belief is that they work together to orchestrate the clotting process, responding and tailoring it to the extent of damage and disease. Regardless of which pathway is involved, they both converge on what was traditionally known as the common pathway, which starts with the activation of factor X.

Haemostasis, thrombus, or clot formation has now been described as three overlapping processes (Hoffman and Monroe 2001).

15.2.1 Activation

Clot initiation begins with activation of factor VII by tissue factor (TF); tissue factor is a receptor that is found on tissues beneath the endothelium (subendothelial), most commonly in the connective tissue layer (Grover and Mackman 2018). Rupturing of the endothelial cell surface during vascular damage exposes the blood (and coagulation proteins) to TF. TF binds to and activates factor VII (FVIIa). In the presence of Ca^{++} Tf-FVIIa forms a complex known as the extrinsic tenase. This complex is termed a tenase because it converts factor X to FXa. FXa then converts prothrombin (FII) into thrombin (FIIa), and it is FIIa that cleaves Fibrinogen (FI) into Fibrin (FIa) to start forming the coagulation mesh (Palta et al. 2014). Apart from other roles in haemostasis, calcium (factor IV) is required as a cofactor to activate all vitamin K-dependent clotting factors (Fig. 15.1).

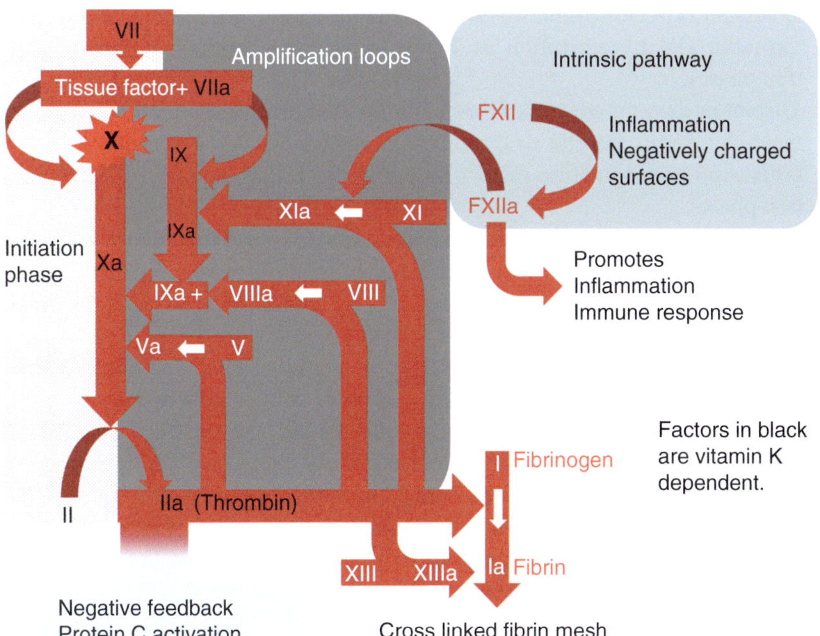

Fig. 15.1 This schematic shows the role of coagulation proteins in initiation and amplification of the coagulation cascade

15.2.2 Amplification

The amount of thrombin formed in the initiation stage is small. However, it has a pivotal role in activating other factors in the extrinsic pathway and indirectly the intrinsic pathway. Activation of these other factors (XIa, Va, and VIIIa) produces positive feedback loops that help amplify the production of Xa, which in turn increases the production of thrombin (IIa) (Fig. 15.1).

Thrombin also activates factor XIII. FXIIIa helps stabilise the fibrin mesh by cross-linking fibrin scaffolding (Fig. 15.1).

15.2.3 Propagation

Propagation of the thrombus or clot is the last stage of the clotting process. Concentration of the extrinsic tenase and the prothrombin-FXa complex on platelet cell surfaces, acts as a production site for large amounts of thrombin, which subsequently produces copious amounts of fibrin to generate a large clot (Hoffman and Monroe 2001; Palta et al. 2014).

15.2.4 Summary

- Coagulation occurs primarily owing to the formation of thrombin (IIa) from prothrombin (II) by activation of the extrinsic and common pathways (initiation phase).
- Thrombin directly converts Fibrinogen (I) to Fibrin (Ia), which then forms the mesh that forms the clot or thrombus. Thrombin activates a feedback loop that utilises other coagulation factors that amplify thrombin production (amplification phase).
- Sustained production of Thrombin and ultimately fibrin is achieved by accumulation of large amounts of key coagulation complexes on platelet surfaces (propagation phase).

A concise account of the anticoagulant elements of the coagulation cascade is now required to help understand certain aspects of anticoagulant pharmacology.

The coagulation system possesses several natural anticoagulant and thrombolytic (clot-dissolving) agents. The most clinically useful are antithrombin III or FXVII and heparin (FXVIII), both inhibit thrombin (IIa), but FXVII also inhibits Xa, amongst others. Initiation and propagation of coagulation is retarded by tissue factor pathway inhibitor (TFPI) (Brodin et al. 2009). Together with these elements, there are two vitamin K-dependent proteins known as protein C (FXIX) and protein S (FXX) that have anticoagulant properties. Protein C is the active anticoagulant, and protein S acts as a cofactor together with thrombin and thrombomodulin to activate protein C (Esmon et al. 1987). Activated protein C modulates coagulation by inhibiting FVa and FVIIIa.

Once the thrombus is formed, it will eventually require dissolution. The breakdown of a clot is known as fibrinolysis. The main fibrinolytic agent in the body is plasmin. Plasmin originates from the zymogen (pro-enzyme) plasminogen. Plasmin activation from plasminogen is mediated by tissue-type plasminogen activator (t-PA) and urokinase-type plasminogen activator (u-PA); these factors, in turn, are inhibited by plasminogen activator inhibitor (Keragala and Medcalf 2021), ensuring the system is finely adjusted and tuned to allow for safe clot dissolution and removal.

15.3 Anticoagulant Medications

Anticoagulants interfere with coagulation protein production and function. The anticoagulants being addressed in this text are anti-vitamin K and direct oral anticoagulants, as well as heparin. These have been selected owing to their common current or increasing clinical use.

15.3.1 Vitamin K Antagonists: (Warfarin)

Possibly the most renowned drug used to inhibit coagulation, warfarin was discovered by Karl Paul Link and Schoeffel in 1941 from research funded by the Wisconsin Alumni Research Fund (WARF), from where the name warfarin is derived (Shehab et al. 2016).

Vitamin K is important in the production of core coagulant proteins, including II, VII, IX, X, together with proteins C and S. There are 2–3 clinically available vitamin K antagonists, and apart from their half-lives, they have very similar pharmacokinetic properties; however, by far the most frequently prescribed anticoagulant medication is warfarin. Indeed, warfarin has been the mainstay anticoagulant medication in clinical use for the last 50 years. It has an indirect mechanism of action. Vitamin K is needed to activate dependent proteins, which leads to vitamin K becoming oxidised. Vitamin K epoxy-reductase reverts vitamin K back to its active (reduced) form (Fig. 15.2). Warfarin inhibits Vit K epoxy-reductase, thereby diminishing the availability of reduced Vit K and consequently core coagulation proteins.

Warfarin also inhibits other vitamin K-dependent proteins, including osteocalcin and matrix gla protein (MGP) (Donaldson and Harrington 2017). Osteocalcin is

Fig. 15.2 This images shows the role of Warfarin's target enzyme, vitamin K epoxy reductase. Vitamin K epoxy reductase reduces oxidised vitamin K to generate its active form. Vitamin K is then involved in formation of the coagulation proteins shown

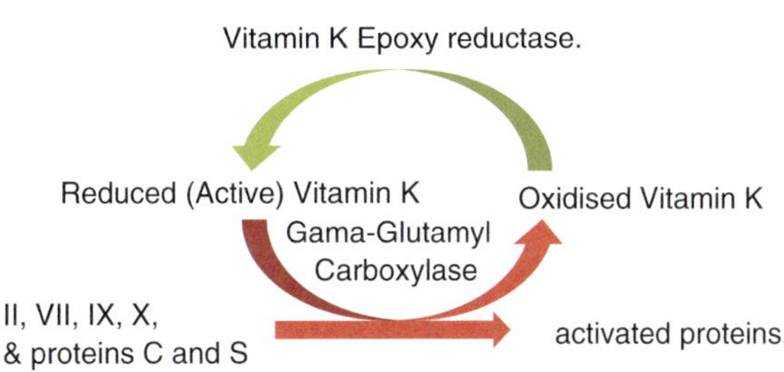

produced and secreted exclusively by bone-forming osteoblasts. The exact nature of ostocalcin's effect on bone formation remains unclear, but it is postulated to have an effect on bone mineralisation and maturation (Zoch et al. 2016). Systemic hormonal effects for osteocalcin have also been suggested; these include contribution to glucose metabolism and Insulin utilisation, effects on cognitive function by influencing brain neurotransmission function, and increasing testosterone levels (Zoch et al. 2016).

MGP, another important Vitamin K-dependent protein, is secreted by bone, chondrocytes, and a number of cells linked to the cardiovascular system, including vascular smooth muscle cells (Bjørklund et al. n.d.). The main function of MGP is to limit calcification in vascular and bone tissue. Inhibition of this protein by administering warfarin may therefore lead to overt calcification of blood vessels and bones (Barrett et al. 2018; Donaldson and Harrington 2017).

15.3.1.1 Warfarin Pharmacokinetics

Warfarin has 97–100% bioavailability, with a half-life of approximately 40 h. It is 99% plasma protein-bound.

Warfarin is available in a combination of two different forms, R-warfarin and S-warfarin. R-warfarin is metabolised by the contribution of several phase I enzymes, including CYP2C8, CYP2C19, CYP1A2, and CYP3A4. Whereas the significantly more potent S-warfarin is mainly metabolised by CYP2C9 (Kaminsky and Zhang 1997). For this reason, warfarin is associated with significant drug–drug interactions that may limit its use. As warfarin targets multiple coagulation proteins and has important CYP interactions, this necessitates coagulation monitoring at appropriate intervals.

Warfarin is mainly eliminated by metabolism, with only a small amount of the drug excreted by the kidneys unchanged. The drug is excreted mainly by the kidney, with 20% being excreted in faeces.

15.3.1.2 Warfarin Monitoring

The effect of anticoagulation provided by warfarin is monitored clinically by a measure known as the international normalised ratio (INR). This ratio uses prothrombin time as the basis of its measure. Prothrombin time measures (in seconds) the time it takes a thromboplastin reagent (a mixture of tissue factor, calcium salts, and membrane lipids) to form a clot in platelet-depleted plasma. An INR presents a patient's prothrombin time as a ratio of the mean normal prothrombin time. This is further corrected for reagent variations by a factor known as the international sensitivity index (ISI) (Dorgalaleh et al. 2021).

A person with a normal prothrombin time has an INR of 1. When using anticoagulants such as warfarin, the aim is to maintain the INR typically between 2 and 3, i.e., 2–3 times more than the normal value of 1, but target INRs will vary according to the cause for anticoagulation.

When initiating warfarin treatment or changing the dosage, the INR may be monitored daily or on alternate days. Then twice weekly, and then weekly. Typically, people taking stable warfarin dosage have their INR measured every 12 weeks, but again this may vary according to; the patient's condition, the drug regimen, any changes to the drug regimen and the risk of bleeding measured by a recognised tool such as HASBLED or CHASDS2-VASc.

15.3.1.3 Adverse Reactions of Warfarin

The main adverse reactions of warfarin are associated with reduced coagulation. The increased bleeding may present in different forms, including black or dark stools, sometimes resembling tar. Dark or brown urine, or unexplained severity and frequency of nose bleeds.

Cerebral bleeds may present as confusion, headache, blurred vision or slurred speech, and loss of consciousness. Movement or sensation may become impaired, and nausea and vomiting may occur. If any of these symptoms occur post head trauma, then it is imperative the person attends emergency care for assessment.

Because of warfarin's inhibitory effects on the MGP, there is a risk of overt calcification in blood vessels with warfarin administration (Harel and Sood 2021). This anomaly, known as calciphylaxis, is a rare but potentially lethal adverse effect of warfarin. Risk factors for this adverse effect are people who have chronic kidney disease (CKD) who are undergoing dialysis, are female, and may also have overactive parathyroid glands (Khudair et al. 2023). Calciphylaxis presents as reddening areas on the skin that develop into black areas, which ultimately form deep ulcerations (Marin et al. 2023).

A similar uncommon adverse effect of warfarin is known as warfarin-induced skin necrosis. This pathology is associated with capillary bed bleeding in the skin that then gives rise to necrosis or death of the skin in that area (Patel and Jain 2022).

15.3.2 Direct Anticoagulant Inhibitors

The arrival of novel oral anticoagulants (NOACS), now termed direct oral anticoagulants (DOACS), has caused a significant change in how orally administered anticoagulation therapies are managed, particularly in primary care. DOACs have specific differences from warfarin and its analogues. These differences overall provide a potentially cheaper and safer alternative to vitamin K antagonists such as warfarin. There are currently 4 DOACs clinically available (Table 15.1). All of these are currently licenced for use in non-valvular atrial fibrillation (AF) to prevent a cardiovascular accident (stroke) or emboli and should be offered when the CHA_2DS_2-VASc is 2 or above. It should be noted that non-valvular primarily means prosthetic mechanical valves and moderate to severe mitral valve stenosis, because these were exclusion criteria in the trials determining the effect of NOACS on reducing thromboembolic events in AF (Steffel et al. 2021). Other indications for use of these medications include prevention of deep vein thrombosis (DVT) and prevention of systemic emboli, including formation of pulmonary emboli.

15.3.2.1 Mechanism of Action of DOACs

Pharmacologically, the first licenced DOAC, dabigatran, inhibits thrombin, while the remaining clinically available DOACs (rivaroxaban, apixaban, and edoxaban) target and inhibit activated factor X (fXa) alone (Table 15.1). The specificity of these drugs

Table 15.1 Novel oral Anticoagulants (NOACs)

Ferri et al. (2022)	Dabigatran	Rivaroxaban	Apixaban	Edoxaban
Target	Thrombin (IIa)	fXa	fXa	fXa
Effect of food	Delayed absorption	Increased absorption	None	None
Vd (L)	60–70	50	21	>300
Half life (h)	12–17	5–9	8–15	8–11
Metabolism	Conjugation	3A4 (18%) 2J2	3A4 (25%), 1A2, 2J2, 2C8, 2C9, 2C19	3A4 < 4%
P-gp Substrate	Yes (prodrug)	Yes	Yes	Yes
Renal elimination	80%	35%	27%	50%

McGrath et al. (2013)

to their individual targets results in very limited spillover effect to other coagulation factors, unlike vitamin K antagonists. This specificity results in a much more measured effect of the drug, negating the need to monitor clotting in most instances.

15.3.2.2 Benefit of DOACS Compared to Warfarin

A number of pivotal trials explored the benefits of DOACs compared to warfarin in preventing strokes in AF, RE-LY (dabigatran vs. warfarin), ROCKET AF & J-ROCKET AF (rivaroxaban vs. warfarin), ARISTOLTE (apixaban vs. warfarin), and ENGAGE AF TIMI (edoxaban vs. warfarin). Overall, these studies (collectively known as the COMBINE AF database) demonstrate a lower bleeding risk while preserving similar clinical anticoagulation benefit for most forms of bleeds except gastrointestinal bleeds.

Interestingly, subgroup analysis of data from these trials evidenced a particular benefit for Asian patients compared to non-Asian patients. This ethnic subgroup experienced a greater reduction in stroke and systemic emboli when compared to non-Asian patients. Asian patients also experienced fewer bleeds, including gastrointestinal bleeds, this suggests the potential for this class of drug to be the drug of choice for Asian patients with AF (Chao et al. 2024).

When reporting safety of antithrombotic medications, it is clear that major bleeds take precedence; however, smaller bleeds may also have a significant impact on care and quality of life. Although there is some disagreement and debate about categorising nonmajor bleeds, Kaatz and colleagues provide a simple working definition; clinically relevant nonmajor bleeds are those that require a face-to-face evaluation, and minor bleeds are more "nuisance" bleeds that may affect a person's quality of life but do not warrant a formal clinical physical evaluation (Kaatz et al. 2015). A systematic review of 19 RCTS involving 85,826 patients rated the risk of minor bleeds and clinically relevant nonmajor bleeds when using VKAs and DOACs (Wang et al. 2023). In both categories, apixaban was found to have the least risk of these nonmajor bleeds.

It is therefore not surprising to see that DOAC prescriptions now account for 62% of all oral anticoagulants prescribed up to 2019 in England, and although warfarin remains the most frequently prescribed single drug (38.1%), Apixaban prescriptions are closing the gap (31%) and are the most widely prescribed DOAC (Afzal et al. 2021).

15.3.2.3 Safety Considerations Related to DOACs

Although the safety profile for DOACs is favourable compared to VKAs, it must be remembered that the safety bar that VKAs such as warfarin present is not particularly high. It is important, therefore, to remain cautious when administering and monitoring the benefits of DOACs. Safety of DOAC prescribing and administration relates to three main factors; Cytochrome P450 metabolism, drug efflux clearance related primarily to P-glycoprotein (Pgp) and to the breast cancer resistance protein (BCRP), and renal function in terms of creatinine clearance. The more factors a particular DOAC is influenced by, the more potential there is for a drug interaction. For example, given the increased frequency of its prescription and its interaction with the most isoforms of Cytochrome P450 (Table 15.1), Apixaban has the potential to experience the most drug–drug interaction in a patient who is receiving polypharmacy. This situation may be further complicated by the inclusion of a Pgp inhibitor in the prescribed drug regimen, such as digoxin or reboxetine.

A systematic review including 71,683 patients from the COMBINE AF database found that standard or low-dose DOACs were more beneficial and safer than warfarin down to a creatinine clearance of 25 mL/min (Harrington et al. 2023). Similar reductions in stroke and systemic embolic and bleeding events were reported regarding the use of DOACs ($n = 1047$) compared to VKAs ($n = 1335$) in patients with stage 4 and 5 chronic kidney disease (creatinine clearance <30 mL/min/1.73 m^2) (Jones et al. 2024).

15.3.2.4 Adverse Reactions of DOACs

As with all medications that interfere with blood clotting, the use of DOACS is associated with an increased risk of bleeding. However, it is increasingly evident that DOACS have a better safety profile related to bleeding when compared to traditional anticoagulants in a number of different disease scenarios, for example; deep vein thrombosis (DVT) (Wang et al. 2023), patients undergoing cardioversion for AF (Troisi et al. 2023), older patients with AF (Doni et al. 2023), liver disease (Zhao et al. 2023; Li et al. 2023) liver cirrhosis, patients with cirrhosis and AF (Hu et al. 2023), and patients with mild to moderate COVID-19 (Tian et al. 2023). DOACS are also reported to have similar rates of thrombotic events (DVT, pulmonary emboli (PE), and major and minor bleeds in a patient with a hip fracture, when compared to low molecular weight heparin (Abatzis-Papadopoulos et al. 2023).

Adverse reactions of DOAC analogues differ slightly; however, some common (1/100) adverse effects include anaemia, urticaria, thrombocytopenia, rash, haematoma, epistaxis, diarrhoea, dyspepsia, gastric reflux, hepatic enzyme increase, alopecia (dabigatran), haematuria (apixaban), dizziness and headache (rivaroxaban & edoxaban), and vaginal haemorrhage (edoxaban).

15.3.3 Heparin

Heparin is a polysaccharide and has no direct anticoagulant properties of its own. It accelerates the effect of Antithrombin (III) Amongst others, Antithrombin inhibits Xa and IIa, two pivotal proteins in the coagulation cascade. In the presence of heparin, this inhibition increases approximately 4000-fold for IIa and around 500-fold for Xa (Olson et al. 1992).

15.3.3.1 Mechanism of Action

The heparin molecule is composed of a polysaccharide chain of varying lengths and a molecular weight ranging from ~3000 to 30,000 Daltons, depending on chain length (Conners and Money 2002).

Heparin's effect is linked to a 5-subunit (pentasaccharide) section of the polysaccharides that binds to Antithrombin, which produces a conformational change in Antithrombin that exposes a reactive site that more effectively binds a selection of coagulation proteins (Kandrotas 1992). The selectivity of heparin to inhibit different coagulation proteins depends upon the heparin chain length. Heparin is available in two main forms, fractionated and unfractionated, depending on the number of units in the polysaccharide chain (Fig. 15.3).

Unfractionated Heparin

Unfractionated heparin (UFH) has a longer chain length with a minimum chain length of 18–20 subunits (Fig. 15.3) (Kandrotas 1992). Owing to the longer chain, UFH can bind a number of different coagulation proteins, including IIa and Xa (Fig. 15.3) as well as other cells, including macrophages and endothelial cells (Kumano et al. 2021). This leads to a significant variation in the pharmacokinetic

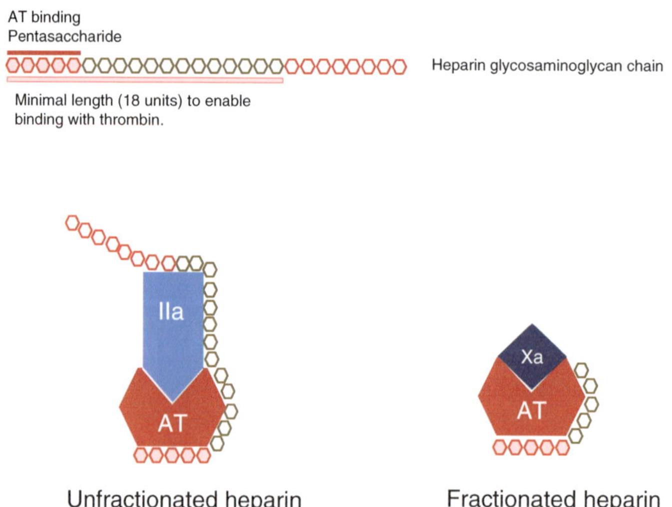

Fig. 15.3 This image shows how the length of the heparin glycosaminoglycan chain affects its binding specificity in unfractionated and fractionated heparin

properties of the medication and thus variability in clinical effect, necessitating monitoring of drug effect. The anticoagulant effect of heparin is monitored using the activated partial thromboplastin time (aPTT). As the actual time measured differs according to which technique is used, it is important to adhere to local hospital policy to ensure the current interpretation of results.

Fractionated or Low Molecular Weight Heparin (LMWH)

Fractionated heparin includes strands of heparin that are below 18 subunits, with a molecular weight between 3000 and 6000 Daltons (Kandrotas 1992). The benefit of this shorter length is that this form of heparin only interacts with the Xa-Antithrombin complex (Fig. 15.3). Also, owing to its shorter length, it has limited nonspecific cell binding, resulting in a predictable therapeutic effect. Therefore, prescription of LMWH is largely based on body weight, although there are special considerations for at-risk groups such as people with cardiovascular disease and people who weigh more than 165 Kg.

15.3.3.2 Pharmacokinetic Characteristics of Heparin

There is significant individual variability in blood levels of UFH. This variability is determined by three main factors;

- The main mechanism that removes heparin from the bloodstream is mediated by a receptor that draws heparin into macrophages and endothelial cells, where it is then broken down. As there is a limited number of receptors that can draw UFH into the cell, this mechanism gets overwhelmed or saturated relatively quickly, at which stage small increases in unfractionated heparin dosage may lead to large increases in blood levels of the drug.
- Renal clearance. This is a slow excretion pathway that is affected by severe renal dysfunction.
- Nonspecific protein binding. This is possibly the most significant factor in determining free UFH in the bloodstream. UFH binds nonspecifically to a large number of plasma proteins. Importantly concentration of these proteins varies significantly in illness, liver damage, and disease, reducing the concentration of these proteins, whereas systemic infections such as sepsis increase the concentration of some plasma proteins. This variability results in a significantly different effect of a given dose of UFH between individuals, necessitating frequent monitoring of drug effect. This is performed by measuring activated partial thromboplastin time (aPPT). Owing to a lack of standard measurement, there is no specific standardised range. Using local laboratory measurements, the aPPT is normally adjusted to 1.5–2.5 of normal as a therapeutic range (Conners and Money 2002).

In comparison to UFH, LMWH is a much smaller molecule that is not removed from the bloodstream via receptor-mediated endocytosis, resulting in the slower renal clearance pathway being its main mechanism of removal from the bloodstream. This provides a longer half-life for the drug. LMWH also has limited nonspecific binding to plasma proteins. Together, this results in a more stable and predictable effect, which enables once or twice daily dosing of the medication subcutaneously.

With a volume of distribution similar to blood volume, LMWH has limited loading into body adipose tissue, and given renal excretion is its main pathway of clearance from the body, caution is needed in renal dysfunction (CR-Cl <30 mL/min).

15.3.3.3 Adverse Reactions of Heparin

The main adverse reaction of UFH and LMWH is bleeding, with UFH heparin causing a higher risk as described.

Heparin can induce a procoagulant state. Heparin-induced or associated thrombocytopenia (HIT or HAT) occurs in two forms (Conners and Money 2002); first a mild Type I form that occurs soon after initiating heparin, which tends to be transient and does not require cessation of heparin administration and is not associated with any significant complications.

The rarer Type II HIT, however, is a serious procoagulant adverse reaction of heparin; again, this is more likely to occur with UFH rather than LMWH. This form of HIT induces an immunogenic response that involves a platelet factor 4 (PF4) interaction with heparin that triggers an IgG immune response. This leads to platelet activation. Activated platelets release more PF4, perpetuating the heparin-related immune response (Mongirdienė et al. 2023). The increased number of platelets causes a hypercoagulant state, which may lead to complications such as disseminated intravascular coagulation (DIC), although together with skin necrosis, DVTs and pulmonary emboli are more common (Fathi, n.d.). Eventually, thrombocytopenia occurs in this procoagulant state because more and more platelets aggregate to form thrombi, and the immune-affected platelets are removed by macrophages. The risk of Type II HIT is higher in surgical patients (1–5%) (Mongirdienė et al. 2023) and in patients with diabetes.

The risk of HIT can be estimated using the 4 T score that includes four criteria, namely, the level of thrombocytopenia, the timing of a fall in platelet count, presence of thrombosis or other consequences of platelet aggregation, and the presence of other causes of reduction in platelet count. A score of 6+ suggests a high risk of having HIT.

Osteoporosis is another rare but problematic risk factor of long-term heparin use. This is because heparin increases osteoclast activity (bone resorption) by inhibiting a protein called osteoprotegrin (Signorelli et al. 2019). Osteoprotegrin normally improves bone density and strength by inhibiting osteoclast activity. The effect of UFH on osteoporosis is more pronounced compared to LMWH.

Having explored the coagulation cascade and its pharmacological manipulation, the role of platelets will now be explained to illustrate how antiplatelet medications act.

15.4   The Role of Platelets in Blood Clotting

Platelets or thrombocytes are small cell fragments devoid of nuclei (enucleate) and are derived from the same progenitor cell that produces all blood cells, the megakaryocyte. Most blood cells are found in the centre of the bloodstream, leaving the peripheral area close to the endothelial cell devoid of cells and thus plasma-rich. Unlike most blood cells, platelets circulate in the plasma-rich zone close to the endothelial cell wall. Platelets normally appear disc-shaped at rest, but on activation, they develop projections (Thomas 2019). Once the platelet is activated, two main events occur; it secretes different substances that encourage platelet adhesion and antiplatelet activity, together with substances that promote inflammation. The other important effect is that glycoprotein (Gp) receptors on the platelet cell surface undergo a structural (conformational) change that enables them to bind different substances, including fibrinogen, collagen, vWF, and others. This enables the platelets to adhere to the damaged vascular wall surface, primarily by binding exposed collagen via the Gp IV receptor (adhesion), and enables platelet to platelet connection via the Gp IIb IIIa receptor that binds fibrinogen allowing platelets to connect and form clumps or aggregates (aggregation) (Fig. 15.4). Many substances can activate platelets including adenosine diphosphate (ADP), thromboxane A_2 (TXA_2), thrombin, and collagen. Platelets, once activated, secrete large amounts of TXA_2 via a COX1-dependent pathway (Bruno et al. 2023), further enhancing platelet aggregation and adhesion. Platelet aggregation and adhesion form an integral and important part of haemostasis and thrombosis, and help localise the thrombus or clot to the site of vascular damage.

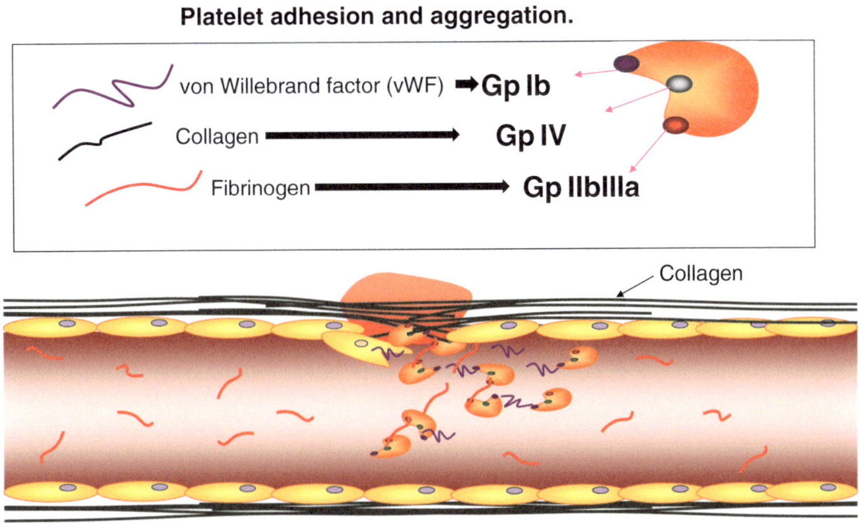

Fig. 15.4 Platelet adhesion and aggregation

An intriguing real-time visual display of the importance of platelets in thrombus formation can be found in (Furie and Furie 2008).

Platelets are therefore a recognised and well-utilised antithrombotic target. Recent research has demonstrated gender-related differences in relation to underlying platelet activity and reactivity to stimuli, with women demonstrating a stronger platelet effect; however, this seems to be somewhat offset by oestradiol-mediated prostacyclin (an antiplatelet product of the COX pathway) production (Gasecka et al. 2023). The clinical relevance of gender differences in platelet activity and its consequent therapeutic and pathological importance remains unclear.

15.5 Antiplatelet Medications

There are two common pharmacological mechanisms that are used to inhibit platelet activity namely, cyclooxygenase pathway inhibition and direct platelet receptor antagonism or inhibition.

Cyclooxygenase and Platelet Activation
The cyclooxygenase (COX) pathway, together with the lipoxygenase and Cytochrome P 450 pathways, are important mechanism by which inflammatory mediators (chemicals) are produced and regulated in the body (Fig. 15.5). The COX pathway produces a number of important eicosanoids (lipids with 20 carbon chains) involved in activating and controlling platelet function. The three main groups of eicosanoids produced by the COX pathway are prostaglandins, prostacyclins, and thromboxanes. Some important functions linked to these eicosanoids are given below.

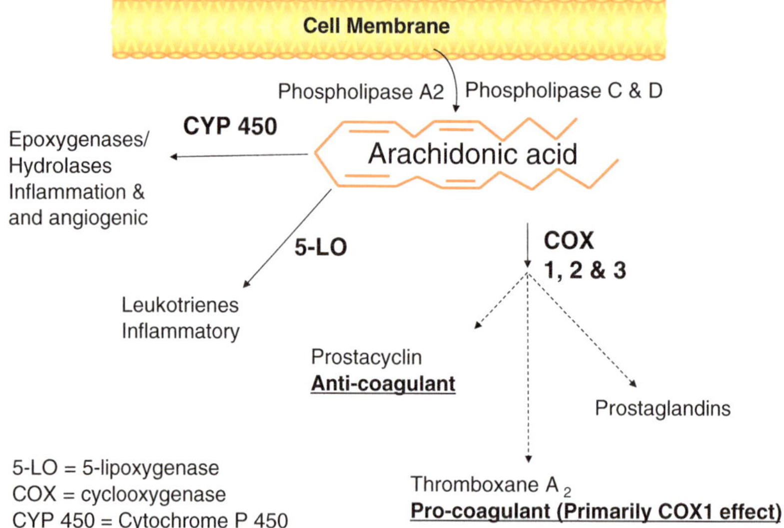

Fig. 15.5 Biochemistry of tissue damage

Prostaglandins
PGE2/PGI$_2$
- Inhibition of gastric acid secretion
- Increase gastric mucosal blood flow
- Cytoprotective characteristics
- Potentiation of inflammatory mediators
- Potent vasodilators influence renal blood flow

Prostacyclin PGI$_2$
- Vasodilatory action
- Increase platelet cAMP (activation)
- Increase platelet disaggregation

Thromboxane A$_2$
- Vasoconstrictor
- increase platelet aggregation

Whereas COX 1 enzymes are always present (constitutive) in all tissues in the body, COX2 is constitutively found in specific organs such as the kidney, gastrointestinal tract, brain, lungs, and thymus (Mitchell and Kirkby 2019). COX2 may be produced (induced) in macrophages and endothelial cells in response to a number of cytokines, bacterial toxins, and growth hormones (Brock et al. 1999). It is this mechanism that is the desired target of nonsteroidal anti-inflammatory drugs (NSAIDs).

Thromboxane A$_2$ (TXA$_2$) is the main platelet active mediator in the COX pathway; this effect is primarily linked to COX1.

15.5.1 COX Inhibitors

All nonsteroidal anti-inflammatory medications inhibit the COX pathway. The most commonly used medication that has this effect is aspirin (acetylsalicylic acid), despite its use spanning back more than 3500 years (Montinari et al. 2019). Its mechanism of action was determined comparatively recently in 1971 by Sune K. Bergström, Bengt I. Samuelsson, and John R. Vane for which they were awarded the Nobel Prize in Physiology or Medicine in 1982. Aspirin is now the commonest antiplatelet medication used globally. Aspirin's reduction in TXA$_2$ is the main mechanism of antiplatelet effect achieved by the irreversible inhibition of COX enzymes.

15.5.1.1 Pharmacokinetics of Aspirin

Aspirin is primarily metabolised in the liver by CYP2C19 and with a possible role for CYP3A4. Aspirin is significantly plasma protein bound (80–90%) and its elimination half-life depends upon the dose given, with low doses (<100 mg) having a half-life of 2–3 h and higher dose between 20 and 30 h (Sostres et al. 2014).

15.5.1.2 Adverse Reactions of Aspirin

Despite its widespread use, aspirin has several adverse reactions that limit its prescription in specific scenarios. Of note are the risks of aspirin exacerbated respiratory disease (AERD), an increased risk of gastric ulceration, and in children, risk of Reyes Syndrome.

Aspirin-Exacerbated Respiratory Disease (AERD)

Since its identification in 1919 by Cooke (Botey et al. 1988), the mechanism of aspirin-induced bronchospasm is described as aspirin and other NSAIDs inhibition of the COX arm of arachidonic acid metabolism that shifts production of inflammatory mediators to the proinflammatory and bronchospasm-promoting 5-LO pathway (Fig. 15.5) (Kim and Cho 2018). Aspirin intolerance in this context is a pivotal component of AERD, also commonly known as 'Samter's triad' following Samter's identification of bronchial asthma, nasal polyps, and aspirin intolerance or sensitivity, as the triad of conditions leading to the condition (Kim and Cho 2018). All patients who have AERD have nasal polyps and intractable sinus disease (Lee and Stevenson 2011). AERD is common (25%) in people with severe asthma. Similarly, aspirin sensitivity or intolerance has been reported in people who have different forms of chronic rhinosinusitis, such as allergic fungal rhinitis (Philpott et al. 2018).

Risk of Gastrointestinal Ulcers

The COX–1 enzyme improves gastrointestinal blood flow, enhances mucous secretion, and reduces hydrochloric acid (HCL) in the stomach. Inhibition of the COX–1 enzyme by aspirin (and other NSAIDs), therefore, increases the risk of gastric and duodenal ulcers. This adverse reaction typically requires coadministration of a proton pump inhibitor with aspirin or other NSAIDs to reduce the risk of GI ulceration. Importantly, an increasing volume of data suggests that gastric and duodenal ulcer risk is greater in new users of low-dose aspirin, compared to people who use it more prevalently (Nguyen et al. 2022), highlighting the need to be vigilant for symptoms of GI bleeds early on when treatment with aspirin starts.

Reye's Disease

Reye's syndrome, although now very rare, is a potentially fatal syndrome that involves encephalopathy together with fatty liver failure. The syndrome is of specific importance in children and teenagers, where use of aspirin in the treatment of common viral infections precipitated the syndrome (Mount and Toltzis 2020). Since its identification in 1963 by Reye, Morgan, and Sydney (Reye et al. 1963), Reye's syndrome and Reye's-like disease was felt to be linked to different forms of genetic errors of metabolism (Schrör 2007). Importantly, high-dose aspirin can be secreted in breast milk, so use of aspirin by a breastfeeding mother is contraindicated (Davanzo et al. 2014). A small number of case studies suggest a low incidence of Reye's syndrome in adults. An analysis of the US Food and Drug Administration (FDA) and the Japanese adverse drug event report databases suggest a diagnosis of Reye's syndrome should be considered in female adults if symptoms are present (Matsumoto et al. 2020).

15.5.2 Platelet $P2Y_{12}$ Receptor Antagonists (Clopidogrel, Prasugrel, Ticagrelor, and Cangrelor)

15.5.2.1 Mechanism of Action of Platelet ADP Receptor Antagonists

The main platelet receptor antagonists used clinically are antagonists of the $P2Y_{12}$ receptor that bind ADP. Activation of this receptor by ADP leads to a release of intracellular calcium that, in turn, causes a conformational change that activates the IIb/IIIa Gp receptor. This receptor enables platelet–platelet binding via fibrinogen (Furie and Furie 2008) thus causing platelet aggregation.

There are currently three generations of oral $P2Y_{12}$ receptor antagonists. The first-generation prototype drug ticlopidine has now been completely superseded by the second-generation drug, clopidogrel, which has been the standard medication for several decades. Newer third-generation medications include prasugrel (approved in Europe and the United States in 2009), and ticagrelor (approved in 2010 in Europe and 2011 in the United States).

15.5.2.2 ADP Receptor Antagonist Pharmacokinetics

All these medications are orally administered and are therefore subject to delays in the time of onset of effect as well as clearance. Clopidogrel and prasugrel are both prodrugs, and in the case of clopidogrel, which has a complex metabolism involving a number of different enzymes (Table 15.2), it is primarily metabolised by CYPC219, and there is considerable variability in the effect of the drug owing to the presence of a number of CYP 2C19 polymorphisms (Galli and Angiolillo 2024). These limitations have led to the development of an intravenous $P2Y_{12}$ receptor inhibitor, cangrelor.

Choice of medication is therefore dependent on their effect and adverse effect profile as well as risk of drug–drug interactions. The aim of this next section is not to recommend a particular medication over another, but to illustrate the considerations that may impact drug choice.

Clinical guidelines, such as the National Institute for Health and Care Excellence (NICE), have issued guidance related to $P2Y_{12}$ receptor antagonists use in acute coronary syndromes (NG185, 2020).

Table 15.2 Pharmacokinetic data for $P2Y_{12}$ receptor antagonists

	Bioavailability	V_d	Protein binding	Metabolism	Half life	excretion
Clopidogrel	50%	39,240 ± 33,520 L	98%	CYPs 2CI9, 3A4/5, 2B6, 1A2, 2C9	6 h	50% urine 46% faeces
Prasugrel	79%	44–68 L	98%	CYP3A4 CYP 2B6	2–15 h Active metabolite	68% urine
Ticagrelor	36%	88 L	>99%	CYP 3A4	8 h parent	~58% faeces ~26% urine
Cangrelor	100%	3.9 L	97–98%	Liver independent	3–5 min	Urine 58% Bile 35%

Data sources (drug bank and eMC)

Currently, all oral $P2Y_{12}$ receptor antagonists are coadministered with aspirin so-called dual antiplatelet therapy (DAPT). Prasugrel and ticagrelor have now superseded clopidogrel in most instances, except when there is a high bleeding risk (Patti et al. 2020). In particular, in populations such as <75-years old and underweight patients (<60 Kg), the use of prasugrel may be harmful and should be used with caution (Clark et al. 2015). When genetic polymorphisms for CYP2C19 may be a consideration or use of proton pump inhibitors is present, again, clopidogrel should be used with caution due to poor metabolism or drug interaction risk (Clark et al. 2015; Schilling et al. 2020). Similarly, although not a main metabolic pathway, coadministration of clopidogrel with strong CYP3A4-inducing drugs can increase the production of the active metabolite of clopidogrel, leading to an increased drug effect. Conversely, administration of a strong CYP3A4 inhibitor may reduce the clopidogrel drug effect owing to a reduction in biotransformation of the clopidogrel prodrug to its active metabolite (Schilling et al. 2020). Finally, owing to its primary metabolism by CYP 3A4, ticagrelor should be used with caution when other medications that have strong interactions with CYP 3A4 and potentially when polypharmacy drug regimens are present. Overall, although renal excretion is not the sole mechanism of excretion (Table 15.2) because of the increased risk of bleeding with DAPT, patients with severe renal dysfunction (<30 mL/min/1.73 m^2) should be prescribed $P2Y_{12}$ receptor antagonists, particularly prasugrel and ticagrelor, with caution and sufficient monitoring (Schilling et al. 2020).

When administration of clopidogrel is indicated, there is potential for point-of-care CYP2C19 polymorphism testing. Bedside testing apparatus such as the Spartan RX has been validated for this purpose (Davis et al. 2020). Although, the use of this system is not currently recommended by NICE. Clopidogrel has also been associated with an increased hypoglycaemic risk in Asian and ageing populations (Chen et al. 2023).

Finally, cangrelor is an effective and useful treatment when short-term antiplatelet activity is required, such as in the case of cardiovascular intervention procedures. Its metabolism is liver independent, so it is not affected by genetic variations and renal dysfunction does not affect its excretion; however, its cost currently prohibits widespread use in the absence of any clear superior clinical benefit.

15.5.2.3 $P2Y_{12}$ Receptor Antagonist Adverse Reactions

All $P2Y_{12}$ receptor antagonists have bleeding as an adverse effect. The consequence of these bleeds depend upon their location but may lead to outcomes such as cerebrovascular accidents, hypotension, arrhythmias haematuria and GI bleeds. Other adverse effects may include precipitation of hyperuricaemia and gout, and for some preparations dyspnoea (Table 15.3).

Table 15.3 Adverse reactions of $P2Y_{12}$ receptor antagonists

Adverse effect	*Clopidogrel*	Prasugrel	Ticagrelor	Cangrelor
Bleeding	x	x	x	x
Sensitivity reactions	x	x		
Anaemia		x		
Hyperuricemia and Gout		x	x	
Dyspnoea			x	x
Dizziness, syncope headache			x	

Summary

Thrombosis is a complex mechanism that involves activation of a series of blood proteins (coagulation proteins) and platelets to form a blood clot. These two mechanisms potentiate each other and contain negative feedback pathways to help regulate the growth of the clot. This process allows for rapid clot formation to help reduce the risk of blood loss from the circulation. Activation of thrombosis by blood vessel disease is a widespread and clinically significant problem that may lead to myocardial infarction, cerebrovascular events, and peripheral vascular disease. Pharmacological manipulation of coagulation proteins and platelet activation gives rise to the two main arms of antithrombotic medications available, namely, anticoagulants and antiplatelets. Whereas warfarin and heparin, and their analogues have been mainstay medications used in clinical practice for decades. Newer and safer medications such as direct oral anticoagulants are now gaining popularity as a replacement for warfarin and its analogues. Many newer antithrombotic medications are safer than previously used medications, as issues related to renal function and polypharmacy are still of concern with some classes of drugs.

Multiple Choice Questions

1. Which coagulation protein is core to the coagulation process
   - (a) IX
   - (b) X
   - (c) XI
   - (d) XII
2. In a blood clot the coagulation mesh is produced by
   - (a) Xa
   - (b) Thrombin
   - (c) Protein C
   - (d) Fibrin
3. Warfarin effects the production of which of these coagulation proteins?
   - (a) Fibrin
   - (b) Factor VIII
   - (c) Factor II
   - (d) Factor XII

4. Which coagulation process occurs on platelets
    (a) Initiation
    (b) Adhesion
    (c) Amplification
    (d) Propagation
5. In addition to bleeding which Type A adverse effect may be caused by warfarin
    (a) Nausea
    (b) Leg pain
    (c) Calciphylaxis
    (d) Liver cirrhosis
6. Epoxide reductase inhibitors are now slowly being replaced by
    (a) Warfarin
    (b) Antiplatelet medications
    (c) Direct oral anticoagulants
    (d) Heparin
7. Heparin may be best described as an
    (a) Inhibitor
    (b) Agonist
    (c) Accelerant
    (d) Competitive antagonist
8. When a patient is required to have an INR to monitor the drug effects on thrombosis. Which medication are they taking
    (a) Heparin
    (b) Warfarin
    (c) Direct oral anticoagulants
    (d) Cyclooxygenase inhibitor.
9. Osteoporosis may occur with which anticoagulant
    (a) Warfarin
    (b) Heparin
    (c) DOACs
    (d) ADP receptor antagonists
10. When a patient is prescribed the antiplatelet medication aspirin, which other medications should they avoid?
    (a) Antacids
    (b) NSAIDs
    (c) Laxatives
    (d) Antipyretics

Answers

1. (b)
2. (d)
3. (c)

4. (d)
5. (c)
6. (c)
7. (c)
8. (b)
9. (b)
10. (b)

References

Abatzis-Papadopoulos M, Tigkiropoulos K, Nikas S, Papoutsis I, Kostopoulou O, Stavridis K, Karamanos D, Lazaridis I, Saratzis N (2023) The effectiveness and safety of direct oral anticoagulants compared to conventional pharmacologic thromboprophylaxis in hip fracture patients: a systematic review and meta-analysis of randomized controlled trials. Orthop Traumatol Surg Res 109(2):103364. https://doi.org/10.1016/J.OTSR.2022.103364

Afzal S, Zaidi STR, Merchant HA, Babar Z-U-D, Hasan SS (2021) Prescribing trends of oral anticoagulants in England over the last decade: a focus on new and old drugs and adverse events reporting. J Thromb Thrombolysis 52(2):646–653. https://doi.org/10.1007/s11239-021-02416-4

Barrett H, O'Keeffe M, Kavanagh E, Walsh M, O'Connor E (2018) Is matrix Gla protein associated with vascular calcification? A systematic review. Nutrients 10(4):415. https://doi.org/10.3390/nu10040415

Bjørklund G, Svanberg E, Dadar M, Card DJ, Chirumbolo S, Harrington DJ, Aaseth J (n.d.) The role of matrix Gla protein (MGP) in vascular calcification. Curr Med Chem 27(10):1647–1660. https://doi.org/10.2174/0929867325666180716104159

Botey J, Navarro C, Marín A, Eseverri JL (1988) Aspirin-induced asthma in children. Allergol Immunopathol 16(3):145–149. http://www.ncbi.nlm.nih.gov/pubmed/3177149

Brock TG, McNish RW, Peters-Golden M (1999) Arachidonic acid is preferentially metabolized by cyclooxygenase-2 to prostacyclin and prostaglandin E2. J Biol Chem 274(17):11660–11666. https://doi.org/10.1074/jbc.274.17.11660

Brodin E, Appelbom H, Østerud B, Hilden I, Petersen LC, Hansen J-B (2009) Regulation of thrombin generation by TFPI in plasma without and with heparin. Transl Res 153(3):124–131. https://doi.org/10.1016/j.trsl.2008.12.004

Bruno A, Tacconelli S, Contursi A, Ballerini P, Patrignani P (2023) Cyclooxygenases and platelet functions. Adv Pharm (San Diego, Calif) 97:133–165. https://doi.org/10.1016/bs.apha.2022.12.001

Bryant JW, Shariat-Madar Z (2009) Human plasma kallikrein-kinin system: physiological and biochemical parameters. Cardiovasc Hematol Agents Med Chem 7(3):234–250. https://doi.org/10.2174/187152509789105444

Chao T, Braunwald E, Palazzolo MG, Antman EM, Carnicelli AP, Connolly SJ, Eikelboom J, Granger CB, Patel MR, Ruff CT, Wallentin L, Giugliano RP (2024) Clinical outcomes in >10,000 Asian vs >61,000 non-Asian race patients with AF randomized to Warfarin vs DOACs: a patient-level meta-analyses from COMBINE AF. Eur Heart J 45(Supplement_1). https://doi.org/10.1093/eurheartj/ehae666.605

Chen S, Qiang J, Zhang Y, Zhao B, Tian R, Yuan T, Li M, Li M, Li Y, Zhu H, Pan H (2023) Hypoglycemia as a potential risk for patients taking clopidogrel: a systematic review and meta-analysis. Front Endocrinol 14. https://doi.org/10.3389/fendo.2023.1091933

Clark MG, Beavers C, Osborne J (2015) Managing the acute coronary syndrome patient: evidence based recommendations for anti-platelet therapy. Heart Lung 44(2):141–149. https://doi.org/10.1016/j.hrtlng.2014.11.005

Conners MS, Money SR (2002) The new Heparins. Ochsner J 4(1):41–47. https://www.ncbi.nlm.nih.gov/pmc/articles/PMC3399228/

Davanzo R, Bua J, Paloni G, Facchina G (2014) Breastfeeding and migraine drugs. Eur J Clin Pharmacol 70(11):1313–1324. https://doi.org/10.1007/s00228-014-1748-0

Davis BH, DeFrank G, Limdi NA, Harada S (2020) Validation of the Spartan RXCYP2C19 genotyping assay utilizing blood samples. Clin Transl Sci 13(2):260–264. https://doi.org/10.1111/cts.12714

Donaldson CJ, Harrington DJ (2017) Therapeutic warfarin use and the extrahepatic functions of vitamin K-dependent proteins. Br J Biomed Sci 74(4):163–169. https://doi.org/10.1080/09674845.2017.1336854

Doni K, Bühn S, Weise A, Mann N-K, Hess S, Sönnichsen A, Salem S, Pieper D, Thürmann P, Mathes T (2023) Safety outcomes of direct oral anticoagulants in older adults with atrial fibrillation: a systematic review and meta-analysis of (subgroup analyses from) randomized controlled trials. GeroScience 46(1):923–944. https://doi.org/10.1007/s11357-023-00825-2

Dorgalaleh A, Favaloro EJ, Bahraini M, Rad F (2021) Standardization of Prothrombin Time/International Normalized Ratio (PT/INR). Int J Lab Hematol 43(1):21–28. https://doi.org/10.1111/ijlh.13349

Esmon CT, Vigano-D'Angelo S, D'Angelo A, Comp PC (1987) Anticoagulation proteins C and S. Adv Exp Med Biol 214:47–54. https://doi.org/10.1007/978-1-4757-5985-3_4

Ferri N, Colombo E, Tenconi M, Baldessin L, Corsini A (2022) Drug-drug interactions of direct oral anticoagulants (DOACs): From Pharmacological to Clinical Practice. Pharmaceutics. 14(6):1120. https://doi.org/10.3390/pharmaceutics14061120

Furie B, Furie BC (2008) Mechanisms of thrombus formation. N Engl J Med 359(9):938–949. https://doi.org/10.1056/NEJMra0801082

Galli M, Angiolillo DJ (2024) Role of the P2Y12 receptor on thrombus formation and evolution in therapeutic strategies. Expert Opin Ther Targets 28(1–2):5–8. https://doi.org/10.1080/14728222.2024.2315017

Gasecka A, Zimodro JM, Appelman Y (2023) Sex differences in antiplatelet therapy: state-of-the art. Platelets 34(1):2176173. https://doi.org/10.1080/09537104.2023.2176173

Grover SP, Mackman N (2018) Tissue factor: an essential mediator of hemostasis and trigger of thrombosis. Arterioscler Thromb Vasc Biol 38(4):709–725. https://doi.org/10.1161/ATVBAHA.117.309846

Harel Z, Sood MM (2021) Is Warfarin being relegated to the pharmaceutical dustbin? Am J Kidney Dis 78(2):174–176. https://doi.org/10.1053/j.ajkd.2021.02.329

Harrington J, Carnicelli AP, Hua K, Wallentin L, Patel MR, Hohnloser SH, Giugliano RP, Fox KAA, Hijazi Z, Lopes RD, Pokorney SD, Hong H, Granger CB (2023) Direct oral anticoagulants versus warfarin across the spectrum of kidney function: patient-level network meta-analyses from COMBINE AF. Circulation 147(23):1748–1757. https://doi.org/10.1161/CIRCULATIONAHA.122.062752

Hoffman M, Monroe DM (2001) A cell-based model of hemostasis. Thromb Haemost 85(6):958–965. http://www.ncbi.nlm.nih.gov/pubmed/11434702

Hu T, Li Y-H, Han W-Q, Maduray K, Chen T-S, Hao L, Zhong J-Q (2023) Direct oral anticoagulants versus vitamin K antagonists in cirrhotic patients with atrial fibrillation: update of systematic review and meta-analysis. Am J Cardiovasc Drugs 23(6):683–694. https://doi.org/10.1007/s40256-023-00598-1

Jones A, Swan D, Lisman T, Barnes GD, Thachil J (2024) Anticoagulation in chronic kidney disease: current status and future perspectives. J Thromb Haemost 22(2):323–336. https://doi.org/10.1016/j.jtha.2023.09.020

Kaatz S, Ahmad D, Spyropoulos AC, Schulman S (2015) Definition of clinically relevant non-major bleeding in studies of anticoagulants in atrial fibrillation and venous thromboembolic disease in non-surgical patients: communication from the SSC of the ISTH. J Thromb Haemost 13(11):2119–2126. https://doi.org/10.1111/jth.13140

Kaminsky LS, Zhang Z-Y (1997) Human P450 metabolism of warfarin. Pharmacol Ther 73(1):67–74. https://doi.org/10.1016/S0163-7258(96)00140-4

Kandrotas RJ (1992) Heparin pharmacokinetics and pharmacodynamics. Clin Pharmacokinet 22(5):359–374. https://doi.org/10.2165/00003088-199222050-00003

Keragala CB, Medcalf RL (2021) Plasminogen: an enigmatic zymogen. Blood 137(21):2881–2889. https://doi.org/10.1182/blood.2020008951

Khudair AD, Khudair AD, Awadh M, Pérez Romano NS, Darwish A (2023) Calciphylaxis: a rare complication with a fatal outcome in end-stage renal disease. Cureus 15(9):e45557. https://doi.org/10.7759/cureus.45557

Kim S-D, Cho K-S (2018) Samter's triad: state of the art. Clin Exp Otorhinol 11(2):71–80. https://doi.org/10.21053/ceo.2017.01606

Kumano O, Akatsuchi K, Amiral J (2021) Updates on anticoagulation and laboratory tools for therapy monitoring of Heparin, Vitamin K antagonists and direct oral anticoagulants. Biomedicine 9(3):264. https://doi.org/10.3390/biomedicines9030264

Lee RU, Stevenson DD (2011) Aspirin-exacerbated respiratory disease: evaluation and management. Allergy, Asthma Immunol Res 3(1):3–10. https://doi.org/10.4168/aair.2011.3.1.3

Li Z, Xu W, Wang L, Chai L, Ageno W, Romeiro FG, Li H, Qi X (2023) Risk of bleeding in liver Cirrhosis receiving direct oral anticoagulants: a systematic review and meta-analysis. Thromb Haemost 123(11):1072–1088. https://doi.org/10.1055/s-0043-1770100

Marin BG, Aghagoli G, Hu SL, Massoud CM, Robinson-Bostom L (2023) Calciphylaxis and kidney disease: a review. Am J Kidney Dis 81(2):232–239. https://doi.org/10.1053/j.ajkd.2022.06.011

Matsumoto K, Hasegawa S, Nakao S, Shimada K, Mukai R, Tanaka M, Satake R, Yoshida Y, Goto F, Inoue M, Ikesue H, Iguchi K, Hashida T, Nakamura M (2020) Assessment of Reye's syndrome profile with data from the US Food and Drug Administration Adverse Event Reporting System and the Japanese Adverse Drug Event Report databases using the disproportionality analysis. SAGE Open Med 8:2050312120974176. https://doi.org/10.1177/2050312120974176

McGrath ER, Eikelboom JW, Kapral MK, O'Donnell MJ (2013) Novel oral anticoagulants: a focused review for stroke physicians. Int J Stroke 9(1):71–78

Mitchell JA, Kirkby NS (2019) Eicosanoids, prostacyclin and cyclooxygenase in the cardiovascular system. Br J Pharmacol 176(8):1038–1050. https://doi.org/10.1111/bph.14167

Mongirdienė A, Liuizė A, Kašauskas A (2023) Novel knowledge about molecular mechanisms of Heparin-induced thrombocytopenia type II and treatment targets. Int J Mol Sci 24(9):8217. https://doi.org/10.3390/ijms24098217

Montinari MR, Minelli S, De Caterina R (2019) The first 3500 years of aspirin history from its roots – a concise summary. Vasc Pharmacol 113:1–8. https://doi.org/10.1016/j.vph.2018.10.008

Mount M, Toltzis P (2020) 50 years ago in the Journal of Pediatrics: Aspirin and Reye syndrome. J Pediatr 222:192. https://doi.org/10.1016/j.jpeds.2020.01.039

Nguyen TNM, Sha S, Chen L, Holleczek B, Brenner H, Schöttker B (2022) Strongly increased risk of gastric and duodenal ulcers among new users of low-dose aspirin: results from two large cohorts with new-user design. Aliment Pharmacol Ther 56(2):251–262. https://doi.org/10.1111/apt.17050

Olson ST, Björk I, Sheffer R, Craig PA, Shore JD, Choay J (1992) Role of the antithrombin-binding pentasaccharide in heparin acceleration of antithrombin-proteinase reactions. Resolution of the antithrombin conformational change contribution to heparin rate enhancement. J Biol Chem 267(18):12528–12538. https://doi.org/10.1016/S0021-9258(18)42309-5

Palta S, Saroa R, Palta A (2014) Overview of the coagulation system. Indian J Anaesth 58(5):515–523. https://doi.org/10.4103/0019-5049.144643

Patel NB, Jain G (2022) Warfarin induced skin necrosis. Postgrad Med J 98(1166):e41–e41. https://doi.org/10.1136/postgradmedj-2021-139988

Patti G, Micieli G, Cimminiello C, Bolognese L (2020) The role of Clopidogrel in 2020: a reappraisal. Cardiovasc Ther 2020:8703627. https://doi.org/10.1155/2020/8703627

Philpott CM, Erskine S, Hopkins C, Kumar N, Anari S, Kara N, Sunkaraneni S, Ray J, Clark A, Wilson A, Erskine S, Philpott C, Clark A, Hopkins C, Robertson A, Ahmed S, Kara N, Carrie S, Sunkaraneni V et al (2018) Prevalence of asthma, aspirin sensitivity and allergy in chronic rhinosinusitis: data from the UK National Chronic Rhinosinusitis Epidemiology Study. Respir Res 19(1):129. https://doi.org/10.1186/s12931-018-0823-y

Reye RDK, Morgan G, Baral J (1963) Encephalopathy and fatty degeneration of the viscera a disease entity in childhood. Lancet 282(7311):749–752. https://doi.org/10.1016/S0140-6736(63)90554-3

Schilling U, Dingemanse J, Ufer M (2020) Pharmacokinetics and pharmacodynamics of approved and investigational P2Y12 receptor antagonists. Clin Pharmacokinet 59(5):545–566. https://doi.org/10.1007/s40262-020-00864-4

Schrör K (2007) Aspirin and Reye syndrome: a review of the evidence. Paediatr Drugs 9(3):195–204. https://doi.org/10.2165/00148581-200709030-00008

Shehab A, Elnour AA, Bhagavathula AS, Erkekoglu P, Hamad F, Al Nuaimi S, Al Shamsi A, Mukhtar I, Ali AbdElrazek AM, Al Suwaidi A, Mandil MA, Baraka M, Sadik A, Saraan K, Al Kalbani NMS, Mahmood AA, Barqawi Y, Al Hajjar M, Shehab OA et al (2016) Novel oral anticoagulants and the 73rd anniversary of historical warfarin. J Saudi Heart Assoc 28(1):31–45. https://doi.org/10.1016/j.jsha.2015.05.003

Signorelli SS, Scuto S, Marino E, Giusti M, Xourafa A, Gaudio A (2019) Anticoagulants and osteoporosis. Int J Mol Sci 20(21):5275. https://doi.org/10.3390/ijms20215275

Sostres C, Gargallo CJ, Lanas A (2014) Aspirin, cyclooxygenase inhibition and colorectal cancer. World J Gastrointest Pharmacol Ther 5(1):40–49. https://doi.org/10.4292/wjgpt.v5.i1.40

Steffel J, Collins R, Antz M, Cornu P, Desteghe L, Haeusler KG, Oldgren J, Reinecke H, Roldan-Schilling V, Rowell N, Sinnaeve P, Vanassche T, Potpara T, Camm AJ, Heidbüchel H, reviewers, E. (2021) 2021 European heart rhythm association practical guide on the use of non-vitamin K antagonist oral anticoagulants in patients with atrial fibrillation. Europace 23(10):1612–1676. https://doi.org/10.1093/europace/euab065

Thomas SG (2019) 3 - The structure of resting and activated platelets. In: Michelson AD (ed) Platelets, 4th edn. Academic Press, pp 47–77. https://www.sciencedirect.com/science/article/pii/B9780128134566000035

Tian Y, Pan T, Wen X, Ao G, Ma Y, Liu X, Liu R, Ran H (2023) Efficacy and safety of direct oral anticoagulants compared with Heparin for preventing thromboembolism in hospitalized patients with COVID-19: a systematic review and meta-analysis. Clin Appl Thromb Hemost 29. https://doi.org/10.1177/10760296231164355

Troisi F, Guida P, Vitulano N, Quadrini F, Di Monaco A, Grimaldi M (2023) Safety and efficacy of direct oral anticoagulants versus vitamin K antagonists in atrial fibrillation electrical cardioversion: an update systematic review and meta-analysis. Int J Cardiol 379:40–47. https://doi.org/10.1016/j.ijcard.2023.03.023

Wang X, Ma Y, Hui X, Li M, Li J, Tian J, Wang Q, Yan P, Li J, Xie P, Yang K, Yao L (2023) Oral direct thrombin inhibitors or oral factor Xa inhibitors versus conventional anticoagulants for the treatment of deep vein thrombosis. The. Cochrane Database Syst Rev 4(4):CD010956. https://doi.org/10.1002/14651858.CD010956.pub3

Zhao Y, Zhu L, Yang Y, Gao H, Zhang R (2023) Safety of direct oral anticoagulants in patients with liver disease: a systematic review and meta-analysis. Acta Clin Belg 78(3):234–244. https://doi.org/10.1080/17843286.2022.2108259

Zoch ML, Clemens TL, Riddle RC (2016) New insights into the biology of osteocalcin. Bone. 82:42-9. https://doi.org/10.1016/j.bone.2015.05.046

Medications Used for Anaesthesia

16

Christoph Schmidt

Learning Outcomes
At the end of this chapter, you will be able to:

- Understand the definition and principles of general anaesthesia.
- Gain knowledge about the core groups of anaesthetic agents used in general anaesthesia and describe their pharmacological properties.
- Recognise the roles of anaesthetists, anaesthetic nurses, and operating department practitioners for the safe delivery of anaesthesia.
- Appreciate the importance of understanding anaesthetic pharmacology for safe and effective delivery of patient care.

16.1 Introduction

Anaesthesia is uniquely positioned at the crossroads between medicine and surgery and is pertinent in delivering perioperative medicine and emergency care throughout the hospital. The practice of anaesthesia is based on the principles of physiology and pharmacology. These subjects are thoroughly taught to preclinical medical students but are often perceived as disconnected from clinical application. Since anaesthesia is one of the largest speciality groups in secondary care, a solid understanding of this field is highly relevant.

A well-performed anaesthetic relies on the complementary skills and knowledge of an anaesthetist and anaesthetic nurse (AN) or operating department practitioner (OPD). All parties are highly skilled members and must understand each other's roles and responsibilities to ensure the safe conduct of anaesthesia. As a team, they

C. Schmidt (✉)
Ashford and St Peter's Hospitals NHS Foundation Trust, Chertsey, UK
e-mail: christoph.schmidt1@nhs.net

© The Author(s), under exclusive license to Springer Nature Switzerland AG 2026
E. Khan, P. Hood (eds.), *Understanding Pharmacology in Nursing Practice*,
https://doi.org/10.1007/978-3-032-03964-4_16

administer general anaesthesia, manage complications during surgery, and provide post-operative care and urgent treatments in the hospital. No matter the scenario, ANs and ODPs must strive to understand the medicines used for each patient to ensure the safe delivery of care.

16.1.1 From a Vague History to Defined Practice

The term 'anaesthesia' (Greek: without sensation) was coined by the philosopher Dioscorides to recount the strictly speaking narcotic (Greek: stuporous, benumbed), effects of the plant mandragora. A similar application of 'sponges soaked with opium and mandragora' for surgical pain relief was described by Italian physician Theodoric of Lucca. This technique is often credited as one of the earliest uses of 'anaesthesia', though it only addressed one of the four principles of general anaesthesia, namely analgesia.

From the early accounts of various pioneers in anaesthesia, the key principles of general anaesthesia can be categorised into the four A's.

Four A's of Anaesthetic Agents

1. The suppression of responses to noxious stimuli: **A**nalgesia
2. The loss of memory of the event: **A**mnesia
3. A state of unconsciousness: Lack of **A**wareness
4. The absence of overt movements (myorelaxation, immobility): **A**kinesia

16.1.2 Modern Definitions of Anaesthesia

The current definitions of anaesthesia, specifically general anaesthesia, are based on these elements. The definitions by bodies including the Royal College of Anaesthetists (RCoA), the American Society of Anaesthesiologists (ASA), the National Institute for Health and Care Excellence (NICE) and the World Health Organization (WHO) all, to varying degrees, define general anaesthesia as:

'A state of medically induced, controlled and reversible unconsciousness with an absence of pain sensation, immobility and unawareness of the procedure allowing for the safe conduct of surgery and diagnostic investigations'.

All-encompassing definitions of anaesthesia also reference spinal, regional, and local anaesthesia with and without sedation. However, these techniques and their respective medicines are beyond the scope of this chapter.

16.1.3 The Role of Nurses in Anaesthesia

In the anaesthetic room, Anaesthetic Nurses (ANs) and Operating Department Practitioners (ODPs) work to create a safe environment. They check equipment, prepare drugs and fluids, assist with procedures, assemble monitoring devices, and provide patient care. The application of their understanding of anaesthetic agents is relevant across all of these duties.

ANs and ODPs must, therefore, understand gases and volatile anaesthetics when working in confined spaces, such as the anaesthetic room or while troubleshooting the anaesthetic machine. They need to be capable of assessing anaesthetic plans when preparing or dispensing intravenous agents and fluids to ensure safety and error prevention. Similarly, they may predict and initiate relevant patient monitoring for invasive anaesthetic procedures to optimise patient comfort and prevent harm. A strong understanding of anaesthetic pharmacology is thus essential.

16.2 General Anaesthetic Agents

This chapter will address the core anaesthetic agents in a typical order of administration for general anaesthesia and divide these medicines into three groups. The first group comprises induction agents that establish general anaesthesia. Inductions are commonly performed using intravenous agents but can be achieved with inhalational agents, usually used for maintenance. Neuromuscular blocking agents (NMBA) are frequently used following an induction and are also discussed. These medications cause muscle relaxation and create optimal conditions for intubation and surgery. The chapter will conclude with a detailed look at the pharmacology of inhalational agents used for maintaining anaesthesia.

16.2.1 Principles of General Anaesthetic Action

Theories on the mechanisms of general anaesthetic action have changed significantly throughout the years, and a definitive explanation for their action has proven enigmatic. While the lack of a clear, unified definition of general anaesthesia has compounded this challenge, any general anaesthetic action must, at the very least, explain a reversible loss of nociception and conscious awareness.

16.2.2 Anatomical Sites of General Anaesthetic Action

General anaesthetic agents most likely target the central nervous system's brain and spinal cord to produce the clinically observed reversible loss of nociception and conscious awareness (explicit memory). Studies on auditory and sensory evoked potentials, measures of electrical activity in the brain in response to sound and touch, have highlighted a region in the brain between the cortex and brainstem, known as the thalamus, in response to general anaesthetic agents. The integrative functions of the thalamus affect sleep, wakefulness, consciousness, memory, and more, and point towards it being the most likely primary anatomical site of action (Fig. 16.1). Other regions in the brain, including the limbic system, have also been

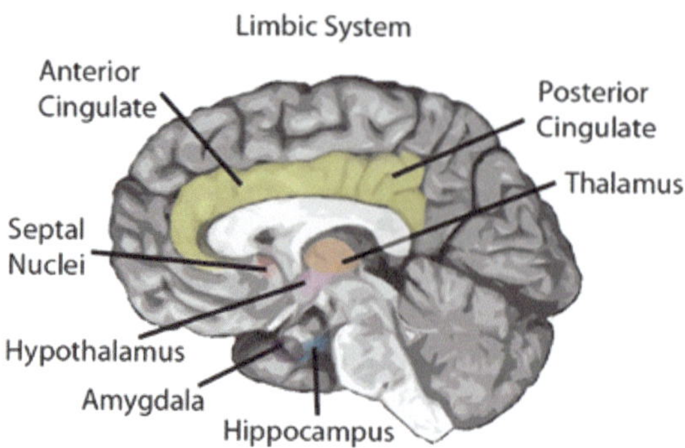

Fig. 16.1 Image of the limbic system (including the thalamus). (With permission from Springer https://doi.org/10.1007/978-3-319-91280-6_208)

implicated as probable secondary sites of action due to their crucial role in memory formation (Fig. 16.1). Furthermore, signal propagation of cortical afferents and peripheral motor efferents appear to be disrupted by general anaesthetic agents through their action at the spinal cord level.

16.2.3 Molecular Theories on General Anaesthetic Action

The initial molecular theory on anaesthetic action stipulated that a non-specific physiochemical property is responsible for the action of anaesthetic agents on account of the linear relationship demonstrated between lipid solubility and potency across a wide range of structurally diverse drugs. Charles Overton and Hans Meyer independently demonstrated the unitary mechanism of general anaesthesia, now known as the Meyer-Overton hypothesis (Kopp Lugli et al. 2009) (Fig. 16.2). However, stereoisomeric pairs of the ketamine, R(+) and S(−), have identical lipid solubility, but only the R(+) isomer has anaesthetic properties. The unitary mechanism proposed based on the Overton–Meyer hypothesis is, therefore, likely relevant but does not fully explain the mechanism of general anaesthetic actions.

Nonetheless, following this remarkable discovery, further research proposed the cell membrane, a highly lipophilic area, as a potential site of molecular action.

One such theory, the critical volume hypothesis, stipulated that anaesthetic agents can change the composition of the phospholipid bilayer, causing it to expand and disrupt the function of membrane receptors and channels. The hypothesis was, however, incomplete as a 1 °C temperature increase resulted in a similar increase in membrane thickness as those caused by general anaesthetic agents without resulting in the same clinical effects.

The most probable mechanism of action of anaesthetics is a modulation of ligand-gated ion channels. This theory stems from molecular research that revealed how anaesthetic agents cause allosteric conformational changes in inhibitory gama amino butyric acid A ($GABA_A$) and glycine, receptors, increasing their activity, and excitatory N-methyl-D-aspartate (NMDA) and nicotinic receptors, reducing their activity.

Fig. 16.2 Meyer-Overton
graph of MAC as a
measure of potency versus
oil:gas partition coefficient
as a measure of lipid
solubility

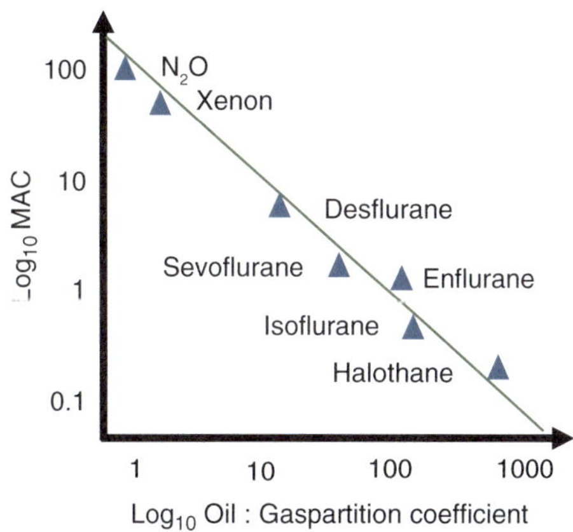

16.3   Intravenous Anaesthetic Agents

Intravenous anaesthetic agents are defined by their action to induce unconsciousness within one arm-brain circulation time. This period refers to the time it takes
from administration of the drug, commonly through a peripheral venous cannula
sited at the hand, to the brain, the target site of action. The ideal intravenous anaesthetic agent would have the following physical, pharmacokinetic and pharmacodynamic properties:

Physical Properties
- High lipid solubility
- Stable in water-soluble formulation
- Stable on light exposure
- Long shelf-life at room temperature
- Minimal environmental impact
- In-expensive

Pharmacokinetic Properties
- Rapid onset (drug in the unionised state; one arm-brain circulation)
- Rapid distribution (to highly vascular tissues)
- Rapid metabolism and clearance (and limited accumulation)
- Absence of active metabolites

Pharmacodynamic Properties
- High therapeutic ratio
- Analgesic at sub-anaesthetic concentrations
- Absence of pain on intravenous injection
- Presence of pain on intra-arterial injection
- Safe profile with inadvertent intra-arterial injection
- Non-irritant on subcutaneous injection

- Absence of thrombophlebitis
- Limited cardiovascular, respiratory or adrenocortical depression
- Absence of emetic effects
- Absence of excitation or emergence phenomenon
- Absence of histamine release and hypersensitivity
- Absence of hangover effect
- Absence of toxicity

No intravenous anaesthetic agent possesses all the ideal qualities, and each drug's properties make it suitable for different circumstances.

16.3.1 Propofol

Physical and Formulation

Propofol is a phenolic derivative (2,6 diisopropyl phenol) (Fig. 16.3). It appears as a white solution and is presented in clear, rubber-topped glass vials that can be stored in light at room temperature.

It is formulated as an isotonic, water-lipid emulsion with a concentration of 10 mg·ml^{-1} (1%) in a mixture of excipients, including soya bean oil, purified egg phosphatides, glycerol, sodium hydroxide, and water. The inclusion of the excipients is required as propofol has minimal water solubility and high lipid solubility. The emulsion is also available in concentrations of 20 mg·ml^{-1} (2%) and 5 mg·ml^{-1} (0.5%).

Application, Administration and Dosage

Propofol is the most commonly used intravenous induction agent, but it may also be used to maintain anaesthesia and sedation. The administration of propofol is intravenous only, and dosages depend on the intended use:

Fig. 16.3 2D chemical structure of Propofol

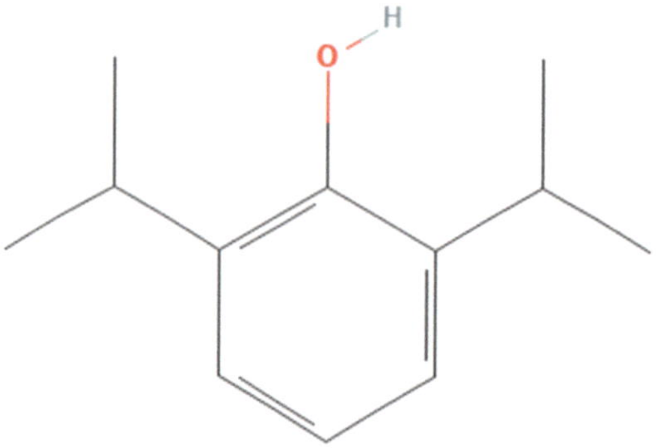

- Induction of anaesthesia: 1–2 mg·kg^{-1} IV as bolus
- Maintenance of anaesthesia: 4–12 mg·kg^{-1}·h^{-1} IV as infusion
- Sedation: 0.5–4 mg·kg^{-1}·h^{-1} IV as infusion

Mechanism of Action

Propofol acts on inhibitory receptors in the brain, mainly GABA, specifically GABA$_A$, but also displays activity on the primary inhibitory receptors of the spinal cord and brainstem, glycine. In binding to the beta subunit of GABA$_A$, a pentameric ion-gated chloride channel, propofol potentiates synaptic inhibition by prolonging the opening time of the chloride channel, resulting in hyperpolarisation (Sahinovic et al. 2018). The resultant decrease in neuronal excitability causes anaesthesia.

Pharmacokinetics

Propofol has a relatively low molecular weight (MW) of 178 Dalton (Da) and a high lipid solubility, which allows it to readily cross the blood–brain barrier (BBB). Consequently, the rate of induction largely depends on the patient's cardiac output (CO) and speed of administration.

The agent is also highly protein-bound; only 1–2% persists as a free drug in plasma. It is also a weak organic acid with a pKa of 11, and on injection, it predominantly exists in the unionised, unbound state, given the physiological pH of 7.4. Furthermore, among intravenous induction agents, propofol has the highest volume of distribution at 4 l·kg^{-1}, secondary to its high lipid solubility. The combination of these features facilitates a rapid onset and offset of action and rapid distribution to well-perfused tissues. The rapid offset continues even during prolonged infusions since the drug is metabolised more quickly than it redistributes from lipid-rich tissues.

The liver predominately metabolises propofol via glucuronidation. This reaction inactivates the drug and increases water solubility. Most inactivated metabolites can be excreted in urine, while a small fraction is excreted in faeces. The drug's clearance rate from the blood is about 2.2 l·min^{-1}, which exceeds hepatic blood flow, indicating an extrahepatic pathway for propofol metabolism. The kidney can contribute up to 30% of propofol metabolism, particularly if hepatic activity is impaired. The drug's terminal elimination half-life ranges from 5 to 12 h, though it can approach 60 h with prolonged continuous infusions over 24 h. This effect may reflect propofol's extensive yet slow redistribution from lipid-rich tissues into the blood (Table 16.1).

Pharmacodynamics

The pharmacodynamic effects of propofol are shown below (Table 16.2):

Special Points

Propofol-related Infusion Syndrome (PRIS) refers to an acute refractory bradycardia leading to asystole that co-presents with metabolic acidosis, rhabdomyolysis or myoglobinuria, lipidemic plasma or an enlarged fatty liver (Hemphill et al. 2019). PRIS is a complication of prolonged, propofol-based sedation for greater than 48 h. The syndrome was initially observed in children but can affect adults.

Table 16.1 Pharmacokinetic profile of propofol

Metric	Value
Molecular weight(MW)	178 Da
pH	6.0–8.5
pKa	11
Protein-bound	98–99%
Volume of distribuition(Vd)	4 $l\cdot kg^{-1}$
Clearence(Cl)	30–60 $ml\cdot kg^{-1}\cdot min^{-1}$
Terminal elimination half-life	5–12 h

MW molecular weight, *Vd* volume of distribuition, *Cl* clearence

Table 16.2 Pharmacodynamic profile of propofol

Organ system	Effect
Central nervous system	Dose-dependent, rapid, smooth cortical depression and anticonvulsive effect with excitatory non-epileptiform movements in 10%, especially with larger doses Reduced Cerebral Blood Flow CBF), Intracranial Pressure(ICP) and Cerebral Metabolic Rate of Oxygen(CMRO)$_2$ Possible anti-emetic effect via Dopamine D$_2$ receptor antagonism
Cardiovascular system	Dose-dependent reduction in vascular tone and myocardial contractility, decreasing sytemic vascular resistance(SVR) and Central Venous Pressure(CVP) and thereby preload, all leading to loss of Cardiac Output(CO) and resultant hypotension Mild effects on Heart Rate(HR); reflex tachycardia is rare; bradycardia is more common
Respiratory System	Reduction in tidal volume and rise in respiratory rate until depressant effect leads to apnea (common) Reduced responsiveness to CO$_2$ Attenuation of laryngeal reflexes reducing risk of laryngospasm or cough
Miscellaneous	Pain on injection; minimised by adding preservative-free lidocaine 1% to propofol 1% 20 mL Rarely green hair and urine

CBF cerebral blood flow, *ICP* intracranial pressure, *CMRO$_2$* cerebral metabolic rate of oxygen, *SVR* sytemic vascular resistance, *CVP* central venous pressure, *CO* cardiac output, *HR* heart rate

16.3.2 Sodium Thiopental

Physical and Formulation

Sodium thiopental, or thiopentone, is a pentobarbital derivative (Fig. 16.4a). The drug appears as a pale yellow powder and is presented in clear, rubber-topped glass vials that can be stored in light at room temperature.

Pentobarbital is a type of oxybarbiturate (Fig. 16.4b). By replacing an oxygen ion of this oxybarbiturate with a sulphur ion, this soluble compound turns insoluble sodium salt sulphur, sodium thiopental, a type of thiobarbiturate.

Barbiturates like this drug have a high lipid but minimal water solubility at physiological pH, and giving their form, readily form crystals in solution. To form a practical preparation for this drug, sodium thiopental is combined with 6% anhydrous sodium carbonate and stored in nitrogen gas instead of air. Both measures reduce the risk of carbon dioxide reacting with the drug's hydrogen ions, preventing

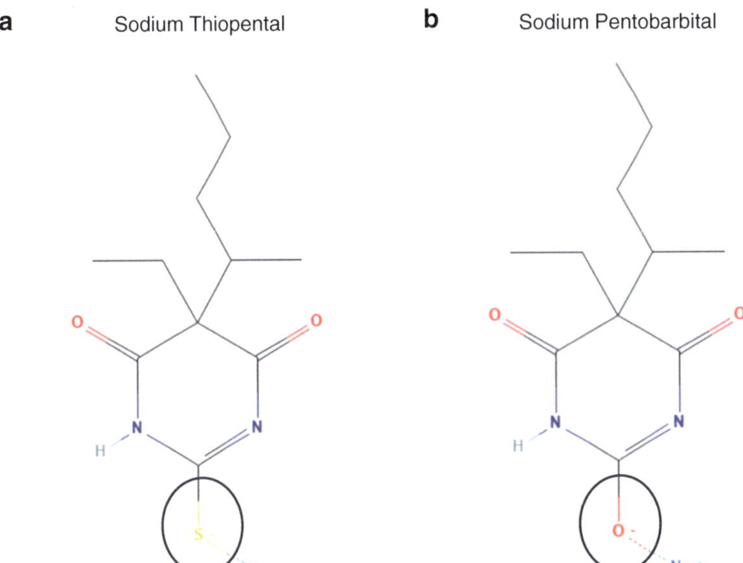

Fig. 16.4 2D chemical structure of sodium thiopental (**a**), a thiobarbiturate, and comparison to the pentobarbital derivative (**b**), an oxybarbiturate

the formation of free acids. This is crucial as sodium thiopental is most soluble in water in an alkaline rather than an acidic pH environment. Reconstituting this drug with sterile water yields a 2.5 mg·ml^{-1} (2.5%) solution that is alkaline in pH at 10.5. Preparing an improperly stored, manufactured or counterfeit drug preparation would likely yield a crystallised solution. This must not be administered as it could cause adverse reactions and an unpredictable clinical effect.

In this formulation, the drug has a pKa of 7.6 and is nearly 100% ionised (inactive). However, when administered intravenously, the physiological pH of 7.4 increases the percentage of unionised drug to 60%. With approximately 60–80% of the drug protein-bound (largely pain-free on administration), 12% of this drug will be in a unionised, free drug state. Despite this small percentage, this form is highly lipid soluble and can rapidly cross the BBB, inducing anaesthesia.

Application, Administration and Dosage

Sodium thiopental is almost exclusively used as an intravenous induction agent but can be administered rectally. This route has a significantly slower onset and was used to treat status epilepticus. The dosage for induction of anaesthesia is as follows:

Induction of anaesthesia: 3–7 mg·kg^{-1} IV as bolus.

Mechanism of Action

Sodium thiopental binds the beta subunits of $GABA_A$ in the brain. Akin to propofol, the drug potentiates synaptic inhibition by prolonging the opening time of the chloride channel. This results in hyperpolarisation and decreased neuronal excitability, which induces anaesthesia. Sodium thiopental also downregulates glutamate-mediated excitatory activity in the brain.

Pharmacokinetics

Sodium thiopental has a MW of 264 Da and high lipid solubility at physiological pH. Therefore, it rapidly traverses the BBB, swiftly inducing anaesthesia. The rate of effect primarily depends on CO as the drug is administered as a slow intravenous injection over 10–15 s only. An equally rapid offset occurs after a single dose of the medication due to its rapid initial distribution in the body, with a Vd of $1.96\ \text{l·kg}^{-1}$, not the drug's metabolism. This contrasts with propofol, where the rapid offset is primarily related to the metabolism.

The liver metabolises Sodium thiopental by oxidation via the cytochrome P450 complex, replacing a sulphur ion with an oxygen ion, reverting the thiobarbiturate to the original oxybarbiturate pentobarbital. This saturable process occurs initially at first-order kinetics but rapidly follows zero-order kinetics. Both unchanged drug and active metabolites are subject to further oxidation and hydroxylation, converting these to inactive metabolites excreted in urine. This process is slow and occurs at 15% per hour, with a clearance rate of $2.7–4.6\ \text{mg·kg}^{-1}\text{·min}^{-1}$, 30% of the drug can remain after 24 h. The terminal elimination half-life is 11 h (Table 16.3).

Pharmacodynamics

The pharmacodynamic effects of sodium thiopental are shown below (Table 16.4):

Table 16.3 Pharmacokinetic profile of sodium thiopental

Metric	Value
MW	264 Da
pH	10.5
pKa	7.6
Protein-bound	60–80%
Vd	$1.96\ \text{l·kg}^{-1}$
Cl	$2.7–4.6\ \text{ml·kg}^{-1}\text{·min}^{-1}$
Terminal elimination half-life	11 h

Table 16.4 Pharmacodynamic profile of sodium thiopental

Organ system	Effect
Central Nervous System	Rapid, smooth cortical depression and anticonvulsive effect Reduced CBF, ICP and $CMRO_2$
Cardiovascular System	Dose-dependent reduction in vascular tone and myocardial contractility, decreasing SVR and CVP and thereby preload, all leading to loss of CO and resultant hypotension Reflex tachycardia is common, particularly in hypovolemic and acidotic with reduced plasma-protein binding
Respiratory System	Dose-dependent respiratory depression and reduced responsiveness to CO_2 Reduced responsiveness to CO_2 Risk of laryngospasm or bronchospasm
Miscellaneous	Antanalgesic at low doses Reduced urine output

Special Points

Sodium Thiopental is safe in hepatic impairment. The drug is contraindicated in porphyria as it may cause an acute porphyric crisis (Hempel 1994).

Intra-arterial injection of the drug can lead to crystal formation as vessels become smaller and the drug less dilute, leading to painful vaso-occlusive ischemia. Similarly, peri-vascular injection is painful and can precipitate severe necrosis.

16.4 Neuromuscular Blocking Agents

NMBAs are routinely administered in general anaesthesia to facilitate endotracheal intubation and establish ideal operating conditions. All types of NMBAs prevent the transmission of neural impulses at the neuromuscular junction. While the mechanisms are diverse, all clinical agents act on the post-junctional nicotinic acetylcholine receptors (nAChR) (Fig. 16.5).

The ideal NMBA would have the following physical, pharmacokinetic and pharmacodynamic features (Stäuble and Blobner 2020); however, no NMBA possesses all these qualities.

Physical Properties
- Stable in water-soluble formulation
- Stable on light exposure
- Long shelf-life at room temperature
- Minimal environmental impact
- Cheap

Pharmacokinetic Properties
- Rapid onset (unionised state; one arm-brain circulation)
- Rapid distribution (to highly vascular tissues)

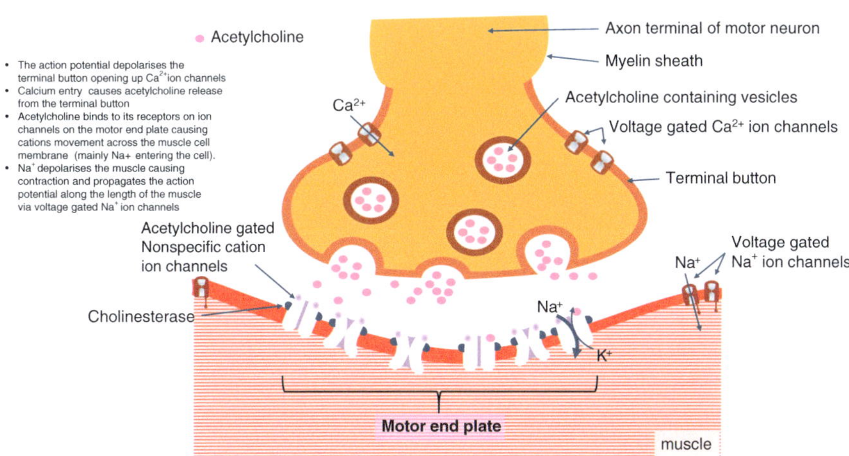

Fig. 16.5 Mechanism of action of neuromuscular blocking agents

- Absence of active metabolites
- Spontaneous predictable reversal
- Short duration of action
- Non-depolarising mechanism of action

Pharmacodynamic Properties
- High potency
- Absence of cardiovascular, respiratory or adrenocortical depression
- Absence of histamine release and hypersensitivity reactions
- Safe in renal and hepatic dysfunction and failure

16.4.1 Suxamethonium Chloride

Physical and Formulation
Suxamethonium chloride, or succinylcholine, is a dicholine ester derivative of acetylcholine (two linked molecules of the endogenous neurotransmitter) (Fig. 16.6) and currently the only clinical depolarising NMBA. The drug appears as a clear, colourless solution and is presented in a clear, rubber-topped glass vial that can be stored in light but must be refrigerated.

It is formulated as an aqueous solution with a pH of 3–5 and is available at a concentration of 50 mg·ml^{-1} (5%). Storage at 4 °C is essential as the NMBA spontaneously hydrolyses in warmer or more alkaline conditions.

Application, Administration and Dosage
Suxamethonium chloride is administered intravenously, producing short-acting, rapid muscle relaxation to facilitate rapid sequence inductions. It has occasionally been used as an intravenous infusion to facilitate muscle relaxation for extended periods.

Fig. 16.6 2D chemical structure of suxamethonium chloride

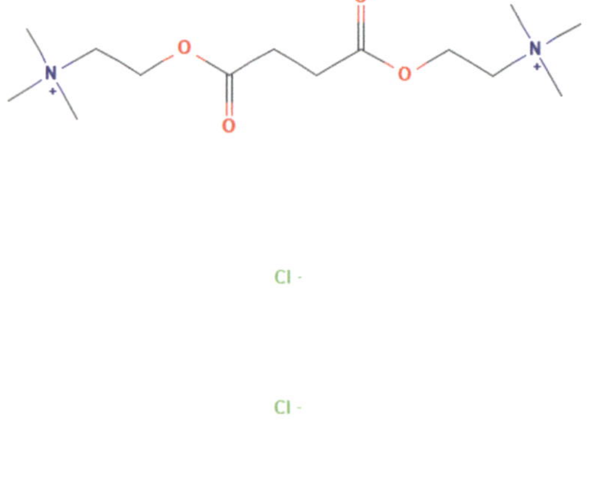

- Rapid muscle relaxation: 0.3–1.1 mg·kg^{-1} IV as bolus
- Continuous muscle relaxation: 2–15 mg·min^{-1} IV as an infusion of 0.1% solution

Mechanism of Action

Suxamethonium chloride is a nAChR agonist that mimics the effects of acetylcholine on the NMJ. However, unlike its endogenous counterpart, suxamethonium chloride is not metabolised by the acetylcholinesterases present at the NMJ. The drug's prolonged presence at the post-synaptic nAChRs leads to continuous membrane depolarisation, preventing repolarisation and rendering the motor end plates refractory to further action potentials. Muscle relaxation occurs after a brief period of stimulation and persists until the drug has adequately diffused away from the NMJ, allowing endogenous acetylcholine to out-compete it. The block is thus reversible and competitive.

The depolarising block following an initial bolus is called a phase I block. If additional boluses are given, the block is referred to as a phase II block, as multiple boluses of the drug exhibit characteristics similar to those of a non-depolarising NMBA (discussed later), although distinct from their mechanism of action.

Pharmacokinetics

The degree of protein binding is unclear as the drug is rapidly metabolised via hydrolysis by plasma-based cholinesterase and pseudo-cholinesterase. Only 20% of the active drug reaches the site of action. Furthermore, the extent and rate of hydrolysis influence the duration of action. The concentration gradient of the NMBA between NMJ and plasma determines the drug redistribution rate and, thus, the spontaneous reversal of the block facilitated by the competitive action of endogenous acetylcholine at the nAChR.

Metabolites comprise inactive choline and weakly active succinylmonocholine, which is further metabolised into inactive choline and succinic acid. Excretion is renal, and due to the rapid metabolism in the plasma, only approximately 10% of the unchanged drug is excreted in the urine. The drug is active within 30 secs of administration and lasts only a few minutes.

Pharmacodynamics

The pharmacodynamic effects of suxamethonium chloride are shown below (Table 16.5):

Special Points

Suxamethonium chloride can cause malignant hyperthermia, a potentially life-threatening complication of the drug that leads to uncontrolled calcium release from the sarcoplasmic reticulum (Pinyavat et al. 2024). This, in turn, causes intense muscle contraction, ATP consumption, and consequently, heat, lactate, and CO_2 release—the effects of this lead to cell breakdown, resulting in myoglobinuria and hyperkalaemia. The condition typically presents through an unexplained rise in end-tidal CO_2: the amount of CO_2 expired (and measured) at the end of each breath, tachycardia, core body temperature and muscle rigidity. Early diagnosis is key to the effective management with dantrolene, the treatment of choice.

Table 16.5 Pharmacodynamic profile of suxamethonium chloride

Organ system	Effect
Central nervous system	Rapid, short-acting neuromuscular blockade
Cardiovascular system	Sinus and nodal bradycardia secondary to mAChR stimulation with hypertension
Respiratory system	Paralysis of respiratory muscles
Miscellaneous	Muscle pain in young males with early ambulation Hyperkalaemia Raised IOP, intragastric pressure, lower oesophageal sphincter pressure

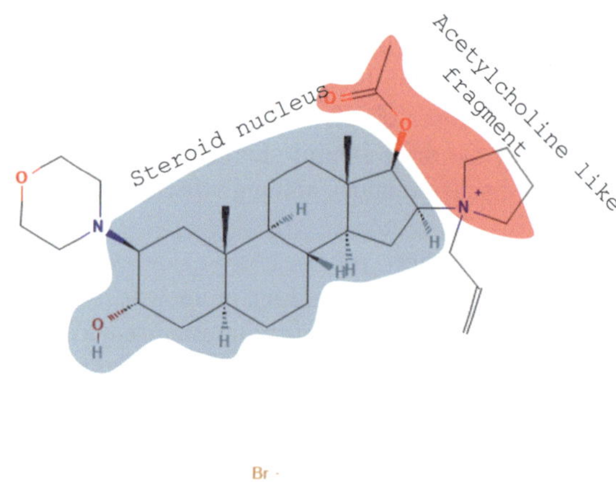

Fig. 16.7 2D chemical structure of rocuronium bromide

The NMBA can also cause histamine release and hyperkalemia, particularly in burns, trauma and renal failure patients, and is therefore contraindicated in these cases.

16.4.2 Rocuronium Bromide

Physical and Formulation

Rocuronium bromide is an aminosteroid consisting of an acetylcholine-type fragment and steroid nucleus (Fig. 16.7). This agent is one of the most commonly used non-depolarising NMBAs. The drug appears as a clear, colourless solution and is presented in a clear, rubber-topped glass vial that should be protected from light and refrigerated.

It is formulated as an aqueous solution and is available in a concentration of 10 mg·ml^{-1} (1%). Storage at 4 °C away from light is essential as the NMBA spontaneously hydrolyses in warmer or brighter conditions.

Application, Administration and Dosage
Rocuronium bromide is administered intravenously and produces moderately long and rapid muscle relaxation within 60–120 s, depending on the dosage.

- Rapid muscle relaxation: 0.5–1.0 mg·kg^{-1} IV as bolus

Mechanism of Action
Rocuronium bromide is a nAChR antagonist that inhibits the action of acetylcholine at the NMJ. The agent's binding to one of two possible sites at the post-synaptic nAChR prevents the binding of at least one of two endogenous acetylcholine molecules. When 75% of nAChRs are drug-bound, contractions fail, and muscle relaxation ensues. This process is competitive and reversible. The block can be overcome as the drug concentration decreases or while the concentration of endogenous acetylcholine increases within the NMJ.

Pharmacokinetics
Only approximately 70% of the agent is free and can reach the target site. The drug is also lipid insoluble owing to its polar nature. It, therefore, has a relatively small volume of distribution of 0.2–0.3 l·kg^{-1}, meaning it does not readily distribute to the lipid-rich tissues. With a relatively low potency compared to other non-depolarising NMBA, rocuronium bromide can be given at larger doses to achieve a faster onset of action.

Rocuronium bromide is mainly unchanged, with a small portion metabolised by deacetylation in the liver and excreted via bile and urine (Radkowski et al. 2024). The resultant clearance rate is 0.25 l·kg^{-1}·hr, and the terminal elimination time is 0.8 h.

Pharmacodynamics
The pharmacodynamic effects of rocuronium bromide are shown below (Table 16.6):

Special Points
Rocuronium bromide is an analogue of vecuronium bromide, another type of non-depolarising NMBA. Although structurally similar, rocuronium bromide has a significantly more 'Rapid Onset' (hence RO-curonium), making it suitable for rapid sequence inductions. It is currently the only licenced non-depolarising NMBA for rapid sequence inductions.

Table 16.6 Pharmacodynamic profile of rocuronium bromide

Organ system	Effect
Central nervous system	None
Cardiovascular system	Minimal increase in HR, CO and BP secondary to vagal block
Respiratory system	Paralysis of respiratory muscles
Miscellaneous	Rare histamine release

16.5 Inhalational Anaesthetic Agents

Inhalational anaesthetic agents with contemporary clinical applications include both anaesthetic gases and volatile agents. While the concept of a gas is straightforward, that of volatile agents can be challenging.

Volatile agents are liquids at room temperature and atmospheric pressure. They are defined by and named for their low boiling points (BP) and high saturated vapour pressures (SVP) relative to water.

The BP is the temperature at which the vapour pressure equals the external pressure surrounding the liquid, causing it to boil. This is similar to a melting point, reflecting intermolecular forces. A higher temperature is needed to evaporate and boil a liquid with stronger intermolecular forces. As a liquid continues to evaporate in a closed space, the pressure of its vapour increases to the point where the evaporated liquid starts to condense. The vapour pressure at which the condensation rate equals the evaporation rate is known as SVP (Fig. 16.8). Simplified, a liquid with a low BP and high SVP has molecules that lift off its surface readily and remain as vapour. These liquids are, hence, more volatile than water.

Nitrous oxide and sevoflurane are the most common clinically used anaesthetic gas and volatile agent, respectively. While nitrous oxide has specific clinical applications, its use is growing out of fashion. This chapter will, therefore, focus on the pharmacology of sevoflurane only.

The ideal volatile anaesthetic agent would have the following physical, pharmacokinetic and pharmacodynamic features. However, no single volatile agent possesses all of these qualities.

Physical Properties
- Liquid at room temperature
- Long shelf-life at room temperature
- Stable on light and heat exposure

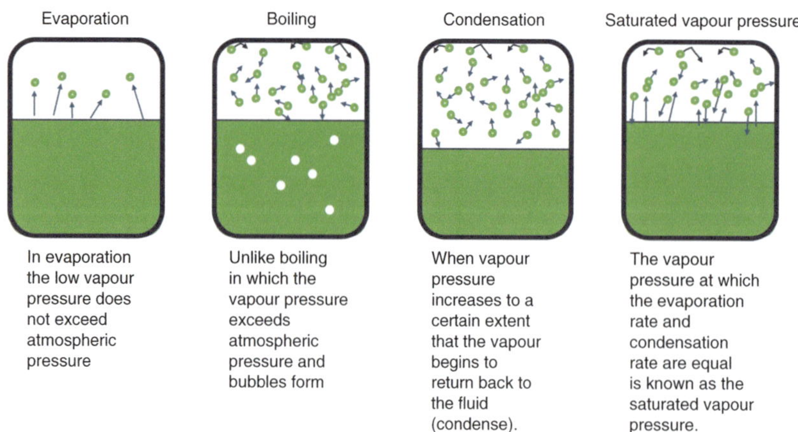

Fig. 16.8 Evaporation, boiling point, condensation and saturated vapour pressure

- Inert when in contact with metal, rubber and soda lime
- Non-flammable or explosive
- Preservative free
- Pleasant odour
- Minimal environmental impact
- Inexpensive

Pharmacokinetic Properties
- Low blood:gas partial coefficient (discussed later)
- High oil:gas partial coefficient and low MAC (discussed later)
- Non-metabolised

Pharmacodynamic Properties
- Specific CNS effect
- Non-toxic
- Non-epileptogenic
- Analgesic effect

16.5.1 Principles of Inhalational Anaesthetic Administration

Anaesthetic gases and volatile agents are delivered to the lung via inhalation (delivery phase) and enter the circulation via the pulmonary capillaries at the alveolar interface (pulmonary phase). From there, the agent gets distributed throughout the body (circulatory phase) via the pulmonary artery.

During delivery, the anaesthetic machine produces a fresh gas mixture that passes through the breathing system. A vaporiser introduces a volatile agent within this system, allowing it to be inhaled alongside the fresh gas mixture.

During the pulmonary phase, lung ventilation leads to a replacement of pre-existing gases in the alveoli. This results in the diffusion of fresh gases and volatile agents across the alveolar membrane. Here, the inspired concentration of the volatile agent directly affects the tension or partial pressure of the anaesthetic in the blood.

The amount of volatile agent needed in the blood and alveolar gas to reach an equilibrium in volume and partial pressure within the two phases is denoted as the blood:gas partial coefficient ratio. This ratio describes the solubility of a volatile agent in blood and determines how readily an agent distributes to the brain and other tissues. Simplified, the blood:gas partial coefficient is comparable to the blood and lipid solubility of intravenous agents. Hence, a low blood:gas partial coefficient indicates that a volatile agent has low blood solubility, and even small amounts will rapidly equilibrate and distribute to the brain during the circulatory phase.

16.5.2 Minimum Alveolar Concentration

Minimum alveolar concentration is a measure of inhalational anaesthetic agents reflecting potency (Aranake et al. 2013). It is defined as the minimum alveolar concentration of an anaesthetic agent at one atmospheric pressure needed to produce immobility in 50% of people subjected to a noxious stimulus, typically a surgical skin incision. Similar to the blood:gas partial coefficient, the oil:gas partial coefficient describes the solubility of the volatile agent in lipid-rich substances. It is a measure of lipid solubility and hence highly related to potency, given that target tissue lies beyond the BBB. Thus, a volatile agent with a high oil:gas partial coefficient requires a relatively low MAC to achieve the same anaesthetic effect as a volatile agent with a low oil:gas partial coefficient and high MAC.

It is important to remember that the key indicator for volatile agents is partial pressure, not concentration. However, volatile agents' concentration and partial pressure are virtually identical at atmospheric pressure when measured in kPa. MAC, therefore, remains an accurate measure of potency as long as atmospheric pressure remains unchanged.

16.5.3 Sevoflurane

Physical and Formulation

Sevoflurane is a polyfluorinated isopropyl methyl ether or simply a halogenated ether. The latter refers to a type of organic compound with an element from group 17 on the periodic table, in this case, fluoride. The wet formulation of the drug appears as a clear, colourless solution with a pleasant odour. It is presented in a yellow, colour-coded, brown glass bottle with a geometric keyed filling system collar that can be stored in light at room temperature. The dry formulation of the drug appears as a powder and is presented and stored differently.

The wet formulation is preservative-free and prepared with 300 parts per million (ppm) of water to prevent the formation of toxic hydrofluoric acid during storage. This excipient is necessary as hydrofluoric acid and other Lewis acids can corrode glass. Preparing an improperly stored, manufactured or counterfeit drug preparation could damage the vapouriser in the anaesthetic machine and must not be administered as it could cause adverse reactions and an unpredictable clinical effect.

Application, Administration and Dosage

Sevoflurane is the most commonly used inhalational anaesthetic agent and is mainly utilised for the maintenance of anaesthesia. Induction of anaesthesia can be achieved but is typically slower than with intravenous agents. The administration of propofol is via the intravenous route only. Dosages depend on the intended use:

- Maintenance of anaesthesia: MAC 1.8–2.0

Mechanism of Action

The exact mechanism of action of sevoflurane has yet to be determined, but the agent likely targets multiple CNS ligand-gated ion channels, potentiating inhibitory $GABA_A$ and glycine receptors while inhibiting excitatory glutamate, acetylcholine, and serotonin receptors (Jabaudon et al. 2022).

Pharmacokinetics

The structure of this halogenated ether gives a lower blood:gas and oil:gas partial coefficient compared to other volatile agents. These properties give the drug a relatively faster onset and offset of anaesthesia but higher MAC given the relatively low oil:gas partial coefficient and thus potency.

Only approximately 5% of sevoflurane is metabolised via the hepatic P450 cytochrome complex. This process generates an inactive yet toxic, inorganic fluoride ion, which is quickly conjugated before it causes liver damage. However, it can reach concentrations high enough to cause kidney damage before this. The majority of sevoflurane is eliminated as an unchanged drug via the lung's ventilation. Depending on the breathing system, exhaled gases, including unchanged sevoflurane, are released directly into the surrounding space or safely vented into the atmosphere outside the hospital via a gas scavenging system. The amount of unscavanged sevoflurane in a room is maintained below 20 ppm through frequent air exchanges to prevent harm from an accumulation of the gas in the air (Table 16.7).

Pharmacodynamics

The pharmacodynamic effects of sevoflurane are shown below (Table 16.8):

Key Points

CO2 absorbers such as soda lime are commonly used in circle breathing systems and help remove exhaled CO2 from the gas mixture that the patient will inhale during the next breath. The soda lime, however, also absorbs and degrades sevoflurane within the breathing system. The type of breakdown products produced is temperature dependent and includes sevoflurane degradation compounds A–E. All five products are generated at higher temperatures, while only compound A and a small proportion of compound B are produced at lower temperatures, as seen in clinical practice. While all five compounds are toxic and can cause hepatic, renal and brain damage, the levels observed in reality are substantially lower than the toxic threshold secondary to a special zeolite-coated soda lime preparation.

Table 16.7 Pharmacokinetic profile of sevoflurane

Metric	Value
MW	200 Da
BP	58.6 °C
SVP	21.3 kPa
Blood: Gas partial coefficient	0.69
Oil: Gas partial coefficient	53
MAC $\approx$ MAP at 1 atm	1.8–2.0% $\approx$ 1–8–2.0 kPa

Table 16.8 Pharmacodynamic profile of sevoflurane

Organ system	Effect
Central nervous system	Rapid anaesthesia No analgesia None epileptogenic
Cardiovascular system	Reduced HR, SVP and BP with stable CO
Respiratory system	Dose-dependent respiratory depression Bronchodilation
Miscellaneous	Potentiated muscle relaxation Uterine relaxation

Sevoflurane can also cause malignant hyperthermia and is, therefore, an absolute contraindication if previously recorded.

Summary

Anaesthetics is a highly specialised branch of clinical practice which utilises an isolated set of medications not typically found in other areas of care. This results in poor exposure or understanding of these medications during typical nurse training. However, to maintain patient safety, an orchestrated effort between the anaesthetist, nurse and if relevant operation department practitioner is important. This chapter provides theoretical underpinnings to the use of common medications used in anaesthetics. This includes intravenous anaesthetic agents, neuromuscular blocking agents and inhalation anaesthetic gases and volatiles. Structurally presented practical information regarding these medications will help the reader understand the choice of medication selection together with general and specific aspects related to drug safety. Together this information will help inform the reader towards safer medication management in clinical areas that utilise anaesthesia.

Multiple Choice Questions

1. The general principles of anaesthesia can be categories into the four A's which are
   Select the correct list
   (a) Analgesia, Ageusia, Amnesia Awareness (lack of)
   (b) Anoxia, Ageusia, Amnesia, Analgesia
   (c) Analgesia, Amnesia, Awareness (lack of), Akinesia.
   (d) Analgesia, Akinesia, Awareness (lack of), Anoxia.

2. In anaesthetics the abbreviation NMBA stands for
   (a) Neuromyoclonic blocking agent
   (b) Neuromuscular blocking agent
   (c) Neuromyalgia blocking agent

   (d) Neuromental blocking agent
3. Which area of the brain is targeted by general anaesthetics
   (a) Corpus callosum
   (b) Blood-brain barrier
   (c) Nucleus Tractus Solitarius
   (d) Thalamus
4. Which drug characteristic is a significant determinant of anaesthetic activity
   (a) Drug size
   (b) Drug water solubility
   (c) Drug fat solubility
   (d) Drug acidity
5. Propofol may be catagorised as
   (a) A chloride ion channel agonist
   (b) A chloride ion channel antagonist
   (c) A glutamine receptor antagonist
   (d) A glutamine receptor agonist
6. Suxamthonium mimics the effect of acetylcholine at the neuromuscular junction to inhibit muscle contraction. It is characterised as a
   (a) Non-depolarising NMBA
   (b) Depolarising NMBA
   (c) Cholinergic receptor antagonist
   (d) Cholinesterase inhibitor.
7. At which percentage of nicotinic acetylcholine receptors (nAChRs) inhibition do you start to see muscle relaxation
   (a) 25%
   (b) 50%
   (c) 75%
   (d) 100%
8. In relation to inhalation anaesthetic gases movement of the agent through the pulmonary artery is known as the
   (a) Pulmonary phase
   (b) Circulatory phase
   (c) Respiratory phase
   (d) Delivery phase
9. Minimum alveolar concentration is a measure of inhalational anaesthetic agents reflecting potency. It is defined as the minimum alveolar concentration of an anaesthetic agent at one atmospheric pressure needed to produce immobility in ________of people subjected to a noxious stimulus, typically a surgical skin incision.
   Fill in the blank from the options below
   (a) 25%
   (b) 50%
   (c) 75%
   (d) 100%

10. The amount of unscavanged sevoflurane in a room is maintained below _____ ppm through frequent air exchanges to prevent harm from an accumulation of the gas in the air.

Fill in the blank from the options below

(a) 5%
(b) 10%
(c) 15%
(d) 20%

Answers

1. (c)
2. (b)
3. (d)
4. (c)
5. (a)
6. (b)
7. (c)
8. (b)
9. (b)
10. (d)

References

Aranake A, Mashour GA, Avidan MS (2013) Minimum alveolar concentration: ongoing relevance and clinical utility. Anaesthesia 68(5):512–522. https://doi.org/10.1111/anae.12168

Hempel V (1994) 60 Jahre Thiopental. AINS - Anästhesiologie · Intensivmedizin · Notfallmedizin · Schmerztherapie 29(07):400–407. https://doi.org/10.1055/s-2007-996770

Hemphill S, McMenamin L, Bellamy MC, Hopkins PM (2019) Propofol infusion syndrome: a structured literature review and analysis of published case reports. Br J Anaesth 122(4):448–459. https://doi.org/10.1016/j.bja.2018.12.025

Jabaudon M, Zhai R, Blondonnet R, Bonda WLM (2022) Inhaled sedation in the intensive care unit. Anaesth Crit Care Pain Med 41(5):101133. https://doi.org/10.1016/j.accpm.2022.101133

Kopp Lugli A, Yost CS, Kindler CH (2009) Anaesthetic mechanisms: update on the challenge of unravelling the mystery of anaesthesia. Eur J Anaesthesiol 26(10):807–820. https://doi.org/10.1097/EJA.0b013e32832d6b0f

Pinyavat T, Riazi S, Deng J, Slessarev M, Cuthbertson BH, Ibarra Moreno CA, Jerath A (2024) Malignant hyperthermia. Crit Care Med 52(12):1934–1940. https://doi.org/10.1097/CCM.0000000000006401

Radkowski P, Krupiniewicz KJ, Suchcicki M, Machoń NJ, Cappello S, Szewczyk M, Wolska JM, Stompór T (2024) Navigating Anesthesia: muscle relaxants and reversal agents in patients with renal impairment. Med Sci Monit 30. https://doi.org/10.12659/MSM.945141

Sahinovic MM, Struys MMRF, Absalom AR (2018) Clinical pharmacokinetics and pharmacodynamics of Propofol. Clin Pharmacokinet 57(12):1539–1558. https://doi.org/10.1007/s40262-018-0672-3

Stäuble CG, Blobner M (2020) The future of neuromuscular blocking agents. Curr Opin Anaesthesiol 33(4):490–498. https://doi.org/10.1097/ACO.0000000000000891

Further Reading

Appiah-Ankam J, Hunter JM (2004) Pharmacology of neuromuscular blocking drugs. Contin Educ Anaesth Crit Care Pain 4(1):2–7. https://doi.org/10.1093/bjaceaccp/mkh002

Clayton T, Ode K (2023) Mechanisms of action of general anaesthetic drugs. Anaesth Intens Care Med 24(4):235–237. https://doi.org/10.1016/j.mpaic.2022.12.031

Khan KS, Hayes I, Buggy DJ (2014a) Pharmacology of anaesthetic agents I: intravenous anaesthetic agents. Continuing Education in Anaesthesia, Critical Care and Pain 14(3):100–105. https://doi.org/10.1093/bjaceaccp/mkt039

Khan KS, Hayes I, Buggy DJ (2014b) Pharmacology of anaesthetic agents II: inhalation anaesthetic agents. Contin Educ Anaesth Crit Care Pain 14(3):106–111. https://doi.org/10.1093/bjaceaccp/mkt038

Lemos CS, Poveda VB (2022) Role of perioperative nursing in anesthesia: a national overview. Rev Esc Enferm USP 56:e20210465. https://doi.org/10.1590/1980-220x-reeusp-2021-0465

Lin T, Smith T, Pinnock CA, Mowatt C (2017) Fundamentals of anaesthesia, 4th edn. Cambridge University Press

Miller KW (2002) The nature of sites of general anaesthetic action. Br J Anaesth 89(1):17–31. https://doi.org/10.1093/bja/aef167

Peck TE, Hill SA (2014) Pharmacology for anaesthesia and intensive care, 4th edn. Cambridge University Press

Ray WT, Desai SP (2016) The history of the nurse anesthesia profession. J Clin Anesth 30:51–58. https://doi.org/10.1016/j.jclinane.2015.11.005

Urban BW, Bleckwenn M (2002) Concepts and correlations relevant to general anaesthesia. Br J Anaesth 89(1):3–16. https://doi.org/10.1093/bja/aef164

Weir CJ (2006) The molecular mechanisms of general anaesthesia: dissecting the GABAA receptor. Contin Educ Anaesth Crit Care Pain 6(2):49–53. https://doi.org/10.1093/bjaceaccp/mki068

The Role of the Nurse and Pharmacology in Practice

17

Tiago Horta Reis Da Silva

Learning Outcomes

At the end of this chapter, you will be able to:

- Appreciate the critical role played by nurses in the management of polypharmacy, performing medication reconciliation, and their involvement in deprescribing programmes.
- Define the professional duty to guarantee psychological safety while also supporting whistleblowers, and explores how assertive communication, along with decision-making skills, benefits patient outcomes.
- Understand the evolving scope of practice for Advanced Clinical Practitioners (ACPs), including their engagement with NICE guidelines, antimicrobial stewardship, and lifelong learning.

17.1 Introduction

Within the clinical setting, the application of pharmacological knowledge to nursing practice is integral to the safe and effective administration of medication. This area of practice necessitates a solid comprehension of pharmacokinetics (the process by which drugs are absorbed, distributed, metabolised, and eliminated) and pharmacodynamics (the process by which drugs affect biological systems) (Reis da Silva 2024a). Nurses must use this knowledge to ensure patient safety and therapeutic effectiveness, as is mandated by the Nursing and Midwifery Council (NMC) Code, with its focus on medication management responsibility and commitment to positive patient outcome (NMC 2018; Nibbelink and Brewer 2018; Liu et al. 2023).

T. H. R. Da Silva (✉)
King's College London, London, UK
e-mail: tiago.horta_reis_da_silva@kcl.ac.uk

E. Khan, P. Hood (eds.), *Understanding Pharmacology in Nursing Practice*,
https://doi.org/10.1007/978-3-032-03964-4_17

With the increasing sophistication of pharmacological therapies, nurses' practice is also becoming more intense, and they require a thorough understanding of pharmacological fundamentals to guide their practice to the greatest extent (Xu et al. 2023; Gao et al. 2023).

Traditionally, a nurse's role with medication management has been confined to the administration of prescribed drugs with little examination of their impact or drug interaction potential (Reis da Silva 2025a). That model no longer applies in today's healthcare, in which collaborative frameworks of healthcare provision place nurses with the scope to make more informed decisions regarding drug management. Practice for nurses today includes contributing to medication reviews, to assess both therapeutic effectiveness and safety prospectively (Taasen et al. 2024; Zainal et al. 2023). Nurses must utilise rigorous critical thinking to individualise medication therapies according to patient need, to assure best therapeutic implications (Reis da Silva 2025b; Oh et al. 2022; Baysal et al. 2018).

Additionally, the wider range of nursing practice anticipates that nurses should achieve competences beyond the administration of medication. Nurses are now anticipated to communicate with patients about their medication effectively, for example, promoting medication adherence and combining pharmacotherapy with lifestyle changes to advance treatment outcomes (Gürsoy et al. 2023; Hoek et al. 2020). Interprofessional practices in multidisciplinary teams also add to the provision of patient-centred care (Reis da Silva 2024b). As nurses engage in collaborative decision-making routines, they can serve as essential bridges between healthcare professionals and patients with direct implications for therapeutic care and the enforcement of the ethical standards outlined in the NMC Code (2018). Undertaking this approach, nurses can substantially minimise healthcare disparities and facilitate patient involvement (Şahin and Başak 2022; Savcı et al. 2021).

The legal and professional frameworks guiding nursing practice also significantly shape nurses' involvement in medication management (Reis da Silva 2024a). The NMC Code requires ongoing professional learning and education in pharmacology, with a call for nurses to stay updated on developments in drug therapies and their application in clinical practice (NMC 2018; Silva et al. 2022). This preparatory measure is needed, especially in light of the increasing emphasis on individualised medicine, which is often based upon genetic foundations that can alter patient responses to medications (Tume et al. 2017; Novalia et al. 2022). For example, pharmacogenomic research has shown how genetic polymorphisms can influence the pharmacokinetics and pharmacodynamics of many medications, which consequently will increasingly require that nurses implement such information in clinical practice (Rababa et al. 2022).

Understanding pharmacokinetics and pharmacodynamics in nursing practice cannot be overstated since these principles directly impact therapeutic effects (Reis da Silva 2024a). Nurses' consideration of a patient's age, gender, and comorbid illness in relation to drug absorption and metabolism, once more demonstrates the complexity of drug therapy (Batran et al. 2022; Abdelhadi et al. 2020). With therapeutic drug monitoring (TDM), nurses can monitor patient responses, titrating treatment according to prescribed parameters, especially for vulnerable populations such as the older person and people with long-term conditions (Anton et al. 2021; Yun et al. 2024). Such vigilant practice reduces the risk of adverse reactions and promotes safe and efficacious pharmacologic treatments for patients (Reis da Silva 2024c).

Ethical consequences of medication management should be considered, especially where polypharmacy is a concern, which exposes patients to excessive risks of adverse reactions (Reis da Silva 2025c). It has been confirmed that effective medication management may reduce these risks by improving communication among healthcare professionals and patients (Alnjadat et al. 2024; Sari et al. 2018). Recognising nurses as central agents, not only with the administration of medication but also with the medication decision-making process, highlights the need for a more integrated and knowledgeable approach to healthcare delivery (Park et al. 2022).

Additionally, ongoing education and research processes for nurses highlight the importance of staying abreast of current pharmacological practice and knowledge. Current research highlights that ongoing pharmacology training enables nurses to work effectively with contemporary medication regimens and helps to enhance patient care (Cook 2024; Hackman et al. 2024). As the therapeutic landscape continues to change, new modalities of therapy like monoclonal antibodies and biologics require a continuous process of education in their pharmacokinetic and pharmacodynamic profiles (Hidayat et al. 2021; Turfi and Al-Jubouri 2022).

The incorporation of informatics and technology into drug management is established in nursing practice (Reis da Silva 2025d). The ability to use electronic health records (EHRs) and clinical decision-support systems enhances the safety and effectiveness of drug administration by providing rich patient information that informs clinical decisions (Reis da Silva 2025d; Gassas et al. 2024; Aliakbari et al. 2020).

Advanced pharmacokinetic modelling software enables simulations that forecast drug response in heterogeneous populations, enabling more personalised treatment regimens to be created (Reis da Silva 2025e; Daungsupawong and Wiwanitkit 2024). In the future, nurses may have a role in interpreting and applying information from these systems, keeping medication management in line with the latest best practice guidelines.

17.2 Nurses and Prescription Safety

A nurse's function in questioning the safety of prescriptions is high on the agenda within the contemporary complex healthcare environment (Reis da Silva 2025c). Medication error is one of the primary reasons for adverse patient outcomes, making it necessary for nurses to be vigilant with the medication process (Reis da Silva 2025e). Nurses must be aware and competent in active medication management, such as identifying potential drug–drug interactions and contraindications, identifying adverse drug reactions (ADRs), and if necessary, questioning inappropriate prescribing (O'Donovan and McAuliffe 2020).

To undertake these responsibilities, nurses need extensive knowledge of pharmacological principles. This involves knowledge of mechanisms of action, pharmacokinetics (absorption, distribution, metabolism, and excretion), and legal and ethical considerations of drug administration (Reis da Silva 2024a). Nurses also need clinical decision-making skills, which involves the assessment of drug options in relation to patient-specific considerations and therapeutic goals. Nurses also need communication skills, which enable them to communicate effectively about medications with patients and healthcare providers (Reis da Silva 2024d). These skills are not only necessary in safeguarding patient health but also in ensuring that nursing practice is in accordance with regulatory requirements (Reis da Silva 2024c; Schwappach and Richard 2018; Alingh et al. 2018).

The 'speaking up' for safety theme has gained momentum in healthcare organisations, and it supports an open and accountable culture among clinicians (Hunt et al. 2021). The model is applicable in how it supports a culture where practitioners are not afraid to report unsafe practice and medication errors without fear of retribution. Whistleblower protection policies are increasingly implemented to safeguard nurses who 'speak up' about unsafe medication practice, hence improving the quality of patient care (Hunt et al. 2021; Mawuena and Mannion 2022).

## 17.3	'Prescriber Ready' Upon Completion of Registration Programme

Both educational and regulatory authorities recognise the need to prepare nursing graduates with the competence to perform these roles. Newly registered nurses need to be competent in medication management at the time of completion of registration courses, although they are not independent prescribers (Lainidi et al. 2023). This foundation knowledge is needed to enable safe delegation, administration, and evaluation of pharmacotherapy, and so educational curricula need to include pharmacological knowledge and patient safety as core components (Ahn and Kim 2024; Lainidi et al. 2023). Nurses' willingness to 'speak up' regarding patient safety is a direct function of the safety culture of their organisations. A psychological safety culture encourages nurses to 'speak up', increasing the likelihood of the detection and prevention of medication errors (Reis da Silva 2025f). Evidence indicates that in organisations with such a culture, healthcare professionals are more likely to use assertive communication regarding safety concerns and challenge inappropriately prescribed medicines (Bell et al. 2018; Passariello and Tarrant 2024).

Consideration must be given to possible barriers that may prevent 'speaking up' about patient safety. Hierarchical structures, conflict avoidance, and lack of support are some of the reasons why nurses might be discouraged from 'speaking up' (Reis da Silva 2025f). Research has established that the reinforcement of communication channels and the provision of professional training can easily reduce such barriers, paving the way for the notion that effective 'speaking up' behaviour is an imperative to ensure patient safety (Li et al. 2024; Rauwolf and Jones 2019). Barriers to effective communication also resonate with the necessity for formal programmes that allow nurses to question and critically evaluate prescriptions. Training programmes to explore team dynamics, assertive communication, and empowerment can possibly create a safety and awareness culture in healthcare organisations (Reis da Silva 2025f). The emphasis on active involvement not only improves patient outcomes but also job satisfaction and professional development among nurses (Pattni et al. 2019; Lee et al. 2023).

The connection between patient safety programmes and psychological safety within the healthcare team cannot be overstated. Research indicates that a culture of safety where healthcare workers can 'speak up' without fear of retribution is central to enhancing patient outcomes. Developing a model that welcomes feedback and fosters trust among teams can avoid medication errors and enhance the quality of care (Lyndon et al. 2017; Martínez et al. 2017). As nurses transition into these positions, they must be aware of the ethical component of their practice. Nurses are patient advocates, and this means questioning unjustified or possibly erroneous orders that can harm patients (Landgren et al. 2016). Nursing programmes must include ethical decision-making in clinical practice scenarios to equip graduates to navigate challenging moral ground when questioning medical decisions (Padash et al. 2023; Landgren et al. 2016).

To implement these complex changes effectively, continuous education, professional development, and mentoring sessions are essential (Fitzpatrick et al. 2023). These should be directed towards increasing nurses' skill for careful review of prescriptions and encouraging safe medication practices. Newly registered nurses may gain from practising with experienced practitioners and participating in interprofessional teams to build confidence and competence in voicing concerns when necessary (Ambanwala 2022; Lawson et al. 2017).

Institutional support for programmes aimed at creating a culture of concern is of crucial importance. Organisations need to prioritise patient safety through protective actions that allow nurses to raise concerns without fear of reprisals (Hunt et al. 2021). Various safety programmes that support open communication and institute continuous feedback mechanisms are important in improving practice environments and ensuring better outcomes in patient care, as described in academic literature (Schwappach and Niederhauser 2019). Involvement of nurses in quality and research activities may also encourage their critical evaluation of medication safety. Providing access to updated evidence and pharmacological practice-related guidelines empowers nurses to make informed decisions that support optimal practices and standards, ensuring patient safety (Reis da Silva 2025a). These collective actions reinforce nurses' professional accountability in medication administration and surveillance, leading to beneficial patient outcomes (Nacioglu 2016).

Since the complexity of nursing duties continues to escalate, it is important that the educational processes enabling these developments are recognised and addressed. Content-rich educational platforms that emphasise greater comprehension of pharmacology, ethical awareness, and patient safety skills are core to the development of competent nursing professionals (Reis da Silva 2024d; Friary et al. 2024; Jeong and Kim 2023). Finally, the value placed on nurses in making definitive judgments on medication safety is of utmost importance. To expand this role requires: a strong educational foundation, a workplace environment that encourages voicing concerns, and dedication to establishing a culture of safety in healthcare organisations (Reis da Silva 2024d). Through advancing their pharmacological knowledge and enhancing patient safety, nurses can significantly minimise the danger of medication errors and improve the quality of care given to inpatient and outpatient groups in diverse settings (Lee et al. 2022; Tear et al. 2020).

17.4 The Role of the Advanced Nursing Practitioner Prescriber

The relevance of Advanced Nursing Practitioners (ANPs) in relation to secure prescribing practices becomes increasingly critical in today's healthcare environments, mainly driven by a heightened demand for skilled medication management (Dumbreck et al. 2015). Through the evolutionary process of healthcare toward greater complexity, the demand for advanced practice professionals, embodied by the ANPs, who bring together clinical practice and prescribing responsibilities, grows ever greater. ANPs operate amid the fields of nursing, having the skills needed to ensure safe and effective prescribing, hence playing a significant role in outcomes in acute healthcare settings (Dumbreck et al. 2015).

To maintain the integrity of prescribing, Advanced Nursing Practitioners can opt to thoroughly and comprehensively train in independent and supplementary prescribing module. Underpinning their professional practice, this initial training enables them to practice in defined parameters and follow national prescribing principles, including those set by the National Institute for Health and Care Excellence [NICE] (2018). NICE guidelines (2018) are important reference guides to ensuring the effectiveness and safety of medications in diverse settings of practice (National Guideline Centre 2018; Yarnall et al. 2017).

A core duty of the Advanced Nursing Practitioner (ANP) prescriber is conducting proper assessment of the patient before any pharmacologic treatments are instituted. These assessments allow the ANP to customise treatment modalities to meet the unique needs of individual patients. Before dispensing any pharmaceutical agents, an ANP considers the medical history of the patient, their current medication intake, and potential contraindications (Mensah et al. 2019). These assessments are essential in identifying potential drug interactions and ensuring that therapy follows best practices and evidence-based practice recommendations. Such a proactive approach not only assists in medication errors prevention but also develops co-operative care, enhancing healthcare professionals' and patients' trust (McCann et al. 2023).

The assessment of patient therapeutic response after the administration of pharmacological interventions forms a critical aspect of safe pharmaceutical practice. ANPs prescribers have a core responsibility in monitoring the response of the patient to pharmacotherapy and adapting dosing or interventions appropriately. Monitoring continuously is important in ensuring optimal therapeutic outcomes while avoiding medication-associated adverse reactions, which remain a foremost risk to patient safety (Maramba et al. 2024). Secondly, the participation of ANPs prescriber also plays a critical role in the domain of antimicrobial stewardship, especially in tackling the growing global problem of antibiotic resistance (O'Flaherty and Ali 2024). Prescribing of antimicrobial agents requires a prudent approach, thus necessitating that ANPs prescribers are well-versed in detailed aspects of indications for antibiotic therapy, regimen of treatments, and alternative disease management options (Luo et al. 2023). Implementation of antimicrobial stewardship through judicious prescription of antimicrobial agents not only safeguards individual patients from inappropriate pharmacotherapy but also greatly enhances public health programmes in addressing antibiotic resistance (O'Flaherty and Ali 2024).

The need for lifelong professional development is essential in the sphere of safe prescribing practise. ANPs prescribers need to regularly assess their capabilities and engage in educational programs to stay up-to-date with developments in pharmacology and evidence-based clinical procedures (Vuuren et al. 2023). Emphasis on lifelong learning is important in ensuring that they can provide well-informed therapeutic options and make safe medication-related decisions, thereby enhancing the outcomes of patient care. Training institutions need to organise regular programmes involving refresher courses and competency reviews specific to ANPs prescribers (Hajj et al. 2020). Several studies identify the critical need for extensive education and the encouragement of a favourable environment friendly to the practice of ANPs prescribers. Efficacy in collaboration between professionals enhances the importance of collaboration among nurse prescribers as well as the overall multidisciplinary health team (McCann et al. 2023). An interprofessional strategy leads to a decrease in medication errors and improved outcomes of the patient, thus affirming the important role of the ACP in the sphere of medication management (Patel et al. 2019).

In addition, there is strong evidence that suggests that poorly developed support systems and insufficient training may impede the successful application of care plans in settings where medications are managed. As a result, healthcare institutions need to continuously reinforce support and training programmes for ANP prescribers in a way that ensures these professionals gain the necessary resources and knowledge needed to discharge their duties efficiently (Wang et al. 2022). Apart from basic clinical skills, the study of legal and ethical aspects is increasingly allocating importance to the tasks and duties related to advanced care plans in pharmaceutical management. It is the responsibility of an advanced care practitioner to navigate complex healthcare laws and ethical principles in relation to pharmaceutical treatments (Chen et al. 2022; Reis da Silva 2025c). The Royal Pharmaceutical Society lays clear standards identifying the skills and expectations of non-medical prescribing positions, directing advanced care practitioners prescribers to ensure consistent practice (Mortensen et al. 2022; Royal Pharmaceutical Society 2022).

17.5   Monitoring Polypharmacy in Comorbidities and Medication Review: Deprescribing

The problem of polypharmacy, which involves the simultaneous use of various pharmacologic agents, represents a problem of considerable importance in the healthcare system, especially among those with long-term health conditions and among individuals of various comorbidities (Reis da Silva 2025d). Even though there are specific clinical contexts in which polypharmacy is needed, it is important to explore the associated risks (Reis da Silva 2024a). These risks include the potential for harmful drug–drug interactions that can lead to adverse reactions, reduced maintenance of treatment regimens due to the complexity of polypharmacy, and diminished functional capacity in susceptible populations, including older persons' communities (Naughton and Hayes 2016; Mardani et al. 2020). Since nurses are often the first point of contact in healthcare settings, their involvement in coordinating polypharmacy, supporting integrated medication assessment, and orchestrating deprescribing initiatives is indispensable in ensuring the protection of the health of patients (Reis da Silva 2024d).

Efficacious management of polypharmacy requires a critical investment in the regular reconciliation of medications to ensure that all related records of medications are accurately recorded and up-to-date. Such a practice is critical as it allows for the identification of medications that are likely to be in excess or duplicative in nature, in turn enhancing the risk of adverse reactions (Reis da Silva 2024c). Mardani et al. (2020) point to the critical role of nurses in the reconciliation of medications in their study, noting that nurses engage in collaboration with pharmacists and physicians in the tracking of medication changes from admission to discharge in the inpatient environment. Through teamwork, nurses are in a position to identify discrepancies and ensure continuity of care, in turn ensuring the safety of the patient. Further, using concrete criteria, including the STOPP/START tool, is a systematic approach to the identification of inappropriate medications among the older population. The combination of the Screening Tool of Older Person's potentially inappropriate Prescriptions (STOPP) and the Screening Tool to Alert doctors to Right Treatment (START) equips the clinician with the ability to assess pharmacologic management using evidence-based guidelines, in turn confirming appropriateness of medication among patients presenting with polypharmacy (Aly and Elsayed 2022). Finally, application of support systems in clinical environments in nursing practice shows a potential for reducing the occurrence of drug-related complications (Aly and Elsayed 2022).

Involvement of nurses in the shared decision-making model is critical to the successful management of polypharmacy. It is critical that nurses talk to patients in terms of the rationale for each medication and how it may affect their overall health and well-being (Aly and Elsayed 2022). Not only does this empower the patient, but it also enhances medication adherence through their inclusion with the individualised care plan. Empirical evidence suggests that when patients acknowledge that they are participants in the medication decision-making process, the likelihood of following their medication regimen and their satisfaction with care increases (Cheng et al. 2023; Zoromski and Frazier 2023). It is the responsibility of nurses to work together with prescribing healthcare professionals and pharmacists to ensure that pharmacotherapy is managed optimally (Reis da Silva 2024d). Through this cooperative strategy, health professionals can collectively scrutinise the need for medications, discontinue those that are redundant, and safely stop them when appropriate. As noted by Rohde and Domm (2017), active nurse involvement in medication management is instrumental in the prevention of medication errors, with prescriptions drawn in accordance with established standards of best practice.

Deprescribing strategies are very important steps that seek to reduce the risks of medication use. Unlike the absolute withdrawal of medication intake, deprescribing utilises a systematic and individualised approach that weighs the benefits and shortcomings of the cessation of a specific medication based on the individual's preferences and level of well-being (Reis da Silva 2025c). Empirical evidence suggests that engaging patients in the deprescribing process is often associated with better health outcomes and the reduction of adverse reactions, especially among older people, who are often at higher risk of the adverse reactions of polypharmacy (Naughton and Hayes 2016; Crowe 2020; Reis da Silva 2025c). To ensure the maximisation of the efficacy of deprescribing strategies, it is critical that nursing staff undergo continuous professional upgrading in medication management skills. In addition, nurses should be appropriately equipped with extensive knowledge of current best practice standards, together with knowledge of the pharmacokinetics and pharmacodynamics of medications and the implications of polypharmacy (Reis da Silva 2024a). Equipped with such extensive knowledge, nurses are in a better position to identify scenarios where polypharmacy is unjustifiable and initiate medication reviews that lead to the deprescribing pathway (Vaismoradi et al. 2024).

In clinical settings, there exist several barriers that undermine the efficient management and discontinuation of medication in patients presenting with polypharmacy and multi-morbidity (Wouters et al. 2019). Some of the identified barriers are system-related in nature, including lack of allocation of adequate clinic appointment time, poor communication among the interdisciplinary teams, and differences in knowledge of deprescribing principles among prescribers (Wouters et al. 2019; Reis da Silva 2024d). Qualitative studies have highlighted the importance of a culture that empowers nurses to challenge current medication regimens and argue in favour of their patients' viewpoints (Wouters et al. 2019). In addition, support for recommendations by interprofessional professional organisation guidelines was found to boost medication management practices greatly, including efforts aimed at deprescribing (Reis da Silva 2025c). Through collaborative working alongside pharmacists and other professionals, nurses can play a key role in carrying out comprehensive medication reviews, which in turn encourages extensive medication management among patients presenting with polypharmacy (Shahzeydi et al. 2024; Halvorsen et al. 2019). Interprofessional working leads to better outcomes in addition to opening the gateway to professional growth and teamwork-based care in healthcare settings (Reis da Silva 2025d).

Summary
The study of pharmacology is critical to providing care that is safe, effective, and focused on the patient. As nurses take on greater responsibilities in medication management, their ability to critically review prescriptions, engage in pharmacological decision-making, and contribute to ensuring safe prescribing becomes progressively important. Increased advanced clinical practitioners' involvement underscores the need for advanced prescribing skills. As polypharmacy is a significant challenge, it

is crucial that medication reviews and deprescribing programmes are supported by nurses in a way that maximises therapeutic effects. Through a lifelong learning approach, nurses can remain leaders in best practice in pharmacology, ultimately enhancing patient safety and quality of care.

Multiple Choice Questions

1. What is the main focus of pharmacokinetics in nursing practice?
   (a) Drug effects on biological systems
   (b) Drug prices and market regulation
   (c) Absorption, distribution, metabolism, and excretion of drugs
   (d) Psychological effects of medication
2. According to the NMC Code (2018), what is a key responsibility of UK nurses regarding medications?
   (a) Diagnosing conditions
   (b) Prescribing independently
   (c) Ensuring safe administration and effectiveness
   (d) Monitoring pharmacy inventory
3. What role do nurses play in lifestyle-related pharmacological interventions?
   (a) Diagnosing diseases
   (b) Promoting adherence and integrating lifestyle advice
   (c) Only administering medication
   (d) Dispensing drugs
4. What tool helps nurses reduce medication-related risks through structured documentation?
   (a) Blood pressure monitor
   (b) Patient survey
   (c) Electronic Health Records (EHRs)
   (d) Clinical thermometer
5. A key responsibility of nurses in the prescription process is to:
   (a) Approve new drugs
   (b) Develop marketing strategies
   (c) Identify contraindications and drug interactions
   (d) Write electronic prescriptions independently
6. What concept supports nurses in reporting unsafe practice?
   (a) Chain of command
   (b) Psychological safety and 'speaking up' culture
   (c) Top-down leadership
   (d) Medication advertising
7. Which UK body provides protection for whistleblowers in healthcare?
   (a) The Home Office
   (b) Royal College of Surgeons
   (c) Nursing and Midwifery Council (NMC)
   (d) Department for Transport

8. Which UK body to report concerns about care provided by an organisation?
    (a) Care Quality Commission (CQC)
    (b) Royal College of Nursing
    (c) Nursing and Midwifery Council
    (d) Royal College of Physicians
9. A nurse suspects a prescription error. What should they do first?
    (a) Ignore it
    (b) Inform a pharmacist or prescribing clinician
    (c) Post about it on social media
    (d) Contact the patient directly without documentation
10. What does 'prescriber ready' mean for UK newly registered nurses?
    (a) They can independently prescribe controlled substances
    (b) They understand medication principles and safety
    (c) They automatically join NICE
    (d) They bypass supervised practice
11. Psychological safety in healthcare teams leads to:
    (a) Increased conflict
    (b) Suppression of dissent
    (c) Improved patient safety through open communication
    (d) Less collaboration
12. What training supports nurses in challenging unsafe prescriptions?
    (a) Political science training
    (b) Assertive communication and team dynamics
    (c) Financial audit training
    (d) Public relations seminars
13. Mentoring and supervision post-registration help new nurses:
    (a) Prescribe medications independently
    (b) Avoid documentation
    (c) Transition into safe medication practices
    (d) Take over physician duties
14. Which of the following is a responsibility of ANPs in prescribing?
    (a) Legal prosecution
    (b) Political campaigning
    (c) Conducting thorough patient assessments
    (d) Hospital maintenance
15. What principle underpins antimicrobial stewardship by ANPs prescribers?
    (a) Reducing use of antiseptics
    (b) Encouraging self-medication
    (c) Rational antibiotic use to prevent resistance
    (d) Avoiding microbial testing
16. Lifelong learning is critical for ANPs prescribers because:
    (a) Laws rarely change
    (b) Drug markets are static
    (c) Pharmacological knowledge evolves rapidly
    (d) They need accounting knowledge

17. What is polypharmacy?
    (a) Taking vitamins regularly
    (b) Using over-the-counter drugs
    (c) Concurrent use of multiple medications
    (d) Avoiding prescriptions
18. Why is polypharmacy a concern in older adults?
    (a) They dislike medication
    (b) They rarely seek care
    (c) Risk of drug interactions and adverse effects
    (d) Medications are more effective
19. What is the goal of deprescribing?
    (a) Stopping all medications
    (b) Saving healthcare costs
    (c) Reviewing and reducing unnecessary medications
    (d) Switching to herbal therapies only
20. What tool helps clinicians identify inappropriate medications in older adults?
    (a) WHO antibiotic checklist
    (b) STOPP/START criteria
    (c) Pain scale
    (d) Maslow's hierarchy
21. Nurses support deprescribing by:
    (a) Refusing all patient medications
    (b) Making solo decisions
    (c) Collaborating with prescribers and involving patients
    (d) Delegating only to junior staff
22. Nurses who are engaged in medication management are better able to:
    (a) Challenge inappropriate prescriptions
    (b) Avoid patient contact
    (c) Conduct lab tests
    (d) Fill out hospital tax forms

Answers

1. (c)
   Rationale: Pharmacokinetics refers to how drugs move through the body, which is essential for safe dosing and administration.
2. (c)
   Rationale: The NMC Code emphasises accountability in medication safety and effectiveness.
3. (b)
   Rationale: Nurses enhance outcomes by integrating pharmacological treatment with health education.
4. (c)
   Rationale: EHRs facilitate access to current medication data and reduce errors.

5. (c)
   Rationale: Vigilance for safety issues is central to nursing responsibilities in the UK.
6. (b)
   Rationale: A psychologically safe environment encourages open communication and accountability.
7. (c)
   Rationale: The NMC supports whistleblowing in accordance with professional standards.
8. (a)
9. (b)
   Rationale: Interprofessional communication is key to safe resolution.
10. (b)
    Rationale: Nurses are not independent prescribers but are expected to have foundational knowledge of pharmacology.
11. (c)
    Rationale: Teams that feel safe to raise concerns perform better and make fewer errors.
12. (b)
    Rationale: Communication and teamwork skills are essential for safe clinical practice.
13. (c)
    Rationale: Support structures help newly qualified nurses consolidate safe practice.
14. (c)
    Rationale: ACPs assess patients to determine safe and effective treatment plans.
15. (c)
    Rationale: Prudent prescribing supports public health and limits antibiotic resistance.
16. (c)
    Rationale: Continuous development ensures safe, updated clinical practice.
17. (c)
    Rationale: Polypharmacy typically involves five or more medications and poses risks.
18. (c)
    Rationale: Older adults are vulnerable to medication-related harm.
19. (c)
    Rationale: Deprescribing improves outcomes by minimising inappropriate polypharmacy.
20. (b)
    Rationale: STOPP/START helps guide appropriate prescribing and deprescribing.
21. (c)
    Rationale: Shared decision-making improves adherence and patient safety.
22. (a)
    Rationale: Pharmacologically informed nurses advocate for patient safety.

References

Abdelhadi N, Drach-Zahavy A, Srulovici E (2020) The nurse's experience of decision-making processes in missed nursing care: a qualitative study. J Adv Nurs 76(8):2161–2170. https://doi.org/10.1111/jan.14387

Ahn S, Kim D (2024) Adaptation and validation of a Korean version of the speaking up about patient safety questionnaire (KSUPS-q). BMC Nurs 23(1). https://doi.org/10.1186/s12912-024-01891-3

Aliakbari F, Ghaedamini M, Deris F, Masoudi R (2020) Relationship between nurses' decision-making style and their disaster response competencies. Disaster Med Public Health Prep 16(1):19–24. https://doi.org/10.1017/dmp.2020.225

Alingh C, Wijngaarden J, Voorde K, Paauwe J, Huijsman R (2018) Speaking up about patient safety concerns: the influence of safety management approaches and climate on nurses' willingness to speak up. BMJ Qual Safe 28(1):39–48. https://doi.org/10.1136/bmjqs-2017-007163

Alnjadat R, Al-Momani E, Hadid L, Al-Omari A, Fraihat A (2024) Confounding factors affecting the clinical decision-making of nursing and midwifery students post-pandemic covid-19: cross-sectional study in Jordan. BMC Nurs 23(1). https://doi.org/10.1186/s12912-024-02108-3

Aly R, Elsayed B (2022) Application of world health organization's five moments for medication safety tool: an intervention towards medication without harm. Egypt J Health Care 13(4):1737–1752. https://doi.org/10.21608/ejhc.2022.284378

Ambanwala A (2022) Likelihood of speaking up by health professionals in emergency setting: a descriptive study. J Ruhunu Clin Soc 27(1):17–26. https://doi.org/10.4038/jrcs.v27i1.121

Anton N, Hornbeck T, Modlin S, Haque M, Crites M, Yu D (2021) Identifying factors that nurses consider in the decision-making process related to patient care during the covid-19 pandemic. PLoS One 16(7):e0254077. https://doi.org/10.1371/journal.pone.0254077

Batran A, Al-Humran S, Malak M, Ayed A (2022) The relationship between nursing informatics competency and clinical decision-making among nurses in west bank, Palestine. Cin Comput Inform Nurs 40(8):547–553. https://doi.org/10.1097/cin.0000000000000890

Baysal E, Sarı D, Erdem H (2018) Ethical decision-making levels of oncology nurses. Nurs Ethics 26(7-8):2204–2212. https://doi.org/10.1177/0969733018803662

Bell S, Roche S, Mueller A, Dente E, O'Reilly K, Lee B et al (2018) Speaking up about care concerns in the ICU: patient and family experiences, attitudes and perceived barriers. BMJ Qual Safe 27(11):928–936. https://doi.org/10.1136/bmjqs-2017-007525

Chen Y, Gao Y, Zhang J, Niu M, Liu X, Zhang Y et al (2022) Quality and clinical applicability of recommendations for incontinence-associated dermatitis: a systematic review of guidelines and consensus statements. J Clin Nurs 32(11-12):2371–2382. https://doi.org/10.1111/jocn.16306

Cheng C, Yu H, Wang Q (2023) Nurses' experiences concerning older adults with polypharmacy: a meta-synthesis of qualitative findings. Healthcare 11(3):334. https://doi.org/10.3390/healthcare11030334

Cook G (2024) Commentary: exploring the moderating role of health-promoting behaviours and self-compassion on the relationship between clinical decision-making and nurses' well-being. J Res Nurs 29(7):582–583. https://doi.org/10.1177/17449871241276866

Crowe E (2020) Deprescribing in chronic disease: perspectives of nurse prescribers. Prescriber 31(3):29–31. https://doi.org/10.1002/psb.1831

Daungsupawong H, Wiwanitkit V (2024) Role of a generative ai model in enhancing clinical decision-making in nursing. J Adv Nurs 80(11):4750–4751. https://doi.org/10.1111/jan.16145

Dumbreck S, Flynn A, Nairn M, Wilson M, Treweek S, Mercer S, Guthrie B (2015) Drug-disease and drug-drug interactions: systematic examination of recommendations in 12 UK national clinical guidelines. BMJ 350(mar11 2):h949–h949. https://doi.org/10.1136/bmj.h949

Fitzpatrick JM, Bianchi LA, Hayes N, Da Silva T, Harris R (2023) Professional development and career planning for nurses working in care homes for older people: a scoping review. Int J Older People Nursing 18:e12519. https://doi.org/10.1111/opn.12519

Friary P, McAllister L, Martin R, Purdy S, Barrow M (2024) Allied health new graduates' voice behavior – new perspectives using realist synthesized narratives. J Health Organ Manag 38(7):1050–1071. https://doi.org/10.1108/jhom-06-2023-0199

Gao Y, Liu J, Liu J, Duan T (2023) Influence of job burnout on decision-making and coping with stress among nurses. Holist Nurs Pract 37(6):E83–E91. https://doi.org/10.1097/hnp.0000000000000609

Gassas R, Ahmed M, Asloob M (2024) Ethical decision-making confidence and professional values among nurse leaders. J Nurs Admin 54(6):353–360. https://doi.org/10.1097/nna.0000000000001438

Gürsoy E, Sağlam H, Başaran F, Atay E, Yavuz N (2023) Turkish nurses' leadership orientations and clinical decision-making skills. Leadersh Health Serv 36(3):402–417. https://doi.org/10.1108/lhs-08-2022-0090

Hackman P, Häggman-Laitila A, Hult M (2024) Prioritization decision-making of care in nursing homes: a qualitative study. Nurs Ethics 32(1):42–55. https://doi.org/10.1177/09697330241230513

Hajj M, Jaam M, Ali S, Saleh R, Awaisu A, Paravattil B et al (2020) Critical appraisal of tobacco dependence treatment guidelines. Int J Clin Pharm 43(1):85–100. https://doi.org/10.1007/s11096-020-01110-4

Halvorsen K, Stadeløkken T, Garcia B (2019) A stepwise pharmacist-led medication review service in interdisciplinary teams in rural nursing homes. Pharmacy 7(4):148. https://doi.org/10.3390/pharmacy7040148

Hidayat A, Kongsuwan W, Nilmanat K, Siwi A, Alivian G (2021) Phenomenological study of Muslim nurses' experience during end-of-life decision making. Jurnal Keperawatan Soedirman 16(3). https://doi.org/10.20884/1.jks.2021.16.3.1716

Hoek D, Thodé M, Jongerden I, Laarhoven H, Smets E, Tange D et al (2020) The role of hospital nurses in shared decision-making about life-prolonging treatment: a qualitative interview study. J Adv Nurs 77(1):296–307. https://doi.org/10.1111/jan.14549

Hunt D, Bailey J, Lennox B, Crofts M, Vincent C (2021) Enhancing psychological safety in mental health services. Int J Ment Heal Syst 15(1). https://doi.org/10.1186/s13033-021-00439-1

Jeong J, Kim S (2023) South Korean nurses' experiences of speaking up for patient safety and incident prevention. Healthcare 11(12):1764. https://doi.org/10.3390/healthcare11121764

Lainidi O, Jendeby M, Montgomery A, Mouratidis C, Paitaridou K, Cook C et al (2023) An integrative systematic review of employee silence and voice in healthcare: what are we really measuring? Front Psych 14. https://doi.org/10.3389/fpsyt.2023.1111579

Landgren R, Alawadi Z, Douma C, Thomas E, Etchegaray J (2016) Barriers of pediatric residents to speaking up about patient safety. Hosp Pediatr 6(12):738–743. https://doi.org/10.1542/hpeds.2016-0042

Lawson C, Predella M, Rowden A, Goldstein J, Sistino J, Fitzgerald D (2017) Assessing the culture of safety in cardiovascular perfusion: attitudes and perceptions. Perfusion 32(7):583–590. https://doi.org/10.1177/0267659117699056

Lee S, Dahinten V, Ji H, Kim E, Lee H (2022) Motivators and inhibitors of nurses' speaking up behaviours: a descriptive qualitative study. J Adv Nurs 78(10):3398–3408. https://doi.org/10.1111/jan.15343

Lee S, Dahinten V, Kim E, Lee S, Han S, Kim P et al (2023) A safety huddle intervention in in-patient surgical units: a mixed-methods study. J Nurs Manag 2023:1–8. https://doi.org/10.1155/2023/8929993

Li Z, Yang Y, Wang Q, Zhang M, Luo C, Zhu L et al (2024) Association between abusive supervision and nurses' withholding voice about patient safety: the roles of impression management motivation and speak up-related climate. BMC Nurs 23(1). https://doi.org/10.1186/s12912-024-01921-0

Liu M, Zhang T, Chen L, Liu Y, Yin A, Xu M et al (2023) Intensive care unit nurses' attitudes toward truth-telling, life-sustaining treatment, and decision-making intention for end-of-life patients. J Hosp Palliat Nurs 26(2):E46–E54. https://doi.org/10.1097/njh.0000000000000989

Luo Z, Tao L, Wang C, Zheng N, Ma X, Quan Y et al (2023) Correlations between moral courage, moral sensitivity, and ethical decision-making by nurse interns: a cross-sectional study. BMC Nurs 22(1). https://doi.org/10.1186/s12912-023-01428-0

Lyndon A, Wisner K, Holschuh C, Fagan K, Franck L (2017) Parents' perspectives on navigating the work of speaking up in the NICU. J Obstet Gynecol Neonatal Nurs 46(5):716–726. https://doi.org/10.1016/j.jogn.2017.06.009

Maramba I, Lim E, Menzies J, Nijman R, Zhou S, Latour J (2024) Signs and symptoms of serious illness in infants aged up to 6 months: rapid review of clinical guidelines. BMJ Paediatr Open 8(1):e002737. https://doi.org/10.1136/bmjpo-2024-002737

Mardani A, Griffiths P, Vaismoradi M (2020) The role of the nurse in the management of medicines during transitional care: a systematic review. J Multidiscip Healthc 13:1347–1361. https://doi.org/10.2147/jmdh.s276061

Martínez W, Lehmann L, Thomas E, Etchegaray J, Shelburne J, Hickson G et al (2017) Speaking up about traditional and professionalism-related patient safety threats: a national survey of interns and residents. BMJ Qual Safe 26(11):869–880. https://doi.org/10.1136/bmjqs-2016-006284

Mawuena E, Mannion R (2022) Implications of resource constraints and high workload on speaking up about threats to patient safety: a qualitative study of surgical teams in Ghana. BMJ Qual Safe 31(9):662–669. https://doi.org/10.1136/bmjqs-2021-014287

McCann C, McCauley C, Harkin D (2023) Barriers and facilitators to opioid deprescribing among advanced nurse practitioners: a qualitative interview study. J Adv Nurs 80(6):2500–2511. https://doi.org/10.1111/jan.15995

Mensah G, Ham-Baloyi W, Rooyen D, Jardien-Baboo S (2019) Guidelines for the nursing management of gestational diabetes mellitus: an integrative literature review. Nurs Open 7(1):78–90. https://doi.org/10.1002/nop2.324

Mortensen M, Tybjærg-Hansen A, Nordestgaard B (2022) Statin eligibility for primary prevention of cardiovascular disease according to 2021 European prevention guidelines compared with other international guidelines. JAMA Cardiol 7(8):836. https://doi.org/10.1001/jamacardio.2022.1876

Nacioglu A (2016) As a critical behavior to improve quality and patient safety in health care: speaking up! Safe Health 2(1). https://doi.org/10.1186/s40886-016-0021-x

National Guideline Centre (2018) Physician extenders. In: Emergency and acute medical care in over 16s: service delivery and organisation. National Institute for Health and Care Excellence (NICE)

Naughton C, Hayes N (2016) Deprescribing in older adults: a new concept for nurses in administering medicines and as prescribers of medicine. Eur J Hosp Pharm 24(1):47–50. https://doi.org/10.1136/ejhpharm-2016-000908

Nibbelink C, Brewer B (2018) Decision-making in nursing practice: an integrative literature review. J Clin Nurs 27(5-6):917–928. https://doi.org/10.1111/jocn.14151

Nursing and Midwifery Council [NMC] (2018) The code. Available at: https://www.nmc.org.uk/standards/code/

Novalia A, Rachmi S, Yetti K (2022) Clinical decision-making of bachelor and clinical internship (professional) nursing students in Indonesia. J Public Health Res 11(2). https://doi.org/10.4081/jphr.2021.2735

O'Donovan R, McAuliffe É (2020) A systematic review exploring the content and outcomes of interventions to improve psychological safety, speaking up and voice behaviour. BMC Health Serv Res 20(1). https://doi.org/10.1186/s12913-020-4931-2

O'Flaherty D, Ali K (2024) Recommendations for upper limb motor recovery: an overview of the UK and European rehabilitation after stroke guidelines (2023). Healthcare 12(14):1433. https://doi.org/10.3390/healthcare12141433

Oh S, Gu M, Sok S (2022) A concept analysis of nurses' clinical decision making: implications for Korea. Int J Environ Res Public Health 19(6):3596. https://doi.org/10.3390/ijerph19063596

Padash M, Miri S, Forouzi M, Jouparinejad S, Farokhzadian J (2023) The effect of clinical risk management training on patient safety competency and related aspects in nursing students. J Patient Safe Risk Manag 28(4):170–176. https://doi.org/10.1177/25160435231190198

Park M, Gu M, Sok S (2022) Path model on decision-making ability of clinical nurses. J Clin Nurs 32(7-8):1343–1353. https://doi.org/10.1111/jocn.16292

Passariello M, Tarrant C (2024) Psychological safety in an ECMO retrieval team: a qualitative study to inform improvement. BMJ Open Qual 13(2):e002706. https://doi.org/10.1136/bmjoq-2023-002706

Patel H, Aguiar P, Pessoa A, Storpirtis S, Long P (2019) Identifying quality of life indicators to improve outpatient pharmacy services for prostate cancer patients: a comparison between Brazilian and British experiences. Int Braz J Urol 45(3):435–448. https://doi.org/10.1590/s1677-5538.ibju.2018.0553

Pattni N, Arzola C, Malavade A, Varmani S, Krimus L, Friedman Z (2019) Challenging authority and speaking up in the operating room environment: a narrative synthesis. Br J Anaesth 122(2):233–244. https://doi.org/10.1016/j.bja.2018.10.056

Rababa M, Bani-Hamad D, Hayajneh A, Al-Mugheed K (2022) Nurses' knowledge, attitudes, practice, and decision-making skills related to sepsis assessment and management. Electron J Gener Med 19(6):em420. https://doi.org/10.29333/ejgm/12556

Rauwolf P, Jones A (2019) Exploring the utility of internal whistleblowing in healthcare via agent-based models. BMJ Open 9(1):e021705. https://doi.org/10.1136/bmjopen-2018-021705

Reis da Silva TH (2024a) Pharmacokinetics in older people: an overview of prescribing practice. J Prescrib Pract 6(9):374–381. https://doi.org/10.12968/jprp.2024.6.9.374

Reis da Silva TH (2024b) Chapter 12 – Emotional intelligence in integrative medicine: enhancing patient-centred care through humanised technology. In: Tikadar S, Liu H, Bhattacharya P, Bhattacharya S (eds) Humanizing technology with emotional intelligence. IGI Global Scientific Publishing, pp 263–280. https://doi.org/10.4018/979-8-3693-7011-7.ch012

Reis da Silva TH (2024c) Chapter 6 – Navigating healthcare complexity: integrating business fundamentals into nursing leadership. In: Sedky A (ed) Resiliency strategies for long-term business success. IGI Global, pp 145–168. https://doi.org/10.4018/979-8-3693-9168-6.ch006

Reis da Silva TH (2024d) Chapter 11 - Integrating business essentials into gerontological nursing: enhancing care for older adults in diverse settings. In: Sedky A (ed) Resiliency strategies for long-term business success. IGI Global, pp 283–316. https://doi.org/10.4018/979-8-3693-9168-6.ch011

Reis da Silva TM (2025a) Quality assurance strategies in nursing education for the care of older adults. In: Naim A, Saklani A, Khan S, Malik P (eds) Global perspectives on quality management and accreditation in higher education. IGI Global Scientific Publishing, pp 25–48. https://doi.org/10.4018/979-8-3693-9481-6.ch002

Reis da Silva TH (2025b) Chapter 11 - Integrating artificial intelligence in geriatric care: enhancing physical and mental health outcomes. In: Jermsittiparsert K, Marzo RR (eds) Physical health, mental health, and human well-being in the age of AI. IGI Global Scientific Publishing. https://doi.org/10.4018/979-8-3693-6190-0.ch11

Reis da Silva TH (2025c) Chapter 8 - Promoting emotional well-being in older adults: the role of AI in supporting emotional intelligence and mental health. In: Jermsittiparsert K, Marzo RR (eds) Physical health, mental health, and human well-being in the age of AI. IGI Global Scientific Publishing, pp 137–167. https://doi.org/10.4018/979-8-3693-6190-0.ch8

Reis da Silva TH (2025d) Chapter 10: emotional intelligence and AI in geriatric nursing: bridging technology and compassionate care. In: Jermsittiparsert K, Marzo RR (eds) Physical health, mental health, and human well-being in the age of AI. IGI Global Scientific Publishing. https://doi.org/10.4018/979-8-3693-6190-0.ch10

Reis da Silva TM (2025e) Integrative approaches to geriatric care: enhancing physical and mental health through AI-driven insights. In: Jermsittiparsert K, Marzo R (eds) Physical health, mental health, and human well-being in the age of AI. IGI Global Scientific Publishing, pp 113–136. https://doi.org/10.4018/979-8-3693-6190-0.ch007

Reis da Silva TMH (2025f) The role of emotional intelligence in promoting mental peace, healthy work environments, and emotional well-being among entrepreneurs. In: Tunio MN (ed) Supporting psychological and emotional wellbeing among entrepreneurs. IGI Global Scientific Publishing. https://doi.org/10.4018/979-8-3693-3673-1.ch21

Rohde E, Domm E (2017) Nurses' clinical reasoning practices that support safe medication administration: an integrative review of the literature. J Clin Nurs 27(3-4). https://doi.org/10.1111/jocn.14077

Royal Pharmaceutical Society (2022) A competency framework for all prescribers. https://www.rpharms.com/Portals/0/RPS%20document%20library/Open%20access/Prescribing%20Competency%20Framework/RPS%20English%20Competency%20Framework%203.pdf?ver=mctnrKo4YaJDh2nA8N5G3A%3d%3d. Access 17/03/2025

Şahin G, Başak T (2022) Is virtual patient simulation superior to human patient simulation. Cin Comput Inform Nurs 41(6):467–476. https://doi.org/10.1097/cin.0000000000000957

Sari D, Baysal E, Çelik G, Eşer İ (2018) Ethical decision making levels of nursing students. Pak J Med Sci 34(3). https://doi.org/10.12669/pjms.343.14922

Savcı C, Akıncı A, Keles F (2021) Anxiety levels and clinical decision-making skills of nurses providing care for patients diagnosed with covid-19. Electron J Gener Med 18(6):em322. https://doi.org/10.29333/ejgm/11300

Schwappach D, Niederhauser A (2019) Speaking up about patient safety in psychiatric hospitals – a cross-sectional survey study among healthcare staff. Int J Ment Health Nurs 28(6):1363–1373. https://doi.org/10.1111/inm.12664

Schwappach D, Richard A (2018) Speak up-related climate and its association with healthcare workers' speaking up and withholding voice behaviours: a cross-sectional survey in Switzerland. BMJ Qual Safe 27(10):827–835. https://doi.org/10.1136/bmjqs-2017-007388

Shahzeydi A, Dianati M, Kalhor F (2024) Clinical simulation in nursing students' safe medication administration: a systematic review. Iran J Nurs Midwifery Res 29(5):522–529. https://doi.org/10.4103/ijnmr.ijnmr_323_23

Silva G, Santos I, Conceição M, Góis R, Santos A, Amestoy S et al (2022) Influencing factors in the nurses' decision-making process in Ibero American university hospitals. Rev Lat Am Enfermagem 30. https://doi.org/10.1590/1518-8345.5648.3527

Taasen S, Kvam F, Blytt K, Messaoudi E (2024) Pharmacology knowledge among nurses working in nursing homes in Norway: a cross-sectional study. Sage Open Nurs 10. https://doi.org/10.1177/23779608241303482

Tear M, Reader T, Shorrock S, Kirwan B (2020) Safety culture and power: interactions between perceptions of safety culture, organisational hierarchy, and national culture. Saf Sci 121:550–561. https://doi.org/10.1016/j.ssci.2018.10.014

Tume L, Kneyber M, Blackwood B, Rose L (2017) Mechanical ventilation, weaning practices, and decision making in european picus*. Pediatr Crit Care Med 18(4):e182–e188. https://doi.org/10.1097/pcc.0000000000001100

Turfi M, Al-Jubouri M (2022) Effect of moral distress on decision making among nurses in intensive care units. PJMHS 16(3):915–918. https://doi.org/10.53350/pjmhs22163915

Vaismoradi M, Mardani A, Lillo-Crespo M, Logan P, Sak-Dankosky N (2024) An integrative systematic review of nurses' involvement in medication deprescription in long-term healthcare settings for older people. Ther Adv Drug Safe 15. https://doi.org/10.1177/20420986241289205

Vuuren A, Rensburg J, Hanekom S (2023) Practitioner's knowledge, attitudes, beliefs and practices towards urinary incontinence. South African. J Physiother 79(1). https://doi.org/10.4102/sajp.v79i1.1860

Wang Y, Wang Q, Peng Y, Zhang Y, Li N (2022) Dissemination of acupuncture-moxibustion clinical practice guidelines among clinical practitioners: a systematic review of quality assessment studies. Evid Based Complement Alternat Med 2022:1–12. https://doi.org/10.1155/2022/8334397

Wouters H, Foster J, Ensink A, O'Donnell L, Zuidema S, Boersma F et al (2019) Barriers and facilitators of conducting medication reviews in nursing home residents: a qualitative study. Front Pharmacol 10. https://doi.org/10.3389/fphar.2019.01026

Xu Q, Li D, Dong Y, Wu Y, Cao H, Zhang F et al (2023) The relationship between personality traits and clinical decision-making, anxiety and stress among intern nursing students during covid-19: a cross-sectional study. Psychol Res Behav Manag 16:57–69. https://doi.org/10.2147/prbm.s387682

Yarnall A, Sayer A, Clegg A, Rockwood K, Parker S, Hindle J (2017) New horizons in multimorbidity in older adults. Age Ageing 46(6):882–888. https://doi.org/10.1093/ageing/afx150

Yun J, Seong M, Cho Y, Sok S (2024) Influences of nursing professionalism, empathy, and clinical decision-making ability on shared decision-making awareness among hemodialysis nurses. J Nurs Manag 2024:1–9. https://doi.org/10.1155/2024/2518065

Zainal N, Musa K, Rasudin N, Mamat Z (2023) Multilevel modeling of individual and group level influences on critical thinking and clinical decision-making skills among registered nurses: a study protocol. Healthcare 11(8):1169. https://doi.org/10.3390/healthcare11081169

Zoromski L, Frazier S (2023) Nurses' role in promoting medication adherence. Nursing 53(1):39–44. https://doi.org/10.1097/01.nurse.0000902956.76232.93

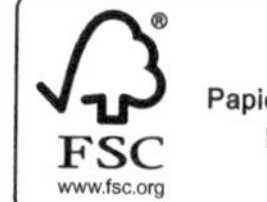